ISCHAEMIC HEART DISEASE AND EXERCISE

Ischaemic Heart Disease and Exercise

ROY J. SHEPHARD

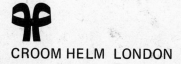

CROOM HELM LONDON

W. SUSSEX INSTITUTE
OF
HIGHER EDUCATION
LIBRARY

©1981 Roy J. Shephard
Croom Helm, 2-10 St John's Road, London SW11

British Library Cataloguing in Publication Data

Shephard, Roy J
    Ischaemic heart disease and exercise.
    1. Coronary heart disease
    2. Exercise − Physiological
    effect
    I. Title
    616.1'23   RC685.C6

    ISBN 0-7099-0325-1

Typeset by Leaper & Gard Ltd, Bristol
Printed in Great Britain by offset lithography by
Billing & Sons Ltd, Guildford, London and Worcester

CONTENTS

Preface

1. Pathology of Ischaemic Heart Disease 13

2. The Current Epidemic of Ischaemic Heart Disease 23

3. Ischaemic Heart Disease and the Risks of Exercise 49

4. Exercise and the Primary Prevention of Ischaemic Heart Disease 66

5. Exercise and the Secondary Prevention of Ischaemic Heart Disease 91

6. Exercise and the Tertiary Prevention of Ischaemic Heart Disease 130

7. Non-invasive Assessment of the Heart and Coronary Circulation 158

8. Heart and Coronary Circulation in Exercise 199

9. Exercise Prescription and Ischaemic Heart Disease 232

10. Adjuvants to Exercise 261

11. Psycho-social Considerations 279

12. Miscellaneous Topics 293

13. Epilogue: The Bottom Line 305

Bibliography 324

Index 419

PREFACE

Exercise in the prevention and treatment of ischaemic heart disease remains a controversial issue. Exercise enthusiasts insist blindly that vigorous physical activity will both prevent and cure cardiac disease. If they commit their ideas to writing, it is usually in popular format, a lurid jacket spelling out a concept such as 'exercise and your heart'. At the other extreme are conservative physicians who know little of exercise, but argue with an aura of great dignity that statistical proof of the value of physical activity is lacking. If they choose to write, it is in sombre medical prose, a dark-blue spine carrying the gold-leaf lettering that spells the end of a patient's productive life — 'ischaemic heart disease' — period.

The present title — 'ischaemic heart disease *and* exercise' — reflects the author's personal philosophy. The book navigates carefully the treacherous strait that separates the Scylla-like temptations of euphoric popular commendation of exercise from the Charybdic whirlpool of cold statistical disdain. The voyage is charted from the perspective of varied and multidisciplinary ventures. After a period as cardiac research fellow at Guy's Hospital under the legendary Maurice Campbell, founder of the *British Heart Journal*, I gained broad experience in applied physiology, working in England, the US and Canada. More recently, I have served as professor to the Department of Preventive Medicine and Biostatistics at the University of Toronto. Now I find myself with a larger office, a carpet and the title of Director of the School of Physical and Health Education. The 'stress' of this somewhat chequered career has probably shortened my personal lifespan by several years, but at least it has provided insight into the respective viewpoints of exercise enthusiasts and agnostics. As in most arguments, the truth lies somewhere between the opposing factions. The present short volume sets on record the views I have formed in mediating many heated discussions. It attempts a careful, balanced and up-to-date review of both the advantages and the dangers of physical activity in cardiac disease.

A natural starting point is found in a brief description of the underlying pathology of cardiac disease. This is discussed in simple terms for the benefit of those who lack an extensive medical background. Attention is then focused on factors responsible for the waxing and

waning of the 'cardiac epidemic', and the question is posed as to
whether changing patterns of daily activity have contributed to this
intriguing phenomenon of twentieth-century medicine. A critical
look is then taken at the hazards of exercise, particular attention being
directed to the possibility that physical activity will precipitate
myocardial infarction and sudden death. Evidence that physical
activity has therapeutic value is next discussed in the context of the
primary, secondary and tertiary prevention of ischaemic heart disease.
Possible beneficial effects of exercise are reviewed, and details of
current therapeutic trials are carefully examined. Normal and pathological reactions of the heart to exercise are considered in the light of
modern non-invasive diagnostic procedures – the electrocardiogram,
echocardiography and the use of radionuclides. Practical principles
of exercise prescription are related to the needs of hospital, outpatient
and home phases of treatment. Mediators of the exercise response
are discussed, and some important contraindications to exercise are
noted. Drugs commonly taken by the cardiac patient are examined
with particular reference to their impact upon stress testing and
training patterns. Psycho-social variables are reviewed, including the
influence of mood upon two key measures of successful treatment –
return to normal employment and full sexual activity after myocardial
infarction. Special problems of patients with angina, by-pass operations
and peripheral vascular disease are covered, and comment is made upon
particular features of cardiac disease in the female patient. A final
chapter examines the topical issue of cost-benefit analyses from the
standpoint of the patient, the physician and the community.
Such a broadly ranging book is intended to attract a broad
readership, spanning the spectrum of medical and paramedical workers
with an interest in the prevention and treatment of ischaemic heart
disease. The text is written with a minimum of technical jargon, to
accommodate a multidisciplinary audience. Nevertheless, all
propositions are founded on sound medical, scientific and (where
necessary) statistical discussion. Further research is facilitated by a
bibliography of more than 1,300 recent references selected from the
world literature.

As in previous writing, I must acknowledge with warm thanks my
profound debt to many teachers, colleagues and students who have
helped in shaping my present views. I still remember the crowded
outpatient department of the early 1950s, with Dr Maurice Campbell
vividly demonstrating simple clinical methods of distinguishing angina
from benign chest pain. More recently, it has been a great pleasure to

work closely with my good friend Dr Terence Kavanagh as physiological consultant to the Toronto Rehabilitation Centre. I have rejoiced in the practical triumphs of his innovative pattern of treatment, as new hope has come to some 2,000 'post-coronary' patients. I have shared Dr Kavanagh's excitement, as some of the patients from the Centre have completed marathon events in a little over three hours. Above all, I have had the total cooperation of Centre and patients in realising the tremendous research potential afforded by this programme. Such material is identified in this monograph as Toronto Rehabilitation Centre data. The past decade has also seen a most fruitful collaboration with Dr Peter Rechnitzer of the University of Western Ontario, and a distinguished group of investigators involved in the Southern Ontario multicentre exercise-heart trial. The team has included Drs G. Andrew, C. Buck, D. Cunningham, N. Jones, T. Kavanagh, N. Oldridge, J.C. Parker, P. Rechnitzer (director), S. Sangal and M. Yuhasz. Where not specifically attributed to one or more of these authors, such material is identified as Southern Ontario multicentre data. Again, this has brought budget, research material and above all a tremendous cross-fertilization of ideas. Several trained graduate students — Veena Pandit, Ken Sidney, Veli Niinimaa, Don Paterson, Mike Cox and Tony Verde — have greatly helped forward the departmental programme of cardiac research. Three decades of reading and scientific meetings have also played their part in the writing of this book. Where possible, I have acknowledged the sources of my information; however, material is sometimes absorbed almost subconsciously and, if a debt has been overlooked, I trust the donor will accept my apology.

The book poses a very practical question. Should we recommend that the coronary-prone and the cardiac patient become involved in vigorous exercise? The reader must judge how far an answer is given. Possibly, as he reads the final page a larger question mark will be forming in his brain. However, this is preferable to a facile and intellectually dissatisfying endorsement of exercise. At least the unanswered problems about physical activity will have been brought into focus. If confusion remains, it is a clearer confusion! This is the first step on the road towards definitive answers. If the book has done no more than facilitate the search for knowledge, I shall feel well rewarded as an author.

Roy J. Shephard
October 1980

1 PATHOLOGY OF ISCHAEMIC HEART DISEASE

I am in anguish! I writhe with pain!
Walls of my heart!
My heart is throbbing!

(Jeremiah 4[19], Jerusalem translation)

Ancient literature contains many passages that could be interpreted as describing manifestations of coronary vascular disease. Thus it is conceivable that the prophet Jeremiah personally experienced the anguish of anginal pain, and translations such as the Jerusalem Bible interpret his warning of a northern invasion of Israel in the tragic poetry of a cardiac analogy. The Ebers Papyrus from ancient Egypt likewise gives a clear account of cardiac failure: 'When the heart is diseased, its work is performed imperfectly; the vessels proceeding from the heart become inactive, so that you cannot feel them' (J.B. Hurry, 1926); however, there is no direct indication that coronary disease was responsible for the pathology thus described.

Hippocrates reported the pain of angina (strangling) as 'extending from the collar-bone', 'like a weight in the forearm'. 'It causes very great pain and orthopnoea; it may suffocate the patient even on the first day' (A.M. Katz & Katz, 1962). Other descriptions in the Hippocratic literature are less characteristic of angina pectoris, and we must conclude that Greek physicians had not fully differentiated this condition from such diseases of the throat as acute tonsillitis and diphtheria. Nevertheless, suggestive evidence that ischaemic heart disease led to occasional fatalities is provided by the messenger Pheidippides, who died suddenly after running 40.0 kilometres to bring the news of victory from Marathon to Athens; the modern Marathon race covers a distance of 42.2 km.

Many more recent authors have shared in the confusion of terminology as they have discussed problems of cardiac oxygen lack (ischaemia). In particular, they have failed to differentiate the primary effects of anoxia (angina, myocardial infarction and sudden death), the immediate reaction to tissue destruction (myocardial fibrosis) and later consequences of such scarring and chronic hypoxia (persistent dysrhythmia, abnormal motion of the cardiac wall and pump failure). To avoid this problem, we will start our review of ischaemic heart disease and exercise with a brief discussion of terminology and the underlying pathology.

Atherosclerosis and Ischaemic Heart Disease

Atherosclerosis

Atherosclerosis is a general condition of the arteries in which the lumina are partially blocked by an accumulation of fat, complex carbohydrates, blood and blood products, fibrous tissue and calcium deposits in their walls, with associated medial changes (World Health Organization, 1958).

The build-up of lipids in arterial lesions has been recognised since R. Virchow (1856). The earliest changes probably occur in the arterial endothelium (M.D. Haust, 1970). One hypothesis is that injurious 'factors' from within the lumen of the blood vessels, either blood-borne chemicals or haemodynamic stresses (M. Texon, 1971), increase the permeability of the endothelium. This allows an 'insudation' of blood constituents into the intimal tissue of affected vessels, disturbing the metabolism of both cells and fibres. Alternatively, the injurious 'factors' may pass through the endothelium without causing initial harm, but resultant changes in the metabolism of the intimal cells lead to secondary effects upon the permeability of the endothelium, with resultant insudation. In either event, there is an increase in the muco-polysaccharide content of the tissue and an extracellular deposition of lipid, particularly cholesterol; accumulation of the latter substance probably reflects both more ready penetration of the intima and an increased retention due to changes in intimal metabolism (E.P. Smith, 1977). As the fatty plaques develop, they bulge into the arterial lumen and become enlarged by inflammation, haemorrhage and thrombus formation.

The first manifestation of coronary atherosclerosis is a fatty streaking of the major vessels; this can be detected in quite young children dying of inter-current disease (G.R. Osborn, 1963; D. Jaffé & Manning, 1971). Studies of young men killed in battle, air crashes and automobile accidents often reveal substantial (although clinically silent) atheroma (W.F. Enos *et al.*, 1953; J.C. Geer & McGill, 1967; H.H. Clarke, 1979). In one study of 20-year-old subjects, 40 per cent of the sample showed atherosclerosis, and in 15 per cent there was more than 75 per cent blockage of a main coronary artery (R. Gorlin, 1976). The disease process advances progressively with age (E.B. Smith *et al.*, 1967), and in many subjects eventually gives rise to symptoms.

Atherosclerotic changes within the coronary arteries predispose to such manifestations of ischaemic heart disease as angina, myocardial infarction and electrical failure of the heart.

Arteriosclerosis

Arteriosclerosis may co-exist with atherosclerosis, but should be distinguished from it (T.R. Harrison & Reeves, 1968). The arteriosclerotic blood vessel shows a progressive loss of elasticity and a hardening of its walls, often with radiologically visible calcification. Many older people are affected to some degree by arteriosclerosis. If severe, it can cause a substantial increase of systolic blood pressure, a narrowing or incompetence of the cardiac valves and ultimately a weakness of the vessel walls.

Plainly, such changes can contribute to and complicate the picture of ischaemic heart disease. The coronary vessels become narrow and rigid, with little potential for dilatation during exercise, while the valvular changes increase the work-load of the heart. However, many older authors have attributed almost every case of cardiac failure occurring in a man over the age of 50 years to arteriosclerotic heart disease, with the result that the term now lacks scientific precision.

Ischaemic heart disease

Ischaemic heart disease is a composite term referring to the several possible manifestations of relative oxygen lack in the myocardium (T.R. Harrison & Reeves, 1968). It is currently preferred to its apparent rival atherosclerotic heart disease.

Although the latter term is sometimes used as a synonym for ischaemic heart disease, the two rubrics do not encompass identical pathologies. Atherosclerosis may be present for many years without the development of clinically recognisable ischaemic heart disease. Clinical manifestations await a second, triggering factor. This may be haemorrhage into a plaque, lodgment of a thrombus at a point of vascular narrowing, coronary vascular spasm (R.C. Schlant, 1974), an unusual myocardial oxygen demand or some metabolic abnormality of the myocardium (T.W. Anderson, 1978a). Furthermore, if the immediate cause of death is ventricular fibrillation or myocardial infarction due to increased cardiac work rather than a specific blockage of the coronary vessels, post-mortem evidence of atherosclerosis may be rather slight. Finally, there are a number of non-atheromatous causes of ischaemic heart disease. These are uncommon, but nevertheless are well documented, including congenital abnormalities of the coronary vessels (H.A. Blake *et al.*, 1964), obstruction of the coronary ostium by syphilitic aortitis or a dissecting aneurysm (T.R. Harrison & Reeves,

1968), various types of aortic arteritis, vascular obstruction by non-atheromatous emboli (air, fat or tumour fragments) and pathological increases in the work-load of the left or right ventricle (for example, aortic stenosis or pulmonary hypertension; J.D. Woods, 1961). This substantial conglomerate of cardiac disorders is conveniently encompassed by the term ischaemic heart disease.

Angina

The classical clinical description of angina was furnished by W. Heberden (1772). He noted the sense of strangling, 'a painful and most disagreeable sensation in the breast, which seems as if it would extinguish life, if it were to continue'; it developed while the patient was 'walking (more especially if it be uphill and soon after eating) . . . but the moment they stand still, all this uneasiness vanishes.' It was plainly a harbinger of sudden death – if 'the disease go on to its height, the patients all suddenly fall down and perish almost immediately.' It also responded in some measure to regular exercise – 'I knew one who set himself a task of sawing wood for half an hour every day and was nearly cured.'

Despite this clear description of the clinical features, Heberden and his contemporaries were unaware of the pathological basis for the disorder. John Hunter drew attention to a bony hardening of the coronary arteries when conducting an autopsy of a patient with angina, but this contribution was ignored by nineteenth-century cardiologists. Laennec considered angina as a type of neuralgia, while William Osler listed angina among the cardiac neuroses. C.S. Keefer & Resnick (1928) seem the first authors to have recognised clearly that angina was due to a *relative* oxygen lack in the myocardium; this could reflect coronary narrowing, an increase of cardiac work-rate or a combination of these two factors.

The oxygen lack of an anginal attack is usually of insufficient duration to cause death of the myocardial tissue (A. Kattus & MacAlpin, 1969), but metabolic changes during the period of anoxia ('accumulation of a P substance'; R.C. Schlant, 1974) can sometimes be acutely painful. In earlier stages of the disease, there may be no more than a mild sense of oppression in the chest or a tightness of the throat which is difficult to diagnose. As the syndrome advances, its features become more characteristic. The patient is gripped by a severe, vice-like

pain the midline of the chest, often radiating upwards into the root
of the neck, or extending along the inner aspect of the left arm.
There is usually a clear precipitating cause — anxiety, or a walk uphill
(particularly in cold weather, when cutaneous vasoconstriction is
maximal and nerve endings within the airway are stimulated by cold,
dry air). Symptoms last no longer than two minutes, and do not cause
general collapse; rest and medication such as glyceryl trinitrate help
in providing rapid relief.

Myocardial Infarction and Fibrosis

Myocardial infarction

This is the usual cause of the 'coronary attack' of popular parlance.
For one of the various reasons discussed when dealing with ischaemic
heart disease (see above), an area of heart wall becomes starved of
blood for sufficient time (five to ten minutes) to cause irreversible
tissue damage. If the affected segment of the myocardium is large, the
immediate or early demise of the patient is likely. Death results from
an abnormality of cardiac rhythm (the irregular and ineffective pattern
of ventricular contraction known as ventricular fibrillation), asystole
(a complete cessation of cardiac contractions) or the onset of cardiac
failure. Overall, 30–40 per cent of patients die before medical attention
is received, and a further 30–35 per cent succumb while in hospital
(W.B. Kannel *et al.*, 1971a, b; Council on Rehabilitation, 1973).
Nevertheless, a proportion of patients, particularly younger individuals,
those with less severe disease (C.K. Friedberg & Unger, 1967; H.I.
Russek & Zohman, 1971; D.G. Julian, 1973) and those receiving early
first-aid treatment (L. Cobb *et al.*, 1975; D.A. Chamberlain, 1978a;
P. Siltanen, 1978) survive the immediate insult. In such cases the
infarcted area (infarcted means literally 'stuffed with blood') is replaced
by dense scar tissue over a period of some three months. The prognosis
for conservatively treated patients is summarised in Table 1.1. The
five-year death rate is at least ten times that indicated by standard
life-assurance tables. Nevertheless, the normal function of the heart
can be restored partially or completely by an extended programme of
physical rehabilitation.

Papers describing the importance of the coronary circulation to the
nutrition of the heart were published by Marshall Hall, Adam Hammer
and George Dock among others, but J.B. Herrick (1912) gave the first
detailed account of four possible clinical presentations:

Table 1.1: Five-year Mortality Following Recovery from Acute
Myocardial Infarction

Year of study	Sample size	Five-year mortality (%)	Authors
1920–30	162	51	Richards *et al.* (1956)
1932–41	285	33	Cole *et al.* (1954)
1934–6	–	29	Metropolitan Life (1953)
1935–52	224	45	Juergens *et al.* (1960)
1935–54	389	34	Biorck *et al.* (1957)
1940–9	286	42	Helander & Levander (1959)
1940–55	202	17	Dimond (1961)
1950–2	503	31	Beard *et al.* (1960)
1950–4	348	39	Honey & Truelove (1957)
1952–9	120	21	Little *et al.* (1965)
1956–61	932	26	Pell & D'Alonzo (1964)
1961–8	407	22*	Weinblatt *et al.* (1968)
1966–74	2,789	21	Coronary Drug Project (1975)

*   4½ years.

Source: Based on data collected by C.K. Friedberg & Unger (1967); P. Rechnitzer *et al.* (1971); T. Kavanagh & Shephard (1973b); and D.H. Paterson (1977). See original papers for details.

(i)   sudden and unanticipated death;
(ii)   severe pain, with profound shock and death in a few minutes;
(iii) anginal pain without a precipitating cause, usually lasting longer than two minutes; and
(iv)   pictures intermediate between (ii) and (iii).

Diagnosis became more certain with the development of precordial electrocardiographic leads by F.N. Wilson (1944), and the demonstration of increases in certain serum enzymes such as glutamic oxaloacetic transaminase (SGOT), lactic dehydrogenase (LDH) and creatine phosphokinase (CPK) (J.S. La Due *et al.*, 1954; L. Cohen, 1967). The electrocardiographic changes include displacement of the ST segment and abnormal Q and T waves, these signs evolving in the first few hours following symptoms. The elevation of serum enzyme concentrations begins some twelve hours after infarction, peaks in two to three days, and persists for 14-21 days.

Anatomical features influencing the extent of a myocardial infarct and the likelihood that the patient will recover include the volume of tissue to which the normal arterial pathway has been interrupted, and the extent of anastomotic connections between the two main coronary vessels (collateral circulation).

Myocardial fibrosis

If an infarct is small, the clinical symptoms may be mistaken for indigestion or even overlooked. Nevertheless, a segment of the heart wall dies and is replaced by scar tissue. Thus a series of such 'silent' infarcts can lead to a progressive fibrosis of the myocardium, with a deterioration in pump function.

Sudden Death

Ischaemic heart disease is the commonest cause of sudden death in a middle-aged or older individual (G.E. Burch & De Pasquale, 1965; L. Kuller, 1966; V. Manninen & Halonen, 1978). In 80-90 per cent of cases where death occurs within an hour of the onset of symptoms, the problem is of cardiovascular origin, but if the definition of 'sudden' death is extended to include all fatalities occurring within 24 hours of the primary complaint, the proportion of cases attributable to cardiovascular disease drops to 50-60 per cent. Some 90 per cent of cardiovascular deaths are in turn attributable to coronary atherosclerosis, although there are other possible pathologies, including acute left-ventricular failure due to aortic stenosis, aortic insufficiency or coarctation of the aorta, right-ventricular failure due to pulmonary hypertension, a dysrhythmia precipitated by a viral myocarditis and rupture of a dissecting aneurysm of the aorta or a berry aneurysm in the circle of Willis at the base of the skull. In one series of 1,348 deaths due to coronary atherosclerosis, 26 per cent had known coronary disease, 33 per cent had undiagnosed symptoms and in 41 per cent the condition had remained silent until immediately before death (R.J. Myerburg & Davies, 1964).

The immediate reason for death in the patient with ischaemic heart disease is thought to be ventricular fibrillation or asystole. However, few electrocardiograms are available except from severely ill patients dying in intensive care units. M.W. Stroud & Feil (1948) noted that, of 16 such cases, seven showed ventricular fibrillation and nine ventricular standstill. J.S. Robinson *et al.* (1965) found 24 examples of ventricular fibrillation and 14 episodes of ventricular asystole. Both reports noted that 'instantaneous' deaths tended to be associated with ventricular fibrillation, while a more prolonged period of shock and poor myocardial function led to ventricular standstill.

The explanation for the early episodes of ventricular fibrillation lies in the pathology of this condition. The abnormal rhythm is often provoked and usually maintained by a unidirectional blockage in transmission of the electrical impulse through an ischaemic portion of the myocardium. This situation allows re-entry of the impulse into a region of the myocardium that is capable of re-excitation, and a vicious cycle of abnormal electrical pathways is established (Figure 1.1; Y. Watanabe & Dreifus, 1972). Within 15~20 minutes of the development of coronary occlusion, the majority of the ischaemic cells have become totally unresponsive, and can no longer participate in re-entrant circuits (D. Durrer *et al.*, 1978).

Figure 1.1: To illustrate how an ischaemic, unidirectional block in transmission of the cardiac impulse can allow an abnormal ('re-entrant') impulse to re-excite an area of the myocardium (Y. Watanabe & Dreifus, 1972)

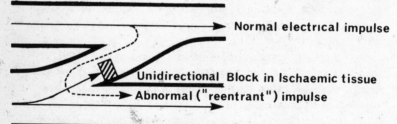

Later Complications

Cardiac failure

A non-fatal episode of myocardial infarction is usually followed by an acute failure of the cardiac pump (D.E. Harken, 1972; H.O. Hirzel *et al.*, 1973). About a third of patients show shock within six hours, a half within 24 hours and two thirds by 36 hours (S. Scheidt *et al.*, 1970). The minimum recorded systemic blood pressure gives an indication of the severity of this reaction.

After the formation of scar tissue, the effectiveness of the cardiac pump may still be handicapped by various types of abnormal motion in the affected portion of the ventricular wall. M.V. Herman *et al.* (1967) distinguish *akinesis* (a total lack of movement in a part of the heart wall), *asyneresis* (diminished motion), *dyskinesis* (paradoxical expansion of the wall) and *asynchrony* (a disturbed temporal sequence of contraction).

Occasionally, there may be rupture of a bulging (aneurysmal) area of the heart wall (R.A. Van Tassel & Edwards, 1972). However, an aneurysm is in itself rather uncommon among patients referred for exercise rehabilitation (14 of 610 cases in the series of R.J. Shephard *et al.*, 1980), and rupture is an even rarer event.

Ventricular fibrillation

The risk of ventricular fibrillation is greatest in the first 24 hours after infarction. Nevertheless, even after many months of apparently successful rehabilitation, the person who has sustained an infarct remains at an increased risk of death from dysrhythmia relative to an age-matched control. There is sometimes a premonitory phase, an increase in the frequency of multifocal premature ventricular contractions occurring during the 'vulnerable' part of the cardiac cycle (the R wave of the premature beat being superimposed on the preceding T wave of the electrocardiogram), but in 25–50 per cent of cases ventricular fibrillation develops without warning (M.G. Wyman & Hammersmith, 1974; K.I. Lie *et al.*, 1975; D.G. Julian *et al.*, 1978).

Extension of disease process

Development of a myocardial infarction is commonly a warning of advanced disease of the coronary vasculature and, unless the clinical episode serves to induce a dramatic change in the lifestyle of the patient, a further extension of the atherosclerotic process is likely.

Recurrent attacks of ischaemia lead to a progressive deterioration of myocardial function. A stage may be reached where exercise induces a decrease of stroke volume and a fall rather than a rise of systemic blood pressure, such phenomena being harbingers of recurrence of the infarction and of death (R.J. Shephard, 1979a). In such patients there is a real danger that exercise may provoke acute cardiac failure with a fatal waterlogging of the lungs, and for this reason exercise rehabilitation may be unwise for the individual with severe exercise-induced angina (J.O. Parker *et al.*, 1966).

International Classification of Diseases

It will be useful in concluding this chapter to relate the various conditions discussed to the International Classification of Disease (World Health Organisation, 1968). Unfortunately, the scheme of classification has undergone several changes over the years, as diagnoses have become more precise; for example, the 1968 revision increased the apparent incidence of coronary deaths by a factor of 1.146 (W.J. Walker, 1977).

The rubrics cited here refer to the eighth (1971) revision of the classification.

Acute ischaemic heart disease: angina pectoris, sudden death, coronary thrombosis and acute myocardial infarction (410, 411, 413).

Chronic ischaemic heart disease: fatty heart, myocardial degeneration (412).

Heart failure, cause unspecified (427-9).

Valvular heart disease (390-8, 421, 424).

2 THE CURRENT EPIDEMIC OF ISCHAEMIC HEART DISEASE

A stimulating popular book entitled *The Medical Runaround* (A. Malleson, 1973) exposes many medical fallacies. One trend for which British physicians had claimed great credit was the drop of suicides in the United Kingdom, from a peak of 5,600 per year in the early 1960s to just over 4,000 per year in 1970. Unfortunately for this piece of self-congratulation, careful analysis of the statistics disclosed that the overall decrease in suicides was the result of two opposing trends — a decrease in deaths from domestic coal-gas poisoning (as the Gas Council replaced coal gas by natural gas), and an increase in suicides by the use of medicaments over which the physicans supposedly had complete control.

The epidemic of ischaemic heart disease has given rise to much similar loose speculation. We will therefore scrutinise closely not only the extent of the epidemic, but also its origins and likely course.

Extent of the Epidemic

Incidence and prevalence

At first inspection, it might seem a simple matter to calculate the incidence and prevalence of ischaemic heart disease in a given community. Thus:

$$\text{Incidence rate} = \frac{\text{number of new cases of disease}}{\text{population at risk}}$$

over a specified period of time such as one year, while

$$\text{Prevalence rate} = \frac{\text{number of existing cases of disease}}{\text{total population}}$$

at any given time.

In practice, there are a number of complications to the derivation of such statistics.

Criterion of disease

It is first necessary to decide upon a criterion of disease. This could be the onset of cardiac symptoms such as anginal pain, the appearance

of an abnormal electrocardiogram, the development of a frank
'coronary' attack or a 'cardiac' death. Each of these various approaches
has its own inherent uncertainties.

Anginal pain. The patient may confuse anginal pain with indigestion or
the discomfort of an arthritic shoulder. Further, the threshold for the
reporting of the symptom varies greatly with the personality of the
patient and the level of physical activity that he habitually undertakes.
One reason why angina pectoris is more frequent in London bus
conductors than in the drivers (J.N. Morris *et al.*, 1953) is that the
former are more likely to undertake a sufficient rate of physical work
to reveal an impairment of their coronary blood supply.

Ischaemic exercise electrocardiogram. The exercise electrocardiogram
shows much day-to-day variation. In the Saskatoon experiment
(D.A. Bailey *et al.*, 1974), a randomly selected sample of adults were
cleared for exercise by a medically supervised sub-maximal stepping
test; nevertheless, when the same physician carried out a sub-maximal
cycle-ergometer test on these subjects a few days later, he found it
necessary to halt the test in four per cent of individuals because of
electrocardiographic abnormalities. The exercise electrocardiogram is
also liable to substantial inter-observer differences of interpretation.
H. Blackburn (1968) commented that the frequency of 'positive'
diagnoses in a set of exercise electrocardiograms varied from five to 55
per cent when interpretations were made by 14 different 'experts'!
Interestingly, technical personnel were more consistent and as accurate
as cardiologists in classifying ischaemic abnormalities of the electrocardiogram. Lastly, there are numerous physiological reasons for the
development of a falsely positive ischaemic appearance in the exercise
electrocardiogram (A.M. Katz, 1977; Table 7.4).

Clinical diagnosis. A severe 'coronary' attack is usually diagnosed fairly
readily, but minor infarcts are difficult to distinguish from other
medical problems, even if there is assistance from objective data such
as serial electrocardiograms and serum enzyme determinations
(Chapter 1).

It might be thought that the diagnosis of sudden death would leave
little room for uncertainty. However, in practice it is often difficult to
find reliable witnesses who can describe the time of onset of discomfort
or the exact minute of death.

The completion of death certificates provides an apparent wealth of information, but unfortunately the details given are notoriously imprecise, with much scope for both temporal and regional fashions when recording the principal cause of death. Interpretation of death rates is further complicated by successive changes in the International Classification of Diseases (Chapter 1).

Survey methods

Having decided upon the criterion of disease, it is then necessary to determine its incidence or prevalence. It is plainly impractical to wait for the patient himself to make a complaint. K.L. White & Ibrahim (1963) estimated that 150 of each 1,000 people in the United States had diagnosable cardiac disease, but that only 60 of the 150 would report their illness. Possible approaches are to conduct household, laboratory or community surveys.

Household surveys. In the usual form of household survey, a suitably trained nurse or health visitor visits randomly selected homes, questioning those encountered about cardiac disease or carrying out a simple exercise test (J. Murphy, 1980; R.J. Shephard, 1980a). If but one call is made to each home, the selected householder may be absent, and there is a danger that the sample will become unduly weighted by those who are confined to their homes. Particular care must be taken to include an appropriate proportion of individuals who live permanently in institutions (old people's homes, hospitals, prisons and the armed services), along with those who are frequent travellers (transport workers, business men and commercial representatives) or shift workers. Cooperation may be refused, questions may be misunderstood and, if an exercise test is performed a lack of habituation to the observer and the test procedure may give a high pulse rate, a high blood pressure and an unusually large secretion of catecholamines (R.J. Shephard, 1969).

Laboratory surveys. If randomly selected subjects are invited to attend a laboratory for a diagnostic procedure, attrition of the intended test population is even more dramatic than with a household survey. D.A. Bailey *et al.* (1974) carried out a fitness survey in the city of Saskatoon by taking names at random from the telephone directory. This approach immediately excluded those with unlisted telephone numbers, the poor who could not afford a telephone and the majority of those living in institutions. Of respondents (Table 2.1), about a third were frankly unwilling to attend the laboratory, and a further third made

Table 2.1: To Illustrate Sample Attrition When Subjects for a 'Fitness Test' are Selected Randomly from the Telephone Directory

Initial exclusions:	Institutionalised subjects	
	No telephone	
	Unlisted number	
Initial sample:	2648	telephone responses
	118	judged as unsuitable for testing
	982	refused test
	649	stated test time inconvenient or similar excuse
	49	failed to report for testing
	72	excluded by screening physician
	778	undertook fitness test

Source: Based on data of D.A. Bailey *et al.* (1974).

some excuse or failed to appear for testing at the appointed time. The group finally examined was thus a slender 32 per cent of the original telephone sample.

Community surveys. A final possibility is a community survey. In a small town, one may attempt to examine the entire population, while in a medium-sized city attention is directed to all citizens of a specific age group (such as all men born in 1913). Such approaches have been adopted with considerable success in Tecumseh, Michigan (H. Montoye, 1975), Framingham, Mass. (W.B. Kannel *et al.*, 1971a,b), Göteburg (L. Wilhelmsen *et al.*, 1972) and Malmö (N.H. Sternby, 1977). Close personal contacts with the population allow a much higher response rate in a small-town setting; for example, Montoye and his associates were able to examine 88 per cent of the 9,500 people living in Tecumseh in 1959-60, and to repeat examinations on 82 per cent of the population between 1961 and 1965.

The main disadvantage of a small-town survey is uncertainty concerning the relevance of the results to the modern metropoli in which most people currently live.

National differences

Keeping in mind these limitations of household, laboratory and community surveys, it is interesting to compare figures for the incidence of

Table 2.2: Age-standardised Average Yearly Incidence of Ischaemic Heart Disease Manifestations in Seven Countries, Expressed as Annual Incidence Rates per 10,000 Men Aged 40–59 Years, Free of Disease at Beginning of Study and Followed up for Five Years

Nation	Deaths	Myocardial infarctions	Angina	Other manifestations of ischaemic heart disease
Japan	9	between 15 and 20*		
Greece	8	8	1	15
Yugoslavia	11	8	18	16
Italy	12	18	30	40
Netherlands	27	33	23	56
US railways	37	28	67	45
Finland	26	31	71	70

* Documentation of non-fatal episodes for Japan is imprecise.

Source: A. Keys (1970).

ischaemic heart disease in different parts of the world (Table 2.2). In almost all nations, ischaemic heart disease is a major cause of disability and death, although there is a several-fold gradient in the occurrence rate for new events between countries such as Japan and Greece (where the incidence is relatively low) and Finland and the United States (where the incidence is particularly high). Some authors (for example, A. Keys, 1970) have attempted to correlate these differences with the average level of such risk factors as the percentage of energy taken in the form of saturated (animal) fat among the populations concerned.

Economic implications

The World Health Organisation (1976) noted that in 29 technologically advanced countries in 1967, cardiovascular disease accounted for 39 per cent of deaths among men aged 25 to 64 years, some three quarters of this total being due to ischaemic heart disease. In the US, cardiovascular disease accounts for 53 per cent of all deaths in men and women, 'coronary' attacks being responsible for 65 per cent of this total (R.A. Bruce, 1974).

The Canadian Government has assessed the economic impact of various health problems in terms of 'lost productive years.' The calculation is made noting deaths that occur after the age of one but

Table 2.3: Annual Loss of Productive Years in Canada through Deaths Occurring between the Ages of One and 70 Years, Based on Data for 1971

Cause of death	Annual loss of productive years	
	Men	Women
Ischaemic heart disease	157,000	36,000
Motor-vehicle accidents	154,000	59,000
Other accidents	136,000	43,000
Respiratory diseases	90,000	50,000
Suicide	51,000	18,000

Source: Lalonde (1974).

before the age of 70 years, each death being multiplied by the number of years that would have elapsed if the individual in question had lived to the age of 70 years (M. Lalonde, 1974; Table 2.3). On this criterion, ischaemic heart disease is the main health problem of Canadian men, and is an important consideration in women also.

Source of the Epidemic

Antiquity of the disease

Many people have viewed ischaemic heart disease as purely a twentieth-century epidemic, associated in some way with the 'evils' of modern civilisation. This concept has been supported by superficial comparisons of the incidence of the disease between the 'developed' and less-developed nations of our day.

Possibly in previous generations the problem was confined to an over-fed and pampered upper class of society. However, the writings of classical and neo-classical physicians (Chapter 1) leave little doubt that, since ancient times, a proportion of the human race has suffered from such manifestations of ischaemic heart disease as angina and sudden death. What has emerged over the past half-century has been a recognition by physicians of the symptoms and signs associated with acute myocardial infarction.

Twentieth-century trends

Although the disease process is not new in itself, vital statistics have shown a dramatic increase in most manifestations of ischaemic heart

Figure 2.1: Annual death rate for age-specific groups of the English and Welsh populations, based upon an analysis of the Registrar-General's statistics for 1931–48. Line (a) shows deaths from acute ischaemic heart disease (coronary arterial disease plus angina, including coronary atheroma — or atherosclerosis — and coronary, ischaemic — or arteriosclerotic — heart disease, particularly the syndrome of thrombosis, occlusion, and infarction and its variants). Line (b) shows chronic myocardial diseases (including late deaths from myocardial infarction). Line (c) is the sum of (a) and (b).

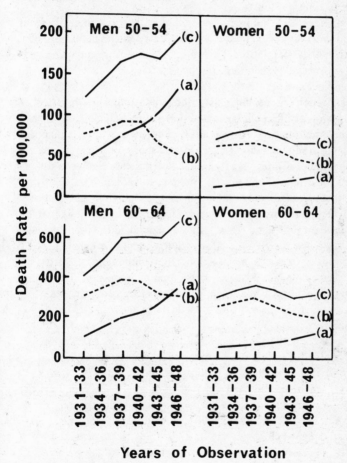

Source: J.N. Morris (1951).

disease over the first half of the present century. J.N. Morris (1951) examined figures for England and Wales, taken from the Registrar General and covering the period 1931-48. Data for men aged 50-4 years and 60-4 years showed a progressive increase in deaths attributed to ischaemic heart disease, this trend being attributable to acute rather than to chronic manifestations of the disorder (Figure 2.1). Among women of comparable age, deaths due to coronary vascular disease were less frequent, but nevertheless they also showed an increase of 'acute' deaths. Subsequent analyses from the United States and Canada revealed similar trends.

It could be argued that part, if not all, of the increase in deaths from ischaemic heart disease is an artefact, reflecting changes in fashions of diagnosis and the completion of death certificates. Some authors have alleged that previous generations of physicians were wont to ascribe sudden and unexpected deaths to vague, non-specific causes such as 'acute indigestion', 'apoplexy' and 'chronic myocardial degeneration'. T.W. Anderson and his colleagues thus devoted considerable effort to establishing that the epidemic was a real phenomenon. An examination of vital statistics for the Province of Ontario showed them an increase in certification of deaths from ischaemic heart disease similar to that described for Britain (Figure 2.2; T.W. Anderson & Le Riche, 1970). They next studied figures for sudden deaths, the majority of which are attributable to ischaemic heart disease (Chapter 1); again they observed a progressive upward trend. Lastly, they re-examined the original death certificates, re-interpreting the information where this seemed appropriate. Contrary to previous suggestions, they found no deaths from 'acute indigestion', and few deaths attributed to 'apoplexy'. The revised statistics thus confirmed that there was a large increase in the death rate due to ischaemic heart disease, particularly between 1931 and 1961.

As a further check upon the reality of the epidemic, death rates were compared for men and for women (T.W. Anderson, 1976; T.W. Anderson & Halliday, 1979; M. Halliday & Anderson, 1979). It was reasoned that if there had been a change of diagnostic fashion, statistics for men and women would have been affected by approximately the same extent. However, in practice the sex ratios for heart disease (all types) remained close to unity until the mid-1920s, when there was a dramatic increase of disease in the men, similar in timing and in magnitude for Canada, the United States and England and Wales (Figure 2.3). Furthermore, there was no decrease in the sex ratio for other conditions that might have been confused with cardiac disease

Figure 2.2: Deaths from ischaemic heart disease in the Province of Ontario. The figure illustrates official mortality data for ischaemic heart disease — angina pectoris, coronary thrombosis, myocardial infarction and arteriosclerotic heart disease — in men aged 45-64 years, the probable incidence of ischaemic heart disease deaths (based upon the authors' reinterpretation of the death certificates; probable ischaemic heart disease includes ischaemic heart disease and non-specific heart disease — heart failure, cardiac dropsy, organic heart disease, myocarditis, etc.), and the incidence of sudden death (adjusted to allow for certificates with no information on duration of illness). Note that, in contrast to the graphs of J.N. Morris (Figure 2.1), a logarithmic scale has been used upon the ordinate.

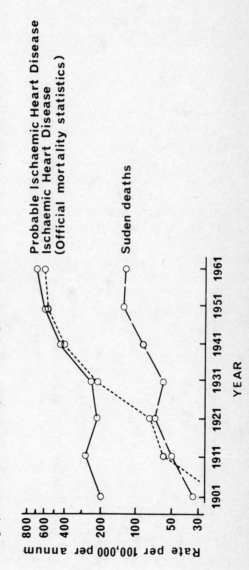

Probable Ischaemic Heart Disease

Ischaemic Heart Disease
(Official mortality statistics)

Suden deaths

Source: Based on an analysis of T.W. Anderson and Le Riche (1970).

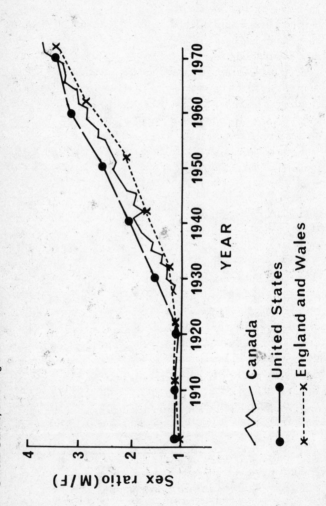

Figure 2.3: The sex ratio (male/female) for all forms of heart disease in subjects aged 45 to 64 years. Data for Canada, United States, and England and Wales.

Source: T.W. Anderson (1976).

(other diseases of the circulation, nephritis, indigestion, asthma and diabetes mellitus). There must therefore have been a true increase of ischaemic heart disease deaths among the men, or (much less likely) a decrease among the women, over the period of inquiry.

Calculation of the sex ratios revealed two other interesting facets of the cardiac epidemic. Firstly, although one might consider coronary atherosclerosis as but one manifestation of a general vascular disorder, there was no evidence of a time-related change in the sex ratio for other vascular conditions such as cerebral vascular accidents; T.W. Anderson (1976) thus suggested that some local factor had increased the vulnerability of the myocardium over the period of observation. Secondly, there had been a progressive change in the social characteristics of those affected by ischaemic heart disease (M. Halliday & Anderson, 1979). In the 1920s, ischaemic heart disease was a problem of the gentry, the rise of sex ratio occurring largely in British social class one (the professional workers). More recently, the disease has extended progressively to blue-collar groups, with a rapid rise in the sex ratio for social class five (the manual labourers).

Factors associated with the current waning of the epidemic are dicussed in the next section of this chapter.

Risk factors and diseases

A number of 'risk factors' (Table 2.4) increase an individual's chances of developing ischaemic heart disease (J. Truett *et al.*, 1967; W.B. Kannel *et al.*, 1971a, b; G.F. Fletcher & Cantwell, 1971, 1974; R.A. Bruce, 1974; J.P. Strong, 1977). Some of these variables, such as age, sex, race, geographic location and the mineral content of the drinking water, are largely outside of personal control, but other factors are strongly related to lifestyle. In the latter context, we may note specifically hypertension, cigarette smoking, physical inactivity, a high serum cholesterol, diabetes and obesity.

It is interesting to search for a parallel between changes to the population levels of these various risk factors and the onset of the current epidemic of ischaemic heart disease, although in so doing we are handicapped by limitations in the data available and uncertainties concerning the time lag between the development of a given risk factor and the appearance of overt disease.

Hypertension. There are many causes of high blood pressure, including some factors over which the hypertensive individual has no control. Nevertheless, population levels of systemic blood pressure are affected

Table 2.4: Risk Factors Predisposing to Ischaemic Heart Disease*

Cigarette smoking/impaired pulmonary function/carboxyhaemoglobin

Hypertension

Blood lipid abnormalities/hereditary hypercholesterolaemia

Physical inactivity/high resting heart rate

Excess body mass

Heredity/family history of 'heart attacks'/blood group other than O

Personality and behaviour patterns/socio-economic status/'stress'

Abnormal ECG

Carbohydrate intolerance/diabetes

Increased serum uric acid/gout

Softness of drinking water

Disorders of blood coagulation

Hypothyroidism

Diet (excess animal fat/sucrose/heavy meals)

Male sex (especially before menopause)

Age

---

* Note that: (1) many of these factors are inter-related (American Heart Association, 1972; R. Paffenbarger, 1977; W.B. Kannel, 1979); (2) a given risk factor has more predictive value in some populations than in others (A. Keys, 1975); and (3) it is by no means proven that the risk of developing clinical disease can be changed by modifying these factors (Council on Rehabilitation, 1973; Hickey *et al.*, 1975).

by lifestyle, particularly the dietary intake of table salt, and the extent of exposure to 'stress'.

Historic details of salt consumption are limited. In some parts of Africa and Asia where salt is still in short supply, the incidence of hypertension is much lower than in Europe and North America (I. Maddocks, 1964). It might be thought that the western use of salt was greater before the general availability of fresh foods and refrigeration. H. Kaunitz (1956) noted that wars were fought over sources of salt, and for centuries its trade was more important than that of any other material. However, B. Friend *et al.* (1979) estimated that in the US an increased consumption of processed food increased the average daily sodium intake by 14 per cent from 1909-13 to 1976.

The 'stress' associated with the life of the modern city dweller is still keenly debated (R.S. Eliot, 1974). H.I. Russek & Russek (1977) reported that one in twenty of US workers had two jobs, and some had three; further, among coronary victims 25 per cent had been holding

Table 2.5: Prevalence of Coronary Disease by Age and Arbitrary Assessment of Occupational Stress

Occupational stress	Prevalence of disease (%)		
	Age 40-9 years	Age 50-9 years	Age 60-9 years
Low: Dermatologists, orthodontists, patent lawyers, periodontists	0.70	5.42	7.38
Moderate: Oral surgeons, other lawyers, pathologists, security analysts, trial lawyers	2.09	6.42	13.46
High: Anaesthesiologists, general practice dentists, general practice lawyers, general practice physicians, security traders	4.20	11.40	19.43

Source: Based on data of H.I. Russek & Russek (1977).

down two jobs, and a further 46 per cent had been working 60 or more hours per week prior to the onset of symptoms. Likewise, T. Kavanagh & Shephard (1973a) noted that in the year prior to a coronary attack business problems had been increased in 71 per cent of their patients, were normal in 27 per cent and decreased in only two per cent, a very different pattern of response from that reported by control subjects from the same occupations. H.I. Russek & Russek (1977) further observed a gradient in the occurrence of ischaemic heart disease that was correlated with the pre-judged stressfulness of 20 different occupations (Table 2.5).

Such views are by no means novel. William Osler (1896) noted that the typical case of angina pectoris was a 'keen and ambitious man, the indicator of whose engines is always set "full speed ahead" ', and others have repeatedly reiterated this assessment (for example, J.A. Arlow, 1945; C. Kemple, 1945). There is clearly some association between the time-oriented, competitive ('Type A') personality and an increased risk of hypertension and ischaemic heart disease (M. Friedman & Rosenman, 1974), although many coronary victims do not show the classical 'Type A' picture of excessively rapid movement, tense musculature, explosive conversation, excessive gesturing and a general air of impatience (H.I. Russek & Zohman, 1958).

It is possible that present-day society encourages the development of 'Type A' characteristics in the 'successful' executive. Several authors have pointed to an association between urban living and hypertension (for example, J. Stamler *et al.*, 1967). However, other investigators have emphasized that not everyone reacts to modern city living in the same manner. Thus L.E. Hinckle & Wolff (1962) found more hypertension in young business executives with only a high-school education than in those who were university graduates; they concluded that business was stressful only for those who were upwardly mobile. Likewise, C. Hames (1975) observed a correlation between the prevalence of coronary disease and the recent acquisition of status symbols such as education and ownership of property. The two points of view may be reconcilable, since it can be argued that the 'Type A' person is the most aggressive in climbing the ladder of success.

Sceptics have claimed that the main stresses faced by many business men are over-large lunches, too frequent cocktails and a lack of physical activity! Certainly, there is no strong evidence that the pressures of daily life have increased over the last 50 years. Furthermore, Japan has had a very high incidence of hypertension over this period, but it has only recently begun to experience the cardiac epidemic (C.P. Wen & Gershoff, 1973). It thus seems unlikely that a salt- or stress-induced outbreak of hypertension is the prime cause of the increase is ischaemic heart disease over the present century.

Cigarette smoking

Cigarette smoking is a much stronger candidate habit for explanation of the cardiac epidemic. It is thought to have a long-term influence upon the course of atherogenesis (N. Wald *et al.*, 1973), hypoxia of the blood vessel walls associated with carboxyhaemoglobin formation and a shift of the oxygen dissociation curve both favouring the formation of atherosclerotic plaques (P. Åstrup *et al.*, 1966; P. Åstrup, 1977; H.C. McGill, 1977). Smoking also has more immediate effects upon myocardial irritability and the dimensions of the coronary vasculature, increasing the frequency of premature ventricular contractions (H.J.L. Marriott & Myerburg, 1974) and speeding the development of exercise-induced angina (W.S. Aronow *et al.*, 1968).

The first cigarette-rolling machines appeared about 1870, and the habit rapidly gained ground in the early 1900s, becoming epidemic among the generation of young men serving in the first world war (Figure 2.4). There is thus a fairly close temporal relationship between

Figure 2.4: Percentage of US men currently smoking cigarettes. Data for 1955, 1966 and 1970, shown in relation to age at time of survey and birth cohort. Note that cigarette smoking first becomes epidemic in the cohort reaching manhood during the first world war.

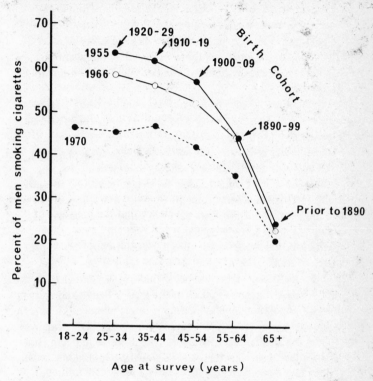

Source: Based on data in *The Health Consequences of Smoking, 1974* (US Dept. of Health, Education and Welfare, Washington, DC).

the development of cigarette consumption in the western world and the appearance of an increased number of male cardiovascular deaths.

In women, smoking first became widespread during the second world war, and over the period 1921 to 1971 the increase in incidence of ischaemic heart disease among women remained relatively small (T.W. Anderson & Halliday, 1979): if we are to accept the hypothesis that cigarette consumption contributed to the male epidemic, we must therefore postulate that other factors have intervened to protect women from the consequences of a similar lifestyle.

Habitual physical inactivity

Daily activity fell progressively over the first half of the present century. One significant change was in the amount of energy used for personal transportation. This can be documented in terms of motor vehicle registrations. In the US, the number of cars rose from a very small number in 1900 to a peak about 1928, this being surpassed only in the 1950s. Since 1950, the main increase has been in the number of families owning two or more cars (Table 2.6), with about a sixth of the population (the poor, the disabled and the elderly) still not owning a car.

Until the recent renaissance of recreational cycling, rising sales of cars were linked with corresponding mass closures of factories manufacturing bicycles.

The ever-increasing industrial and domestic power consumption suggests that automation has also reduced the energy demands of occupational and domestic pursuits over the present century, although O.G. Edholm (1970) has advanced the provocative hypothesis that new technology has increased the output of goods per worker, leaving the energy cost of his daily activity unchanged.

The overall food consumption of the US population showed a per capita decline of some 1.25 Megajoules (MJ) per day from 1930 to 1960 (Table 2.7); although there has been some recovery of energy usage in the 1970s, if account is taken of the greater height and mass of the present-day population, energy consumption would need to have increased by about 0.6 MJ per day in order to sustain the level of daily activity seen in the 1930s. Part of the observed decrease in energy usage could be attributed to such factors as ageing of the population (basal

Table 2.6: Car Ownership in the United States (per family)

Year	No car (%)	One car (%)	Two or more cars (%)
1950	41	52	7
1955	30	60	10
1960	23	62	15
1965	21	55	24
1970	21	50	29
1974	18*	49	33

* But two per cent have some form of light truck, leaving only 16 per cent without personal transportation.

Table 2.7: Daily per Capita Food Consumption in the United States

Year	Total energy value (MJ)	Carbohydrate (g)	Fat (g)	Protein (g)
1930	14.4	474	134	93
1940	14.0	429	143	93
1950	13.6	402	145	94
1960	13.1	375	143	95
1965	13.1	372	144	96
1970	13.8	380	157	100
1975	13.6	377	152	99
1977	14.1	391	159	103

metabolism decreases with age) and an increased use of processed food (with a decrease of kitchen wastage). However, casual observation suggests that the wastage of food has increased rather than decreased as the population has become more affluent. The data therefore strongly suggest that there has been a decrease of physical activity, particularly between 1930 and 1960.

Nevertheless, the contribution of physical inactivity to the cardiac epidemic is probably rather small. In terms of motor-car usage, relatively few citizens of the United Kingdom owned vehicles before world war II, and during the war most civilians were unable to obtain petrol for the operation of personal transportation. However, the cardiac epidemic was well established in 1946-8 (Figure 2.1), and indeed the male/female ratio increased with only slight retardation relative to US statistics (Figure 2.3). Automation is also unlikely to have been a major factor, since in the Britain of J.N. Morris's study there had been little attempt to modernise industry or to reduce the physical demands upon the worker. Even patterns of leisure activity had shown little change in Britain by 1948; although public television broadcasting was introduced in 1936, the majority of the population did not purchase television sets until the mid-1950s.

We must conclude that, while habitual activity has undoubtedly undergone changes over the present century, the pace of change has shown quite large differences between North America and western Europe, without parallel differences in the time course of the cardiac epidemic.

Serum cholesterol

Much of the serum cholesterol is normally manufactured in the liver (H.S. Sodhi *et al.*, 1977). Nevertheless, there is some evidence that the level of serum cholesterol is influenced by the balance between habitual activity and the dietary intake of animal fat. J.J. Groen *et al.* (1959) noted low cholesterol levels in Trappist monks who did not eat fish, meat, eggs or butter. Likewise, Somali camel-herders (V. Lapiccirella *et al.*, 1962) and the East African Masai (G.V. Mann *et al.*, 1965) seem relatively free of ischaemic heart disease despite a diet rich in dairy fat, presumably because they counter their adverse diet by a much higher level of physical activity than is usual in western man.

Many western peoples have increased their fat consumption over the present century, but this is due more to an increase in the consumption of salad oil, cooking oil and margarine than to an increased intake of other forms of fat (Table 2.8). If the present intake of animal fat is undesirably high, it would seem that this situation was already established in the early part of the present century, at least in the United States.

An interesting contrast is provided by data for occupied Europe during world war II. Between 1942 and 1946, the diet dropped to a total energy input of 3.4–4.2 MJ per day, with some 5–10 g in the form of fat. The mean body mass was 10–15 kg below normal, and the serum cholesterol fell from a pre-war average of around 200 $mg \cdot dl^{-1}$ to about 140 $mg \cdot dl^{-1}$. Given this drastic modification of national diets, atherosclerotic deaths due to conditions such as myocardial infarction

Table 2.8: Patterns of Fat Consumption in the United States, 1909-13 to 1976

Year	Total fat consumed (g)	Salad oil, cooking oil and margarine (g)	Other fat (g)
1909-13	125	3.4	121.6
1935-9	132	10.9	121.1
1947-9	140	14.7	125.3
1957-9	143	22.5	120.5
1965	144	27.5	116.5
1970	156	33.6	122.4
1976	157	38.5	118.5

Source: Based on data of B. Friend *et al.* (1979).

were substantially reduced relative to pre-war statistics (Malmros, 1950; G. Schettler, 1977).

Refined carbohydrate and diabetes

A second major historical change of diet has involved a progressive increase in the consumption of sucrose and other refined carbohydrates. Early statistics suggest that there was an annual per capita usage of 5 lb (2.3 kg) of sucrose in 1750 and 25 lb (11.4 kg) in 1850. More recent US data (B. Friend *et al.*, 1979) show a further rise from 75 lb (34 kg) in 1909–13 to a peak of 104 lb (47 kg) at the time of prohibition. Subsequent consumption has hovered just under 100 lb per year, with a peak of 102 lb (46 kg) in 1973 (probably due to the ban on the sale of cyclamates), and a decrease in 1974 (probably related to a substantial rise in world sugar prices).

The increased sugar intake could influence cardiovascular health at least indirectly. Diabetes is a well-recognised risk factor for ischaemic heart disease, and the likelihood of maturity-onset diabetes is influenced by the balance between habitual activity and the dietary intake of sucrose. However, the chain of events is somewhat tenuous, and again the increase of sugar consumption began long before the onset of the cardiac epidemic.

Obesity

The epidemiological significance of obesity is still a matter of some controversy. A Keys *et al.* (1972) claimed that an excessive body weight was not a risk factor for ischaemic heart disease if prior allowance was made for the associated risks of high systemic blood pressure and a high serum cholesterol level. Such computer analyses are interesting, but unfortunately they cannot prove whether hypertension or obesity is the primary disorder. There is certainly an association between gross obesity and death from cardiovascular disease (Society of Actuaries, 1959). In men aged 15–69 years, the mortality due to diseases of the heart and circulation is 131 per cent of standard for those 24 kg above the ideal mass, rising to 155 per cent with 33 kg excess mass, and 185 per cent with 42 kg of excess mass. Furthermore, there is good evidence that a reduction of excess mass will reduce both hypertension and cholesterol (F.W. Ashley & Kannel, 1974). Thus in a practical sense, if there has been an increase in the proportion of obese individuals in a country, this could have contributed to the appearance of a cardiac epidemic.

Historical information on obesity is limited, and inter-survey comparisons are complicated by (i) the secular trend to an increase of standing height, and (ii) uncertainties concerning the adjustments that investigators have made for the mass of clothing and the height of shoes when reporting their data. Portrait galleries from previous centuries suggest that many of the wealthy were quite obese. In contrast, in poor and underdeveloped societies, a low incidence of ischaemic heart disease today remains coupled with extremely low skinfold readings, and a body mass that is often 10–15 kg below the actuarial ideal value (R.J. Shephard, 1974a, 1978a).

Many Europeans are currently much heavier than their counterparts were during world war II. Thus the Birmingham workers of 1960 studied by T. Khosla & Lowe (1967) were 6–7 kg heavier than the men of wartime Britain (W.F.F. Kemsley, 1951–3), even when the two sets of data were standardised to a common height of 175 cm. Nevertheless, such increases of body mass do not parallel the time course of the cardiac epidemic in England and Wales (Figure 2.1).

Conclusion

The cause or causes of the cardiac epidemic have yet to be identified with certainty. Cigarette smoking is one major aspect of lifestyle that does appear to have changed in parallel with the epidemic, but its influence is not strong enough to account for the entire phenomenon. Heavy smoking approximately doubles the risk of a fatal coronary attack (R. Paffenbarger, 1977) and, since some 50 per cent of men developed a heavy cigarette habit over the period in question, smoking could have increased the attack rate by about 50 per cent. In fact, there was at least a three- to four-fold increase of mortality between the early 1900s and 1960 (Figures 2.1–2.3). We must thus presume that smoking interacted with other risk factors yet to be delineated. On the statistics of R. Paffenbarger (1977), the entire increase might be explained by a combination of smoking, low energy output and hypertension secondary to obesity.

Recent Course of Epidemic

The downturn

Epidemiologists in the United States and Canada have been fascinated to note that over the past 15 years the trend to an increase of ischaemic heart disease deaths has been reversed (T.W. Anderson, 1978b; Figure 2.5). In Britain, mortality only began to decrease in 1974 (Du V.C. Florey *et al.*, 1978), but the North American epidemic apparently

Figure 2.5: Course of ischaemic heart disease epidemic 1950–76. Data for Canadian and US 'white' subjects aged 55–64 years, adjusted to allow for the change in classification of ischaemic heart disease (1968, USA; 1969, Canada).

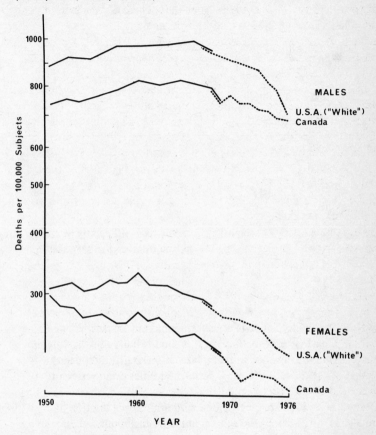

Source: T.W. Anderson (1978b).

peaked about 1967, and 'cardiac deaths' among middle-aged adults have subsequently fallen by about 25 per cent (Table 2.9). The decrease has occurred equally in 'white' and 'non-white' groups, but it has been some four per cent larger in those with recorded hypertension than in those without this sign, while the improvement of prognosis for acute myocardial infarction (the first eight weeks after the attack) has been almost twice as large as for those dying of chronic ischaemic heart

Table 2.9: Decrease in Age-specific Coronary Mortality of US Citizens, 1963–75, Adjusted for Changes in Eighth Revision of International Classification of Disease

Age (years)	Decline of age-specific coronary mortality (%)
35–44	27.2
45–54	27.4
55–64	23.5
65–74	25.3
75–84	12.8
Over 85	19.3

Source: W.D. Walker (1977).

disease. It has been less clearly established that the incidence of non-fatal attacks has changed.

Naturally, many groups, ranging from exercise enthusiasts to cardiac surgeons, have been eager to claim responsibility for this favourable trend of vital statistics.

Improved treatment

A part of the reduction in 'coronary' deaths is probably due to recent advances in the medical and surgical treatment of ischaemic heart disease. In particular, it could be argued that fewer young and middle-aged patients who sustain 'heart attacks' are dying of their disease.

In the past, a large number of cardiac fatalities occurred before the patient could reach hospital, and it might thus be inferred that the improved prognosis was related to the widespread instruction of ambulance crews and of the general public in techniques of cardiac resuscitation (L. Cobb *et al.*, 1975; D.A. Chamberlain, 1978a; J.R. Hampton & Nicholas, 1978; A.F. MacKintosh *et al.*, 1978; P. Siltanen, 1978). Over a third of the Seattle population, for example, is now qualified to undertake such emergency treatment. While gains are to be anticipated from such training, in fact they have yet to be realised. P. Siltanen (1978) found that the specially trained ambulance crews reached about a half of the cases of cardiac arrest where medical aid was summoned before death had occurred, but they were able to treat less than five per cent of all cases of unexpected cardiac arrest. Perhaps because of fears generated by arrival of the special 'cardiac' ambulance, the early mortality for mobile coronary care units has also equalled or slightly exceeded that for patients transported by normal ambulance (J.R. Hampton & Nicholas, 1978; P. Siltanen, 1978).

It might be anticipated that a large reduction of 'coronary' mortality would have resulted from the introduction of expensively equipped intensive-care wards. However, again possibly because of fears aroused by the special treatment, controlled trials have shown that the acute coronary care unit offers little advantage of prognosis relative to treatment in the patient's own home (J.D. Hill *et al.*, 1978).

Early trials of β-adrenoceptor antagonists had disappointingly little influence upon mortality following myocardial infarction (R. Balcon *et al.*, 1966; J. Clausen *et al.*, 1966; Multicentre Trial, 1966; R.M. Norris *et al.*, 1968), but it has been suggested that the dose of propranolol used was too small. D.A. Chamberlain (1978b) has now presented evidence that large doses of cardio-selective β-blocking drugs such as practolol and alprenolol reduce the number of cardiac deaths in the period one month to one year post-infarction, although the effect observed (a halving of events) would reduce the overall mortality from ischaemic heart disease by about two per cent rather than 25 per cent.

By-pass surgery may also improve prognosis in selected cases (Table 2.10), particularly patients with multiple-vessel disease (A.V.G. Bruschke, 1977) or left-main-stem coronary-artery disease (M.H. Frick *et al.*, 1978). Frick *et al.* comment that 'in no report has the surgical treatment been inferior to medical management' but that 'data analyzed do not strongly favor surgical therapy as a means of reducing the rate of sudden death nor death in general for that matter.'

We must thus conclude that the overall contribution of improved treatment to the decline in mortality has been relatively small, and certainly much less than 25 per cent.

Increased physical activity

Voluntary leisure-time physical activity has undoubtedly increased in popularity among North Americans over the past 15 years. In one survey of Harvard alumnae, R. Paffenbarger *et al.* (1978) observed that the proportion of physically active individuals had increased from 35 per cent to 70–80 per cent over the course of a longitudinal study. Sales of recreational bicycles, cross-country skis and other equipment for endurance activity have increased vastly since the early 1960s. Nevertheless in North America, as in Scandinavia (S. Stensassen, 1978), this

Table 2.10: Influence of Surgical Treatment on Survival Following Myocardial Infarction

Type of disease	Period of follow-up (years)	Medical treatment (%)	Surgical treatment (%)
Single-vessel disease	5	89.0	94.6
Two-vessel disease	5	70.0	94.1
Three-vessel disease	4	65.0	92.7
Aneurysm	4	59.0	84.1
Diffuse myocardial impairment	3	23.9	33.0

Source: Based on data of A.V.G. Bruschke (1977).

change of attitude is predominantly a middle-class phenomenon, and the great mass of lower-class Americans have yet to turn from their sedentary lifestyle.

Among the telephone sample of the Saskatoon population (D.A. Bailey *et al.*, 1974), 60 per cent of men and 64 per cent of women were still taking only one session or less of endurance activity per week. On the limiting assumptions that (i) a half of the remaining 38 per cent were new converts to exercise, and (ii) that such exercise halved the chances of a fatal heart attack (R. Paffenbarger, 1977; R. Paffenbarger *et al.*, 1978), the maximum reduction in mortality from this cause would be ten per cent.

Cigarette smoking

The proportion of male cigarette smokers in the coronary-prone age categories has dropped steadily over the period of inquiry. The US sample reached a peak of about 63 per cent smokers in 1955 (Figure 2.4), dropping to about 46 per cent in 1970. Figures for Canada are similar, with 44 per cent of continuing smokers in 1973 (*Smoking in Canada*, 1973).

On the basis that smoking doubles the risk of sudden death (Framingham Heart Study, 1966), this change of behaviour would in itself account for a twelve per cent decrease in deaths from ischaemic heart disease. Many of the fatalities in continuing smokers are sudden deaths due to the onset of ventricular fibrillation. The contribution of reduced smoking to the waning of the epidemic is thus supported by the greater relative reduction of acute than of chronic deaths.

Table 2.11: Change in Per Capita Consumption of Tobacco and Fat
(US Citizens, 1963 to 1975)

Product	Change in per capita consumption (%)
Tobacco (all forms)	− 22.4
Animal fat and oils	− 56.7
Vegetable fat and oils	+ 44.1
Butter	− 31.9
Milk and cream	− 19.2
Eggs	− 12.6

Source: Based on an analysis by W.D. Walker (1977).

Intake of animal fat

North Americans have shown a substantial increase in the intake of
supposedly unsaturated fat over the present century (Tables 2.8 and
2.11). However, the trend was initiated at a time when the incidence
of ischaemic heart disease was still rising steeply. A long lag period
between fat intake and disease must thus be postulated if the recent
decline in mortality is to be attributed to the dietary change. Such is
indeed possible. A reduced intake of animal fat probably does little
to reverse established atherosclerotic lesions, but it may well prevent
the formation of the initial fatty plaques in younger individuals who
as yet have healthy arteries.

Conclusion

Much of the decrease in deaths from ischaemic heart disease over the
past fifteen years can apparently be attributed to favourable changes
in the lifestyle of the average North American (Table 2.11). There is
prima facie evidence that a combination of reduced cigarette smoking
and enhanced physical activity account for over 20 per cent of the
observed change, with the remaining five per cent possibly due to long-
term changes in eating habits and improved patterns of treatment for
established disease.

   This conclusion is particularly encouraging for those concerned
with preventive medicine. Until recently, cynics have insisted that
human behaviour cannot be changed. They have pointed out that gains
from health education seem few and short-lived. For example, the
massive report of the US surgeon-general on *Smoking and Health*

(1964) apparently produced no more than a five per cent decrease of US cigarette consumption, which disappeared over the next one to two years. Nevertheless, graphs such as Figure 2.4 show that in a more long-term sense the efforts of the health educators are modifying human behaviour, and this in turn is now having a positive influence upon the health of the North American population.

3 ISCHAEMIC HEART DISEASE AND THE RISKS OF EXERCISE

Newspapers frequently publicise fatalities involving well-known athletes, particularly if death has occurred during physical activity. R. Medved *et al.* (1973) describe a 29-year-old member of the Yugoslavian national soccer team who died suddenly, soon after competition, with narrowing of the aorta as a possible contributory cause. K.S. Zakopoulos (1973) collected histories of seven such episodes in Greek soccer players over the course of twenty years; one 24-year-old man died of cardiac arrest, and another man aged 29 died of acute myocardial infarction. Personal experience of this type of incident includes an apparently healthy 23-year-old university student who died after hanging for several minutes from the parallel bars in the gymnasium, and a middle-aged janitor who died while rushing up several flights of stairs to attend to a broken water-main. The latter individual had completed a multistage stress test some weeks previously; the laboratory exercise had been symptomless, but the electrocardiogram had shown marked ST segmental depression and multiple abnormalities of cardiac rhythm as maximum effort was approached (see Chapter 8).

Before proceeding to consider the possible therapeutic value of exercise, it is thus necessary to examine the alternative hypothesis that physical activity increases the immediate mortality of seemingly normal adults, of the 'coronary-prone' and of patients with established clinical ischaemic heart disease. After noting the basic risk of a coronary attack in the average adult, we shall look at the patho-physiology of those dying during exercise, epidemiological data and the experience gained through exercise testing and prescription. The issues of more general injury and infection attributable to exercise will be discussed briefly in Chapter 9.

The Basic Risk of Myocardial Infarction and Sudden Death

Even if physical activity was not a precipitating factor, a certain number of 'coronary' events would be anticipated in exercising subjects as a matter of chance. The likely statistics can be calculated

49

from the incidence of ischaemic heart disease (Chapter 2). In an older man of working age, for example, the risk of developing a heart attack in any given year is about one chance in three hundred, and only about a third of these cases will die during the acute episode.

Given that the average bout of voluntary exercise lasts about 30 minutes, the chances that the attack will occur during this specific session are about two in ten million, with the risk of a fatality about six in 100 million. Figures for women are only about a third as large. Statistics can be further improved if training programmes educate the general public in the techniques of cardiac resuscitation (Chapter 2).

On the other hand, if exercise is repeated 150 times per year, there is a corresponding increase in the *a priori* likelihood that an attack will occur while the individual is physically active.

Patho-physiology of Sudden Death during Exercise

Possible mechanisms

E. Jokl (1958) and more recently E. Jokl & McClellan (1971) have maintained that exercise never causes the death of a normal heart, at least in a temperate climate. Likewise L.E. Hinckle *et al.* (1969) suggested that, if abnormalities of cardiac rhythm were provoked by ordinary physical activity, there was usually some underlying cardiac disease. While such views are probably correct, they are not particularly helpful in elucidating the dangers of exercise, for as we have already noted there is evidence of atherosclerosis in the hearts of most North Americans from a relatively early age (W.F. Ebos *et al.*, 1955; D. Jaffé & Manning, 1971).

Sudden death has many patho-physiological connotations, particularly if statistics are extended to include all patients dying within 24 hours of the onset of symptoms. However, if interest is restricted to the first one or two hours, ventricular fibrillation or asystole is largely responsible (Chapter 1; H.K. Hellerstein & Turrell, 1964; H. Grendahl, 1967; T.N. James, 1972). There are several possible mechanisms whereby an increase of physical activity could enhance myocardial irritability and thus provoke fibrillation or asystole.

The cardiac work-rate may be augmented four- or five-fold by increases in: (i) heart rate; (ii) systolic pressure; and (iii) myocardial contractility (Chapter 8). A combination of shortened diastole and increase of systolic pressure restricts perfusion of left-ventricular muscle, increasing the chances that a relative oxygen lack will develop. The sub-endocardial tissue is particularly vulnerable, and hypoxia may persist in this region during the recovery period. At this stage, a catastrophic fall of blood pressure and thus coronary perfusion may arise from passive standing in a humid changing room or use of an excessively hot shower (R.A. Bruce *et al.*, 1968), while slowing of the heart rate enhances the danger of re-entry of the electrical impulse (Chapter 1). The excitability of the myocardium is further disturbed by alterations of the balance between sodium and potassium ions across the cell membranes of the myocardium, as potassium ions leak from skeletal and cardiac muscle (R.J. Shephard & Kavanagh, 1975) and fluids with an excessive content of potassium ions are administered (T. Kavanagh & Shephard, 1978). If the patient becomes anxious, hyperventilation and an increased liberation of catecholamines add to the irritability of the heart.

Ventricular premature contractions are generally held to be of two types (G. Bourne, 1927; R.H. Mann & Burchell, 1952). One is present at rest and becomes less frequent during exercise. This form of dysrhythmia is quite common (for example, R.G. Hiss & Lamb, 1962, found a prevalence of 0.8 per cent among 122,000 asymptomatic Air Force personnel aged 16 to 50 years). It appears to be relatively benign (J.M. Clarke *et al.*, 1976; M. Brodsky *et al.*, 1977). The other type of premature ventricular contractions is aggravated by exercise or appears for the first time during exercise (B. Lown *et al.*, 1969; H. Blackburn *et al.*, 1973; J.M. Atkins *et al.*, 1976), and becomes even more apparent in the recovery period. This second type of dysrhythmia is an accompaniment of otherwise symptomless atheroma in the middle-aged person and, particularly if of multifocal origin, it is associated with both ischaemic depression of the ST segment of the electrocardiogram and progression to sudden death from ventricular fibrillation or asystole (B. Chiang *et al.*, 1969; L.E. Hinckle *et al.*, 1969; J.A. Vedin *et al.*, 1972).

Exercise may also contribute to the development of a frank myocardial infarct. This could arise from a relative ischaemia of the myocardium, due to the various factors discussed above. Alternatively, an exercise-induced increase of coronary blood flow or an enhanced movement of the ventricular wall could precipitate haemorrhage into a pre-existing atheromatous plaque (A.C. Burton, 1965) or lead to the breaking away of an embolic fragment of plaque and overlying clot which becomes impacted in a more distal branch of the coronary arterial tree. There are thus good patho-physiological grounds for suggesting that exercise can sometimes precipitate death through dysrhythmia, asystole or myocardial infarction.

Post-mortem findings

E. Jokl (1958) collected post-mortem reports on 76 cases of sudden death during exercise. The majority date from the period prior to world war II, but nevertheless the material is of some interest in indicating the commonest pathological findings.

Coronary insufficiency or occlusion was noted in 34 cases. Rupture of the heart or a major blood vessel occurred in 22 instances, although two of these episodes associated with advanced tuberculosis and one related to tertiary syphilis would be unlikely in a more recent series; 4 of the lesions developed in the heart wall, eleven in the aorta, five in cerebral blood vessels and two in the pulmonary vessels. Cardiac rupture is often associated with an unsuspected myocardial infarction. The diagnosis is sometimes missed because of a psychosis (W.W. Jetter & White, 1944), but even in psychiatrically normal individuals up to 25 per cent of infarctions pass unrecognised under such guises as a self-medicated 'attack of indigestion' (W.B. Kannel *et al.*, 1970). Cardiac failure was blamed in 17 of the 76 deaths discussed by E. Jokl, eight being examples of chronic infection or degenerative conditions and five acute viral or bacterial infections. We have noted the decrease in popularity of chronic myocardial degeneration as a descriptor of the cause of death (Chapter 2). Nevertheless, degeneration can develop with repeated small infarcts, or as a consequence of malnutrition (for example, in alcoholics and in many of the patients from under-developed countries). Acute infections may sometimes account for the general malaise that is a frequent precursor of myocardial infarction. Congenital lesions (four cases) were a relatively infrequent diagnosis, while in three of the 76 reports the cause of death was not clearly established.

About a third of the 76 cases presented a history of sustained isometric effort before death. Examples included 'weight-lifting', 'carrying heavy luggage', 'cranking a motor-car', 'lifting a heavy couch' and 'killing animals with a 25 pound hammer'. However, some deaths had been preceded by more moderate activities such as walking, and the remaining third had been associated with sustained rhythmic activities such as long-distance running, cycling, games of football, tennis and swimming.

Several other pathological reports point to similar conclusions. L. Schmid & Hornof (1973) described 76 deaths in Czechoslovak athletes. The average age was 31.2 years, and (probably as a consequence of relative participation rates) 94.7 per cent of the sample were men. In 30 of the 76, coronary disease was implicated, and in 20

Table 3.1: Activities Undertaken by 174 Athletes Sustaining
Cardiovascular Deaths while Exercising

Baseball	1	Quoits	1
Basketball	17	Riding	1
Bowls	2	Running	57
Boxing	2	Shot-put	4
Climbing	2	Skiing — downhill & Nordic	13
Cricket	2	Skipping	1
Curling	4	Softball	1
Cycling	4	Squash	1
Dancing	4	Swimming	8
Football (rugby, soccer & US)	25	Wrestling	3
Golf	4	Weight lifting	1
Gymnastics	3	Yachting	2
Hockey	1		
Judo	3		
Pentathlon	1		

Source: Data compiled from the reports specified in the text.

of the remainder other cardiac disorders were held to be responsible.
N.D. Graievskaia & Markov (1973) reported on the deaths of five
Russian athletes; they thought it significant that all of the fatalities
occurred in individuals who were training irregularly (although it is
arguable that this may have been an effect rather than the cause of
their problem). I. Vuori (1975) examined details of deaths during
20-90-km cross-country skiing events; unfortunately, autopsy reports
were available for only seven of ten fatalities, three of the seven being
acute myocardial infarctions. J. Moncur (1973) obtained reports of
63 deaths in Scottish sportsmen; 43 were due to environmental
exposure or trauma, but twelve of the remaining 20 were attributed
to coronary occlusion. In West Germany, a Documentation Centre has
recorded 110 sports deaths over ten years (H. Munscheck, 1980); 40
of 85 organic disorders were coronary atherosclerosis, and a further ten
were instances of myocarditis. One somewhat divergent report was
from the US Armed Forces Institute of Pathology (B.J. Maron, 1980);
among 19 competitive atheletes who died suddenly, the commonest
anatomic lesion (six cases) was said to be hypertrophy. Nevertheless,
severe coronary atherosclerosis was seen in three cases, and congenital

coronary arterial anomalies in a further three cases.

Information on the nature of the sport being undertaken is available from a total of 174 reports (E. Jokl, 1958; T.N. James *et al.*, 1971; T. Izeki, 1973; R. Medved *et al.*, 1973; K.S. Zakopoulos, 1973; R.J. Shephard, 1974b; I. Vuori, 1975; B.J. Maron, 1980). Interpretation is hampered by the specific interests of many of the investigators, and by differences in the average ages of competitors in different sports. Nevertheless, almost no type of sporting activity seems immune from such attacks (Table 3.1).

Epidemiological Data

General considerations

If physical activity contributes significantly to myocardial infarction and sudden death, as the above data suggest, one should find a differing incidence of 'coronary' episodes during the parts of the day devoted to sleep, employment (usually sedentary or light physical activity) and leisure (when most of the intense and unusual expenditures of energy are undertaken).

Unfortunately, a simple epidemiological analysis of this sort is rarely possible. Published reports commonly suffer from a dilution of the data. Information on attacks in the middle-aged and relatively healthy wage-earner is often confounded with data for very elderly patients (for example, R. Kala *et al.*, 1978) and, as W.M. Yater *et al.* (1971) have noted, the proportion of coronary victims dying at rest increases with their age. Even among the middle-aged, the consequences of physical activity could well be masked by statistics for that 70–90 per cent of the population who take little physical activity either at work or in their leisure hours (R.J. Shephard, 1976a; R.J. Shephard *et al.*, 1968c; D.A. Bailey *et al.*, 1974). Any activity that is undertaken is usually of brief duration, and the allowable latent period between exercise and death is uncertain. In one of the cases cited by E. Jokl (1958), twelve weeks had elapsed between the supposedly unusual exercise and death! A maximum of six hours should probably be allowed, and the evidence is most convincing if death occurs during or within 15 minutes of the completion of exercise. R. Kala *et al.* (1978) found that strenuous activity was more than twice as common during or immediately before an attack as on the preceding day.

A further problem is that data are usually collected retrospectively, and there is then a risk that relatives will have searched vigorously for a 'cause' of death, attaching excessive importance to some trivial incident. Death is usually ascribed to a 'coronary attack' or 'ischaemic heart disease', without distinguishing the several possible pathologies (ventricular fibrillation, relative ischaemia, haemorrhage into an atheromatous plaque, lodgement of an embolus or cardiac failure following progressive thrombosis of a major coronary vessel). Whereas the first four of these conditions could be precipitated by exercise, the last seems more likely to arise while the coronary blood flow is sluggish (for example, during sleep). R. Kala *et al.* (1978) noted that physical activity was 2.4 times more common in subjects dying instantaneously than in their total sample of 'coronary' deaths.

A final difficulty is that the classification of activity may be inadequate if not misleading. Bed rest, for example, may be a modest description which hides a substantial number of attacks brought about by sexual activity.

Previous investigations

C.K. Friedberg (1966) has summarised much of the older literature on this topic. C. Phipps (1936) assembled a series of 437 cases. Deliberate physical exercise was noted in 13 per cent, and moderate or unusual exertion in a further 18 per cent, while only eight per cent of subjects were sleeping at the time of attack. A.M. Master (1946) apparently set out to disprove the association between disease and exertion, and claimed to have substantiated his argument when only two per cent of 1,108 cases gave a history of unusual exertion. However, a surprising 16 per cent were walking, and another nine per cent were engaged in moderate activity, bringing the total who were exercising to 27 per cent of his series. G. Fitzhugh & Hamilton (1933) found 24 per cent of their population had been involved in violent exertion, and 33 per cent in moderate activity. Other of the older authors repeat this story. Unusual exertion was noted in 17 per cent (W.B. Cooksey, 1939), 33 per cent (A.J. French & Dock, 1944) or even 60 per cent of patients (C. Smith *et al.*, 1942). W.M. Yater *et al* (1971) looked at 'coronary attacks' in young soldiers, and commented that during physical effort the incidence was twice the anticipated figure for resting conditions. G. Fitzhugh & Hamilton (1933) observed that the critical episode was often associated with fatigue, inadequate sleep and emotional strain. This point is well illustrated by Werkmeister's patient, who died while walking to college on his examination day (E. Jokl, 1958). A.J. French & Dock (1944) provided examples of the type of daily activity associated with myocardial infarction — cranking a car in cold weather, lifting a heavy trunk, pushing a stalled car and long walks uphill. They emphasised that many of the individuals concerned had either not attempted these tasks previously, or at least had not carried them out for many years.

A.R. Moritz & Zamcheck (1946) looked at the antecedents of sudden and unexpected death in soldiers. Their subjects were presumably younger and in better physical condition than the average coronary victim, yet the number of sudden deaths occurring during vigorous activity was about twice the anticipated figure. L. Adelson (1961) found that 55 per cent of his sample were engaged in light activity, five per cent in strenuous activity and only 21 per cent were asleep at the time of attack. However, his population was atypical, consisting largely of 'alcoholics and vagabonds'. D.M. Spain & Bradess (1960a) examined episodes of sudden 'coronary' death in Westchester County, New York; they reported that 14 per cent of those with atherosclerotic lesions and 16 per cent of those with thrombotic lesions had been involved in unusual activity at the moment of attack. A. Armstrong *et al.* (1972) noted that, of 226 medically unattended sudden deaths, a surprisingly large proportion (19 per cent) occurred 'on the street'. B. Wikland (1971) scrutinised all medically unattended fatal cases of ischaemic heart disease in a defined population; he observed that 27 per cent of the men and 25 per cent of the women were walking at the time of attack. Only four per cent of the men and six per cent of the women in his sample were asleep, but a relatively large percentage (52 per cent of the men and 56 per cent of the women) were said to be resting.

Against this long list of reports stressing the association between physical activity and attack, S. Pell & D'Alonzo (1964) stated that 60 per cent of ischaemic heart disease in wage-earning men occurred during sleep or rest, while L. Kuller *et al.* (1967) found no relationship of sudden death to time of day, season, place, occupation or activity. As already noted, some of the discrepancy in conclusions is related to the suddenness of death (R. Kala *et al.*, 1978). M. Friedman *et al.* (1973) distinguished sudden death (within 24 hours of the onset of symptoms) from instantaneous death (within 30 seconds of the onset of symptoms). The latter type of fatality was almost always due to a dysrhythmia, and in more than a half of cases it developed during or immediately after physical exertion.

E. Simonson & Berman (1972) have summarised the experience of Russian investigators. Findings seem much as in the west. Myocardial infarction is by no means a rarity in young Russians. The male/female ratio is much higher for young than for older patients, and excessive physical effort — vigorous bouts of running, skiing, athletic games and the lifting of heavy loads — seems the commonest cause of attack in the young.

The antecedents of coronary attacks in women have received relatively little study. C. Bengtsson (1973) reported that two per cent of women were under mental stress, and 15 per cent were physically active at the time of attack. M. Romo (1972) compared the activity patterns of men and women dying suddenly from ischaemic heart disease. Some six per cent of the men were actually engaged in strenuous physical activity, and a further nine per cent presented such a history immediately prior to attack (items cited included formal sports, snow-shovelling and the carrying of heavy loads). However, perhaps because such activities were infrequent among the women of Helsinki in 1972, only one per cent of the females had been engaged in vigorous work at the time of attack. As in most other studies, both sexes showed a small deficit of cases between midnight and 6 a.m.

To summarise previous epidemiological data, most authors have found some relationship between physical activity and sudden death, at least in men. On the other hand, the strength of the association has varied widely from one study to another, being greater for near-instantaneous deaths than for episodes where some hours had elapsed between the onset of symptoms and death.

The Toronto study

T. Kavanagh & Shephard (1973a) made a further study of the antecedents of myocardial infarction in relatively young coronary victims (average age 45 years) who had survived the acute episode and were attending an exercise-centred rehabilitation programme.

Events were reviewed for one year, one week and one day prior to attack. By way of control, the same questionnaire was administered to healthy colleagues of the 'post-coronary' sample. Data were available from 203 primary and 30 recurrent non-fatal attacks. In the year preceding the primary episode, 79 of the 203 men noted an increase in body mass, and only 16 a decrease; however, 28 of 57 controls also reported a gain in body mass. Physical activity was regarded as 'normal' by most of the coronary group, but 130 of the 203 reported an increase of business problems, and only three men a decrease ($P < 0.001$); 61 also noted increased social and domestic problems, and only two a decrease ($P < 0.001$).

One week before attack, there was still no change in physical activity, but business problems (increased in 106/203, decreased in 8/203) and social or domestic problems (increased in 42/203, decreased in 4/203) were again perceived as important. Only nine of the 203 patients identified a clear-cut fever or upper respiratory infection, but 73 felt vaguely 'unwell' in the week preceding the attack (compared with eleven who noted an improvement of health; $P <$ 0.001). In about two thirds of the group, the complaints could perhaps be interpreted as incipient myocardial oxygen lack, but the remainder merely complained of tiredness, nervous tension or depression. In some instances, an accumulation of business worries may have led to excessive smoking, an abnormally large intake of coffee, loss of physical condition or an increase in body mass. In other cases, acute infection or a disturbance of electrolyte balance may have had a more direct impact upon myocardial irritability.

On the day prior to attack, information was incomplete for two individuals, 85 of 201 felt unwell, vigorous physical activity was noted by 51/201 and heavy lifting by 47/202. In contrast, unusual annoyance (41/203), business problems (40/203) and social or domestic problems (25/203) were less common than in the entire year preceding the attack. Humid heat was reported by 35/203; the association between heat stress and cardiac deaths is well recognised in the United States (G.S. Berenson & Burch, 1952). Fresh, wet snow was reported by 25/202, cold or very cold weather by 87/203, and snow-shovelling by 9/203. Despite frequent newspaper headlines in northern cities, snow-shovelling is a relatively infrequent antecedent of heart attacks. This is partly because the total number of minutes devoted to shovelling is relatively few in any given year, and partly because the cardiac work-load varies widely with such variables as the depth and wetness of the snow, the chill factor and the possible physiological and psychological strains of rapid shovelling immediately after breakfast.

Among the control sample, complaints of increased business worries were made by only 16 of 57 subjects at one year, 14 of 57 at one week, and four of 57 at one day prior to completion of the questionnaire. Likewise, social and domestic problems were increased in only 14 of 57 at one week, and two of 57 on the day prior to questioning. Only eight of the 57 noted annoyance on the preceding day, and only four of 57 a deterioration of health in the preceding week. It would thus appear that business and social problems along with a general malaise are common features of the period before a frank coronary attack. Nevertheless, it remains arguable that the perception of such problems has been heightened by the critical experience of the acute episode.

Perhaps the most intriguing comparison is between the activities actually reported at the time of attack and the anticipated daily activity

pattern of the average Toronto business man. We expected, for
example, about 7.7 hours of sleep per day, which would have yielded
81 sleep-related attacks among our total sample of 233 primary and
recurrent episodes; however, in fact there were only 48 such attacks.
Likewise, at least 70 attacks should have occurred at the place of
employment, but there were only 30 such incidents. In contrast, odd
jobs and sports should not have accounted for more than five cases
apiece, yet the totals were 21 and 30 cases, respectively. Walking also
accounted for 13 rather than the anticipated three cases. Other
significant concentrations were for running (eight cases), various
sports (13 cases, including one in the shower area), snow-shovelling
(nine cases), various other heavy domestic chores (15 cases) and
sexual intercourse (two cases). In a number of instances, the physical
activity closely followed a heavy meal, or was associated with
emotional stress (for instance, defending a curling championship).
Other episodes were related to the patient's aggressive 'Type A'
behaviour, for example determination to beat an opponent at tennis
after some years away from the courts, and reluctance to admit
exhaustion (well illustrated by a politician entered in a long-distance
charity run). A number of histories referred to unusual isometric
activity, such as a professor who had spent a whole day moving 25 kg
cartons of mineral specimens after a sabbatical leave, and a 'cottager'
who had carried his canoe for almost 1 km when closing his summer
home for the season.

Several incidents occurred while attending a hospital or a doctor's
office, apparently for treatment of an unrelated condition. It is possible
that the premonitory malaise of a coronary attack had contributed to
the decision to undergo medical examination, but it is also arguable
that anxiety associated with the examination precipitated the attack.
The latter viewpoint has two practical corollaries — effort should be
given to making medical examinations a less frightening experience,
and over-zealous medical supervision may on occasion provoke the
calamity it is trying to avoid.

Because of the location of the Toronto Rehabilitation Centre, the
majority of our patients are 'white-collar' workers. It is thus possible
that more employment-related episodes might be encountered in other
communities where physical labour was the norm. In Brisbane, the
State Compensation Board accepts some 500 cases per year (about a
third of the total coronary victims among employed males in Queens-
land) as being caused or aggravated by daily work. Usually, the work
accepted for purposes of compensation is of a physical nature, although

occasional episodes have been attributed successfully to unusual mental stresses that have arisen in the course of employment.

Both the Toronto and the Brisbane statistics support the view that exercise increases the immediate risk of myocardial infarction. Adverse features include activity that is unusual for the patient, is excessive relative to his level of physical fitness, and is accompanied by emotional stress.

Experience during Exercise Testing and Prescription

Another possible tactic is to review the experience of exercise test facilities and gymnasia. The problem with such an approach is that we are dealing with an infrequent occurrence. Even a very busy laboratory hardly accumulates enough data to yield accurate statistics. If the test facility is in a hospital, the population examined is usually biased in the direction of the middle-aged and the coronary-prone, and performance of the test involves not only vigorous exercise, but also anxiety concerning the test result.

Exercise testing

J.R. McDonough & Bruce (1969) set the hazard of clinical exercise testing at one attack of ventricular fibrillation for every 3,000 maximum-effort tests, and one attack for every 15,000 sub-maximum tests. Many of their cases of ventricular fibrillation were successfully resuscitated, partly because the coronary vasculature of those tested was adequate for rest if not for maximum effort, and partly because a well-trained emergency team was always close at hand.

P. Rochmis & Blackburn (1971) found 16 fatal incidents in pooled data from 72 North American laboratories. It was estimated that the investigators concerned had carried out a total of about 170,000 maximum or sub-maximum tests. Thirteen of the fatal episodes began within one hour of exercise, an attack rate of one in 13,000; all were patients with known cardiac disease, but unfortunately there were no means of determining how many of the 170,000 individuals who were tested also fell into this 'high-risk' category.

Other researchers have had a somewhat similar experience. L. Brock (1967) encountered three fatal episodes in a series of 17,000 work evaluation tests. M. Ellestad *et al.* (1969) had no deaths in 4,000 symptom-limited maximum tests, but about 0.9 per cent of his patients developed ventricular tachycardia. A. Kattus & McAlpin

(1968) reported two attacks of ventricular fibrillation (one fatal) in 500 treadmill tests, while B. Phibbs *et al.* (1968) noted 'three major complications including a massive current of injury and ventricular flutter' in 787 tests.

There is some evidence that the Master two-step exercise is less hazardous than maximum exercise; three series (A.J. Brody, 1959; L.E. Lamb & Hiss, 1962; G.P. Robb & Marks, 1964) observed no significant dysrhythmias other than one evanescent tachycardia in a total of 4,266 cases.

The attack rate of P. Rochmis & Blackburn is equivalent to 674 attacks per 1,000 man-years, even neglecting the effect of the three subjects who died in the period between one and 24 hours after testing. If we assume that the base population was mainly male, half being average middle-aged adults with a coronary risk of 3.5 attacks per 1,000 man-years, and half 'coronary' patients with a recurrence rate of 25 attacks per 1,000 man years, the observed frequency of attacks during exercise would be 47 times the anticipated figure. Conclusions of a similar order can be drawn from the other reports concerning maximum and sub-maximum exercise tests.

Operation of gymnasia

Anecdotal reports suggest that vigorous physical activity can have appreciable risk for middle-aged adults. Thus S. Fox (personal communication) noted that, over a one-year period, eight deaths of men wearing jogging clothes occurred in Orange County, California.

The mass ski contests of Scandinavia provide sufficient man-hours of exercise to allow risk calculations. P.O. Åstrand (personal communication) comments that two large cross-country events in Sweden have attracted about 10,000 entrants for each of 50 years, with only two fatalities, both in 1971. The Finnish experience is similar. I. Vuori (1975) found ten fatalities in twelve million man-hours of cross-country skiing. Between a half and three quarters of the villagers participated in the events that he examined, and he estimated that the death rate was about four times that of a comparable population under resting conditions. Uncertainties include the impact of conditioning and competition, but this is probably a minimum estimate of the danger of sustained exercise, since the unhealthy members of a community would tend to avoid the ski races. A further imponderable is the relationship between brief and extended activity. Many of the harmful effects of exercise, such as the rise in systemic blood pressure and the secretion of catecholamines, are cumulative phenomena, so that the hazard of a six-hour ski race might be much greater than a 30-minute 'work-out' in a gymnasium; on the other hand, there are specific risks associated with the warm-up (R.J. Barnard *et al.*, 1973) and the warm-down (J.R. McDonough & Bruce, 1969), and in this sense a number of short bouts of activity create more danger than one long race.

Almost a quarter of the patients attending the Toronto Rehabilitation Centre perceived their 'coronary' attacks as occurring during exercise (T. Kavanagh & Shephard, 1973a). It is unlikely that the average member of this group was spending more than 30–60 minutes per day in such physical activity prior to infarction, and on this basis we would estimate that the risk of a non-fatal coronary incident was increased between six- and twelve-fold during exercise. The patients studied were of course a high-risk group, heavy smokers, with a high serum cholesterol, 'Type A' personalities and other disadvantages of the 'coronary-prone' person.

A few years ago, calculations based on reports reaching Toronto newspapers suggested that the attack rate in unsupervised gymnastic programmes for the coronary-prone middle-aged male might be as high as one in 2,500 man-hours (Shephard, 1971). Subsequent to publication of this pessimistic statistic, admission criteria were greatly tightened in Ontario and elsewhere, and the frequency of such episodes decreased dramatically. More recent figures refer to patients with known ischaemic heart disease. H.R. Pyfer *et al.* (1975) have experienced one episode of cardiac arrest for every 7,000 man-hours of supervised training, all patients being successfully resuscitated. W.L. Haskell (1978) collected data on 949,568 man-hours of exercise from 86 exercise programmes. Considering all available information, the risk of cardiac arrest was one in 29,674 man-hours, but in recent years a more cautious approach to operation of the clubs had apparently reduced the risk to one in 268,922 man-hours. Ten years' experience in Toronto has yielded similar statistics. T. Kavanagh and I have now accumulated 242,420 hours of supervised and 700,840 hours of unsupervised activity, with a total of eight incidents (four of which were successfully resuscitated); our attack rate is thus one in 117,907 man-hours of exercise. This is low, but is nevertheless equivalent to an annual rate of 7.43 per cent, more than four times the overall coronary recurrence rate for our particular sample of patients.

The Southern Ontario multicentre exercise-heart trial has followed 750 post-coronary patients prospectively for a total of four years. About a quarter of the recurrent infarctions in this group were associated with exercise (R.J. Shephard, 1979a). Even taking account of substantial exercise prescriptions, the attack rate during physical activity was at least six times as large as expected.

Conclusions

Available data suggest that in normal subjects, coronary-prone individuals and post-coronary patients exercise increases the immediate risk of a 'coronary attack' by a factor of between four and twelve. Statistics of this order show the need for individualised exercise prescription, with avoidance of excessive competition and unusual activity for which a person is ill prepared; in patients, there must also be a careful monitoring of the training response, with a graded progression and avoidance of isometric effort.

Some reports indicate a risk of group exercise that is between 10- and twenty-fold greater than the currently accepted North American figure. It is not clear how far this can be explained simply by factors of patient selection. One adverse factor may be emotional stress, whether due to the task itself (for example, a crucial competition), the outcome of the exercise (a stress test) or some unrelated circumstance of business or domestic life.

Paradoxically, such figures are not an argument against advising people to exercise. Although exercise may precipitate a 'coronary' attack, it is serving mainly to reveal the presence of a badly damaged coronary arterial tree. The affected individual is likely to succumb to ischaemic heart disease over the next few months, and it is preferable for the critical incident to develop in a gymnasium where help is at hand, rather than in some remote area of the countryside. Furthermore, our analysis has to this point merely focussed on the brief period of the day when the victim has been active, and a complete examination of prognosis must consider whether the chances of a critical event are reduced in the intervals between exercise bouts. A four-fold worsening of prognosis during one hour of activity could well be counteracted by a 13 per cent improvement of prognosis for the remaining 23 hours of the day!

Avoiding Exercise-induced Catastrophes

There are unfortunately few specific clues to the individual who will develop cardiac arrest, fibrillation or infarction while he is exercising. An analysis of 230 episodes in patients referred to the Toronto Rehabilitation Centre (R.J. Shephard & Kavanagh, 1978a) noted that those individuals who were active at the time of attack were less likely to have detected an abnormal cardiac rhythm or a general malaise than those who were inactive, but were more likely to have been aware of nervous tension or depression. It also seems likely that they approached exercise in a more competitive spirit, since their subsequent training response was marked by a larger gain of aerobic power (21 per cent, compared with 13.5 per cent), and a small decrease (0.5 kg) as compared with a small gain (0.6 kg) in body mass. After the attack, the blood pressure of the two groups showed no difference, either at rest or during graded exercise; however, it is probable that blood pressures were modified by the acute episode, and in any event there are considerable differences between a laboratory stress test and participation in competitive sports.

In the Southern Ontario multicentre exercise-heart trial, the main features that distinguished patients who developed a recurrence of their infarction while exercising (Table 3.2) were persistent resting ECG abnormalities, a poor exercise compliance and an ST segmental depression of more than 0.2 mV during exercise stress testing (R.J. Shephard, 1980b). Sequential testing further established that immediately prior to reinfarction a number of patients showed an impaired cardiac response to exercise, with a low stroke volume and cardiac output, plus a compensatory broadening of the arterio-venous oxygen difference (R.J. Shephard, 1979a).

Despite this limited information, certain general suggestions can be made to increase the safety of both exercise testing and subsequent exercise prescription. Within the doctor's office or laboatory, care must be taken to allay anxiety. Unnecessary apparatus should be removed from the room, and staff should cultivate a relaxed, non-authoritarian manner. It is often helpful to carry out a brief preliminary practice of the test, deferring formal assessment to a second visit. The safety of the test is increased by a careful preliminary medical examination (K.H. Cooper, 1970; K.L. Andersen *et al.*, 1971), the continuous monitoring of blood pressure and electrocardiograms during the tests with rigid criteria for halting an investigation and the presence of an efficient, well-trained and well-equipped resuscitation team.

If a significant dysrhythmia or ST segmental depression develops during the laboratory test, the heart rate corresponding to this occurrence should be noted, and the prescribed activity so arranged that the intensity of effort falls just below this danger level. Particularly when dealing with the post-coronary patient, close adherence to the exercise prescription should be stressed. Individual class members should be taught to count their pulse rate and to recognise such

Table 3.2: A Comparison of Patients Sustaining a Recurrence of Myocardial Infarction during Exercise with Those Sustaining Attack at Other Times

Variable	Recurrence during exercise (%)	Recurrence at other times (%)	P
Exercise compliance (average attendance at sessions over previous 3 months)	38.4	62.4	0.2 > P > 0.1
Current smoking	60.0	64.5	n.s.
Angina	60.0	58.1	n.s.
Systemic hypertension (resting pressure > 150/100 mm Hg)	0	11.1	n.s.
Serum cholesterol (> 270 mg/100 ml)	0	9.1	n.s.
Persistent resting ECG abnormalities	83.3	53.3	0.2 > P > 0.1
Exercise ST segmental depression > 0.2 mV	50.0	22.6	0.1 > P > 0.05
Ventricular premature beats	0	4.9	n.s.

Source: Based on preliminary data from Southern Ontario multicentre exercise-heart trial (R.J. Shephard, 1979a).

symptoms as angina and premature ventricular contractions. They should be advised to train regularly, avoiding both peaks of unusual activity and intense competition. Further, they should be warned to reduce their prescription temporarily in any unfavourable situation, be it climatic (very hot or very cold weather), medical (the sensing of ischaemic prodromata) or psychological (mental tension or depression).

Despite such precautions, some risks will remain. This may seem a negative conclusion to the committed exercise enthusiast. However, it is important to credibility that exercise scientists admit this hazard. And to set the matter in perspective, I would finally endorse the view (P.O. Åstrand & Rodahl, 1977) that, while physical activity carries some small risks, there is evidence (Chapter 4) that a careful medical examination is even more necessary for the person who plans to take no further exercise!

4 EXERCISE AND THE PRIMARY PREVENTION OF ISCHAEMIC HEART DISEASE

Textbooks of epidemiology distinguish the primary, secondary and tertiary prevention of disease (J.S. Mausner & Bahn, 1974). Primary prevention will be the main focus of this chapter. It is applied in the phase of susceptibility, and operates through a change of exposure to disease-causing agents or a reduction in the susceptibility of the individual. Since the initial changes of atherosclerosis develop at an early age (Chapter 1), exercise can have no role in primary prevention if it is not applied from childhood. Certain principles of secondary prevention will also be introduced, to be discussed more fully in Chapter 5. Secondary prevention involves the early detection and treatment of disease, usually while it is in the pre-clinical stage. In the context of ischaemic heart disease, we face the typical situation of the middle-aged adult who becomes involved in an exercise programme. Tertiary prevention, discussed in Chapter 6, is concerned with the restoration of effective function after clinical manifestations of disease have appeared. A typical example is the patient who has sustained a non-fatal myocardial infarction, and subsequently joins an exercise rehabilitation programme with a view to speeding his return to normal life and minimising his chances of a second infarction.

A comprehensive scheme of primary prevention involves both general measures of health promotion and specific action to protect the individual. Relevant techniques for the encouragement of physical activity in the community and the individual will be covered in Chapter 9. The present chapter will review normal reactions to regular endurance training, will consider the possible relevance of such changes to the prevention of ischaemic heart disease and will finally examine the fate of animals encouraged to exercise for long periods of their lives.

Normal Responses to Endurance Training

General considerations

The pattern of exercise most widely suggested as a means of preventing ischaemic heart disease is endurance training. Definitions vary somewhat from one investigator to another, but the usual implication is activity at 60–70 per cent of the individual's maximum oxygen intake, carried out in bouts of 30 minutes' duration or longer three or more times per week (R.J. Shephard, 1977a). In the context of primary prevention, the training must begin in childhood, and continue throughout the lifetime of the subject.

Physiological responses to endurance training were at one time inferred from cross-sectional comparisons between endurance athletes and the general public. This approach has the advantage that the activity considered has been intense and followed for a number of years. However, conclusions are hampered by the fact that top athletes represent a highly selected population sample; probably between a half and two thirds of their unusual ability is due to genetic endowment rather than endurance training (R.J. Shephard, 1978a, 1980c). Much current data is thus drawn from longitudinal studies. Often exercise is initiated as a young adult rather than as a child, and the period of observation is short in the context of chronic disease prevention; nevertheless, a number of interesting physiological changes can be demonstrated over a typical two-to-three month study. Appropriate control groups are an important precaution, since the exercise response can also be altered by habituation to the test environment (R.J. Shephard, 1969), learning of the test procedure (R.J. Shephard *et al.*, 1968a; R.J. Shephard & Lavallée, 1977), seasonal changes in fitness levels (R.J. Shephard *et al.*, 1978b), and long-term trends in the lifestyle of a community (for example, the acculturation of primitive societies to western patterns of diet and inactivity; R.J. Shephard, 1978a).

Recent reports have emphasised the specificity of training. While there is little dispute that the effects of 'weight' training are not the same as those induced by regular distance running, there are also differences in response to different types of endurance exercise, particularly if the total mass of muscle involved in the activity is fairly small. Gains of performance developed on the treadmill are largely transferable to cycle-ergometer exercise, but the reverse is not necessarily true. J.P. Clausen *et al.* (1973) found that some 50 per cent of the response to regular cycle-ergometer training was transferred to an arm-ergometer task, but that arm-ergometer training did little to improve the response to leg ergometry. Likewise, I. Holmér & Åstrand (1972) reported that a trained swimmer showed a larger difference of maximum oxygen intake from her twin sister when swimming than when exercising on an arm ergometer.

Many body systems are modified by regular endurance training

(A. Steinhaus, 1933; P.O. Åstrand & Rodahl, 1977; R.J. Shephard, 1980c). We will consider specifically changes in the heart and cardio-vascular system, the respiratory system, metabolism and body composition (Table 4.1), along with one convenient overall index of endurance fitness, the maximum oxygen intake (R.J. Shephard, 1977a). The average gain of maximum oxygen intake when a sedentary adult undergoes endurance training is about 20 per cent (R.J. Shephard, 1965a, 1977a), but the increase can be much larger if the exercise programme is both heavy and sustained (B. Saltin *et al.*, 1968; R.J. Shephard, 1979b); Dr T. Kavanagh and I have observed one middle-aged man develop from a value of 27 ml·kg^{-1}·min^{-1} immediately after myocardial infarction to about 65 ml·kg^{-1}·min^{-1} five years later (R.J. Shephard, 1979b). Individual responsiveness is modified by many variables, particularly initial fitness and the intensity of training (R.J. Shephard, 1968a, 1975a; M.L. Pollock, 1973). Gains are further augmented if the subject has been 'deconditioned' by a preliminary period of two to three weeks' bed rest (H.L. Taylor *et al.*, 1949; B. Saltin *et al.*, 1968; T. Fried & Shephard, 1969). Suggestions that older subjects train less readily than children or young adults (for example, B. Saltin, 1969) seem a fallacy, caused by judging initial fitness levels in terms of maximum oxygen intake without adjusting this variable for normal age-related changes. If the increase in maximum oxygen intake with training is expressed as a percentage of the initial value, the response of a sedentary 65-year-old adult is at least as large as that observed in his 25-year-old counterpart (K.H. Sidney & Shephard, 1978; R.J. Shephard, 1978b).

The deconditioning experiments illustrate the truth that fitness cannot be stored; indeed, much of the advantage of the endurance athlete is dissipated by a few weeks of inactivity (P.S. Fardy, 1969; M. Katila & Frick, 1970; W. Siegel *et al.*, 1970; Z.B. Kendrick *et al.*, 1971; Å. Kilböm, 1971; M.H. Williams & Edwards, 1971; B. Drinkwater & Horvath, 1972).

Cardiovascular changes

The most obvious cardiovascular response to endurance training is a decrease of heart rate at rest and during sub-maximum exercise (R.J. Barnard, 1975). Whereas the resting heart rate of a sedentary person is 70–80 beats·min^{-1}, that of a superbly conditioned athlete can be 30 beats·min^{-1} or less. The maximum heart rate is reached at a higher oxygen intake after training, and the peak heart rate may show a small (5–10 beats·min^{-1}) decrease (C.T.M. Davies, 1967; R.J. Shephard, 1980c).

Table 4.1: A Comparison of Physiological Variables between a Sedentary Normal Individual, a Trained Normal Individual and a World-class Endurance Athlete

Variable	Sedentary normal Rest	Sedentary normal Maximum	Trained normal Rest	Trained normal Maximum	Endurance athlete Rest	Endurance athlete Maximum
Cardiovascular						
Heart rate (beats•min $^{-1}$)	71	185	59	183	36	174
Stroke volume (ml)	65	120	80	140	125	200
Cardiac output (l•min $^{-1}$)	4.6	22.2	4.7	25.6	4.5	34.8
Blood pressure:						
systolic (mm Hg)	135	210	130	205	120	210
diastolic (mm Hg)	78	82	76	80	65	65
Heart volume (ml)	750		820		1,200	
Blood volume (l)	4.7		5.1		6.0	
Respiratory						
Resp. min. volume (l•min $^{-1}$ BTPS)	7	110	6	135	6	195
Frequency of respiration (breaths•min $^{-1}$)	14	40	12	45	12	55
Tidal volume (l)	0.5	2.75	0.5	3.0	0.5	3.5
Vital capacity (l)	5.8		6.0		6.2	
Residual volume (l)	1.4		1.2		1.2	
Metabolic						
Oxygen intake (ml•kg $^{-1}$•min $^{-1}$)	3.5	40.5	3.7	49.8	4.0	76.7
Blood lactate (mg•dl $^{-1}$)	10	110	10	125	10	185
Arterio-venous oxygen difference (ml•dl $^{-1}$)	6.0	14.5	6.0	15.0	6.0	16.0
Body composition						
Body mass (kg)	79.5		77.3		68.2	
Fat mass (kg)	12.7		9.7		5.1	
Lean mass (kg)	66.8		67.6		63.1	
Relative fat (%)	16.0		12.5		7.5	

Source: J.H. Wilmore & Norton (1974).

There is also an increase in the stroke volume of the heart at rest and in sub-maximal exercise (B. Saltin *et al.*, 1968; R. Simmons & Shephard, 1971a), while output per beat is better maintained in maximum effort (V. Niinimaa & Shephard, 1978). Consequently, the maximum output of the heart is increased roughly in proportion to the gain of maximum oxygen intake (B. Ekblom *et al.*, 1968; R. Simmons & Shephard, 1971a).

Oxygen delivery is further facilitated by a widening of the maximum arterio-venous oxygen difference (B. Saltin *et al.*, 1968; R. Simmons & Shephard, 1971a; H. Roskamm, 1973a). Each litre of blood that is pumped by the heart may yield 160 rather than 140 ml of oxygen to the tissues. This reflects a redistribution of blood flow away from the regions of limited oxygen extraction such as the skin (R. Simmons & Shephard, 1971a) and the viscera (L.B. Rowell, 1974), with a possible increase of oxygen extraction in the working muscles. During sub-maximum exercise, muscle perfusion may be reduced (F.G.V. Douglas & Becklake, 1968; F. Treumann & Schroeder, 1968; J.P. Clausen *et al.*, 1973), but in maximum effort the flow to the muscles is increased (R.H. Rochelle *et al.*, 1971; H. de Marées & Barbey, 1973). The latter change may reflect in a part a strengthening of the working muscles, so that they contract at a small fraction of their maximum force during vigorous effort; this in turn reduces the impedance to their perfusion (C. Kay & Shephard, 1969).

As training proceeds, the drive to the heart from the sympathetic nervous system diminishes both at rest and during exercise. This affects not only the heart rate, but also the myocardial contractility (J. Crews & Aldinger, 1967; S. Penpargkul & Scheuer, 1970). At rest, such indices of myocardial contractility as the maximum rate of rise of intraventricular pressure are the same in sedentary and in trained individuals, but in maximum effort the rate of pressure rise is decreased by training (B.D. Franks & Cureton, 1969; J.F. Wiley, 1971; H. Roskamm, 1973a, b).

Most (L.H. Hartley *et al.*, 1969; Å. Kilböm *et al.*, 1969; J. Chrastek & Adimirova, 1970; H.A. de Vries, 1970; J.S. Hanson & Nedde, 1970; E. Jokl *et al.*, 1970; G. Choquette & Ferguson, 1973) but not all (M.H. Frick *et al.*, 1963; B.S. Tabakin *et al.*, 1965; B. Ekblom *et al.*, 1968) reports have indicated that regular physical exercise lowers the resting systemic blood pressure, both in hypertensive individuals and in those with 'normal' pressures. Blood-pressure readings may also be reduced at a given sub-maximal rate of working. On the other hand, the maximum attained blood pressure may be increased, particularly in hearts where there was difficulty in sustaining stroke output at high work rates prior to training (R.J. Shephard, 1978b).

Hypertrophy of the rat heart is more readily induced in young than in older animals (A.S. Leon & Bloor, 1970; R.J. Tomanek, 1970). In the dog, both the mass and the thickness of the ventricular wall can be increased by as little as twelve weeks of endurance training (H.L. Wyatt & Mitchell, 1974). Cardiac hypertrophy can also occur in human hearts (for example, children with congenital valvular abnormalities), and endurance athletes typically have large hearts (H. Reindell *et al.*, 1966); however, attempts to induce hypertrophy by the moderate endurance training of adolescents and young adults have had far from uniform success (H. Roskamm & Reindell, 1972; J. Cermak, 1973; H. Roskamm, 1973a; R.A. Bruce *et al.*, 1975).

The cardiac work-load comprises effort expended against friction and turbulence in the blood stream, internal work needed to develop and maintain tension in the ventricular walls and smaller energy losses associated with the basal metabolism of the heart muscle, activation of the myocardial fibres and internal friction as the fibres shorten (G. Blomqvist, 1974; E.F. Blick & Stein, 1977; C.R. Jorgensen *et al.*, 1977). Considering only the two main components, the rate of working $\dot{W}$ of each ventricle is approximated by the equation:

$$\dot{W} = (\int_{V_d}^{V_s} P_v \, \delta V + \alpha \int_0^t T \, \delta t) f_h$$

where P_v is the ventricular pressure, integrated between diastolic and systolic volumes; δV is the instantaneous change of ventricular volume; T is the tension in the ventricular wall integrated over the systolic phase of the cardiac cycle; δt is the instant of time at which a specific value of T is recorded; α is a constant to convert the tension integral to units of work; and f_h is the heart rate. The first term of the equation corresponds to frictional and turbulent work, and the second to tension work. Common non-invasive indices of cardiac work rate are: (i) the heart rate; (ii) the product of systolic pressure and heart rate, sometimes called the double product or the tension-time index; and (iii) the triple product (systolic pressure × heart rate × duration of systole). Heart rate (Y. Wang, 1972; C.R. Jorgensen *et al.*, 1977) is proportional to cardiac work rate only if ventricular pressure, stroke volume and cardiac contraction time all remain constant. The tension-time index depends on the constancy of stroke volume and contraction time. During exercise, the second variable changes less than the first and, fortunately for the index, the tension item is by far the largest component of cardiac work; perhaps for this reason the tension-time index is said to correlate well with direct measurements of myocardial oxygen consumption (C.R. Jorgensen *et al.*, 1977). The triple product is theoretically more precise, but in practice its use is limited by the difficulty in making non-invasive measurements of cardiac contraction times.

Training modifies several components of the cardiac work load.

There may be a small fall in systemic pressure, particularly at rest and in sub-maximum exercise. At the same time, the trained heart tends to empty more completely than the untrained heart, so that the radii of the heart tend to decrease. The relationship between ventricular pressure P_v and tension T is approximated most simply by the law of Laplace for a thin-walled structure:

$$T = (R_1 + R_2)P_v$$

where R_1 and R_2 are the principal radii of the heart; plainly, a decrease of mean dimensions leads to a drop in wall tension. With more sustained conditioning, the cardiac dimensions may be increased by hypertrophy; while this increases the overall tension, the thickening of the ventricular wall further lessens the force exerted by unit cross section of muscle. Heart rate is decreased mainly by a lengthening of the diastolic phase; the term relating to frictional and turbulent work is affected relatively little, since stroke volume per beat is increased, but the slow heart rate greatly diminishes the work performed against intramural tension. Finally, the work rate is modified by any changes of myocardial contractility that develop with training.

In the context of ischaemic-heart-disease prevention and treatment, much importance attaches to the delicate balance between the rate of working of the heart and the myocardial blood flow. Oxygen extraction from the coronary blood is relatively complete even at rest, so that the oxygen needs of exercise demand an increase of flow. The left ventricle is more vulnerable to ischaemia than is the right, as it has a heavier work rate and the coronary vessels are exposed to much greater external forces from the myocardium. Flow to the left side of the heart wall occurs mainly during diastole (D.E. Gregg & Fisher, 1963), and the training-induced lengthening of the diastolic phase of the cardiac cycle aids myocardial perfusion. The diastolic pressure may be reduced somewhat by training, but this is offset by a reduction of intramural vascular compression, since wall tension is reduced by a decrease of cardiac size and a thickening of the ventricular wall. Substantial anastomoses occur between the two main coronary arteries, particularly at the apex of the heart. Such collaterals are important in reducing the area of heart muscle subject to infarction if flow through the normal pathway fails to satisfy metabolic demand. Some authors have postulated that regular exercise provides a 'hypoxic' stimulus that encourages the opening up of potential anastomotic pathways. Experiments in dogs exercised after surgically induced narrowing of the coronary vessels

have sometimes shown such an effect (R.W. Eckstein, 1957; V.F.
Froehlicher, 1972; but not F.R. Cobb *et al.*, 1968). The coronary
arterial tree is also enlarged (J. Tepperman & Pearlman, 1961; J.A.F.
Stevenson, 1967), and the capillary/muscle-fibre ratio is increased
at least in experimental animals (R.J. Tomanek, 1970; R.L.
Rasmussen *et al.*, 1978). On the other hand, primary prevention
(exercise prior to occlusion) does not seem to protect animals against
subsequent blockage of their coronary vessels (J.J. Burt & Jackson,
1965; E. Kaplinsky *et al.*, 1968; T.M. Sanders *et al.*, 1978). Observations in man have been limited to tertiary exercise therapy for anginal
and 'post-coronary' patients. In general, no collateral formation has
been observed (A. Kattus & Grollman, 1972; R.J. Ferguson *et al.*,
1974; M.H. Ellestad, 1975; H.K. Hellerstein, 1977; T. Semple, 1977;
N.K. Wenger, 1977). However, it could be objected that: (i) the
technique used in man (coronary angiography) only detects vessels
larger than 100 μ; and (ii) caution of the patients or their physician
leads to exercise of insufficient intensity to stimulate collateral
formation.

Respiratory system

The respiratory system has only a modest influence upon the oxygen
transport of a healthy adult (R.J. Shephard, 1977a, 1978a). Nevertheless, endurance training modifies a number of respiratory variables. The
respiratory minute volume is reduced both at rest and during sub-
maximum effort, and the ventilatory equivalent (the ventilatory volume
in litres BTPS per litre SPTD of oxygen intake) diminishes towards a
limiting value of 25 litres per litre. This reflects partly the adoption
of a slower and deeper pattern of breathing, and partly an increase of
the threshold work-rate for anaerobic effort (with its associated disproportionate hyperventilation; J. Karlsson *et al.*, 1972). The ventilation
attained during maximum effort is increased with training. This is
due in part to a strengthening of the respiratory muscles, and in part to
an increase in pulmonary blood flow; the latter change augments the
critical respiratory minute volume at which the oxygen cost of
breathing exceeds the added oxygen intake derived from a further
increase in ventilation (A.B. Otis, 1964; R.J. Shephard, 1966a).

Vital capacity shows a moderate correlation with athletic performance (T. Ishiko, 1967), even after allowance for body size (K. Sidney
& Shephard, 1973) or body mass (T. Ishiko, 1967). This is attributable
partly to selection, and partly to a strengthening of the chest muscles
by exercise (L. Delhez *et al.*, 1967–8); modest gains of vital capacity

can sometimes be observed after training (Table 3.1).

In the context of ischaemic heart disease, W.B. Kannel (1967) reported an association between a low vital capacity and both attacks of angina and coronary heart disease deaths:

	Anginal attacks (% expected)	Coronary heart disease deaths (% expected)
Low vital capacity	116	171
Normal vital capacity	95	82

Kannel interpreted vital capacity as one indicator of habitual activity, although it is possible that the coronary deaths and the low vital capacity also had a mutual association with cigarette smoking.

Recent research (V. Niinimaa *et al.*, 1980) has established that most subjects augment nose breathing by the oral inhalation of air when the respiratory minute volume exceeds 35 $l \cdot min^{-1}$ BTPS. This leads to a significant deterioration in the 'conditioning' of inspired air. The impingement of cold, dry air on the tracheal mucosa not only tends to provoke bronchospasm, but may also lead to an increase in systemic blood pressure and a reflex reduction in coronary blood flow (Bezold-Jarisch reflex). If training reduces the ventilatory cost of a given activity below the oral augmentation point, this may thus lead to an appreciable improvement in the balance between the cardiac work rate and the oxygen supplied via the coronary vessels.

Metabolism

Much effort has been directed to exploring the metabolic conse-quences of habitual activity. If the exercise is of sufficient vigour, there is an increase in the mitochondrial fraction of skeletal muscle (K.H. Kiessling *et al.*, 1973). On the other hand, myocardial enzyme activity usually remains unchanged (L. Oscai *et al.*, 1971), and some authors have observed mitochondrial degeneration in the heart muscle of the rat following strenuous exercise (J.C. Arcos *et al.*, 1968; E.E. Aldinger & Sohal, 1970; E.W. Banister *et al.*, 1971).

Animal experiments and human biopsies of skeletal muscle both show augmented activity of enzymes concerned in glycogen synthesis and breakdown, glucose breakdown, pyruvate oxidation and the coupling of chemical energy to muscle proteins (B. Saltin, 1973; J.O. Holloszy, 1973; A.W. Taylor, 1975). While there are also 'central' (cardiovascular and nervous) responses in the child and young adult, it has been argued that much of the training response in middle-aged adults and 'post-coronary' patients is of the peripheral type (J.P. Clausen *et al.*, 1971). Evidence advanced to support this view includes: (i) an apparent correlation between gains of maximum oxygen intake and measures of mitochondrial function such as increased enzyme activity; and (ii) a supposed increase in peripheral oxygen extraction as indicated by a widening of the arterio-venous oxygen difference.

The increase in enzyme activity is not in fact a strong argument, since much larger changes of enzyme activity are induced by isometric or anaerobic than by endurance training (P. Gollnick & Hermansen, 1973). Furthermore, the increase in enzyme activity usually develops more rapidly than the gain in maximum oxygen intake. It is also difficult to envisage any great increase in oxygen extraction in the active muscles as a result of increased enzyme activity; L.H. Hartley & Saltin (1969), for example, found that the normal oxygen content of femoral venous blood was only 6 ml of oxygen per litre, while E. Doll *et al.* (1968) noted no difference in femoral-venous oxygen tension between athletes and sedentary subjects. An alternative explanation of the widened arterio-venous oxygen difference is that a trained person directs a larger proportion of his total cardiac output to the working tissues (R. Simmons & Shephard, 1971a); this reflects: (i) an increase in maximum cardiac output; (ii) a reduction in cutaneous blood flow associated with earlier sweating and a loss of subcutaneous fat; and (iii) a possible further reduction in visceral blood flow.

What then is the reason for the doubling of enzyme activity that accompanies endurance training? It can hardly be regarded as a compensation for muscle hypertrophy, for although there are sometimes increases of muscle-fibre dimensions with training, these are roughly matched by an increase in the capillary bed of the muscles (R.E. Carrow *et al.*, 1967; R.J. Tomanek, 1970; L. Hermansen & Wachtlová, 1971; K. Rakusan *et al.*, 1971). One advantage of the increased enzyme concentrations is that the body does not need to go so far into oxygen debt to 'switch on' mechanisms of oxygen transport at the beginning of a bout of vigorous work (B. Saltin & Karlsson, 1971). Perhaps more importantly, the greater enzyme activity encourages the utilisation of fat rather than carbohydrate during physical activity (J.O. Holloszy, 1973); the conservation of glycogen thus realised is of help to the distance athlete, the child avoids excessive fat deposition and the obese middle-aged adult is encouraged by the mobilisation of subcutaneous adipose tissue.

Table 4.2: *In vitro* Release of Free Fatty Acids from Epididymal Tissue of Male Rats Subjected to Habitual Exercise (E), Controls (C) and Hypokinesis (H)

Condition	Age 85 days			Age 125 days		
	E	C	H	E	C	H
Spontaneous release:						
60 min incubation	192	100	80	141	100	84
210 min incubation	183	100	41	174	100	114
After adrenaline:						
100 min incubation	105	100	80	150	100	95

Source: Based on experiments of J. Pařízková (1977).

J. Pařízková (1977) studied the liberation of fat from rat epididymal tissue (Table 4.2). Habitual exercise facilitated both the spontaneous release of free fatty acids from adipocytes and also their response to adrenaline, restoring to old rats a responsiveness that almost matched that of younger animals; in the young, the response to adrenaline was curtailed by hypokinesis but was not greatly increased by added activity, whereas in older animals the reverse was true.

Much of the body cholesterol is synthesised in the liver. One might thus anticipate the blood levels of this 'risk factor' and resultant arterial wall deposition could be controlled by striking an improved balance between the total energy intake and habitual physical activity (Chapter 2). This concept has yet to be tested in the growing child. However, in young adults blood cholesterol levels change little in response to a training programme, provided that the total intake of energy is sufficient to sustain body mass (R.C. Goode *et al.*, 1966). From the viewpoint of atherosclerosis (W.P. Castelli *et al.*, 1977; T. Gordon *et al.*, 1977), the total cholesterol is probably less important than the ratio of high-density to low-density lipoprotein cholesterol. It may be that the HDL cholesterol competes with the LDL at the cell membranes, preventing entry of the more irritant LDL into the cells; alternatively, the HDL may act as a scavenger, carrying excess cholesterol back to the liver before it has opportunity to cause vascular damage (P.D. Wood, 1979). There have been a number of reports indicating that concentrations of HDL cholesterol are positively correlated with regular participation in regular aerobic exercise (for example, L.A. Carlson, 1967; E.B. Altekruse & Wilmore, 1973;

A. Lopez *et al.*, 1974; P.D. Wood *et al.*, 1976; A.S. Leon *et al.*, 1977; G.H. Hartung *et al.*, 1978; A. Lehtonen & Viikari, 1978). However, the magnitude of the response is small (15–18 per cent increase), and no change is observed when middle-aged subjects participate in such moderate activities as a six-month industrial fitness programme (R.J. Shephard *et al.*, 1980b). Triglyceride readings are reduced by a regular daily programme of vigorous activity (R.C. Goode *et al.*, 1966), but it is uncertain how far a high triglyceride reading contributes to the risk of ischaemic heart disease, once allowance has been made for the associated influence of high serum cholesterol levels.

Physical activity has both acute and chronic effects upon the secretion of hormones. During the acute phase of activity, lipid mobilisation is favoured by an increased blood level of growth hormone, but the long-term effect of training seems to be a reduced secretion of growth hormone at any given rate of working (L.H. Hartley *et al.*, 1972; L. Mikulaj *et al.*, 1975; R.J. Shephard & Sidney, 1975). The level of free thyroxine is increased by an acute bout of exercise; regular activity also increases free thyroxine, but decreases total thyroxine, apparently without any effect upon the rate of basal metabolism (R.L. Terjung & Tipton, 1971; R.L. Terjung & Winder, 1975). Vigorous exercise causes an increased output of adrenaline and noradrenaline, particularly if there is associated emotional stress (E.W. Banister & Griffiths, 1972; L.H. Hartley *et al.*, 1972; U.S. Von Euler, 1973; H. Galbo *et al.*, 1975; L.H. Hartley, 1975); the response is less marked after training (L.H. Hartley *et al.*, 1972), but this may be partly because conditioning has diminished both the physical and the emotional stress associated with performance of a given work bout.

Body composition

We have already noted that training may lead to cardiac hypertrophy. Typically, there is also an increase in total blood volume, and some authors such as A. Holmgren (1967) have claimed a close correlation between total blood volume, total haemoglobin and physical working capacity. A muscle-building regimen may lead to some increase in red cell mass per unit volume of blood (R.J. Shephard *et al.*, 1977a), but often other factors such as iron loss in sweat, poor iron absorption, diminished red cell synthesis and an increased rate of haemolysis lead to a low blood haemoglobin level in the endurance-trained individual (J.F. de Wijn *et al.*, 1971; R.J. Shephard, 1980c).

Regular conditioning avoids fat accumulation in the child, and reduces adiposity in the adult, energy balance being adjusted by: (i) the appetite-suppressing effect of vigorous activity (J.A.F. Stevenson, 1967); (ii) the energy cost of the added activity; (iii) the energy cost of muscle building; and (iv) possible energy losses in ketosis (W. O'Hara *et al.*, 1979). Although scorned by many clinicians, vigorous exercise can lead to a rapid and substantial loss of body fat in a sedentary, middle-aged adult, particularly if it is performed in a cold environment (W. O'Hara *et al.*, 1977). Furthermore, once the habit of regular exercise is established, the fat loss is sustained, in marked contrast with the poor long-term effects of most programmes of dietary restriction (K.H. Sidney *et al.*, 1977). Reports that denigrate exercise are usually based on a search for 'weight loss'. In fact, regular daily activity provides an effective means of avoiding fat accumulation, and although body mass often remains unchanged over the course of a training programme, the reason is that excess fat becomes replaced by a similar mass of skeletal muscle. The type of activity most effective in controlling the percentage of body fat is sustained moderate work. There are two main reasons for this: (i) since fat combustion requires oxygen, the proportion of fat that is burnt is greatest at levels of activity that allow full perfusion of all active muscle fibres; and (ii) it is easier to burn a substantial amount of energy through an hour of moderate activity than through five minutes of all-out effort.

The lean body mass generally shows some increase with training, although the response is larger with weight-lifting and isometric programmes than with endurance-type activity. The practical consequence of such hypertrophy is that the muscle groups affected are able to exert a greater maximum force. In some instances, very rigorous programmes of endurance training such as those adopted for marathon and ultra-marathon contests lead to a loss of protein from less active regions of the body including the arms and the upper part of the trunk (R.J. Shephard, 1978a).

Relevance of Training Responses to Prevention of Ischaemic Heart Disease

General changes

Some of the benefits of a regular exercise programme are very general in nature, and arise almost independently of the intensity or amount of activity that is undertaken. The individual becomes health conscious and shares advice on prudent living with fellow enthusiasts; particularly if activity is followed on a group basis, matters such as smoking habits, diet and attitudes to daily work receive frequent discussion (S.M. Fox *et al.*, 1972). Many participants, particularly the women, value the camaraderie that develops in a group setting (R.J. Shephard *et al.*, 1980a), and the resultant psychological support may buttress the individual against life stresses that are a frequent precipitant of cardiac attacks (T.H. Holmes & Rahe, 1967). Class members also speak enthusiastically about an elevation of mood, although this is hard to document by formal psychological tests (K.H. Sidney & Shephard, 1977a). Transient effects probably arise from the increased secretion of catecholamines and the added input to the reticular formation of the brain stem; if so, the mood change would be greater with vigorous than with light effort. There has been much discussion of the possible role of physical activity in the release of tension and pent-up aggression. The concept of catharsis had its origins in ancient Greece (R.J. Shephard, 1978c), where the dramatic portrayal of violence with appropriate punishment of the evil-doer was held to purge an audience of dangerous emotions. Freud applied this concept to physical activity, but in more recent times some sports psychologists have tended to the view that violent games breed as much excitement and aggression as they release (J.E. Kohanson, 1970; M. Gluckman, 1973). However, G. Rivard *et al.* (1977) found that boys participating in an international hockey tournament had above average teacher-ratings for such items as group integration and participation (team work). The contest itself had no immediate effect on frustration scores, whether the participant's team won or lost. Much presumably depends upon the nature of the activity, the manner in which it is pursued and the attitude of team-mates and coach (if any). Non-competitive walking, cycling or jogging is less likely to arouse excitement, tension or hostility than competitive sports such as ice-hockey, tennis or squash. Nevertheless, many coronary-prone individuals have the type of personality that turns any activity into an aggressive act; they are determined to beat their opponent at tennis, and equally insist upon walking further and faster than others of their own age, sometimes to the point of provoking a coronary attack while they are exercising (Chapter 3). E.M. Layman (1970) distinguishes hot-tempered anger, induced by and directed towards an external stimulus ('reactive aggression') and the coldly calculated but equally fierce aggression of a body check ('instrumental anger'). Violence can perhaps restore physiological equilibrium following hot anger, although this seems unlikely to occur if the external stimulus is removed from the sports arena or gymnasium (for example, a problem of home, office or classroom); instrumental aggression, in contrast, seems likely to breed further aggression.

Cardiovascular changes

There is normally a linear relationship between heart rate and oxygen consumption or the equivalent power output of the body during sub-maximal exercise. Training leads to a substantial rightward shift in this relationship, due largely to: (i) the decrease of resting heart rate; (ii) the increased maximum rate of working; and (iii) some decrease of maximum heart rate. Other possible (but less firmly established) contributory factors include: (i) habituation to the various stresses of vigorous activity; (ii) a reduction in skin blood flow (heat dissipation being facilitated by a reduction of subcutaneous fat and an earlier onset of sweating); (iii) other improvements in blood flow; (iv) more ready perfusion of the working muscles (due to an increase in their maximum voluntary force); (v) better maintenance of stroke volume (due to an increase in blood volume and an increase in cardiac contractility; and (vi) an increased arterio-venous oxygen difference (related to an increase in red cell mass, a resultant increase in arterial oxygen content and a reduction in mixed venous oxygen content attributable to either more effective distribution of cardiac output or more complete extraction of oxygen in the active muscles). The net result of the slower heart rate is a considerable decrease in the cardiac work rate at any given level of oxygen consumption, so that, for a given coronary blood flow, myocardial ischaemia is less likely to arise.

The systemic blood pressure is also reduced by training; the resting values show only a minor change, but there are larger decreases during the performance of a given sub-maximal task. The latter changes reflect both alterations in central regulatory mechanisms and also a strengthening of the working muscles, since one function of the exercise-induced hypertension is to sustain the perfusion of muscle fibres that are contracting at more than 15 per cent of their maximum voluntary force (A.R. Lind & McNicol, 1967). The lesser rise of blood pressure during exercise reduces the cardiac work rate required for a given external effort. Moreover, myocardial efficiency is improved, since that component of work performed against tension in the ventricular wall does not contribute to the pumping of blood around the circulation.

Other possible cardiac responses to training could further improve the precarious balance between cardiac work rate and coronary oxygen supply, as follows:

(i)   myocardial hypertrophy might facilitate cardiac perfusion by reducing the tension per unit cross section of ventricular wall;

(ii)   reduction of systolic reserve might, through the LaPlace relationship, reduce wall tension for a given intraventricular pressure;

(iii) lessening of the sympathetic drive to the heart might decrease myocardial contractility and thus myocardial O_2 consumption at any given external work rate;

(iv)   lengthening of the diastolic phase of the cardiac cycle (when left ventricular perfusion occurs) might increase the average coronary blood flow over a cardiac cycle;

(v)   possible widening of the arterio-venous oxygen difference in the coronary circulation (through an increase in red cell mass, or an increase in myocardial enzyme activity) might increase oxygen delivery per unit of coronary blood flow.

The possible impact of endurance training upon the coronary vasculature has already been noted. Animal experiments suggest the potential for both an enlargement of the coronary arterial tree and a development of collateral anastomoses. There have been no related studies of primary prevention in man, although the middle-aged adult apparently fails to respond in this way when he participates in the usual type of mild training programme arranged for his age group. Nevertheless, there are mechanisms whereby regular physical activity can reduce the obstruction associated with partially formed intravascular lesions. Fibrinolysis is promoted, at least in the period immediately after an exercise bout (J.D. Cash & McGill, 1969; B. Berkada *et al.*, 1971; V. McAlpine *et al.*, 1971; T. Åstrup, 1973). There may also be an acute decrease in the stickiness of the platelets (G. Lee *et al.*, 1977), although increases in the platelet count and in some of the plasma clotting factors (A. Pelliccia, 1978) leads to an increase in the coagulability of the blood with exercise (J.R. Poortmans *et al.*, 1971; K. Korsan-Bengtsen *et al.*, 1973). Habitual endurance activity apparently curtails the increase in blood coagulability following a fatty meal (G.A. McDonald & Fullerton, 1958), but it is still disputed whether it can decrease the blood coagulability of fasting subjects (H.J. Montoye, 1960; K. Korsan-Bengtsen *et al.*, 1973).

Respiratory changes

The training-induced increase in anerobic threshold, reduced oxygen cost of breathing and increase in maximum exercise ventilation all tend to improve oxygen transport to the heart and the active muscles. Oral augmentation of breathing may also be avoided during submaximal exercise, on account of the greater efficiency of ventilation;

this lessens the chances of provoking reflex bronchial and coronary arterial spasm in a cold and dry atmosphere.

A sub-normal vital capacity is possibly linked to risk of ischaemic heart disease through a mutual association with cigarette smoking. Endurance training could thus improve both lung function and prognosis by encouraging abstinence from cigarettes. On the other hand, the extent of physical activity necessary to break an established smoking pattern seems to be quite large (P. Morgan *et al.*, 1976).

Metabolic changes

The increase in muscle enzyme activity with conditioning has at least two practical consequences. The ability to metabolise fat during exercise is enhanced; conceivably, this could reduce not only the accumulation of fat in peripheral depots, but also the fatty infiltration of the blood vessels. There is also some possibility of increased oxygen extraction from blood perfusing the working tissues; such a change would diminish the cardiac output needed to sustain a given power output in the active muscles.

A few authors have noted an increase in electron transport in cardiac muscle following endurance training (for example, H. Kraus & Kirsten, 1970; M.J. Hamilton & Ferguson, 1972); unfortunately from the viewpoint of preventing myocardial ischaemia, these findings have not been confirmed by other investigators (L.B. Oscai *et al.*, 1971; P.D. Gollnick & Ianuzzo, 1972; G.L. Dohm *et al.*, 1972).

The blood-lipid profile may be modified by a training programme, particularly if the required exercise is vigorous and prolonged, with a negative energy balance. A high total cholesterol, a high triglyceride level and a low HDL cholesterol are well-accepted risk-factors for the development of ischaemic heart disease; control of blood lipids from early childhood is plainly advantageous, but there is less evidence that correction of the lipid profile in middle age will improve ultimate prognosis.

It is easier to ascribe primary and/or secondary preventive value to some of the hormonal responses to increased physical activity. Excessive blood levels of catecholamines are plainly a factor contributing to ventricular dysrhythmias, and the training-induced reduction of noradrenaline and adrenaline secretion at any given work-rate should thus diminish the likelihood of developing a ventricular tachycardia or fibrillation. Fat deposition is reduced and fat mobilisation is enhanced by both the greater sensitivity of the adipocytes to catecholamines (Table 4.2) and the vigorous secretion of growth hormone during acute bouts of physical activity. The development of maturity-onset diabetes seems linked to lack of exercise, and the condition is often corrected by a programme of progressive activity (B.P. Björntorp et al., 1972); again, the onset of diabetes is recognised as a risk factor for subsequent ischaemic heart disease (F.H. Epstein, 1974), but it is less certain that the late (secondary) control of glucose intolerance will restore a normal prognosis. Lastly, the increase of free thyroxine levels during acute bouts of exercise may help to control fat accumulation by burning excess energy, although any increase of metabolism is of relatively short duration.

Body composition

Cardiac hypertrophy has several conflicting effects upon the relative oxygen supply to the myocardium. Usually, the capillary blood supply increases roughly in proportion with the increase in cross section of the myofibrils. However, if the mean radius of the ventricle is increased, the wall tension is augmented, as would be predicted from the LaPlace relationship. Fortunately, this tendency is offset by the increase in wall thickness, so that the tension per unit of cross section is diminished.

Any rise in red cell mass is also a mixed blessing. While the increase in oxygen carriage per unit volume of blood lessens the cardiac output needed to sustain a given external power output, any large increase in red cell count can lead to a substantial augmentation in both the viscous resistance to blood flow and the coagulability of the blood.

Skeletal-muscle hypertrophy reduces the force that must be exerted by unit cross section of muscle at any given intensity of activity. This lessens the perception of exertion (and associated psychological stress); it also facilitates perfusion of the working muscles, reducing the need for compensatory hypertension with resultant loading of the heart.

A reduction in subcutaneous fat, if associated with a decrease in body mass, increases the relative aerobic power (oxygen transport per kilogram of body mass), and reduces the oxygen cost of most tasks that involve the raising and lowering of body parts. Furthermore, the isometric demands for body support become smaller. All of these changes reduce the cardiac loading for a given external task. Loss of subcutaneous fat also facilitates heat elimination, thus curtailing the skin blood-flow requirement when exercising in a warm environment. It is less certain how far fat loss helps the individual who already has pre-clinical atherosclerotic changes in his blood vessels; observations in patients with wasting diseases and ileal by-pass operations are encouraging (G. Weber, 1978), but if secondary changes have occurred in connective tissue, with clotting and calcium impregnation of fatty plaques, such changes are unlikely to be reversed by an increased consumption of fat.

Required pattern of exercise

The pattern of activity needed in a programme of primary or secondary prevention cannot be fully resolved until there is more agreement on the basis of such prevention. Some of the supposed general benefits of exercise — advice on prudent living, camaraderie, joie de vivre and pleasurable relaxation — stem more from the development of new interests and affiliation to a group of like-minded enthusiasts than from the vigour of the exercise that is undertaken; it is thus arguable that equal benefit could be derived from a class directed to an alternative aspect of health or even to a pleasant but sedentary hobby. Other supposed mechanisms of prevention — reduction in adiposity, control of serum cholesterol and triglyceride levels and correction of glucose intolerance — demand a substantial daily expenditure of energy, but sustained moderate exercise is a more effective method of attaining this objective than brief bouts of very vigorous activity (G. Gwinup, 1975). Intense exercise is the only likely stimulus to enlargement of the coronary arterial tree, development of the collateral circulation and habituation of the individual to the stresses of maximum effort. However, most suggested mechanisms of primary and secondary prevention (S.M. Fox *et al.*, 1972; Table 4.3) require regular endurance-type training.

Primary prevention is easier to institute than secondary prevention, since the child is more ready to learn an active pattern of behaviour than is the middle-aged adult. However, it is important that the activity habit be taught in such a way that it is maintained throughout adult life; certain school programmes with a heavy team emphasis tend to be abandoned rapidly after completion of school or university. Instruction should encompass a wide variety of endurance-type activities, so that the pupil has a chance to find an athletic discipline that is both enjoyable and suited to his body build and motor skills. The emphasis should be upon participation rather than the development of a star performance, with the development of interests that can be carried over into adult life and practised as a family. A minimum of facilities, equipment and fellow participants should be required. Suitable suggestions include distance cycling, swimming, cross-country skiing, jogging, fast walking, hill-climbing and the vigorous performance of non-mechanised household chores such as lawn-mowing and sawing logs.

Table 4.3: Possible Mechanisms by Which Physical Activity May Prevent Ischaemic Heart Disease

Light activity	Moderate activity	Intense activity	Increased energy consumption
Prudent living	Reduced cardiac workload, heart rate, blood pressure, increased myocardial efficiency	Coronary artery size enlarged	Adipose tissue decreased
Camaraderie		Collateral vessels developed	Serum cholesterol reduced
Joie de vivre	Improved O_2 transport, red cell mass, arterial O_2 content, blood volume, blood flow distribution, tissue enzyme activity	Habituation	Serum triglycerides reduced
Relaxation			Glucose tolerance improved
Correction of 'stress'	Hormonal changes, neurohormonal balance, catecholamine secretion, growth hormone, thyroid hormone		
	Blood coagulability, fibrinolysis, platelet stickiness improved		

Source: After S.M. Fox et al (1972), but classified in terms of activity pattern required.

There have been a number of longitudinal studies of exercise programmes in children (for example, T.K. Cureton, 1964; H.H. Clarke,
1971; R. Bauss & Roth, 1977; R. Mirwald *et al.*, 1977; R. Renson *et
al.*, 1977; R.J. Shephard *et al.*, 1977b). Physical condition has generally
improved as a result of training, with gains of maximum oxygen intake,
muscle strength, and physical performance. J. Pařízková (1977) also
observed a reduction in body fat in boys attending a special summer
camp, but other investigators have found surprisingly little effect of
increased classroom activity upon the percentage of body fat in free-
living students (R.J. Shephard *et al.*, 1977b). There is plainly a need for
studies that commence in childhood and continue throughout the adult
life-span. However, practical problems have prevented the initiation of
such a project. Indeed, most of the investigations completed to date
have continued for insufficient time to allow the effects of school-age
programmes upon the health and behaviour of the young adult to be
assessed. One exception is a follow-up study of Swedish female
swimming champions, carried out five years after ceasing competition.
This demonstrated that the physical condition of the swimmers had on
average regressed to the point where the maximum oxygen intakes were
less than in sedentary housewives of the same age (P.O. Åstrand *et al.*,
1963). While the protagonists of exercise programmes must be discouraged by this information, it should be stressed that the individuals
concerned had been obliged to undertake gruelling competitive training.
It thus remains possible that the moderate activity appropriate to a
programme of primary prevention may build up more favourable
attitudes, with permanent acceptance of an active lifestyle.

Animal Experiments

General considerations

In view of the dearth of long-term primary preventive trials in man,
particular interest attaches to the results obtained from longitudinal
animal experiments. Through specific manipulation of diet, physical
activity and hormonal balance, the time course of atherosclerosis can
be accelerated by a factor of 20-30, coronary narrowing can be
surgically induced and specimens can be taken freely for histological
examination. Furthermore, activity and dietary patterns are more
readily controlled than in human studies.

Spontaneous atherosclerosis is a well-recognised feature of zoo and
domesticated animals (M. Sherman, 1964). This is apparently due in
part to an inappropriate diet; 80 per cent of laboratory dogs that are

Table 4.4: Some Characteristics of Animal Models Used in the Study of Atherosclerosis

Model	Characteristics of atherosclerotic model
Dog	Produced by thyroid depression and atherogenic diet. Cardiovascular system, lipid and cholesterol metabolism differ from man
Fowls (chicken, pigeon)	Produced readily by atherogenic diet, but plaques differ from human, as do anatomy, lipid and cholesterol metabolism. Picture sometimes complicated by cholesterol accumulation in reticulo-endothelial system
Rabbit	Produced readily by atherogenic diet, but plaques differ from human, as do topography of lesions, lipid and cholesterol metabolism. Lesions resistant to regression
Monkey	Advanced atherosclerosis readily produced by atherogenic diet; lesions, anatomy and biochemistry similar to man, but animals are expensive, hard to handle and procure
Pig	Plaques difficult to produce without special manipulation but anatomy, physiology and biochemistry similar to man, plaques similar, large size permits arteriography, open heart surgery and measurements of cardiac functions

Source: R.W. Wissler and Vesselinovitch (1977).

fed a commercial dry dog food have a serum cholesterol reading of 200 mg·dl^{-1} or less, whereas 67 per cent of more liberally fed household pets show a cholesterol value of over 200 mg·dl^{-1}, and in ten per cent of animals values are greater than 300 mg·dl^{-1}.

Atherosclerotic lesions can be produced experimentally in a variety of species, including monkeys, pigs, rabbits and fowls (D. Kritchevsky, 1974; M.L. Armstrong, 1976; H.C. Stary *et al.*, 1977; R.W. Wissler & Vesselinovitch, 1977). However, the relevance of such models to human disease has been questioned (H.C. McGill, 1965; E.P. Benditt, 1977). The appearance and distribution of the atherosclerotic plaques sometimes differs substantially from that observed in human ischaemic heart disease, and there are inevitable inter-species differences in vascular anatomy, physiology, biochemistry and lipid metabolism, including the characteristics of the various lipoproteins (Table 4.4). Furthermore, the 'accelerated' lesions that are so convenient for rapid experimentation appear only if the animal is exposed to a markedly atherogenic diet, hormonal manipulation such as thyroid extirpation and/or a severe restriction of physical activity (H. Montoye, 1960).

Primary prevention

The preventive value of exercise is suggested by the fact that athero-sclerosis is more common in domesticated species than in their wild (and presumably more active) counterparts. Among the fowls, for example, atherosclerosis is seen in the turkey and the chicken, but is less evident in birds that fly regularly; certain varieties of domesticated pigeon are markedly affected, but in racing pigeons the condition does not progress beyond a slight fatty streaking of the great vessels (M. Sherman, 1964).

Prospective experimental studies, reviewed by Sherman, have yielded conflicting results (N.H. Warnock *et al*., 1957; A.L. Myasnikov, 1958; F.F. McAllister *et al*., 1959). When cockerels were fed a high-fat diet, exercise corrected elevation of the serum cholesterol (N.H. Warnock *et al*., 1957). On the other hand, hens that were exercised on a treadmill five days per week for twelve weeks showed as much atherosclerosis as non-exercised birds. One study of rabbits suggested that regular physical activity failed to inhibit deposition of cholesterol in the heart and aorta, perhaps because exercised animals ate more than the controls (A.L. Myasnikov, 1958). A second study of the same species noted that exercise decreased the severity and extent of experimental athero-sclerosis without decreasing the serum cholesterol level (S.D. Kobernick *et al*., 1957). It was thus speculated that physical activity in some way hampered the escape of cholesterol from the blood stream.

Studies of longevity have been carried out in rats (D.W. Edington *et al*., 1972). The influence of physical activity upon lifespan apparently depends upon the age at which it is initiated. In young animals, the effect is favourable, but in 'middle-aged' animals (400 days or more from a 600-day lifespan) the prognosis is worsened by a daily training programme.

J.T. Flaherty *et al*. (1972) have emphasised the role of mechanical stress in determining the location of lesions within the vascular tree. In their experiments, lesions were potentiated when blood flow was increased by a surgical arterio-venous anastomosis. Exercise plainly leads to an increase in both aortic and coronary blood flow, and it is thus arguable that wall stress is augmented during the acute phase of physical activity. However, from the viewpoint of atherosclerosis, the crucial information is presumably the average wall stress for a 24-hour period, and there is at present little evidence whether this is increased or decreased by a regular programme of activity.

Secondary prevention

From the viewpoint of secondary prevention, it is encouraging to observe the regression of experimental atherosclerotic lesions when an atherogenic diet is replaced by hypolipidic foods (D. Vesselovitch *et al.*, 1974; G. Weber *et al.*, 1975; M.L. Armstrong, 1976; R.J. Friedman *et al.*, 1976; A.S. Daoud *et al.*, 1977; R.G. De Palma *et al.*, 1977; H.C. Stary *et al.*, 1977). To the extent that physical activity improves the lipid profile, it presumably has a similar effect to the hypolipidic diet.

Coronary circulation

It is difficult to visualise the coronary circulation in man, and much of the evidence concerning exercise and myocardial blood flow is thus derived from animal experiments. Unfortunately, the data are far from consistent. Acute bouts of physical activity can have an adverse effect if they are linked with experimental narrowing of the coronary vessels. P.L. Thompson & Lown (1975) developed a pattern of coronary occlusion that was tolerated by resting dogs. When the same procedure was given to exercising animals, it was often lethal, eight of ten dogs dying of ventricular fibrillation within 24 hours. Occlusion immediately following exercise also worsened prognosis (two sudden deaths and four further deaths among ten animals over a 24-hour period). However, if exercise was undertaken more than one hour after occlusion, the activity did not lead to ventricular fibrillation or death.

Wild species have a better myocardial oxygen supply than their domesticated counterparts (O. Poupa *et al.*, 1970). A regular programme of daily activity enlarges the coronary arterial tree of the rat (J. Tepperman & Pearlman, 1961; J.A.F. Stevenson, 1967), particularly if there is cardiac hypertrophy (A. Kerr *et al.*, 1968; A.S. Leon & Bloor, 1970). It also augments the capillary/fibre ratio of the myocardium (T. Petren *et al.*, 1936; R.J. Tomanek, 1970; R.L. Rasmussen *et al.*, 1978) at least in young animals (where hyperplasia occurs; O. Poupa *et al.*, 1970), but it may decrease the ratio in older animals where there is simple hypertrophy (J. Hakkila, 1955; O. Poupa *et al.*, 1970). Prior training increases survival after experimental narrowing of the coronary vessels (R.W. Eckstein, 1957) or infarction (B.C. Wexler & Greenberg, 1974). On the other hand, regular exercise does not seem to protect an animal against subsequent occlusion of its coronary vessels (J.J. Burt & Jackson, 1965; E. Kaplinsky *et al.*, 1968; T.M. Sanders *et al.*, 1978).

Summary

Animal experiments generally support the view that regular physical exercise will inhibit the development of atherosclerosis, increasing longevity (at least in young animals) and enhancing the formation of coronary collaterals (at least where there is already some narrowing of the coronary vessels). Furthermore, there is some evidence that established lesions can be reversed by a sustained programme of physical activity. Nevertheless, these findings must be accepted with caution, since there are some discordant reports, and in any event there are significant differences in the atherosclerotic process between man and most of the commonly used experimental animals.

5 EXERCISE AND THE SECONDARY PREVENTION OF ISCHAEMIC HEART DISEASE

Evidence concerning the value of physical activity in the secondary prevention of ischaemic heart disease is largely epidemiological in type (J.O. Holloszy, 1973; W.L. Haskell & Fox, 1974; R.J. Barnard, 1975; V.F. Froehlicher, 1976; G.H. Hartung, 1977; H.J. Montoye, 1977). After a brief discussion of the epidemiological method and problems of direct experimentation, we will examine available experimental data. Information garnered from studies of ethnic populations, athletes and groups differing in occupational or leisure activities will then be reviewed in the light of Bradford Hill's postulates for a 'causal' association between two variables.

Epidemiology versus Direct Experimentation

Epidemiology examines associations between events as they occur in free-living populations. The associations observed may have a high level of statistical significance but, unless a direct experimental step is undertaken, it is generally difficult to establish a cause and effect relationship between two variables.

One of the earliest epidemiologists was a physician named John Snow (1855). He practised in the Soho district of London at a time when epidemics of cholera were commonplace. The wisdom of the period attributed this disease to mysterious miasmata, spreading from the creeks of central London during episodes of dense fog. However, John Snow patiently traced the relationship between an outbreak of cholera and the drinking of water from a specific source, the Broad Street pump. Microscopic examination of the water in question showed the presence of many 'animalicules', and further enquiry established that a sailor with obvious symptoms of cholera had taken up residence in a public house adjacent to the pump shortly before the disease became prevalent. The distance separating the privy of the hotel from the well was only a few feet. Cause and effect was indicated more clearly than in many subsequent epidemics, yet the crucial step in John Snow's research was experimental rather than epidemiological — the outbreak of cholera was checked when he removed the handle from the offending pump. (Purists may note that this does not provide categoric proof. In fact, the handle was removed from the pump at a time when the epidemic was waning from natural causes.)

The hypothesis that exercise is of benefit in the secondary prevention of ischaemic heart disease rests largely upon a series of epidemiological associations. The crucial experimental proof is lacking. In essence, no-one has found a way to 'take the handle off the pump'. The problem lies in the area of logistics. Coronary events in normal middle-aged men are sufficiently rare that given a 25 or 50 per cent benefit from an increase in physical activity, the usual experiment with random allocation of subjects to exercise and control groups would require an unmanageably large sample in order to have a reasonable chance of demonstrating a significant effect (Table 5.1). The required number of subjects is further increased by sample attrition (Table 5.2). One pilot trial concluded that, even if attention was focussed upon a population with a number of coronary 'risk factors', the cost of a definitive experiment would be US $31 million, measured in 1962 currency (H.L. Taylor *et al.*, 1966; R.D. Remington & Schork, 1967). The likely drop-out rate would be 50 per cent over the first six months of exercise (J. Ilmarinen & Fardy, 1977), with further defections over the remaining four to five years of observation; the residual sample would thus be small and atypical of the original population from which it was drawn, making valid conclusions impossible. The British Cardiac Society (Joint Working Party, 1976) likewise concluded that while a randomised controlled trial of exercise in the secondary prevention of ischaemic heart disease was a theoretical possibility, it was not practical.

As we shall see in the next chapter, prospective assessments of exercise therapy have been attempted in patients with a recent myocardial infarction. Such individuals have a substantial motivation to increased physical activity from their 'critical event', but even when using this type of population, results are inconclusive because of: (i) a high drop-out rate; (ii) poor compliance with the required exercise programme; (iii) contamination of control subjects with an interest in physical activity (R.J. Shephard & Kavanagh, 1978b); and (iv) simultaneous changes in other health habits.

According to current thinking, lack of physical activity remains one probable risk factor in the causation of ischaemic heart disease, but other variables such as smoking habits, systemic hypertension and serum cholesterol levels are of at least equal importance. Having regard to both the high cost of a definitive trial and the multifactorial nature

Table 5.1: The Size of Random Sample Needed for a 90 Per Cent Chance of Demonstrating a 25 and a 50 Per Cent Reduction in the Incidence of Myocardial Infarction ($P < 0.05$) as a Result of Increased Physical Activity

Age of sample (years)	Annual incidence (5-year study per 1,000 subjects)	Sample size		Annual incidence (10-year study per 1,000 subjects)	Sample size	
		25% reduction	50% reduction		25% reduction	50% reduction
40–49	3.2	14,800	3,200	3.8	6,100	1,300
45–54	4.6	10,200	2,200	5.3	4,300	925
50–59	6.6	7,050	1,550	7.5	3,000	650
55–64	9.5	4,900	1,050			

Source: H.L. Taylor *et al*. (1966).

Table 5.2: The Size of Random Sample Needed for a 90 Per Cent Chance of Demonstrating a 50 Per Cent Reduction in the Incidence of Myocardial Infarction ($P < 0.05$) in Relation to Drop-out Rate and Incidence of Disease in Control Subjects

Incidence in control group (one year, per 1,000)	Sample size versus drop-out rate		
	10% of residue per year	25% of residue per year	50% of residue per year
7.5	2,600	5,500	21,000
10.0	2,000	4,200	15,000
15.0	1,300	2,800	11,000
20.0	1,000	2,100	7,600
40.0	500	1,100	3,900
80.0	260	720	2,100

Source: R.D. Remington & Schork (1967).

of the disease, the present generation of secondary preventive trials are thus adopting the technique of multiple risk-factor modification. Such an approach may well cure the disease without indicating whether an increase in physical activity has made a useful contribution to therapy.

Table 5.3: Changes in Coronary 'Risk Factors' with One-year and Ten-year Participation in a Lifestyle-modification Programme

Variable	One year	Ten years
Participation (%)		
Non-smokers	96.4	71.8
Smokers	92.3	49.7
Energy intake		
(10-year average, % baseline)	–	–25.7
Total fat intake		
(10-year average, % baseline)	–	–19.1
Animal fat intake		
(10-year average, % baseline)	–	–32.4
Cholesterol intake		
(10-year average, % baseline)	–	–48.6
Decrease in body mass		
(%, continuing participants)	– 5.5	– 4.7
Serum cholesterol		
(% change, continuing participants)	–10.8	– 7.3
Diastolic pressure		
(% change, continuing participants)	– 5.0	– 4.3
On-job activity		
(arbitrary units, continuing participants)	+ 0.1	– 0.6
Leisure activity		
(arbitrary units, continuing participants)	+ 0.4	+ 0.5
Cigarette smoking	About a half of continuing participants stopped smoking by 6 years	

Source: J. Stamler (1978).

Experimental Trials of Secondary Prevention

Chicago Programme

In 1957, J. Stamler (1978) initiated a lifestyle-modification programme in central Chicago. His subjects were deliberately selected in terms of coronary risk factors such as a high serum cholesterol level, an excessive body mass relative to actuarial tables, a diastolic pressure higher than 95 mm Hg, non-specific changes in the T wave of the electrocardiogram and cigarette smoking. The retention of study participants was remarkably successful, 71.8 per cent for non-smokers and 49.7 per cent for smokers over a ten-year period of observation (Table 5.3). As in data from Toronto (R.J. Shephard & Cox, unpublished), a seven-day diet recall sheet indicated a suspiciously large reduction in energy, fat and cholesterol intake over the course of the programme. Presumably, the collection of nutritional information led to a temporary

Table 5.4: Influence of Chicago Programme of Lifestyle Modification on Prognosis

	N	Ten-year mortality (per 1,000)	
		All causes	Coronary heart disease
Chicago programme	519	54	23
adjusted data*	519	64	27
US 'Pooling Project'	2,896	85	36
Life insurance standard risk, age 50		119	—
Life table — US white males, age 19-70		134	—

* Adjusted to allow for age and risk factors, relative to data of US 'Pooling Project'.

Source: J. Stamler (1978).

modification of diet during the week of observation. Nevertheless, continuing study participants showed useful changes in a number of risk factors, including a decrease of body mass, serum cholesterol and diastolic pressure, an increase of leisure activity and the cessation of smoking in about a half of those who initially had a cigarette habit.

It is difficult to assess the impact of the programme upon prognosis, since the subjects were volunteers rather than a random sample of the Chicago population. After adjustment for age and the various risk factors observed on entry to the study, the ten-year mortality from coronary heart disease was some 25 per cent below the average for subjects enrolled in five US prospective epidemiological studies (the 'Pooling Project'; D. McGee & Gordon, 1976). However, this could reflect the initial selection of subjects willing to enrol in a ten-year health study rather than a specific response to the subsequent programmed lifestyle modification (Table 5.4).

Other studies in the US

Subsequent prospective studies in the US have examined dietary modification (National Diet-Heart Study Research Group, 1968; L. Mojonnier *et al.*, 1979), reduction in body mass (A. Keys & Parlin, 1966; MRFIT, 1977), control of hypertension (Hypertension Detection Follow-up Programme, cited by H. Blackburn, 1979),

Table 5.5: Changes in Risk Factors over a Prospective Trial of Exercise (Three One-hour Sessions per Week)

Variable	Change over study	
	Exercise group	Control group
Serum cholesterol (mg•dl $^{-1}$)	−5.4	−4.1
Blood pressure		
Systolic (mm Hg)	−3.1	−2.2
Diastolic (mm Hg)	−4.0	−3.6
Quit smoking (number of subjects)	4	4

Source: Based on data of H.L. Taylor *et al.* (1973).

cessation of smoking (MRFIT, 1980) and management of stress (A.P. Shapiro *et al.*, 1977; C.B. Taylor *et al.*, 1977) as possible tactics for the control of ischaemic heart disease.

The Multiple Risk Factor Intervention Trial (MRFIT) is a relatively large-scale experiment which will conclude in 1982 (R.C. Benfari, 1979). The subjects, 12,000 men aged 35–57 years, are at increased risk of ischaemic heart disease due to a high serum cholesterol, a high diastolic blood pressure and cigarette smoking. An attempt is being made to modify each of these variables over a six-year period, using dietary counselling, antihypertensive agents and various smoking cessation techniques. As yet, only a few preliminary results are available (MRFIT, 1977, 1980).

Surprisingly few of the US trials have included deliberate physical activity in their protocol. H.L. Taylor *et al.* (1973) initiated a three-centre study where 'high-risk' middle-aged men carried out three one-hour sessions of supervised exercise per week. Subjects were asked to maintain a normal lifestyle with respect to diet and smoking habits. After twelve months, the exercised group showed a greater reduction of serum cholesterol than the controls, but by 18 months the two groups showed similar small decreases in serum cholesterol, systolic and diastolic blood pressures, and a few members of each group had quit smoking (Table 5.5).

A. Leon *et al.* (1979) had greater success with a sixteen-week exercise regimen. This involved 90 minutes of supervised walking per day at a treadmill speed of 5.1 km•h $^{-1}$ and a slope of 10 per cent. Favourable changes in coronary risk factors included a loss of body fat and body mass, improved glucose tolerance, decrease of serum

Table 5.6: Effects of 16 Weeks of Walking (90 min, Five Days a Week, 5.1 km·h⁻¹, 10 Per Cent Grade) on Obese Young Men Not Subjected to Dietary Restriction

Variable	Change over 16 weeks
Body mass (kg)	− 5.6
Mass of fat (kg)	− 4.8
Mass of lean tissue (kg)	− 0.9
Skinfold readings (mm)	−10.7
Blood-glucose (mg·dl⁻¹)	−39.0
Insulin (μU·ml⁻¹)	−140.9
Plasma cholesterol (mg·dl⁻¹)	− 6.0
Plasma triglycerides (mg·dl⁻¹)	−21.0
HDL/LDL ratio	+ 0.07
Treadmill endurance (min)	+ 2.5

Source: Based on data of A. Leon *et al.* (1979).

Table 5.7: Influence of Hygienic Measures and of Hygienic Measures plus Exercise upon Frequency of Electrocardiographic Abnormalities

Variable	Hygienic measures Initial	After 6 weeks	Hygienic measures plus exercise Initial	After 6 weeks	Control Initial	After 6 weeks
Standard ECG	2.0	2.7	2.8	2.5	2.2	2.4
Isometric test	3.8	5.4	4.4	2.6	4.4	5.0
Treadmill test	2.7	1.9	1.7	3.3	3.2	2.1
Multiple waveform (%)	44	48	20	24	55	35
R on T PVCs (%)	15	15	20	12	28	17
Pairs or runs of PVCs (%)	44	44	32	28	28	31
PVC fusion, beats (%)	19	7	0	16	7	10

Source: H. Blackburn *et al.* (1976).

cholesterol and triglycerides and an increase in the ratio of HDL to
LDL cholesterol (Table 5.6). As in an earlier study by K.H. Sidney
et al. (1977), regular exercise was remarkably successful in controlling
appetite and energy balance, without specific dietetic measures.

H. Blackburn *et al.* (1976) examined the possibility of controlling
premature ventricular contractions by either hygienic measures (for
instance, cessation of smoking, abstinence from coffee, reduced
consumption of alcohol and increased hours of sleep) or a combination
of such measures with a supervised programme of endurance exercise
(one hour of walking and jogging three times per week). Unfortunately,
the trial was concluded after six weeks, but over this period neither of
the two treatment groups showed any striking improvement in their
ECG tracings relative to a control sample drawn from the same
population (Table 5.7).

K.H. Cooper *et al.* (1977) reviewed data for subjects attending the
Aerobics Institute in Dallas, Texas. Of 9,000 men and women tested
since 1971, seven had sustained a fatal myocardial infarction, 11 had
experienced a non-fatal episode, and nine had undergone cardiac
'by-pass' surgery. The 27 cardiac victims were compared with 81
matched controls, chosen for their initial similarity in terms of serum
cholesterol, systemic blood pressure, glucose tolerance, left-ventricular
dimensions and age. It was concluded that a low level of physical fitness
(as indicated by a limited treadmill-endurance time) and an abnormal
stress electrocardiogram each contributed to the detection of subsequent
coronary events independent of the other risk factors isolated.
However, the close correlation between a low treadmill score and the
development of electrocardiographic abnormalities prevented any
assessment of the relative importance of these two variables.

European studies

European centres have embarked upon a number of risk-factor intervention studies (M. Miettinen *et al.*, 1972; L. Wilhelmsen *et al.*, 1972;
P. Puska, 1974; P. Leren *et al.*, 1975; World Health Organization,
1977). However, with the exception of the experiment initiated by the
World Health Organization European Collaborative Group, no attempt
has been made to increase the physical activity of study participants.

The World Health Organization compared entire factories, matched
for size, geographical location and nature of the manufactured product.
In experimental factories, community advice was given on diet,
smoking cessation, reduction in body mass and the treatment of
hypertension, particular attention being directed to high-risk subjects.

Table 5.8: Changes in Risk Factors over Two Years of WHO European Collaborative Trial (E = Experimental Group, C = Control)

Country and sample	Serum cholesterol (mg•dl^{-1}) E	C	Systolic blood pressure (mm Hg) E	C	Cigarettes smoked per day in smokers E	C
Belgium						
Random sample	+ 5.9	+ 20.0	−7	−0.4	− 9	− 4
High-risk sample	−10.0	+ 1.0	−	−	−11	−10
Italy						
High-risk sample	− 3.0	−	−	−	−	−
UK						
Random sample	+ 2.2	+ 5.4	−4	−4	−11	+ 2
High-risk sample	− 6.0	−	−	−	−29	−17

Source: Based on data of World Health Organization (1977).

Over a two-year period of observation, serum cholesterol, systolic blood pressure and the number of continuing smokers all changed favourably relative to workers in the control factories (Table 5.8).

In Europe, as in the US, many studies have been marred by a rapid attrition of volunteers. A participation rate of some 90 per cent was achieved in North Karelia (P. Puska *et al.*, 1978), but in Gothenburg 25 per cent of the population neither answered a mailed questionnaire nor attended an initial screening examination (L. Wilhelmsen *et al.*, 1976). Careful investigation disclosed an excess of immigrants, unmarried and divorced men and cigarette smokers among the non-volunteers (L. Wilhelmsen *et al.*, 1972); non-participants also had an above-average prevalence of alcoholism and chronic disease (L. Wilhelmsen *et al.*, 1976).

P. Teräslinna *et al.* (1969) found that 58 per cent of male executives either did not respond or were unwilling to participate in an exercise training programme. Subjects with a high-risk profile were selected from the 42 per cent of positive respondents. Endurance exercise was carried out for 30-60 minutes three times per week. Over 18 months, the drop-out rate was 14 per cent, with a class-participation rate of 72 per cent; the maximum oxygen intake increased by 20 per cent relative to control subjects, but there was no significant change of serum cholesterol, body mass, systemic blood pressure or smoking habits (K. Pyörälä *et al.*, 1971). Three years after completion of the study, the majority of the subjects had reverted to a sedentary lifestyle (J. Ilmarinen & Fardy, 1977).

Conclusion

Logistics have to date prevented effective long-term trials of exercise in the secondary prevention of ischaemic heart disease. Physical activity of sufficient vigour induces favourable changes in a number of coronary risk factors. However, such a response is not always observed with the relatively mild exercise programme usually arranged for the middle-aged adult. Furthermore, high drop-out rates cast doubt upon the practicality of exercise as a means of secondary prevention in the absence of greater social acceptance of physical activity as a normal component of leisure.

Cross-cultural Comparisons

Rationale

Cross-cultural comparisons identify regional and ethnic populations with coronary risk profiles that differ substantially from those of the typical 'white' North American.

Body fat content

Many 'primitive' people are extremely thin (R.J. Shephard, 1978a). For example, a double fold of skin and subcutaneous tissue measures only 6-7 mm in the Canadian Eskimo, as compared with 12-16 mm in an average 'white' person. On the other hand, measurements of total body fat suggest that the internal stores of the Eskimo are not proportionately reduced (R.J. Shephard et al., 1973). Furthermore, because of a short stature and well-developed musculature, the traditional Eskimo has a substantial excess body mass relative to actuarial standards for the 'white' population. The low percentage of body fat is related to continued acceptance of a traditional lifestyle, and there is a positive correlation between the thickness of subcutaneous fat and indices of 'acculturation' to our western civilisation (R.J. Shephard, 1978a). In Alaska, skinfold readings have increased from six to twelve millimetres over 15 years of urbanisation (P.L. Jamison & Zegura, 1970). Two other indigenous populations with substantial obesity (the Maoris and the Polynesians of Hawai) now show a high prevalence of coronary arterial disease (D.R. Bassett et al., 1966; I.A.M. Prior & Davidson, 1966).

Table 5.9: Lipid Profile of Greenlandic Eskimos and Danes

	Eskimos	Danes
Total lipid $(g \cdot l^{-1})$	6.18	7.15
Cholesterol $(mmol \cdot l^{-1})$	5.91	7.27
Triglyceride $(mmol \cdot l^{-1})$	0.57	1.23
Chylomicrons $(g \cdot l^{-1})$	0.27	0.19
Pre-β-lipoprotein $(g \cdot l^{-1})$	0.43	1.29
β-Lipoprotein $(g \cdot l^{-1})$	4.45	5.21
α-Lipoprotein $(g \cdot l^{-1})$	4.00	5.34

Source: Based on data of H.O. Bang *et al.* (1976).

Blood lipids

When different populations are compared, the rank-order correlation
between the prevalence of atherosclerotic lesions and an elevation of
serum cholesterol levels is as high as 0.76 (N.S. Scrimshaw & Guzman,
1968; A. Keys, 1970). There is little question that the serum cholesterol
is low in most underdeveloped nations, although the relative
contribution of vigorous daily activity and restricted diet to this
situation remains uncertain. Traditional Eskimos have a favourable lipid
profile (Table 5.9) despite a very high fat diet (H.O. Bang *et al.*, 1976;
H.H. Draper, 1976; J. Sayed *et al.*, 1976); nevertheless, much of the
ingested fat may be unsaturated in type (A. Keys, 1975). Somali camel-
herders (V. Lapiccirella *et al.*, 1962) and East African Masai (G.V.
Mann *et al.*, 1965) eat much milk, meat and blood, yet maintain a low
serum cholesterol and a low incidence of ischaemic heart disease.
Although this has been attributed to high levels of daily energy
expenditure, other possible contributory factors include a low total
intake of energy (A. Keys, 1975), efficient inhibition of cholesterol
synthesis (K. Biss *et al.*, 1971) and the presence of a specific cholesterol
inhibitor in fermented milk (G.V. Mann, 1977). Other studies from
Africa (R.F. Scott *et al.*, 1966), Israel (J.H. Medalie *et al.*, 1968), India
(I.J. Pinto *et al.*, 1970) and the Pacific (I.A.M. Prior & Evans, 1970) all
show favourable lipid readings in 'primitive' groups, although there
remains an association between serum cholesterol and the likelihood of
myocardial infarction even when average values for the population are
very low (I.J. Pinto *et al.*, 1970). As a 'western' lifestyle is adopted,
serum cholesterol concentrations increase. Thus Alaskan Eskimos in
general (K. Ho *et al.*, 1972; J.E. Maynard, 1976), Canadian Eskimos

living in Montreal (R. Carrier *et al.*, 1972), and Greenlandic Eskimos living in Denmark (H.O. Bang *et al.*, 1976) all show relatively 'normal' cholesterol readings, with a corresponding increase in cardiovascular disease relative to their counterparts who conserve a traditional life-style (S.A. Feldman *et al.*, 1972; O. Schaefer, 1973; J.E. Maynard, 1976). Even within India, there is a trend to increasing cholesterol values (I.J. Pinto *et al.*, 1970), and much higher figures are encountered in wealthy Indians who have migrated to East Africa (R.F. Scott *et al.*, 1963).

Habitual activity

It has often been suggested that a high level of physical activity is necessary for survival in a 'primitive' community. However, formal measurements of 24-hour pulse rates (L. Hermansen & Ekblom, 1966) and energy expenditures (O.G. Edholm *et al.*, 1973; G. Godin & Shephard, 1973b; R.J. Shephard, 1978a) do not always confirm this supposition. In the pleasant climate of Easter Island, many of the native people undertake very little physical activity (L. Hermansen & Ekblom, 1966). Ugandan farmers work no more than 3½ hours per day (W.H. Boshoff, 1965), and the activity of East African nomads is reported as no more than 'moderate' (A.G. Shaper, 1970). Relatively few 'primitive' people exhibit high levels of energy expenditure or aerobic power (R.J. Shephard, 1978a). The ceremonial runners of the Tarahumara Indians are one notable exception (D. Groom, 1971). High daily energy expenditures are also encountered in traditional Canadian Eskimos (range 10.6-18.6 MJ per day, average 15.3 MJ. 'Acculturated' Eskimos who spend most of their time at wage-earning work in permanent settlements have a lower average energy usage (13.7 MJ per day), with a parallel loss of aerobic power and an increase in skinfold thickness (A. Rode & Shephard, 1971a). There seems to be an increased incidence of ischaemic heart disease with decreasing physical activity, even in underdeveloped nations. V.V. Shah *et al.* (1968) found that ischaemic heart disease was more frequent among sedentary Indian workers than in those with active occupations, while S.G. Sarvotham & Berry (1968) did not find a single case of cardiac disease among Indian heavy manual workers. In general, statistics for ischaemic heart disease favour underdeveloped societies, but it is by no means proven that physical activity is responsible for this advantage; other possible contributing factors (R.J. Shephard, 1974a) include genetic constitution, differing types and intensities of emotional stress, differences in the amount and type of tobacco consumed, differences in blood coagulability, differences in the prevalence of hypertension, differences in diet and drinking water (hard versus soft water) and inherited differences in glucose tolerance.

Apparent ethnic differences

Substantial ethnic differences in the prevalence of ischaemic heart disease have been observed between populations living in the same region. While it is well-recognised that constitutional factors contribute to 'coronary' susceptibility (M.M. Gertler & White, 1954; R. Cederlöf *et al.*, 1967; T.M. Allan & Dawson, 1968), lifestyle factors are probably responsible for many of the apparent ethnic differences. H.C. McGill (1968) compared men of Caucasian and African descent living in New Orleans, São Paulo and Puerto Rico. In each of these locations, post-mortem examination showed that the men of African origin had less coronary arterial stenosis than the Caucasians. Data on men of American Indian ancestry were unfortunately obtained from other cities (Caracas, Calin and Lima), but coronary arterial stenosis in such subjects was less severe than that observed in either Caucasians or Africans.

Studies of migrants

European-born men predominated among Israelis showing scars of myocardial infarction and coronary thrombosis following traumatic death (I. Mitrani *et al.*, 1967). A prospective study of 10,000 male civil-service employees (J.H. Medalie *et al.*, 1968) showed significant differences in the prevalence of angina pectoris, myocardial infarction and ischaemic heart disease according to the area of birth. Age-adjusted rates were highest for Jews from eastern or central Europe, intermediate for those born in Israel or southern Europe and lowest for those from Africa and other parts of the Middle-East (Table 5.10).

The importance of community lifestyle is strongly supported by other studies of migrants. Native-born Australians have a mortality from arteriosclerotic and degenerative heart disease of 1.69/1,000 over the age range 40-9 years. Italians resident in Australia for up to six years have a mortality of only 0.16/1,000 over the same age span; however, with 7-19 years of residence the figure rises to 0.51/1,000, and with more than 20 years of residence it is 1.30/1,000 (Table 5.11). Equally, United Kingdom, Norwegian, Irish and Japanese migrants to the United States have shown an increase in ischaemic-heart-disease mortality, with increased cigarette consumption accounting for only a part of the worsening of prognosis (G. Rose, 1970; M.F. Trulson *et al.*,

Table 5.10: Prevalence of Ischaemic Heart Disease in Migrants to Israel

| Country of birth | Criterion (age-adjusted prevalence, per 1,000) | | |
	Angina pectoris	Previous myocardial infarction	ECG changes (LBBB, probable or possible infarct)
Eastern Europe	40	28	27
Central Europe	37	26	31
Southern Europe	40	15	18
Israel	33	20	20
Middle East	24	7	12
Africa	22	9	17

Source: J.H. Medalie *et al*. (1968).

Table 5.11: Mortality from Arteriosclerotic and Degenerative Heart Disease (ISC 420-2) among Italians Migrating to Australia, Australians, and Italians Remaining in Italy

| Country of birth | Years of residence | Deaths from heart disease (per 1,000 per year) | | |
		Age 40-9 years	Age 50-9 years	Age 60-9 years
Italy	0-6 years (Austrialia)	0.16	1.23	2.60
	7-19	0.51	1.70	3.76
	20	1.30	3.44	7.58
	Resident in Italy*	0.80	2.40	6.80
Australia	Resident in Austrialia	1.69	5.92	14.72

* Those who remain in Italy also have a differing prognosis from early migrants; both existing disease and lifestyle factors probably influence the decision to migrate.

Source: G. Rose (1970).

cited by H.S. Ingraham, 1977).

As in more 'primitive' societies, differences in habitual activity may contribute to inter-population differences in the prevalence of ischaemic heart disease, but there seems no simple method of separating the effect of this variable from other lifestyle-related influences.

Studies of Ischaemic Heart Disease in Athletes

Studies of ischaemic heart disease in athletes have two principal attractions — the individuals concerned have engaged in more rigorous training than could be expected of the general population, and they have maintained this activity for months if not years.

Data on former athletes

Surveys of the incidence of ischaemic heart disease in former athletes (K. Yamaji & Shephard, 1977) have not been particularly helpful in proving or disproving the exercise hypothesis (Table 5.12). Early studies compared former university athletes with the general population, but it was soon realised that the advantage of longevity in ex-athletes was due to their favoured socio-economic status rather than to the physical activity involved in competitive sports. Comparisons were next made between those who represented their university for a particular sport and other members of the same academic community; this approach overcame socio-economic inequalities, but was nevertheless fallible, since it was rarely established that the 'non-athletes' were inactive while at university; some control series were indeed locker-holders in an athletic facility.

P. Fardy *et al.* (1976) found that, in later life, former athletes maintained some advantage of both activity pattern and myocardial function relative to non-athletes. However, other studies noted that many of those classed as athletes ceased to participate in their chosen sport some years before reaching the period of manifest coronary disease (Figure 5.1); when compared with their contemporaries, the so-called athletes were less active, more likely to be regular cigarette smokers and drinkers of alcoholic beverages and more likely to have sustained a large increase in body mass (Figure 5.2; H. Montoye *et al.*, 1956).

Data on continuing athletes

Where athletes have continued with vigorous endurance activity into

Table 5.12: Causes of Death among Former Athletes

Author	Heart and vascular disease	Genito-urinary disease	Cancer and tumours	Influenza, pneu-monia, bron-chitis	Tubercu-losis	Accidents, war, death, homicides, suicides
Wakefield (1944):						
Athletes	16.3		—	10.5	13.8	34.0
Controls	16.3		—	11.5	20.9	17.3
Rook (1954):						
Athletes	36.4	5.2	13.9	8.9	—	12.0
Controls	41.5	7.1	12.8	10.5	—	7.0
Pomeroy & White (1958):						
Athletes	37.9	4.6	12.6	10.3	—	24.1
Controls	49.0	3.7	13.6	4.8	—	7.5
H. Montoye *et al.* (1956):						
Athletes	66.0		12.0	2.0	—	10.0
Controls	56.0		14.0	5.8	—	13.0
Poldenak & Damon (1970):						
Major athletes	38.0	—	12.0	7.2	—	5.4
Minor athletes	42.5	—	12.3	3.9	—	7.4
Non-athletes	40.0	—	9.7	4.8	—	5.0
Schnor (1971):						
Athletes	34.7	5.6	23.6	3.5	—	9.1
Controls	36.7	4.1	25.1	1.2	—	7.7
Poldenak (1972):						
Major athletes	39.6	—	14.4	5.4	—	6.2
Minor athletes	42.6	—	13.3	4.0	—	7.6
Non-athletes	41.7	—	11.7	5.0	—	6.6

Source: Based on data accumulated by K. Yamaji & Shephard (1977).

their middle and later years, they have sometimes lived several additional years relative to (presumably) less active fellow citizens. M.J. Karvonen *et al.* (1974) studied cross-country skiers (mainly participants in the Oulu races of 1889–1930); mortality was compared with the general male population of Finland, using a life-table analysis. On average, the skiers lived 73.0 years, while the longevity of the reference population was 68.7 years. However, there is no proof that there were not initial differences of health favouring the ski champions, and their endurance sport necessarily fostered other health habits, including a

Figure 5.1: Current sports participation of former 'athletes' and 'non-athletes'; note that the sample size is small for the oldest age group.

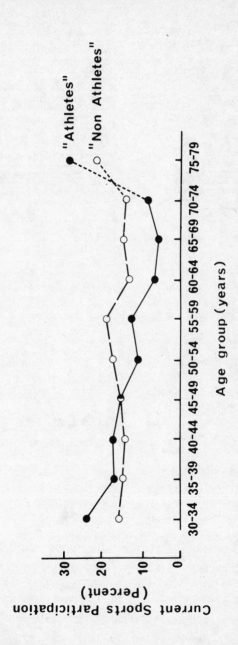

Source: Based on data of H.J. Montoye *et al.* (1957).

Figure 5.2: Percentage of subjects smoking and drinking regularly in middle age in relation to athletic 'letter' earnt while at University.

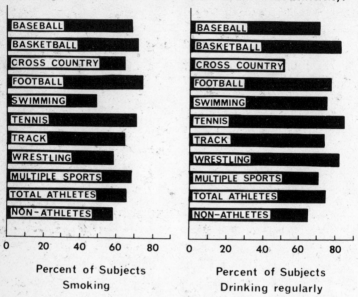

Source: Based on data of H.J. Montoye *et al.* (1957).

lifetime aversion to cigarette smoking. A study of former long-distance runners and champion skiers (K. Pyörälä *et al.*, 1967a, b) revealed a lower blood pressure than in controls (137/87 mm Hg, compared with 147/92 mm Hg); symptoms of ischaemic heart disease were also less frequent, but nevertheless electrocardiographic abnormalities had a similar prevalence in atheletes and non-athletes.

The Bassler hypothesis

T.J. Bassler (1977) has repeatedly advanced the hypothesis that the running of marathon distances protects the heart against what he has described as coronary heart disease, ischaemic heart disease, fatal myocardial infarction, loafer's heart and coronary atherosclerosis. He has attributed the supposed protection in part to the rareness of cigarette smoking in the distance runner, and in part to the metabolic consumption of fat, which is the major fuel used in marathon running. Unfortunately for the Bassler hypothesis, T. Noakes *et al.* (1977) have now described six cases of myocardial infarction in well-trained

Table 5.13: Resting Systemic Blood Pressures (mm Hg) for Participants in Masters' Track and Field Competitions, Compared with Data of A. Master *et al.* (1964) for the General Population

Age group (years)	Masters' athletes						Sedentary normals	
	(T. Kavanagh & Shephard, 1977a)		(M.L. Pollock, 1974)		(K. Asano *et al.*, 1978)		(A.M. Master *et al.*, 1964)	
	Syst.	Diast.	Syst.	Diast.	Syst.	Diast.	Syst.	Diast.
< 40	124	79	—	—	—	—	127	80
40–50	120	77	117	76	117	70	130	82
50–60	127	77	129	81	132	79	137	84
60–70	128	77	122	78	135	82	143	84
> 70	140	83	141	83	157	78	146	82

Source: Based on data collected by T. Kavanagh & Shephard (1977a).

marathon runners, four of the six cases having coronary arterial disease demonstrated by angiography. P. Milvy (1977) has further stressed that the number and age of marathon runners (total sample of 9,958 in the US in 1975) are such that, even if running conferred no protection, no more than one death would be anticipated in any two-year period.

Observations on Masters' athletes

Findings for Masters' athletes have been reviewed by T. Kavanagh & Shephard (1977a). In their study, twelve of 135 Masters' contestants had a heart volume of more than 14 ml·kg^{-1}, compared with the anticipated value of 10–11 ml·kg^{-1} for sedentary men of the same age. The resting systemic blood pressure was also slightly less than in the general population (Table 5.13). Some authors have reported a high prevalence of ST segmental depression in the exercise electrocardiogram of former endurance competitors (A. Holmgren & Strandell, 1959), but others have found a normal or even a low prevalence of abnormalities (K. Pyörälä *et al.*, 1967b; B. Saltin & Grimby, 1968). T. Kavanagh & Shephard (1977a) noted ventricular premature systoles in 17 of 135 competitors at rest, but the abnormal rhythm disappeared during exercise in all except two of the group. Fifteen of 135 tracings showed ST segmental depression of more than 0.1 mV when subjects were exercising at 75 per cent of aerobic power; having regard to their

Table 5.14: Prevalence of Abnormal Electrocardiogram (ST Depression > 0.1 mV) when Exercising at 75 Per Cent of Aerobic Power for Masters' Track and Field Athletes, as Compared with Normal Sedentary Canadians

Age group (years)	Masters' competitors		Sedentary Canadian men
< 40	2/8	(25%)	2%
40–50	4/64	(6.3%)	7
50–60	6/34	(17.6%)	17
60–70	3/18	(16.7%)	30*
70–90	0/4	(0%)	—

* Age 60–5 years.

Source: Data of T. Kavanagh & Shephard (1977a) for Masters' athletes and of G. Cumming (1972) for sedentary Canadians.

advanced age, this was possibly a smaller proportion of abnormal records than would have been anticipated in the general Canadian population (Table 5.14). Possible explanations of any favourable findings in the Masters' athletes include a development of collateral blood flow to the myocardium, a lesser hypokalaemia of effort and a reduction of workload per unit mass of myocardium secondary to hypertrophy and other changes of myocardial dimensions.

The problem of self-selection

Self-selection is perhaps the most serious criticism of all studies of athletes. Almost by definition, the competitor is an atypical member of the population from which he is drawn. He is necessarily in good initial health, and is committed to a health-conscious lifestyle. Selection for specific sports occurs on the basis of body type, and this also is a factor with a powerful influence upon prognosis. The ectomorphic cross-country skier or distance runner is inevitably at a lower risk of ischaemic heart disease than his mesomorphic or endomorphic counterpart, and this explains part of the substantial difference in longevity between endurance athletes and other classes of sportsmen (Table 5.15; K. Yamaji & Shephard, 1977). Finally many reports do not indicate the cause of death, and while heart disease may be less common in athletes than in the general population, this potential advantage is often masked by an increase in violent deaths from accident, suicide, homicide and war (Table 5.12).

Table 5.15: Mean Lifespan of Various Sportsmen, Excluding Those Dying at War or by Accident

Sport	Dublin (1928) (expected)	Rook (1954) (years)	Poldenak (1972) (years)	Largey (1972) (years)
Track & field	91.8	67.4	66.9	71.3
Cricket	–	68.1	–	–
Crew	94.1	67.1	66.8	–
Rugby football	–	68.8	–	–
American football	88.3	–	66.6	57.4
Baseball	98.0	–	65.2	64.1
Boxing	–	–	–	61.6
Two or more sports	78.3	–	67.2	–

Source: Based on data accumulated by K. Yamaji & Shephard (1977).

Such problems make it clear that the exercise hypothesis can be neither proven nor disproven by studies of champion athletes.

Occupational Surveys

Occupational surveys also have the attraction that a given level of physical activity is usually sustained for many years. Historically, the intensity of occupational effort has ranged from completely sedentary employment to tasks demanding quite vigorous physical activity. Epidemiologists were thus quick to compare the cardiac health of workers in jobs that demanded differing levels of energy expenditure (F.G. Pedley, 1942; J.A. Ryle & Russel, 1949; J.N. Morris *et al.*, 1953; O.F. Hedley, 1959).

Types of analysis

Early studies were retrospective in nature, but more recently there have been examinations of disease prevalence (J. Stamler *et al.*, 1960; H.L. Taylor *et al.*, 1962; J. McDonough *et al.*, 1965) and substantial prospective investigations (J.M. Chapman & Massey, 1964; J.N. Morris *et al.*, 1966; R. Paffenbarger & Hale, 1975). Bases of comparison have included: (i) the annual incidence of deaths from ischaemic heart disease; (ii) the annual incidence of sudden deaths; (iii) the annual

Table 5.16: The Influence of Physical Activity upon Various Indices of Ischaemic Heart Disease, Expressed as the Ratio of Incidence for Active and Inactive Populations

Index of ischaemic heart disease	Mean ratio	Range	Number of studies
Myocardial pain	0.48	0.21—0.68	8
Angina pectoris	1.36	0.65—1.98	7
Myocardial infarction	0.56	0.33—0.98	9
Coronary heart disease			
Attack rate	0.60	0.17—1.03	16
Mortality	0.66	0.28—1.22	21
Vascular pathology	0.76	0.51—1.00	7

Source: Based on data accumulated by S. Fox & Haskell (1968a).

incidence of myocardial infarctions; (iv) the annual incidence of freshly diagnosed cases of angina; and (v) some combinations of these statistics. A few authors have also examined the prevalence of electrocardiographic evidence of myocardial ischaemia (J. McDonough *et al.*, 1965; J.N. Morris, 1975) and the extent of pathological changes visible at post-mortem examination (myocardial scarring and fibrosis, coronary atherosclerosis; J.N. Morris & Crawford, 1958; D.M. Spain & Bradess, 1960b; G. Rose *et al.*, 1967).

Typical findings

The majority of surveys (16 of 20 listed by H.H. Clarke, 1972) have shown a higher incidence of deaths, sudden deaths and infarctions among those working in relatively sedentary occupations (Table 5.16). The remaining studies, sometimes described as negative, have generally shown similar trends. Nevertheless, the benefits of exercise have not always been statistically significant, as a result of an inadequate cohort size – a problem in the studies of J. Stamler *et al.* (1960) and of A. Keys (1970); transfer of subjects from active to inactive jobs with the recognition of disease – a problem merely noted in the negative study of H. Kahn (1963), but allowed for in the positive study of R. Paffenbarger *et al.* (1977); and inadequate categorisation of either occupation or infarction (I.M. Moriyama *et al.*, 1958; O. Paul, 1969).

One study of accident victims found that ischaemic changes (calcification, fatty streaking, raised lesions and coronary narrowing) were more common in light than in heavy occupations (V. Rissanen, 1976). However, others report coronary atheromata and narrowing as being equally prevalent in men from all job categories (J.N. Morris & Crawford, 1958; G. Rose *et al.*, 1967). Further, anginal pain is more common among active than inactive workers (J.N. Morris *et al.*, 1953; W.B. Kannel *et al.*, 1971a, b). It has thus been reasoned that, if occupational activity does indeed improve prognosis, this is not by preventing the development of ischaemic heart disease, but rather by making the individual aware of his condition and giving him a greater ability to live with it.

Social class differences

One major problem when interpreting occupational data is an association of the energy requirements of work with social class and related variables such as smoking and drinking habits. The first report from the Gothenburg study of 'men born in 1913' found a significant influence of occupational activity upon the likelihood of subsequent coronary events (L. Wilhelmsen & Tibblin, 1971). A second analysis from the same study (D. Elmfeldt *et al.*, 1976) is sometimes said to 'prove' that occupational activity has no influence upon the likelihood of a subsequent coronary event. In fact, there were differences of income, housing, nutrition and health habits between those tabulated as having 'high' and 'low' levels of occupational activity, and such confounding factors may well have obscured any benefit of exercise. Similar problems have arisen in a number of US studies, some of which have failed to show a significant association between physical inactivity and cardiovascular disease. Manual workers have generally been of a lower social class than sedentary employees, and sometimes there have also been differences of milieu (urban versus rural; H.L. Taylor *et al.*, 1962) or race (J. McDonough *et al.*, 1965) between the two groups. While rural 'blacks' living in the US have less coronary disease than their 'white' counterparts (J. Cassel *et al.*, 1971), the negroes of the urban ghettos (J.M. Chapman & Massey, 1964; J. Stamler *et al.*, 1960) (who preponderate among the blue-collar workers) have a high incidence of ischaemic heart disease, linked to their propensity for obesity and cigarette smoking. J.M. Chapman & Massey (1964) observed no difference in the incidence of ischaemic heart disease with social class, but it may be that in the sample investigated the adverse health habits of the blue-collar workers were counterbalanced by the added energy expenditure of their work. Among studies with a reasonable matching of socio-economic status, we may mention comparisons of

London bus drivers and conductors (J.N. Morris *et al.*, 1953, 1966), postal clerks and mail carriers (J.N. Morris & Raffle, 1954; H. Kahn, 1963), and office and field workers of the Jewish kibbutzim (D. Brunner & Manelis, 1971).

Influence of emotional stress

It has been argued that sedentary employees are exposed to greater emotional stress than those in physically active employment. In the case of the London bus drivers, this hypothesis was explored and rejected through a comparison of men operating city and rural routes (J.N. Morris *et al.*, 1966). Other attempts to demonstrate an effect of occupational stress upon the incidence of ischaemic heart disease have generally been unconvincing (Chapter 2), one exception being managers with upward social mobility (L. Hinckle *et al.*, 1968).

Intensity of occupational activity

Occupations that demand more than two to three times the resting metabolic rate are now a rarity, and a heart rate 'ceiling' of 115 beats·min^{-1} is common for 'heavy' industry. On the other hand, most physiologists suggest that a young adult should reach a minimum heart rate of 140 beats·min^{-1} in order to improve his physical condition (M.L. Pollock, 1973; R.J. Shephard, 1975, 1977a). Even in a 65-year-old worker, conditioning is unlikely with a heart rate of less than 120 beats·min^{-1} (K.H. Sidney & Shephard, 1978). Admittedly, physiologists are still uncertain how to equate 30 minutes of training at a heart rate of 140 beats·min^{-1} and 8 hours of industrial activity at a heart rate of 115 beats·min^{-1}. Nevertheless, it seems likely that the majority of North Americans now find their main source of physical activity outside of their daily employment (H. Montoye, 1975), confounding the whole concept of classifying habitual activity by occupation.

Many retrospective occupational studies have used very 'soft' data. Occupational classifications have been crude, and there has been no guarantee that the small minority sustaining heart attacks were working at a level typical of their category. Reports have often referred to the period immediately prior to the heart attack, ignoring the possibility that warning symptoms such as angina pectoris may have led a man to change from active to sedentary employment. Where occupation has apparently had no effect upon prognosis, this may thus reflect difficulties of classification rather than a true absence of relationship.

Self-selection

As in studies of athletes, the major criticism of occupational surveys is the problem of self-selection. In general, people choose their mode of employment. In a classical paper subtitled 'The epidemiology of uniforms', J.N. Morris *et al.* (1956) showed that, at the time of recruitment to the London Transport bus system, the drivers had a larger average abdominal girth than the conductors. They also had a higher serum cholesterol, a higher systemic blood pressure (J.N. Morris *et al.*, 1956) and a greater body mass (R.M. Oliver, 1967), giving them an increased initial risk of ischaemic heart disease. A large occupational survey from Eire (N. Hickey *et al.*, 1975) showed a similar negative association between heavy work and coronary risk factors at the time of commencing employment.

The bias becomes exaggerated over a longitudinal study, since those with symptoms of ischaemic heart disease leave the labour force or are transferred from the active to the sedentary group (H.L. Taylor *et al.*, 1962; H. Kahn, 1963). This could explain why heavy work seems protective for young but not for older workers (R. Paffenbarger *et al.*, 1970, 1977). One statistical remedy is to reclassify workers annually according to their currently reported job assignment (R. Paffenbarger & Hale, 1975; R. Paffenbarger *et al.*, 1977); however, this tactic is rendered ineffective if the union insists that a worker retain a high-paying job classification even though he is unable to function at the required intensity of effort.

D. Brunner & Manelis (1971) maintained that, in the Jewish kibbutzim, difficulties of self-selection were eliminated, since the type of employment was determined by a central committee. If they are correct in this view, their data has great importance, for the field workers encountered the same diet, income and living conditions as those whose employment involved sitting for at least 80 per cent of the day. The two groups had comparable values for body mass, serum cholesterol and triglycerides, yet the physically active workers had a much lower incidence of ischaemic heart disease. Unfortunately, it is hard to believe that the kibbutz committee was uninfluenced by initial health and physique when assigning an individual's duties. Almost inevitably, such factors must have determined both initial placement and subsequent annual reallocation of jobs; indeed, the medical history probably influenced job selection more than in a free-market economy.

Multivariate analyses

Perhaps the most sophisticated of the occupational surveys is that reported by R. Paffenbarger (1977). He examined 3,686 Californian longshoremen over a 22-year period, from 1951 to 1972. Employment categories were well-defined by the union concerned, and a part of the sample had a very high energy expenditure at work (22-31 kJ·min^{-1}); the intensity was sufficiently high that union regulations limited each hour to 55 per cent labour and 45 per cent rest periods. Note was taken when a fatal heart attack was certified as the underlying cause of death, and the data were sorted into sudden deaths (within one hour of the onset of symptoms) and delayed deaths on the basis that premonitory symptoms might have caused a change of job classification in the latter group of subjects.

Table 5.17: Initial Self-selection of Job Category by Californian Longshoremen, Expressed as Age-adjusted Per Cent of Sample

Variable	Occupational energy expenditure	
	Low	High
Cigarettes (> 1 pack·day^{-1})	39.1*	34.2*
Systolic blood pressure (⩾ mean)	44.3	45.3
Diastolic blood pressure (⩾ mean)	47.2	48.7
Diagnosed heart disease	17.0	18.2
'Weight for height' (⩾ mean)	48.0*	45.9*
Abnormal glucose tolerance	4.1	4.0
Serum cholesterol (⩾ mean)	48.4	42.8

* Significant difference ($P < 0.05$).

Source: Based on data of R. Paffenbarger (1977).

Two factors of initial self-selection were noted (Table 5.17). There were less pack-a-day smokers among the heavy than among the moderate and light workers, partly because the former were not allowed to smoke except in specified 'rest areas'. Also, a smaller proportion of the heavy workers had an above average 'weight for height'. However, Paffenbarger argued that these differences were not sufficient to invalidate his subsequent data analysis.

A lesser energy output at work (6-22 kJ·min^{-1}), the smoking of more than a pack of cigarettes per day and a systolic blood pressure equal to or greater than the mean all made independent contributions

Table 5.18: Relative Risk of Fatal Heart Attack, Adjusted for Age and Other Two Principal Risk Factors for California Longshoremen

Type of death	Low energy output	Cigarettes (≥ 1 pack·day^{-1})	Systolic blood pressure ($\geq$ mean)
Sudden	3.3	1.6	2.7
Delayed	1.6	2.1	1.4
Unspecified	1.7	2.5	2.2
All	2.0	2.1	2.1

Source: Based on data of R. Paffenbarger (1977).

to the risk of cardiac death; in the case of the lower energy output, the effect was much greater for sudden than for delayed deaths (Table 5.18). Serum cholesterol had surprisingly little influence upon risk, possibly because most categories of longshoremen had a higher level of energy expenditure than that required in ordinary modern occupations.

The incidence of deaths from cerebrovascular disease was also related to a lesser energy output at work, but exacerbation of disease was relatively specific to the cardiovascular system; deaths from cancer, accidents and suicides were unrelated to the activity level at work.

Paffenbarger used multivariate statistics to estimate the health benefits that would accrue from a modification of the three prime risk factors that he had identified. Acting singly, an increase of energy output would reduce the cardiac death rate by 31-67 per cent. The smoking of less than a pack of cigarettes a day would reduce the risk 20-36 per cent, while reduction of the systolic blood pressure below the population mean would reduce the risk by 21-37 per cent. If all three changes were effected, the cardiac death rate would drop by a dramatic 70-100 per cent (Table 5.19).

In marked contrast with Paffenbarger, R.H. Rosenman *et al.* (1977) had essentially negative findings in a four-year prospective survey of US Federal employees living in the San Francisco Bay area. Significant differences were seen between those classed as having light, moderate and heavy energy expenditure at work (Table 5.20). However, there was a substantial influence of social class upon smoking habits, relative body mass and serum cholesterol levels (Table 5.21). A multivariate analysis that allowed for socio-economic status revealed no effect of occupational activity upon either risk factors or the

Table 5.19: Hypothetical Reduction in Risk of Fatal Heart Attack with Change of Health Behaviour

Health behaviour modified	Fatal heart attacks per 1,000 man-years with adverse behaviour	Potential reduction in risk (%)	
1. Low energy output	6.97	48.8	(30.6–67.0)
2. Cigarettes ($\geq$ 1 pack·day^{-1})	9.43	27.9	(20.1–35.7)
3. Systolic blood pressure ($\geq$ mean)	8.91	28.8	(20..6–37.0)
4. 1 + 2	9.57	64.7	(44.5–84.9)
5. 1 + 3	9.15	73.5	(56.9–90.1)
6. 2 + 3	16.16	50.3	(39.7–60.9)
7. 1 + 2 + 3	15.19	88.2	(70.2–100.0)

Source: Based on data of R. Paffenbarger (1977).

Table 5.20: Correlations between Intensity of Vocational Activity (Light, Moderate or Heavy) and Other Risk Factors for Ischaemic Heart Disease at Beginning of Prospective Study

Variable	Age 35-9 years Light	Mod.	Heavy	Age 40-9 years Light	Mod.	Heavy	Age 50-9 years Light	Mod.	Heavy
Current smokers (%)	27.9	39.6*	37.0*	26.0	37.7	42.4	35.9	37.3	41.4
Relative body mass (% predicted)	99.8	97.5	106.1*	100.4	101.1	102.6*	100.6	101.5	101.6
Serum cholesterol (mg·dl^{-1})	237	240	253	247	245	260*	247	242	259*
Blood pressure:									
Systolic (mm Hg)	133	133	137	134	135	137	140	141	141
Diastolic (mm Hg)	84	84	87	86	86	87	89	88	89

* Statistically significant difference from light-activity group.

Source: Based on data of R.H. Rosenman *et al.* (1977).

Table 5.21: Influence of Socio-economic Status (High, Medium, Low) upon Level of Risk of Ischaemic Heart Disease at Beginning of Prospective Study

Variable	Age 35–9 years			Age 40–9 years			Age 50–9 years		
	High	Med.	Low	High	Med.	Low	High	Med.	Low
Current smokers (%)	24.2	42.3*	46.2*	31.6	37.4*	44.3*	31.8	37.7*	40.5*
Relative body mass (% predicted)	98.5	99.2	103.6*	99.1	103.0*	102.3*	99.5	103.1*	101.4
Serum cholesterol (mg•dl^{-1})	237	246	244	243	249*	255*	248	238*	251
Blood pressure:									
Systolic (mm Hg)	132	134	136	133	133	138	139	141	142
Diastolic (mm Hg)	83	86	87*	85	86	88*	87	89	89

* Statistically significant difference from high-status group.

Source: Based on data on R.H. Rosenman *et al.* (1977).

incidence of clinical manifestations of ischaemic heart disease. Specific differences from the Paffenbarger experiment included a more hetero-geneous population, a less clear-cut indicator of disease, a lower intensity of physical activity in most of the 'active' population and a less certain categorisation of activity. On the other hand, the adjustment for socio-economic status covered effects of the latter upon cigarette consumption, relative body mass, serum cholesterol level, diastolic blood pressure and non-occupational activity, factors that could have contributed to the apparent association between occupation and disease in the Paffenbarger study.

C.L. Rose & Cohen (1977) made a multivariate analysis of longevity, using as their data-base 500 white male deaths reported to Boston City Hall in 1965. Factors such as age-appearance, smoking habits, mother's age at death, sense of humour, urban-versus-rural residence, intelligence and worries were all related more closely to the age at death than was leisure activity, while this in turn was also a better indicator of longevity than was activity at work. Interestingly, the assessed vigour of activity both on and off the job decreased progressively as the individual became older (Figure 5.3).

Figure 5.3: Influence of age upon mean physical activity scores at work and during leisure

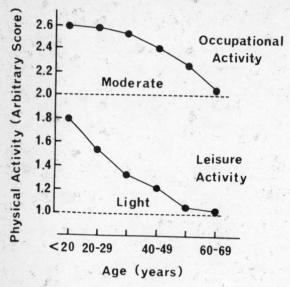

Based on data of C.L. Rose & Cohen (1977).

Conclusion

While some of the evidence from occupational surveys supports the exercise hypothesis, the verdict is by no means unanimous. Interest in organising further studies is waning, since: (a) with increasing automation the city-dweller must look to his leisure hours rather than his work in order to increase his habitual activity; and (b) observations relating occupation to the incidence of ischaemic heart disease can never provide conclusive proof that exercise has preventive value.

Leisure-activity Patterns

Problems of methodology

Problems in surveying leisure activity include the poor reliability of most physical activity questionnaires (W.J. Zukel *et al.*, 1959), and a denial of disability by those who have already suffered a myocardial infarction (V. Froehlicher & Oberman, 1972). If a whole community is studied (for example, D. Elmfeldt *et al.*, 1976), the analysis is further complicated by a positive correlation between vigorous voluntary

Table 5.22: Vigorous Leisure Exercise among Married Men Age 17 and Older Living in London area

Type of activity	Per cent participants by social class		
	I	III	IV & V
Swimming	34	20	8
Football (soccer)	6	8	5
Tennis	8	2	0
Squash	7	2	0
Athletics	2	1	0
Average number of sports	1.1	0.6	0.3

Source: Based on data of M. Young & Willmot (1973).

Table 5.23: Socio-economic Status (High, Medium, Low) and Habitual Physical Activity

Age (years)	Physical activity (h•wk^{-1})					
	Occupational status			Leisure status		
	High	Medium	Low	High	Medium	Low
35-9	4.6	12.6	19.3	8.9	9.4	9.6
40-9	5.3	10.9	17.5	9.3	9.5	8.4
50-9	5.2	11.9	17.1	9.7	8.7	8.7

Source: Based on data of R.H. Rosenman *et al.* (1977).

activity and social class (M. Young & Willmot, 1973; R.H. Rosenman *et al.*, 1977; Tables 5.22 and 5.23). Recent investigations have overcome this problem by focussing upon narrow cross sections of society.

Harvard alumnae study

R.S. Paffenbarger *et al.* (1977) made an extensive prospective study of Harvard graduates, relating the certified causes of death and the incidence of physician-diagnosed ischaemic heart disease to smoking habits and continued participation in various forms of physical activity. The sample size was large (16,936 subjects, 117,680 person-years), and for this reason it was possible to classify participants by athletic discipline (avoiding some of the problems of association between sport selection and body build, discussed above). Substantial protection against ischaemic heart disease (heart attack rate of 1.00 relative to standard figure of 1.64) was seen with an additional overall energy expenditure of 8,000 kJ·wk^{-1}, a figure reminiscent of that deduced from occupational surveys. Furthermore, the age-adjusted cardiac fatality rate showed a steep downward gradient as additional energy expenditure was increased from 2,000 to 10,000 kJ·wk^{-1}. Strenuous sports alone yielded a protection ratio of 1.00:1.38. Subjects who had commenced their sport after leaving university were protected, whereas those who had been athletes at college but subsequently become inactive forfeited their advantage. Protection ratios for the walking of at least one mile per day, and the climbing of fifty stairs per day were 1.00:1.26 and 1.00:1.25 respectively. Protection against a first heart attack was demonstrated in both high- and low-risk segments of the sample (Table 5.24). Paffenbarger's study thus supports the exercise hypothesis. Some criticisms remain with respect to self-selection of the type and vigour of habitual activity, although this source of uncertainty is reduced by the demonstration that sports participation at university has no influence upon prognosis. Again, it can be argued that endurance activity has modified other risk factors such as cigarette consumption (P. Morgan *et al.*, 1976), although protection is seen both in smokers and non-smokers.

British civil servants study

A prospective study by J.N. Morris *et al.* (1973) found a significant reduction in the incidence of ischaemic heart disease (Table 5.25), among British civil servants who engaged in: (a) more than five minutes per day of active recreation, keeping fit or 'vigorous getting about' (near maximum effort); or (b) more than 30 minutes per day of 'heavy' leisure activity (> 31 kJ·min^{-1}). Electrocardiographic abnormalities were also less frequent in the active groups (L. Epstein *et al.*, 1976). The added energy expenditure, no more than 750 kJ·day^{-1}, is substantially less than the figure calculated from eight-hour occupational surveys, and it seems more likely to commend itself to the average sedentary middle-aged person. J.N. Morris and his associates were able to exclude differences of cigarette smoking as an explanation of their data. Nevertheless, it remains conceivable that the chosen criteria (five minutes of vigorous getting about and/or 30 minutes of heavy leisure activity) served as indicators of a general attitude towards exercise and health. The total daily energy expenditure of the active civil servants may thus have exceeded that of

Table 5.24: Protection against First Heart Attack with Additional Weekly Energy Expenditure of 8,000 kJ, All Indices Being 1.00 for the Active Group and a Higher Figure for Those Who Are Less Active

Risk factor	Protection against first heart attack	
	Risk factor present	Risk factor absent
Cigarette smoking	2.22	1.55
Systolic pressure > 130 mm Hg	1.86	1.54
Diastolic pressure > 80 mm Hg	1.36	1.86
Quetelet index (mass $\times 10^3$/height^2) > 34	1.58	1.61
Parent dead	1.63	1.74
No varsity sport	1.59	1.65

Source: R. Paffenbarger *et al.* (1977).

Table 5.25: Frequency of Vigorous Exercise Reported by 239 British Civil Servants Sustaining First Clinical Attack of Myocardial Infarction Relative to Frequency in 476 Matched Controls

Type of activity	Frequency of physical activity	
	Attacked subjects (n = 238)	Matched controls (n = 476)
Active recreation	5	19
Keeping fit	3	16
Vigorous getting about*	1	21
Heavy work*	19	78
Climbing > 450 stairs•day $^{-1}$	0	8
Total reporting activity	25/238	120/476

* See text for definition.

Source: Based on data of J.N. Morris *et al.* (1973).

their sedentary counterparts by a larger margin than 750 kJ, while the choice of (for instance) a vigorous morning walk to the station may have been reflected in other positive health practices. Although active and inactive groups were similar in height, body mass and skinfold thickness, the active group included fewer subjects with a serum cholesterol > 6.4 mmol•l $^{-1}$, more subjects with a blood pressure >

150/90 mm Hg and slightly fewer smokers (26 versus 32 per cent).
Finally, as with similar surveys, we are left with the obstacle of self-
selection. It was the civil servants rather than Dr J.N. Morris who
decided upon their daily activity patterns, and this decision was
undoubtedly influenced both by initial health and constitution.

Other studies

W.B. Kannel (1967, 1979) studied cardiovascular risk factors in
5,127 men and women living in Framingham, Mass. Physical activity
was assessed from a 24-hour history of usual physical activity and
from a number of physiological indices (resting heart rate, vital
capacity, hand grip strength and relative body mass). Coronary heart
disease and mortality were found to be higher in cohorts where a
sedentary lifestyle was inferred, although it was recognised that other
risk factors (a high serum cholesterol, a high systemic blood pressure,
cigarette smoking, glucose intolerance and ECG abnormalities) were
more important determinants of prognosis than was exercise.

R.H. Rosenman (1970) examined the habits of more than 30,000
middle-aged men participating in the Western Collaborative Group
Study. The prime focus of his investigation was psychological.
Nevertheless, he observed a protective effect of regular exercise; this
appeared in 'Type A' men (rates 9.1/1,000 and 15.0/1,000) but not in
those with a 'Type B' personality (rates 5.7/1,000 and 5.3/1,000). He
commented that the protective value of exercise disappeared if subjects
had a high diastolic pressure ($>$ 95 mm Hg), high fasting serum
triglycerides ($>$ 130 mg$\cdot$dl^{-1}), or a low HDL/LDL ratio.

S. Shapiro *et al.* (1969) reported data for men and women aged
35–64 years who were enrolled in the Health Insurance Plan of Greater
New York. Among men, those who were the least active on and off the
job had twice as large an incidence of first myocardial infarctions as
those who were moderately active, but no additional advantage was
gained from further activity. Total infarctions were four times more
frequent in the active group, but the incidence of angina was unrelated
to reported physical activity.

We have noted above that, in the Gothenburg study, occupational
activity had no significant influence upon the development of ischaemic
heart disease. However, when leisure-time activities were explored, there
was a trend towards inactivity in those who subsequently developed
coronary disease (G. Tibblin *et al.*, 1975).

Coronary risk factors

H.J. Montoye (1975) examined the relationships between coronary risk factors and physical activity in 1,696 men living in the small town of Tecumseh, Michigan. When information from leisure and occupational activity was combined, the mean systolic and diastolic blood pressures and serum cholesterol levels were highest in the most sedentary of his subjects.

N. Hickey *et al*. (1975) screened 15,171 Irish workers; they found that heavy leisure activity was associated with a low blood pressure, a low serum cholesterol, a favourable relative body mass and a reduced likelihood of cigarette smoking.

Conclusion

As in the occupational surveys, there is much to support the exercise hypothesis in studies of leisure pursuits. Nevertheless, it is unlikely that conclusive proof will be obtained by further extension of such investigations. Problems arise from the need to average data over a wide range of subject ages and a substantial period of history (in which the epidemic of coronary disease has waned; B.M. Meyer, 1979). Above all, self-selection remains an insuperable obstacle to substantiating the value of physical activity.

The Bradford Hill Criteria

Given the impossibility of experimental proof, an alternative possibility is to exclude spurious and indirect associations, and then to weigh the evidence against nine criteria that A. Bradford Hill (1971) has suggested should be satisfied if a statistical association is to be regarded as causal rather than casual.

Spurious association

Several causes of spurious association must first be excluded. There is the Type I error of the statistical method — given a 0.05 level of probability, there is one chance in twenty that an association is a statistical artifact. The likelihood of such an error is reduced in the case of the exercise hypothesis, since the association has been replicated many times in differing circumstances.

Problems may also arise when one sub-group of a population has unusual characteristics. For example, when exploring leisure activity, the active group is likely to be younger and to have a higher social class than those who are inactive. Such difficulties have been overcome at the expense of some loss of generality by introducing age 'adjustments' and concentrating upon a single social class (for example, the executive category of civil servant in the study of J.N. Morris *et al.*, 1973).

On occasion, bias can be introduced by the methodology or the observer. For instance, in a retrospective survey of activity patterns, an investigator who favoured the exercise hypothesis might be tempted to class people with cardiovascular disease as physically inactive. However, such a bias can hardly have arisen in studies where activity was classified prior to the onset of disease. Bias in the selection of control subjects is least likely in studies where activity patterns have been classified for almost all members of a population. When volunteers have been more widely solicited, it is likely that even the control subjects were more active and more health-conscious than a true random sample of the general population. The observed influence of physical activity upon ischaemic heart disease is thus a conservative measure of the effect that would occur in a truly sedentary population with a poor lifestyle.

Indirect association

An indirect association is possible if both physical inactivity and ischaemic heart disease are linked to a common variable. One possible candidate would be cigarette smoking. Certainly, this influences the likelihood of ischaemic heart disease (P. Morgan *et al.*, 1976), and it may also be linked to physical inactivity. Regular exercise is also related to a healthy lifestyle, and particular sports to a characteristic body build (K. Yamaji & Shephard, 1977). The effect of such indirect associations is largely controlled in recent multivariate analyses of the relationship between physical inactivity and ischaemic heart disease.

Bradford Hill criteria

1. Strength of the association. A causal association is a strong one. The incidence of ischaemic heart disease should thus be low in the presence of physical activity, and high in its absence. In fact, the ratio is probably not much better than 1:2 (S. Fox & Haskell, 1967; R. Paffenbarger, 1977). This is much smaller than for the ratio relating cigarette smoking to lung cancer, but is of the same order as for other cardiac risk factors such as a high systemic blood pressure, an abnormal exercise electrocardiogram and a cigarette habit.

2. Consistency of the association. A causal association is reported by many investigators, studying different populations, and using different techniques. In general, this condition is met for exercise and ischaemic heart disease. Perhaps because of counteracting influences of race and socio-economic class, a few authors have not observed any benefit from physical activity, but there seem no reports of cardiovascular harm from vigorous habitual exercise (H.H. Clarke, 1972). Nevertheless, there remains the possibility of a consistent bias; for instance, most of the investigators concerned have a vested interest in physical activity, and this could have given a spurious unanimity to published reports.

3. Temporally correct association. Exposure to the putative cause must antedate the onset of disease by an appropriate period. As already noted, the latent period for the development of ischaemic heart disease has yet to be clarified. However, in many of the studies we have discussed, the habit of physical activity or inactivity has persisted for a sufficient number of years that this condition is likely to have been satisfied.

4. Specificity of the association. Ideally, existence of the causal variable should lead to occurrence of the disease. However, lack of specificity can occur if a given factor causes more than one disease, or if a condition has a multiple aetiology. In the present context, possible sequelae of inactivity include both obesity and ischaemic heart disease; furthermore, clinical manifestations of a sedentary lifestyle are more likely in a person with a congenital abnormality of lipid meta-bolism than in the absence of this disorder. There are thus reasonable explanations for some lack of specificity in the association between inactivity and ischaemic heart disease.

5. Biological gradient. A graded dose-response relationship is charac-teristic of a causal relationship. Some suggestion of a biological gradient with increasing inactivity can be seen in the comparison of rail clerks, switchmen and sectionmen (H.L. Taylor *et al.*, 1962), in the Framingham study (T. Gordon *et al.*, 1971) and in the comparison between long-shoremen with high, medium and low levels of occupational activity (R. Paffenbarger *et al.*, 1975). On the other hand, some reports postulate a 'threshold dose' of exercise for a protective effect, rather than a smooth activity-related gradient (R.S. Paffenberger *et al.*, 1977).

6. Biological plausibility. There should be at least one plausible patho-physiological mechanism whereby the postulated cause could bring about the disease. In the context of preventing cardiac disease, this question has been well reviewed by S. Fox & Skinner (1964) and by W.L. Haskell (1979). These authors suggest many (almost too many!) reasons why an increase in physical activity could protect an individual against ischaemic heart disease.

7. *Coherence.* The requirement of coherence is closely related to that of plausibility. If the association is causal, the hypothesis advanced should provide a coherent explanation of the data. This condition is unfortunately not well satisfied in the case of exercise and ischaemic heart disease. There are many points in the natural history of the disease yet to be elucidated, including the obvious scarring of the myocardium in physically active patients, and the occasional instance where a myocardial infarction is precipitated by vigorous and unusual exercise.

8. *Experimental verification.* A causal association should be susceptible to experimental proof. We have already reviewed the difficulties that have prevented such a verification of the exercise hypothesis. The suggested treatment cannot be administered in a double-blind fashion, and an increase of activity inevitably changes other health habits. Future randomised controlled trials will probably have a multifactorial basis, rather than testing simply the effects of increased physical activity (H. Blackburn, 1972).

9. *Analogy.* The final criterion of a causal association is that of analogy. It can be illustrated in terms of the relationship between cigarette smoking and lung cancer. The causal viewpoint is given credence because individual constituents of tobacco smoke induce analogous carcinogenic changes at the cellular level. However, there is as yet little evidence that some component of the exercise response has cellular effects that offer protection against ischaemic heart disease.

Conclusion

We must conclude that several of Bradford Hill's criteria of a causal relationship remain unsatisfied with respect to exercise and the secondary prevention of ischaemic heart disease. As. P.O. Åstrand has pointed out (1967), it may well take 100 years to obtain a proof of the exercise hypothesis that will satisfy statisticians. But in the meantime, we have a potential remedy that is both agreeable and non-addictive, with few serious complications. 'Moderate activity is part of balanced, satisfying living and is the safe and hygienic prescription of the thoughtful physician for his patients, the high risk and the healthy alike' (H. Blackburn, 1974).

6   EXERCISE AND THE TERTIARY PREVENTION OF ISCHAEMIC HEART DISEASE

Since the early observations of V. Gottheiner (1960, 1968), J.J. Kellerman & Kariv (1968) and H.K. Hellerstein (1968), many authors have assumed that a programme of exercise rehabilitation improves the prognosis of the patient who has already sustained a myocardial infarction. In this chapter, we shall look critically at existing information drawn from both simple longitudinal studies and randomised controlled trials, seeking answers to the following questions.

(1)   Does a regimen of progressive endurance exercise reduce the likelihood of recurrent infarction and/or a fatal heart attack?
(2)   If so, does exercise therapy improve prognosis for all post-coronary patients, or is there a category of individuals who should be warned against taking additional physical activity?
(3)   If exercise indeed has an effect, does it act in its own right, or is it merely modifying other risk factors?

Early Longitudinal Studies

Studies in Israel

Findings from early longitudinal studies are summarised in Table 6.1. V. Gottheiner (1960, 1968) was probably the first physician to undertake a systematic programme of exercise therapy for coronary victims. His patients were advanced cautiously through a graded activity schedule. This culminated in selected sports, including an 11 km race around Mount Tabor. The competitive nature of his programme was regarded as useful in maintaining patient interest. The average death rate over five years of observation was 0.88 per cent per year; this was much less than the figure of 4.8 per cent per year for physically inactive but otherwise comparable patients who were attending myocardial infarction clinics in other parts of Israel. Gottheiner originally recruited 1,500 subjects, but only 1,103 continued to exercise for the full five years. It could thus be argued that the drop-out process biased the residual sample towards patients with minor infarctions.

J.J. Kellerman & Kariv (1968) rehabilitated 'post-coronary' patients attending the Tel-Hashomer Hospital through a hospital-based activity

Table 6.1: Some Estimates of the Value of Exercise in the Tertiary Prevention of Ischaemic Heart Disease, Derived from Cross-sectional Comparisons

Follow-up period (years)	N	Exercised group			Control group			Author
		Recurrence rate (%/yr)	Death rate (%/yr)	Cardiac death rate (%/yr)	Recurrence rate (%/yr)	Death rate (%/yr)	Cardiac death rate (%/yr)	
1.0	64	9.4	3.1	–	25.0	10.9	–	D. Brunner (1968)
5.0	1,103	–	0.88	0.72	–	4.8[1]	–	V. Gottheiner (1968)
2.0[2]	41	2.5[2]	–	–	6.9[2]	–	–	E.M. Heller (1968)
2.7	254	–	2.0	–	–	4.5–6.0[3]	–	H.K. Hellerstein (1968)
6.0[4]	150	–	–	3.3[4]	–	–	10.6[4]	J.J. Kellerman & Kariv (1968)
2.7[5]	71	2.1	0.5	–	10.5	0.8	–	E.M. Heller (1972)
5.0[6]	77	(1.0)[6]	(0.8)[6]	–	(7.3)[6]	(2.4)[6]	–	P. Rechnitzer et al. (1972)
7.0[7]	68	5.0	3.6	–	14.3	9.0	–	Ibid.

1. Controls followed up for one to four years at other clinics.
2. Estimate of average follow-up (some subjects were followed up for up to four years). 'Controls' were 36 'drop-outs' who failed to enter programme; twelve of the 36 showed cardiovascular complications.
3. Estimated experience of other patients in Cleveland area.
4. Apparently not true annual mortality rates.
5. Subjects followed up for 0.5–5.0 years; 2.7 years is estimated average period of follow-up. Sample of 71 patients included six cases with acute coronary insufficiency.
6. Not all subjects were followed up for the full five-year period. Death rates are thus underestimates of the true values. Controls drawn from a larger city.
7. Not all subjects were followed up for the full seven-year period. Data adjusted to an average study duration of 2.1 years, assuming a linear relationship between follow-up period and death rate. Controls taken from other hospitals in the same city.

programme; breathing and relaxation exercises, the lifting of light weights and calisthenics were undertaken for 45-60 minutes three times per week. The overall regimen brought physical working capacity from 57 to 83 per cent of the age-related normal value. J.J. Kellerman & Kariv (1968) further claimed that the cardiac death rate for their sample was much lower than that for patients who did not receive active rehabilitation. Nevertheless, it was accepted that a selected series had been observed: 'no patients with acute cardiac or coronary insufficiency or severe arrhythmias were admitted to the exercise program' (J.J. Kellermann *et al.*, 1970).

D. Brunner (1968, 1973) exercised his patients on a cycle ergometer twice per week for four months. Individual training sessions were conducted in an interval fashion, bouts of activity lasting three to six minutes at loadings of 25-100 W being alternated with rest intervals of four to eight minutes. The exercised group included cases of both myocardial infarction and angina pectoris; 80 patients were admitted to the programme, but only 64 completed the four-month study. The 'control' series were the next 40 patients attending Dr Brunner's clinic; they were treated with isosorbide dinitrate, 10 mg three times per day, and over the next year they encountered much more recurrent disease than those who had exercised.

Studies in USA

H.K. Hellerstein (1968) was an early advocate of exercise for the patient with ischaemic heart disease. His report described 254 patients who remained in a gymnasium-based exercise programme for an average of 2.7 years. Over this time, eleven patients died, giving a death rate of 2.0 per cent per year. Hellerstein argued that this mortality rate compared very favourably with the usual figure of 4.5-6.0 per cent per year for 'post-coronary' patients receiving conventional treatment in the Cleveland area. However, Hellerstein's programme included not only exercise but also a deliberate campaign against other risk factors through an anti-atherogenic diet, abstinence from cigarettes and reduction of body mass. Furthermore, patients who could not tolerate the exercise programme were necessarily excluded from the group. It is thus difficult to compare his sample with the general experience of Cleveland clinics.

Early Canadian studies

E.M. Heller (1968, 1972) referred 'post-coronary' patients to the YMHA for a paramedically supervised programme of progressive endurance exercise. It is not possible to calculate precise recurrence rates from his reports, since the follow-up period varied from one individual to another, but nevertheless the exercised subjects were apparently at a substantial advantage relative to those who for various reasons did not enter the YMHA programme.

P. Rechnitzer *et al.* (1972) enrolled their patients in biweekly sessions of progressive endurance activity; this regimen was supplemented by mild daily home exercises and the walking of one to two miles per day. The first comparison was made between these patients, who were living in the medium-sized city of London, Ontario (population about 200,000) and other, conservatively treated patients who were living in metropolitan Toronto (population over two million). Critics immediately objected that conditions of life were very different in the two cities. For this reason, Rechnitzer and his associates went on to compare their data with results for patients treated at other hospitals in the London area. Both comparisons indicated that recurrence and death rates were considerably lower for the exercised than for the conservatively treated groups.

Early longitudinal studies thus suggested that exercise rehabilitation had a favourable influence upon prognosis. However, none of the reports cited were able to rule out the possibility that the apparent benefit of increased physical activity has arisen because subjects with less extensive disease were selected for exercise-rehabilitation programmes.

A Non-randomised Trial in Toronto

The Toronto trial was based upon a consecutive series of 688 patients who were referred to the exercise rehabilitation programme of the Toronto Rehabilitation Centre. Subjects attended the Centre for a period varying from one to eight years (an average of three years) over the period 1967-76 (T. Kavanagh *et al.*, in preparation). The data is unusual with respect to the intensity of the prescribed exercise, the compliance rate and success in obtaining 100 per cent follow-up information with respect to fatal and non-fatal reinfarctions plus deaths from other causes.

Patient selection

All of the sample had been referred to the Centre by their personal physicians following a myocardial infarction. The diagnosis was verified by the presence of at least two out of three criteria (classical chest pain, a significant rise in serum enzymes and serial electro-cardiographic changes). Over the period of observation, 80 patients received coronary arterial 'by-pass' operations; two of the eighty died, and to avoid all possibility of bias these two individuals were included in our sample. The other 78 'by-passed' patients were excluded from the study, leaving a total of 610 otherwise unselected referrals.

Exercise programme

Admission to the programme occurred a minimum of two months and an average of eight months following myocardial infarction. The programme of progressive supervised exercise was based on walking and jogging, the goal being to cover three miles in 30 or 36 minutes, depending upon age. For the first two years, the patient attended the Centre once per week, and trained four times a week on his own, using a personalised prescription that specified distance, pace and frequency of exercise. Thereafter, attendance was once in eight weeks, with repeat exercise tests once per year. Of the group, 22 continued to attend the Centre more frequently, and progressed to the point of running in marathon events (T. Kavanagh *et al.*, 1974b; T. Kavanagh *et al.*, 1977a); one patient covered the 42.1 km in as little as 190 minutes. Altogether, 428 of the patients (70.2 per cent) visited the Centre as scheduled. Although irregular in their attendance, many of the remaining patients persisted with their prescribed exercise; 505/610 (82.8 per cent) engaged in at least three sessions of training per week throughout the study, and even at the end of our investigation only a very small number of subjects (27/610; 2.8 per cent) were taking no training at all. Acceptance of the programme was indicated by substantial gains of maximum oxygen intake. The average improvement was 22.6 per cent over the three years, and there was a 77 per cent increase in readings for marathon participants.

Fatalities

A total of 35 patients died over the follow-up period. Of these fatalities, 23 were plainly a consequence of ischaemic heart disease (19 recurrences, one complicated by viral myocarditis, and four 'electrical' deaths). One patient died during coronary angiography, so that his death might also be regarded as due to cardiac disease, but the remaining eleven cases died of other causes (including four cerebro-vascular accidents). Recurrences rates were as follows:

| Time subsequent to | Recurrence rates | | | Number of |
infarction	Non-fatal (%/yr)	Fatal (%/yr)	Total (%/yr)	subjects
Year one	0.96	2.15	3.11	610
Year two	1.19	1.39	2.58	503
Years three to five	1.05	0.45	1.50	227
Years six to eight	0.00	0.81	0.81	41

In contrast with many series of conservatively treated patients, the recurrence rate diminished progressively with time subsequent to infarction. Since there was a 100 per cent follow-up, this cannot be attributed to attrition of the sample; either there was a change in the pattern of referrals as the study continued, or the beneficial effect of exercise developed progressively over the period of observation. Of the 23 patients who sustained a fatal recurrence, eight had been attending the exercise class for six months or less, and one man had participated in only one exercise session. In all, ten were exercising regularly at the time of their fatal recurrence, two were exercising sporadically, and eleven had ceased to participate in the programme. In only four of the non-exercisers was there a medical reason for non-participation. Of the 23 episodes, eight were sudden deaths, seven of which were unassociated with physical exertion. One man died while he was exercising away from the Centre; he was apparently recovering from a bout of influenza and, despite warnings to the contrary, had continued activity, even exceeding his normal exercise prescription.

Non-fatal recurrences

A total of 21 cases developed a non-fatal recurrence over the follow-up period. Three of those affected had been exercising for less than six months. Five were exercising regularly, four were participating in a sporadic fashion and twelve were not exercising at all. In only three cases were there medical reasons for non-participation (all of these men had exertional angina).

Comparison with HIP data

The results of the Toronto trial can be compared with published information for 745 male patients enrolled in the Health Insurance Plan of New York (E. Weinblatt *et al.*, 1968, 1973). The New York group had survived an average of six months following a first myocardial infarction or diagnosis of angina without infarction. There are obvious differences between Toronto and New York. Nevertheless, the HIP

data was selected for reference rather than results from the larger
Coronary Drug Trial (J. Stamler, 1975) because the prognosis of the
New York sample was specified in terms of a number of commonly
accepted primary risk factors, acting singly and in various combinations.

E. Weinblatt *et al.* (1968, 1973) cite smoothed cumulative
probabilities of death for the period 0.5–3.0 years after infarction in
relation to three prognostic factors (persistent abnormalities of the
resting electrocardiogram, hypertension and elevation of serum
cholesterol). In order to compare results with data from the 36.5-
month Toronto study, all probabilities of death were multiplied by
36.5/30.0; this adjustment is acceptable, since the overall mortality
rate in the New York study was very similar for 30 months (4.01 per
cent per annum) and for 54 months (3.88 per cent per annum). The
association between the several variables and the likelihood of death
is shown in Table 6.2, along with the expected number of fatalities.
If our sample had behaved in the same manner as the New York
population, there would have been 89 rather than 35 deaths;
furthermore, in Toronto only 66–8 per cent of deaths were attributable to a recurrence of cardiac disease, whereas the proportion of
recurrences was 81 per cent in New York.

Alternative hypotheses

It is particularly striking that the prognosis of the Toronto group
improved coincidently with the development of cardio-respiratory
conditioning. However, before postulating a causal association, several
alternative hypotheses must be weighed.

Information was necessarily collected on patients referred to the
Toronto Rehabilitation Centre, and it is possible that, because
vigorous exercise therapy was offered, a low-risk category of patient
was seen. In partial support of this view, a subsequent randomised trial
showed an annual rate of reinfarction of only 1.5 per cent per
annum in a low-intensity-exercise (control) group attending the
Toronto centre.

The average time of entry into our exercise programme was eight
months after infarction, but some patients were recruited as soon as
two to three months after the acute episode. Since mortality is
greatest in the first six months after infarction, this factor should have
increased rather than decreased the mortality in the Toronto series.

Treatment undoubtedly evolved between the New York study
(1961–5) and the Toronto experiment (1968–76). Some ten per cent

Table 6.2: A 'Risk-factor' Prediction of Death Rate for 610 'Post-coronary' Patients Treated by Vigorous Exercise Rehabilitation in Toronto

Cholesterol[1],[2] (≥ 270 mg·dl[-1])	Risk factor present Hyper-tension[1],[3] (≥ 150/100 mg Hg)	Persistent abnormalities of resting ECG[4]	Number of cases with specified characteristics	Anticipated deaths in sample of 610 subjects followed up 36.5 months
Yes	Yes	Yes	15	2.5
Yes	Yes	No	0	0
Yes	No	Yes	30	2.1
Yes	No	No	0	0
No	Yes	Yes	121	32.1
No	Yes	No	5	0.6
No	No	Yes	427	51.1
No	No	No	12	0.6
			Total	89.0

1. In order to make a conservative estimate of risk for the Toronto population, the table excludes from the high-risk category eleven patients merely reported as having a 'high' serum cholesterol and seven patients noted only as 'hypertensive'.

2. The methodology used in Toronto was internationally standardised. The proportion with a high serum cholesterol was less than in New York, probably as a result of an increase in dietary modification at the time of the Toronto study.

3. The Toronto subjects were well-habituated to the observer, and the diastolic criterion (100 mm Hg) was higher than in New York (165/90 mm Hg); the prevalence of hypertension thus tended to be underestimated relative to the comparison series.

4. Abnormal resting ECGs were more frequent in Toronto (97.2 per cent) than in New York (62.1 per cent); this reflects our more stringent requirement of myocardial infarction before admission to the trial.

Source: Based on data of E. Weinblatt *et al.* (1968, 1972) and T. Kavanagh *et al.* (in preparation).

of the Toronto group were receiving β-blocking drugs, although almost none were receiving anticoagulants. In any event, changes in treatment can hardly account for the improved prognosis of the Toronto group, since most studies suggest that β-blocking agents, anticoagulants, dietary modification and other forms of therapy have only marginal effects on late prognosis (S.H. Rinzler, 1968; O. Turpeinen *et al.*, 1968; S. Dayton *et al.*, 1969; J. Stamler, 1975; D.A. Chamberlain, 1978b).

Sample attrition cannot account for the favourable prognosis in the Toronto population, since all 610 patients were included in the data

Table 6.3: Potential Adjustments in a 'Risk-factor' Prediction of Death Rate for 610 'Post-coronary' Patients Treated by Vigorous Exercise Rehabilitation in Toronto

Variable	Adjustment made	Predicted deaths	
		Number over 36.5 months	Annual rate (%)
Serum cholesterol, hypertension and electro-cardiogram	See Table 6.2	89.0	4.80
Age	48.1 ± 7.3 years (six years younger than Weinblatt series)	64.2	3.46
Diabetes	1.6% of Toronto series taking insulin, 11.6% 'diabetics' in Weinblatt series	63.5	3.42
Blue-collar/ Jewish	Greater in Weinblatt series	No adjustment	
Cigarette smoking	35.8% of sample (compared with 38.4% in series of S. Tominaga & Blackburn, 1973)	No adjustment	
Angina	34.3% of sample had angina on admission to rehabilitation, compared with 17.8% of Weinblatt series	No adjustment	
By-pass surgery	3.9% of Toronto group (omitted from series, with exception of 2 fatalities; see text)	No adjustment	

Source: Based on data of E. Weinblatt *et al.* (1968, 1972) and T. Kavanagh *et al.* (in preparation).

analysis, irrespective of whether they had persisted with the required exercise programme.

A final possibility is that risk factors other than those noted in Table 6.2 were more prevalent in the New York than in the Toronto series (Table 6.3). In Toronto, almost all subjects were white-collar employees, whereas in New York about a half were blue-collar workers, with a high proportion (50 per cent) of Jewish subjects; however, recent Ontario data (P. Rechnitzer *et al.*, unpublished) suggests that, if other factors are equal, reinfarction rates for white-collar workers who enrol in an exercise programme should be almost identical with those for a mixture of white- and blue-collar workers who do not exercise. The age of the Toronto sample was some six years younger than the HIP group, and 1.6 per cent of the Toronto series were taking insulin, compared with 11.6 per cent of 'diabetics' in New York. Allowing for these two important differences, but neglecting a larger proportion of subjects with angina in the Toronto series, the anticipated death rate of our sample would drop to 3.42 per cent per year; this must be compared with the observed overall rate of 1.88 per cent per year for the Toronto series (1.29 per cent per year due to cardiac events), and the even lower figure of 0.67 per cent cardiac and non-cardiac deaths per year for the third to the eighth year of rehabilitation.

Conclusion

There remain considerable uncertainties when attempting to compare patients living in Toronto and New York. Nevertheless, the apparent advantage of our exercised group is sufficient to encourage a further application of this approach, drawing exercised and control subjects from the same city and applying rigorous adjustments for all of the factors known to modify prognosis after myocardial infarction.

Randomised Controlled Studies

General considerations

A large-scale randomised controlled trial is theoretically the best method of deciding whether exercise rehabilitation improves the prognosis of the 'post-coronary' patient. However, in practice, the trials conducted to date have proved inconclusive, as a result of poor compliance with the required regimen, an inadequate duration of rehabilitation and correspondingly limited gains of physiological function.

Sample attrition is an inevitable source of difficulty. The health experience of the 'drop-outs' is usually averaged with, and dilutes, any response in programme adherents. Some studies have had many drop-outs from the exercised group, and controls have become contaminated by unauthorised participation in 'keep-fit' programmes. It could be argued that a high 'drop-out' rate is itself an argument against the practicality of exercise treatment. However, the Toronto experience (above) illustrates that good compliance can be sustained in a large group of patients for several years if the programme is well-organised.

Because sample attrition is a cumulative phenomenon, many authors have been content to report studies of relatively short duration. Interpretation of data is then complicated by the averaging of early mortality (where increased physical activity has not had time to produce an effect) and later mortality (where a beneficial response to exercise is conceivable). Most authors (E. Kentala, 1972; H. Sanne *et al.*, 1972; T. Kavanagh *et al.*, 1973b; L. Wilhelmsen *et al.*, 1975; T. Kavanagh *et al.*, 1977a) are agreed that relatively little training of the post-coronary patient is accomplished during the first few months of attendance at a rehabilitation centre; indeed, dramatic gains of maximum oxygen intake may not appear until the patient has been exercising for some years (Figure 6.1). This is in marked contrast to the response of healthy subjects, and it may reflect fear on the part of the patient, his family or his medical advisors. Plainly, it is unrealistic to expect a benefit from exercise until some training effect has occurred, and there may be a further lag period before the full potential health gains of the increased activity pattern are realised.

Large numbers of both patients and staff are required for a random-ised controlled trial. There are corresponding difficulties in ensuring consistent and effective exercise and control regimens at all cooperat-ing centres. Partly for this reason, and partly because of fears of over-exertion, many so-called 'exercise' classes for the 'post-coronary' patient have been essentially homoeopathic, producing no real training response (Table 6.4).

Finally, even if a sufficient sample of subjects can be both recruited and retained over a random trial, constraints of practicality still leave a substantial 'beta error' (the chance of a falsely negative conclusion); this is commonly as large as ten or even 20 per cent (Table 5.1).

Gothenburg study

The Gothenburg study (H. Sanne *et al.*, 1972; L. Wilhelmsen *et al.*, 1975) was based on 315 patients under 58 years of age who sustained a myocardial infarction between 1968 and 1971. Although some 90 per cent of available patients were recruited for the investigation, the sample was nevertheless rather small to prove or disprove the exercise hypothesis. Both test and control subjects were given a general recommendation to increase their physical activity, but three months after infarction a randomly selected half of the sample were invited to attend the hospital three times per week for a 30-minute programme of calisthenics, cycling and interval running.

Unfortunately, only 73 per cent of the intended experimental group began training, and the drop-out rate was also high. After one year, only 39 per cent of the experimental group were attending the hospital, with a further 21 per cent continuing some training at home or at work.

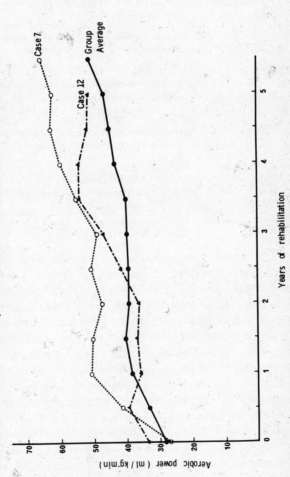

Figure 6.1: Time course of the increases in directly measured maximum oxygen intake with vigorous training. Data of T. Kavanagh & Shephard for 13 post-coronary runners who finally participated in marathon events, along with individual curves for two subjects who made substantial gains in aerobic power.

© 1979, Houghton Mifflin Professional Publishers, Boston.

Source: Reprinted from Roy J. Shephard, 'Cardiac Rehabilitation in Prospect' in *Heart Disease and Rehabilitation*, edited by M.L. Pollock and D.H. Schmidt, by permission of the publisher.

Table 6.4: Changes of Exercise Tolerance in Selected 'Post-coronary' Rehabilitation Programmes

Author	Change of exercise tolerance
E. Kentala (1972)	20% improvement of maximal working capacity *but* seen equally in experimental and control subjects; 56% gain of maximal working capacity in sub-sample attending more than 70% of training sessions
L. Wilhelmsen *et al*. (1975)	24 W gain of working capacity in experimental subjects with no change in controls; three quarters of changes in heart-rate responses to sub-maximal exercise not significantly different in experimental and control subjects
D.A. Cunningham *et al*. (1977)	average decrease of heart rate at $\dot{V}_{O_2}$ = 1.25 $l \cdot min^{-1}$ 13.1 $beats \cdot min^{-1}$ in experimental and 0.6 $beats \cdot min^{-1}$ in control subjects; *but* subjects divisible into four roughly equal groups — 15% and 5% decrease of heart rate in experimental subjects and 3.6% decrease and 2.7% increase in control subjects
T. Kavanagh & Shephard	22.6% gain of predicted $\dot{V}_{O_2}$ (max) over 3 years (average for 610 patients); 77% gain over five years in marathon participants (Figure 6.1)

There was a 24-W increase in the maximum tolerated work-load of the experimental group, with no significant change in the maximum performance of the control subjects. However, the heart-rate response to sub-maximum exercise decreased both in exercise and control groups, and in three of four comparisons the difference between experimental and control subjects was not statistically significant. This reflects in part a contamination of the control group by an interest in exercise, and in part limited compliance of the experimental subjects with the intended exercise programme. Whereas the one-year gain of maximum working capacity for the entire exercise group was 14 per cent, in those 'adequately trained' it was 22 per cent.

H. Sanne *et al*. (1972) and L. Wilhelmsen *et al*. (1975) commented specifically on the issues of study duration and compliance. Over a four-year follow-up period, the mortality and morbidity were very similar for their two groups of patients — 28 deaths and 25 non-fatal myocardial infarctions in the exercised group, with 35 deaths and 28 non-fatal infarctions in the control group. Separating out patients who had participated in the study for six months or longer, H. Sanne *et al.* (1972) observed eight deaths in the training group and 19 in the control series, the difference being significant at the five per cent level of probability. When the 'six-month' patients were followed up for a total of four years, corresponding figures were 19 and 29 deaths ($P = 0.18$); this probably reflects differences in compliance since, among those who adhered to the programme for at least one year, the mortality (five of 67, seven per cent) was only half of that seen in the controls (20 of 141, 14 per cent). Interpretation of the data is complex, since more of the 'drop-outs' than the continuing exercisers were smokers (L. Wilhelmsen *et al.*, 1975).

The overall death rate for the exercise group was 3.48 per cent per annum, more than five times the figure found in the Toronto trial for post-coronary patients who were exercising hard (see above). This may reflect in part a more complete sampling of the post-coronary population in the Gothenburg study, and in part absence of an exercise response in Gothenburg due to the extensive defections from the experimental programme.

Helsinki study

E. Kentala (1972) carried out a similar study in Helsinki. Severely diseased patients were excluded from his sample but, with this proviso, 158 consecutively acutely infarcted patients younger than 65 years were allocated randomly to experimental and control groups. Again, the sample size was less than that required for conclusive examination of the exercise hypothesis.

The planned intervention was a 30-minute session of exercise conducted three times per week at the local hospital. However, after one year only ten of 79 patients were attending the exercise sessions, while a further 16 claimed to be exercising on their own. At least eleven of the control series were also exercising quite vigorously. It is thus hardly surprising that one year after the myocardial infarction there was no difference in physical working capacity between experimental and control groups.

Subjects were followed up for two years, and over this time there was no difference in either total mortality or in new ischaemic heart disease events between the supposed exercise and control groups; such findings were hardly surprising in view of the poor compliance with the intended regimen.

Oulu study

I. Palatsi (1976) initiated a home-training experiment in the Oulu region of Finland. His subjects were male and female patients under 65 years of age; those judged as having severe disease or poor motivation were excluded from the sample. A total of 180 cases (mainly city dwellers) were allocated to the training regimen, and 200 cases (mainly those living in rural areas) served as controls.

The plan involved 30 minutes of home exercises per day, reinforcing visits being made to the hospital once every month. At the end of one year, about a half of the exercisers reported that they were training between six and seven times per week, and two thirds of the group attended the last hospital session. However, the intended experimental subjects showed no improvement in physical working capacity relative to the control series.

Over a 2.5-year period of observation, twelve per cent of the exercise group and 15 per cent of the controls suffered a reinfarction, with respective mortality rates of 7 and 14 per cent.

World Health Organization study

A study initiated by the European Office of the World Health Organization (1977) involves modification of a number of risk factors including physical inactivity (Chapter 5, p. 98). Control patients are treated by their personal physicians. Analysis of one segment of this data (V. Kallio, 1978) suggests that the experimental subjects gain some protection against sudden death and coronary mortality, particularly over the first year. However, the total number of reinfarctions is higher in the exercised group.

Canadian experiments

One early controlled trial was carried out in Toronto (T. Kavanagh *et al.*, 1973b). The primary objectives were physiological, and the total sample size (31 cases) was therefore small. Over the first year of observation, patients allocated to an exercise regimen fared little better than a control group who received equal physician contact through a hypnosis class. During the second year, a proportion of the exercised group who had progressed to long-distance running showed substantial physiological and electrocardiographic gains with respect to the hypnosis group, but others, apparently those who were older and had more severe disease, still had a comparable status to the hypnotherapy controls. Over the two-year study, the recurrence rate was 2.3 per cent per annum for the exercise group, and 5.0 per cent for the controls, but the reinfarctions in the exercise group were fatal, whereas those in the hypnotherapy group were non-fatal.

A more definitive trial of morbidity and mortality was planned by P.A. Rechnitzer *et al.* (1975). A sample size of 750 patients was chosen to give a 90 per cent chance of showing a 50 per cent reduction of recurrences in the exercised group, with a probability of 0.05; this calculation was based on a recurrence rate of 23 per cent over a four-year period, with a sample attrition of 35 per cent or less. Subjects under 55 years of age were recruited three to twelve months following a well-documented attack of myocardial infarction. They were allocated in a stratified random fashion to either a regimen of vigorous and progressive endurance-type exercise, or a homeopathic recreational-exercise programme. Stratification was in terms of angina, hypertension, blue- or white-collar occupation and personality type (Friedman & Rosenmann Type A or B).

According to popular belief, the drop-out rate from an exercise programme is greatest in the first few months, and some studies have thus given their subjects several preliminary months of physical activity prior to randomisation (J. Naughton, 1978). The preliminary results of the Southern Ontario multicentre trial to date do not altogether support this view; if attrition rates are calculated as a percentage of the residual sample, losses seem at least as great in the third and fourth as in the first two years of observation; furthermore, we are now anticipating that the overall drop-out rate for the four-year study may be 60·5 per cent rather than the intended 35 per cent (R.J. Shephard, 1979c). Medical problems account for only 22 per cent of defections (N.B. Oldridge, 1979), and almost a half of these are non-cardiac problems. A further 25 per cent of subject losses are unavoidable, as a result of such factors as change of employment, leaving 42 per cent attributable to psycho-social factors and 11 per cent to other causes. The worst experience has been with blue-collar employees engaged in light work who are also smokers and inactive in their leisure time; 95 per cent of such subjects have dropped out of the study within two years. We have noted a two-fold intercentre difference in sample attrition; this seems to be related to methods of recruitment (physician referral, 43 per cent attrition, versus the combing of cardiac wards, 55 per cent attrition), socio-economic factors and differences in the personality of the clinical staff and their degree of involvement in the rehabilitation process.

The Southern Ontario trial monitored the response of subjects to training in terms of the heart rate at a directly measured or closely interpolated oxygen consumption of $1.25 \ l \cdot min^{-1}$ STPD. On this criterion, the experimental model worked rather better than in a number of the other studies reviewed above; the heart rate decreased in those who received high-intensity exercise, but showed no significant change in the control group; nevertheless, it was possible to distinguish a substantial sub-sample of the high-intensity-exercise group who (because of poor compliance or a relatively high initial fitness level) showed little change of exercise heart rate. There was also a sub-sample of the low-intensity-exercise group who became contaminated by an enthusiasm for vigorous activity, with corresponding reductions in the exercise heart rate (D.A. Cunningham *et al.*, 1979).

As an ethical safeguard, the supervising statistician monitored cardiac events by the technique of sequential analysis (A. Wald, 1947). It was planned to halt the experiment if either the initial hypothesis was proven, or the proportion of reinfarctions in the high-intensity-exercise group exceeded 67 per cent of the sample. The sample of 750 patients was successfully recruited. A preliminary analysis of data showed that of the first 50 recurrences, 20 occurred within twelve months of recruitment (Table 6.5). It could be argued that none of these patients had been trained for sufficient time to realise the possible benefits of exercise. Theoretically, fourteen of the remaining thirty patients with recurrent disease were still enrolled in the trial. However, many were, for practical purposes, drop-outs. While the effects of training are largely dissipated by a few weeks of inactivity, it takes a minimum of two to three months to probe a patient's excuses and realise that he has dropped out of the study. Even if this problem is ignored, we have to date only 14 critical events among programme participants, ten in the high-intensity-exercise group and four in the low-intensity-exercise group. Repeated laboratory data were available for ten of these 14 subjects. An improvement in physical condition was seen in five of the six high-intensity exercisers, but there was also a significant decrease of exercise heart rate in two of the four low-intensity exercisers. As with other randomised trials, such numbers are far too small to prove or disprove the exercise hypothesis.

The statistics cited refer to the first twenty months' operation of the Southern Ontario trial, and numbers will be approximately doubled when the four-year follow-up of all patients is completed. Nevertheless, incomplete compliance with the required exercise regimen, a high attrition rate, some contamination of the control group, a slow onset of the training response and a lower frequency of reinfarction than anticipated may leave the experiment short of the statistical proof originally envisaged.

Table 6.5: Non-fatal and Fatal Recurrences among Patients Enrolled in Southern Ontario Multicentre Exercise-heart Trial; A Preliminary Analysis of Data in Subjects Followed for an Average Period of 20 Months

Event	Patient status	High-intensity-exercise group		Low-intensity-exercise group	
		Number of events	Reported compliance* (%)	Number of events	Reported compliance* (%)
Non-fatal recurrences	Participant > 12 months	9	76	4	83
	Participant < 12 months	9	85	5	76
	'Drop-out'	6	16	5	6
Fatal recurrences	Participant > 12 months	1	100	0	—
	Participant < 12 months	2	78	4	78
	'Drop-out'	3	8	2	0
Total recurrences	Participant > 12 months	10	78	4	83
	Participant < 12 months	11	84	9	77
	'Drop-out'	9	13	7	4

* Attendance reported for three months preceding recurrence.

Source: R.J. Shephard (1979c).
Note: A report covering the full four year study is currently being prepared by Dr P. Rechnitzer and the Southern Ontario research team.

Conclusion

Given that all of the randomised controlled trials completed to date have been inconclusive, what are the options for the future? To accept empirical evidence from non-randomised trials is scientifically unsatisfactory. Attempts to merge data from the several existing controlled studies are also unlikely to succeed, because of differences in populations and protocol. It is thus necessary to contemplate a larger trial. It will be necessary first to explore carefully the factors influencing exercise compliance, and then to recruit at least 4,000 patients willing to participate in a randomised experiment. In view of the large sample size and the resultant cost of the investigation, this will succeed only if organised on an international basis.

Possible Contraindications to Exercise Rehabilitation

Once infarction has occurred, the usual 'coronary' risk factors such as a high serum cholesterol, systemic hypertension and diabetes seem of less importance to prognosis. Adverse features now include a prior history of angina, a poor left-ventricular function, a wide resting arterio-venous oxygen difference, various types of dysrhythmia and left-atrial enlargement as indicated by a negative terminal force in the P wave of the electrocardiogram (E.H. Estes, 1974; E. Kentala & Sarna, 1976).

Do these 'tertiary' risk factors apply to the patient who is under-going exercise rehabilitation? In particular, are there contraindications to deliberate exercise as shown by an increase of risk ratio relative to more conservative treatment? Information relating to these questions is available from both non-randomised and randomised trials of exercise therapy.

Non-randomised trials

T. Kavanagh *et al.* (1977c) examined factors related to fatal and non-fatal recurrence of infarction in a group of 610 'post-coronary' patients who were participating in a vigorous exercise rehabilitation programme for an average of 36.5 months. During this time, the group sustained 21 non-fatal recurrences and 23 fatal recurrences (p. 133). Calculating risk ratios (Table 6.6), the most useful indicator of a poor prognosis

Table 6.6: Method of Calculating Risk Ratios for Population of 610 'Post-coronary' Patients with 44 Non-fatal and Fatal Recurrences

Clinical status	Present	Presumed risk factor Absent	Row total
Recurrence	$(R + F)$	$44 - (R + F)$	44
No recurrence	C	$566 - C$	566
Column total	$(R + F) + C$	$610 - (R + F + C)$	610

Predictive value of positive test (P) = $(R + F)/(R + F + C)$

Predictive value of negative test (N) = $44 - (R + F)/610 - (R + F + C)$

Risk ratio = P/N

Sensitivity of risk factor = $(R + F)/44$

Specificity of risk factor = $[610 - (R + F + C)] - [44 - (R + F)]/566$

Table 6.7: Indicators of Non-fatal and Fatal Recurrence of Myocardial Infarction among 610 Patients Participating in Programme of Vigorous Exercise Rehabilitation

Variable	Frequency in subjects with recurrence Non-fatal (n = 21; %)	Fatal (n = 23; %)	Frequency in subjects free of recurrence (n = 566; %)	Predictive value of positive (P, %)	Predictive value of negative (N, %)	Risk ratio (P/N)
Exercise non-compliance	57.1	47.8	0.7	85.2	3.60	23.7[4]
Medications:						
Anti-dysrhythmics	42.9	39.0	30.2	9.5	6.17	1.54
Diuretics	19.0	34.8	15.9	11.8	6.30	1.87[2]
Digitalis	9.5	39.0	11.7	14.3	5.82	2.46[2]
Still smoking[1]	47.6	43.5	34.9	10.3	5.78	1.78[2]
Angina	33.3	52.2	30.6	9.9	5.98	1.66
Initial test	14.3	42.9	14.8	12.5	6.22	2.01[2]
Final test	4.8	13.0	3.71	16.0	6.83	2.34[2]
Enlarged heart	0.0	8.7	2.12	14.3	7.04	2.05
Aneurysm	23.8	21.7	23.1	7.09	7.25	0.98
Hypertension (≥ 150/100 mm Hg)	14.3	13.0	6.89	13.3	6.72	1.98[2]
Blood cholesterol (> 270 mg•dl⁻¹)						
Electrocardiogram:						
Resting abnormalities	100.0	95.6	98.9	7.25	5.88	1.23
Horizontal or downsloping exercise ST ≥ 0.2 mV	38.1	43.5	33.4	12.4	5.59	2.22[3]
Unifocal exercise VPBs	4.8	0.0	8.8	1.96	7.69	0.25
Multifocal exercise VPBs	4.8	8.7	4.4	10.7	7.04	1.52

1. No data on 66 patients.
2. P < 0.05.
3. P < 0.01.
4. P < 0.001.

Source: T. Kavanagh et al. (1977c).

Table 6.8: Odds Ratios Comparing Non-compliant and Exercise-compliant Patients Enrolled in a Vigorous 'Post-coronary' Exercise Rehabilitation Programme

Risk indicator	Non-fatal recurrences	Odds ratio[1] Fatal recurrences	All recurrences
Smoking history			
Continued	∞	5.79	7.87
Reduced	13.90	–	13.89
Stopped	4.13	6.06	4.78
Never smoked	0.99	5.05	3.34
Combined odds ratio	(5.19)[2]	5.44	5.86
Z score[3]	3.65	3.52	5.37
Angina			
Both tests	2.88	9.23	5.87
Initial test	19.00	2.82	7.67
Final test	0.00	6.33	3.00
Neither test	4.13	5.23	4.91
Combined odds ratio	5.06	5.43	5.85
Z score	3.57	3.86	5.57
ST depression			
ST < 0.2 mV	3.51	13.57	7.48
ST > 0.2 mV	7.97	1.82	4.12
Combined odds ratio	4.82	(5.44)[2]	5.86
Z score	3.44	4.19	5.73
Complications			
Nil	4.66	4.51	5.00
Enlarged heart	∞	8.00	16.00
Aneurysm	–	∞	∞
Combined odds ratio	(5.12)[2]	(5.73)[2]	(5.99)[2]
Z score	3.61	3.99	5.70

1. Odds ratio = [(number of recurrences in non-compliant group)/(number without recurrence in non-compliant group)] × [(number without recurrence in compliant group)/(number of recurrences in compliant group)].

2. It is not strictly possible to calculate a mean for this category because of sample heterogeneity.

3. A Z score of 1.96 would have a chance probability of 0.05.

Source: R.J. Shephard *et al*. (1979a).

Table 6.9: Relationship between Exercise Compliance and Other Risk Factors

Variable	Exercise compliance				Significance
Smoking habits	Continued 70.5%	Reduced 84.2%	Stopped 85.5%	Never 83.2%	n.s.
Angina	Both tests 73.5%	Initial test 80.0%	Final test 83.3%	Neither 86.0%	(0.05)
ST depression	> 0.2 mV 80.1%	< 0.2 mV 84.2%			n.s.
Complication	Enlarged heart 73.9%	Aneurysm 69.2%	Nil 84.0%		n.s.

Source: Based on data of R.J. Shephard *et al.* (1979a).

was failure to comply with the prescribed exercise regimen (Table 6.7). Among the 27 subjects who had ceased exercising at the end of the study, the risk of recurrence was 23.7 times the standard figure ($P <$ 0.001). Furthermore, there was some evidence for the view that lack of exercise was responsible for the progression of disease rather than the converse. Of the 27 non-compliers, 15 were uninterested in exercise or had encountered family opposition, three had been told not to exercise by their family physicians and only nine had a medical reason for stopping exercise (angina, orthopaedic problems, mental disorders and alcoholism). Taking data for a larger group of 105 subjects who finally were exercising less than three times per week, the 'odds ratio' for either a fatal or a non-fatal recurrence was five or six to one when such poorly compliant subjects were compared with the 'compliant'. This disadvantage was independent of smoking habits, but was obscured in subjects with ST segmental depression of more than 0.2 mV during exercise at a target rate equal to 75 per cent of aerobic power (Table 6.8; R.J. Shephard *et al.*, 1979a). There was a slight suggestion that a poor exercise compliance was linked to continued smoking, the presence of angina at both tests, ST segmental depression of more than 0.2 mV and complications such as enlarged heart or an aneurysm; however, with the available sample of 46 recurrences, the only significant trend was for angina (Table 6.9).

The risk ratios of Table 6.7 suggest an adverse prognosis with several other findings, including persistent cigarette smoking, the use of digitalis or diuretics (both presumably indicators of cardiac failure), the presence of angina at the final exercise test, radiographic evidence of cardiac enlargement, a horizontal or downward-sloping depression of the ST segment of the exercise electrocardiogram and a serum cholesterol greater than 270 mg·dl^{-1}. The majority of the items noted had a fair sensitivity but (with the exception of exercise non-compliance, persistent cigarette smoking and exercise ST segmental depression) a rather low specificity; for calculation of sensitivity and specificity, see Table 6.6.

We may thus conclude that many of the secondary and tertiary risk factors encountered in sedentary individuals still apply in the 'post-coronary' patient who is engaged in vigorous physical activity.

It is now necessary to make a comparison between the risk ratios for active and sedentary individuals (Table 6.10). In many instances, the statistics are surprisingly similar. However, the risk ratio is some 50 per cent greater for active patients who have an exercise-induced ST segmental depression, and the question thus arises as to whether this

Table 6.10: A Comparison of Simple Risk Ratios for Active and
Sedentary 'Post-coronary' Patients

| Variable | Risk ratios* | | Authors of data for sedentary patients |
	Physically active patients	Sedentary patients	
Exercise non-compliance	74.9	—	R.J. Shephard *et al.* (1980)
Continued smoking	1.30	2.00	L. Wilhelmsen *et al.* (1975)
Angina (final exercise test)	1.93	1.93	S. Tominaga & Blackburn (1973)
Aneurysm	2.05	1.80	A.V.G. Bruschke *et al.* (1973)
Enlarged heart	2.40	2.32	S. Tominaga & Blackburn (1973)
Serum cholesterol ≥ 270 mg$\cdot$dl^{-1}	1.98	1.49	S. Tominaga & Blackburn (1973)
		0.80	E. Weinblatt *et al.* (1973)
		1.09	S. Tominaga & Blackburn (1973)
Hypertension $\geq 150/100$ mm Hg	0.98	2.55	E. Weinblatt *et al.* (1973)
Persistent resting ECG abnormalities	1.02	2.47	E. Weinblatt *et al.* (1973)
Exercise ST depression ≥ 0.2 mV	1.82	1.23	J.R. Margolis *et al.* (1975)
Polyfocal VPBs (> 3 in 10 seconds' exercise	1.53	1.61	S. Tominaga & Blackburn (1973)
		~1	E. Kentala & Sarna (1976)

* Events in group with abnormality relative to events in group without
abnormality.

Source: Based on data accumulated by T. Kavanagh *et al.* (1979).

group should be cautioned against participating in an exercise-centred
rehabilitation programme. J.O. Parker *et al.* (1966) have described how
exercise can induce cardiac failure in the ischaemic myocardium.
Nevertheless, in the Toronto series the overall fatality rate for the
exercisers was so low that the absolute prognosis was apparently
improved relative to conservative tretament, even in those patients who

exercised despite ST segmental depression (recurrence rate for this group 4.08 per cent per annum, cardiac fatality rate 2.27 per cent per annum).

Randomised controlled trials

Similar investigations are being carried out on patients enrolled in the Southern Ontario multicentre randomised controlled trial of exercise rehabilitation. After an average of 20 months observation, 51 of 751 participants had sustained a recurrence. Some 24 per cent of the new cardiac episodes were closely associated with various types of physical activity, and in a further 22 per cent of recurrences vigorous exercise (sometimes of an unusual nature) was noted a few hours prior to reinfarction (R.J. Shephard, 1979a). These findings could not have arisen by chance unless the subjects were physically active for six hours per day. The majority of patients had sedentary forms of employment, so that even allowing for the effect of the prescribed activity, a more reasonable expectation would have been 1½ hours of activity per day. It would thus appear that physical activity increased the immediate likelihood of reinfarction by a factor of at least four.

Since a half of the group were enrolled in a high-intensity-exercise programme, and the other half were undertaking homeopathic recreational activity, it was possible to make a comparison of 'risk factors' between the two groups (Table 6.11). The importance of continued cigarette smoking and recent angina as determinants of prognosis was confirmed. Some 36.5 per cent of the overall sample were smokers, but percentages of 55.5 and 73.6 per cent were observed among members of the high- and low-intensity groups who developed a recurrence. Likewise, 25.6 per cent of the overall sample showed angina of effort, but figures were 50.0 and 71.4 per cent for those of the high- and low-intensity-exercise groups who sustained a recurrence. There was a slight suggestion that the high-intensity-exercise programme protected continuing smokers and those with recent angina against non-fatal recurrences. On the other hand, there was a suggestion that a high serum cholesterol level was a greater risk factor for those who exercised vigorously, and as in the non-randomised trial an exercise ST segmental depression of more than 0.2 mV was significantly associated with the likelihood of a fatal recurrence in the vigorously exercised group.

Data from this survey were analysed further in the search for characteristics of those who developed a recurrence of their disease during physical activity (Table 3.2). The main features of those who

Table 6.11: Risk Factors in Post-coronary Rehabilitation — A
Comparison between Patients Allocated to a Progressive High-intensity-
Exercise Programme and Patients Allocated to a Homeopathic
Recreational Programme

Risk factor and type of recurrence	Incidence of risk factor in patients with recurrence		Significance
	High-intensity-exercise programme (%)	Recreational-exercise programme (%)	
Smoking habits			
Current smokers:			
Non-fatal recurrence	47.6	76.9	$0.1 > P > 0.05$
Fatal recurrence	83.3	66.7	
All recurrences	55.5	73.6	
Former smokers:			
Non-fatal recurrence	90.9	100.0	
Fatal recurrence	100.0	100.0	
All recurrences	92.8	100.0	
Recent angina			
Non-fatal recurrence	43.5	73.3	$0.1 > P > 0.05$
Fatal recurrence	71.4	66.7	
All recurrences	50.0	71.4	$0.2 > P > 0.1$
Hypertension (> 150/100 mm Hg)			
Non-fatal recurrences	4.8	14.3	
Fatal recurrences	0	20.0	
All recurrences	3.7	15.8	
High serum cholesterol (> 270 mg·dl $^{-1}$)			
Non-fatal recurrences	5.2	0.0	
Fatal recurrences	28.5	0.0	
All recurrences	11.5	0.0	$0.2 > P > 0.1$
Abnormal resting ECG			
Non-fatal recurrences	52.9	72.7	
Fatal recurrences	28.5	75.0	$0.2 > P > 0.1$
All recurrences	47.8	73.3	$0.2 > P > 0.1$
Exercise ST segmental depression > 0.2 mV			
Non-fatal recurrences	17.3	26.7	
Fatal recurrences	71.4	16.7	$P < 0.05$
All recurrences	30.0	23.8	
Ventricular premature beats			
Non-fatal recurrences	4.3	6.7	
Fatal recurrences	0	0.0	
All recurrences	3.3	4.8	

Source: Based on preliminary data from Southern Ontario multicentre exercise-
heart trial, published by R.J. Shephard (1979a).

succumbed during exercise were a poor exercise compliance, and a greater likelihood of an abnormal resting and exercise electrocardiogram.

As in the primary episode (Chapter 3), socio-economic factors sometimes contributed to the critical event. One man commented on a large promissory note that he was unable to finance, and another was experiencing serious family troubles. One patient was attending the funeral of a friend, and three attacks occurred during or shortly after evening parties.

Other preliminary data from the Southern Ontario multicentre trial suggest that socio-economic factors interacted with the response to added exercise. In particular, 'blue-collar' workers with a 'Type B' personality fared significantly worse in a high- than in a low-intensity-exercise programme (P.A. Rechnitzer *et al.*, report in preparation). This may reflect an unfavourable lifestyle in the lower socio-economic groups. It is also conceivable that some of the blue-collar employees obtained sufficient physical activity at work, without an additional prescription for their leisure hours. However, this is at variance with what would be predicted from the low fitness levels of heavy workers as a class (J.G. Allen, 1966).

Implications for therapy

The frequency of recurrences during physical activity is sufficient to indicate the need for a cautious approach to exercise-centred rehabilitation. Nevertheless, more detailed analysis of individual histories suggests that the majority of cardiac episodes occurred with unsupervised effort in those who were failing to fulfill their prescription on a regular basis. An adverse response to irregular and excessive exercise is predictable, and does not necessarily prove that regular and carefully graded physical activity is harmful.

It may still be that data from a larger sample of patients will establish that exercise has an unfavourable effect upon immediate prognosis. However, at most it will be shown that physical effort has localised the timing of an impending infarction to the gymnasium session. Such an observation is quite compatible with an unchanged or even an improved overall prognosis for those who participate faithfully in an exercise programme. Furthermore, if reinfarction is imminent, it is an advantage to bring the myocardial ischaemia to the attention of an observer, so that surgical treatment can be considered. If a recurrence is unavoidable, it is also better that this develops in a gymnasium where resuscitation can be undertaken, rather than in some situation where the patient is unable to obtain assistance.

Patients with severe exercise-induced ST segmental depression may form a specific sub-group for whom vigorous and infrequently supervised exercise is contraindicated. Unfortunately, such patients have a marked impact upon the overall mortality of the post-coronary population, to the point where any benefit of exercise to the remaining subjects in a clinical trial may be obscured (R.J. Shephard, 1980d).

Exercise and Risk-factor Modification

If it is eventually established that exercise has a beneficial effect upon the overall prognosis following myocardial infarction, it is conceivable that the effect will be indirect, through a modification of the various risk factors already discussed. In these circumstances, we would need to weigh the merits of exercise therapy against other, possibly more powerful, methods of changing lifestyle.

However, current evidence gives little support to the concept of benefit through risk-factor modification alone. Over a three-year period of observation, the proportion of cigarette smokers among 'post-coronary' patients attending the Toronto Rehabilitation Centre remained almost constant at 36 per cent, only a little below the figure reported for subjects enrolled in the coronary drug trial (S. Tominaga & Blackburn, 1973), the latter being a programme that did not include deliberate exercise. Likewise, the Toronto patients showed negligible changes in body mass and skinfold thicknesses over the three-year study. The resting systolic pressure decreased slightly, possibly due to a progressive habituation to the test laboratory, but there was a small increase in the maximum systolic pressure developed during exercise as myocardial contractility improved (T. Kavanagh *et al.*, 1977c).

Two comments should be made with regard to these findings. Firstly, the typical patient who is recruited a few months after a myocardial infarction is no longer an obese individual with a high consumption of cigarettes and animal fat. Such faults of lifestyle have already been corrected while in hospital. Secondly, although exercise produces no further changes in such controllable risk factors, this is not entirely a negative conclusion. In matters of diet and smoking, recidivism is commonplace, and the ability of exercise to conserve the improved health habits established in a hospital setting is itself a major accomplishment that undoubtedly improves the prognosis for a post-coronary patient.

The family physcian must often rely on clinical assessments of exercise tolerance. Objective scales such as those proposed by the British Medical Research Council (Table 7.1) and the American Heart Association (Table 7.2) improve the reliability of patient responses to questioning, but do not overcome the limitation that sensations are reported within the framework of the patient's habitual activity patterns and current anxiety level. There has thus been an aggressive search for simple non-invasive techniques to examine the performance of the heart and coronary circulation during graded exercise.

Before considering normal cardiac responses to physical activity and training, we shall make a brief review of these non-invasive procedures. Topics to be discussed include the measurement of overall cardiac output, regional myocardial function, overall and regional coronary blood flow, the electrocardiogram and exercise stress tests.

Cardiac Output

Direct Fick principle

The standard technique against which non-invasive measurements of cardiac output are evaluated involves a direct application of the 'Fick principle'. The usual procedure requires the steady-state measurement of oxygen intake ($\dot{V}_{O_2}$), with the collection of corresponding blood samples from a peripheral artery (oxygen content C_{a,O_2}) and the pulmonary arterial trunk (mixed venous oxygen content $C_{\bar{v},O_2}$). The cardiac output $\dot{Q}$ is then given by:

$$\dot{Q} = \dot{V}_{O_2}/(C_{a,O_2} - C_{\bar{v},O_2})$$

The catheterisation of a peripheral artery is not to be undertaken lightly, particularly during exercise. Occasional complications include haemorrhage, thrombosis and even gangrene of the distal part, such risks being greatest when the procedure has been undertaken in subjects with vascular disease. Catheterisation of the pulmonary artery is also best avoided unless necessary for clinical management. Among potential

Table 7.1: Classification of Exercise Tolerance

Grade	Clinical status
0	Breathing as good as other people of same age and build at work, walking and on climbing hills and stairs
1	Breathing probably as good as other people of same age and build at work, walking and on climbing hills and stairs
2	Able to walk with people of same age and build on the level, but unable to keep up on hills or stairs
3	Unable to keep up with people of same age and build, but can walk 1.6 km at own speed
4	Unable to walk more than 50-70 m without a stop
5	Obviously breathless on talking or undressing, or unable to leave home because of breathlessness

Source: J.C. Gilson & Hugh-Jones (1955).

Table 7.2: Functional Classification of Cardiac Patients Proposed by the New York Heart Association

Class	Clinical status	Likely maximum oxygen intake $(ml \cdot kg^{-1} \cdot min^{-1})$
I	Patients with heart disease, but no symptoms. Ordinary physical activity does not cause fatigue, palpitations, dyspnoea or anginal pain	> 21
II	Patients comfortable at rest, but symptoms with ordinary physical activity	13-21
III	Patients comfortable at rest, but symptoms with less than ordinary physical effort	3.5-12
IV	Patients with symptoms at rest	< 3.5

Source: Criterion Committee of the New York Heart Association (1964); American Heart Association (1972).

complications of this procedure, we may note bacterial endocarditis, perforation of the heart wall, fracture of the catheter and provocation of a dysrhythmia. Again, risks are higher in the patient with ischaemic heart disease than in an individual with a normal heart (R.J. Corliss, 1979).

Because of these problems, it is usual to make indirect determination of cardiac output in the patient with ischaemic heart disease. However, opportunity for direct measurements may arise if there is angiography of the coronary circulation as a prelude to possible by-pass surgery or cardiac catheterisation to assess the function of sclerosed aortic valves.

Dye-injection techniques

Cardiac output can be assessed by the injection of a marker substance that is rapidly removed from the circulation (W.F. Hamilton, 1962). The dye indocyanine green is commonly used for this purpose. A relatively non-invasive assessment is possible at rest; the dye is injected into a peripheral vein, and its passage through the circulation is monitored by means of a photocell attached to the ear lobe. However, during leg exercise the blood flow through the arm veins is insufficient to allow a satisfactory ('square-wave') injection of dye, and a catheter must be advanced into the right atrium before dye-concentration curves are adequate to calculate cardiac output. Furthermore, exercise leads to changes in thickness of the ear lobe and mechanical displacement of the photocell; an intra-arterial catheter is thus needed to record dye concentrations accurately. The dye method then has little advantage over use of the direct Fick principle.

Foreign-gas methods

The Fick equation may be applied to the pulmonary uptake of a very soluble foreign gas such as acetylene or nitrous oxide.

The acetylene technique was originally introduced by A. Grollman (1929), and early results underestimated the true cardiac output. The necessary gas analysis has been facilitated by the introduction of gas chromatography (R. Simmons & Shephard, 1971b) and mass spectrometry (J.H. Triebwasser *et al.*, 1977). It is now possible to use low (one per cent), relatively pleasant and non-explosive concentrations of acetylene; the modern techniques yield results that have a probable error of less than three per cent and agree well with other methods (R. Simmons & Shephard, 1971b).

While acetylene is the preferred gas (L. Cander & Forster, 1959), nitrous oxide is a possible alternative. Gas concentrations are then determined by either infrared or gas-chromatographic analysis (M. Rigatto, 1967; B. Ayotte *et al.*, 1970).

Most investigators have based their calculations upon the few (eight to ten) seconds before significant recirculation of the foreign gas occurs. Open-circuit procedures have been described (T. Hatch & Cook, 1955; R.J. Shephard, 1959; M. Becklake *et al.*, 1962), but these are cumbersome and of doubtful validity during exercise.

Carbon-dioxide rebreathing

Carbon-dioxide concentrations are very readily determined by 'breathe-through' infrared cells. For this reason, the commonest non-invasive method of cardiac-output determination applies the Fick equation to the exchange of carbon dioxide:

$$\dot{Q} = \dot{V}_{CO_2} / (C_{a,CO_2} - C_{\bar{v},CO_2})$$

The steady-state output of carbon-dioxide ($\dot{V}_{CO_2}$) is measured by an open-circuit method, any given intensity of exercise testing being sustained until the expired CO_2 concentration remains constant for two successive minutes. The arterial carbon-dioxide concentration (C_{a,CO_2}) can be estimated in specimens of 'arterialised' capillary blood, collected from the heated fingertip or ear lobe. Alternatively, the arterial carbon-dioxide tension can be estimated from a continuous record of CO_2 concentration during a rapid expiration. At rest, the concentration seen in the final portion of the expirate coincides rather closely with the arterial value, but in exercise there are substantial variations of alveolar CO_2 concentration over the breathing cycle (R.J. Shephard, 1968b); mainly for this reason, the best approximation to the arterial CO_2 tension of an exercising subject is given by the average of mid- and end-tidal readings (G. Matell, 1963). A third option is to calculate the alveolar CO_2 concentration from the expired reading by means of the Bohr equation, using a formula of N. Jones *et al.* (1966) for dead space (V_D):

$$V_D = 138.4 + 0.077(V_T)$$

where V_T is the subject's tidal volume.

The mixed venous CO_2 reading is usually obtained by rebreathing from a bag containing between five and 15 per cent carbon dioxide. In the Defares method (J.G. Defares, 1956; A. Amery *et al.*, 1977), the subject takes one breath per second. A graph relating the CO_2 content of the nth to the $(n+1)$th breath is extrapolated to the line of identity. It is assumed that at this point the bag would have reached equilibrium with the mixed venous concentration, causing CO_2 elimination to cease.

An alternative approach (N.L. Jones *et al.*, 1975) selects a re-breathing mixture close to the anticipated mixed venous gas content. If an appropriate mixture is chosen, CO_2 is neither eliminated nor absorbed. After a few oscillations, the CO_2 concentration at the mouth reaches a 'plateau' value close to that of mixed venous blood; this is disturbed when recirculation of blood with higher CO_2 content causes an upward movement of the record (after eight to ten seconds in vigorous exercise). For reasons that are still not fully understood, the plateau reading overestimates the true mixed venous value, particularly during exercise. N.L. Jones *et al.* (1967) thus proposed 'correcting' the bag reading (P_{bag,CO_2}) according to the equation:

$$P_{\bar{v},CO_2} = P_{bag,CO_2} - [(0.24 P_{bag,CO_2}) - 1.47]$$

Unfortunately, the necessary correction may modify the estimate of arterio-venous CO_2 difference by as much as 25 per cent, and this brings the absolute determination of cardiac output into serious question. On the other hand, the CO_2 rebreathing technique is quite satisfactory for following the progress of an individual, and also for comparing his performance with that of other patients tested by the same procedure. At rest, the arterio-venous carbon-dioxode tension difference is only about 6 torr, but it rises to 30-40 torr during vigorous exercise. Since both arterial and venous CO_2 tensions have an error of 1-2 torr, the CO_2 rebreathing procedure is better suited to the measurement of cardiac output when subjects are exercising than when they are under resting conditions.

Neither foreign-gas nor CO_2 rebreathing procedures work particularly well in patients with chronic chest disease, since the permissible rebreathing period (eight to ten seconds) is too short to establish an equilibrium between poorly ventilated regions of the lungs and the rebreathing bag. There thus remains scope for the development of a non-invasive procedure that will allow the measurement of cardiac output in patients with poor gas-mixing.

Regional Myocardial Function

Cine-angiography

Direct estimates of both regional function and cardiac stroke volume can be obtained by injection of a radio-opaque dye and filming the cardiac chamber in the postero-anterior and lateral planes (S.H. Bartle & Sanmarco, 1966; J.W. Kennedy *et al.*, 1966). Computer technology now permits very sophisticated three-dimensional analysis of angiographic videotapes (P.H. Heintzen *et al.*, 1974; S.A. Johnson *et al.*, 1974; H. Sandler & Dodge, 1974), but the technique involves substantial x irradiation and the injection of a dye that occasionally precipitates cardiac arrest. Furthermore, trunk movements make it difficult to apply cine-angiography during more than very light exercise.

Ultrasound

Ultrasound has potential as a method for the estimation of cardiac stroke volume during rest and light exercise (E.I. Edler, 1965; D.H. Bennett & Evans, 1974; H. Feigenbaum, 1974; R.S. Rennemann, 1974; P. Bubenheimer *et al.*, 1980; J.L. Laurenceau *et al.*, 1980; A. Venco *et al.*, 1980). However, to the present it has been used most frequently to detect portions of the ventricular wall with weakened or paradoxical motion.

High-frequency sound waves (2-10 MHz) are directed through the chest and reflected from the ventricular walls. The relative positions of various intracardiac structures are then deduced from transit times for the sound waves. Light exercise can be performed if the subject remains supine or semi-supine. Cardiac output can be estimated from the stroke volume and heart rate, but if the arterio-venous oxygen difference is to be calculated from cardiac output and oxygen intake it is important to await a 'steady state', since the exercise 'on transients' differ for these last two variables.

Nuclear cardiology

Both non-invasive and invasive applications of nuclear cardiology are used in the management of patients with ischaemic heart disease. A static image may be obtained following the injection of technetium pyrophosphate in order to localise and determine the size of a recent myocardial infarction; the marker is selectively retained by infarcted tissue for eight to ten days following the acute episode (R.W. Parkey *et al.*, 1974).

Injection of the thallium radioisotope ^{201}Tl is a second possible static-imaging technique. A low thallium uptake indicates a zone with poor myocardial perfusion or prior scarring (J. Leppo *et al.*, 1979; D.H. Schmidt *et al.*, 1979). The method can be used to diagnose infarction, to assess the viability of tissue, and to document regional perfusion.

Dynamic studies use either a 'gated' camera, or the 'first-pass' approach. The gated camera records radioactivity at the end of systole and the end of diastole (R.D. Burrow *et al.*, 1977). The 'first-pass' method employs a multiple-crystal camera with a fast counting rate and a short dead time; this allows a bolus of radioactive material to be followed from the moment of its injection into a peripheral vein until it has completed a first passage through the heart. Transit times and ejection fractions can thus be calculated for both ventricles (R.C. Marshall *et al.*, 1977; N. Schad, 1977). Estimates of ejection fraction correlate quite well ($r = 0.91$) with measurements made by contrast ventriculography (D.H. Schmidt *et al.*, 1979), and assessments of regional wall motion have a 75 per cent inter-observer agreement. Further developments of this technique allow semi-quantitative determinations of cardiac output both at rest and during moderate exercise (J.S. Borer *et al.*, 1977; S.K. Rerych *et al.*, 1978).

Left-ventricular function

Direct measurements of left-ventricular function are sometimes made by catheterisation before and after coronary arterial surgery (J.C. Manley, 1979). Note is taken of the left-ventricular stroke work index (the product of ventricular stroke index, ml per beat per m^2 of body surface area, and the difference between mean aortic pressure and the left-ventricular end-diastolic pressure). This index is examined in relation to left-ventricular end-diastolic pressure. Improvement of condition following by-pass surgery may be reflected in a greater capacity to increase left-ventricular stroke work, or a lesser associated rise of end-diastolic pressure during exercise. Attempts to assess myocardial performance through resting measurements of maximum shortening velocity ($\dot{V}_{max}$), mean systolic ejection rate and maximum rate of pressure rise (dp/dt) have proven relatively unsuccessful.

Indirect assessments of cardiac contractility can be derived from angiography, echocardiography and nuclear cardiology, as noted above. More simply, data can be taken from simultaneous recordings of the electrocardiogram, heart sounds and carotid pulse wave (G.R. Cumming & Edwards, 1963; W. Raab, 1966; W.S. Harris, 1974). Possible measurements include the total duration of ventricular systole (from the Q wave of the electrocardiogram to the second heart sound, QS_2), the left ventricular ejection time (from the beginning of the carotid pulse wave to its dicrotic notch, LVET) and the pre-ejection period (PEP = QS_2 − LVET). Since such data vary with heart-rate-related changes of contractility, they are commonly 'corrected' to a standard heart rate (H. Montoye *et al.*, 1971; G.M.A. Van der Hoeven *et al.*, 1977). The best simple index of contractility seems to be the ratio PEP/LVET; this is reduced by training, and increased by myocardial disease. Unfortunately, it is difficult to record the carotid pulse wave during vigorous exercise; measurements are thus made immediately after cycle-ergometer work, or during isometric handgrip contractions

(W.F. Jacobs *et al.*, 1970; C. Kivowitz *et al.*, 1970; C.B. Mullins *et al.*, 1970; R.H. Helfant *et al.*, 1971; D.S. Bloom & Vecht, 1978).

Coronary Perfusion

Coronary angiography

Direct visualisation of the coronary vessels by the injection of radio-opaque materials is the standard technique against which other assessments of myocardial perfusion are compared. The contrast medium outlines vessels down to a size of some 110 microns, and local narrowing by atheromatous plaques can also be seen. The status of individual arteries is commonly reported (for example, 50 per cent obstruction of the left anterior descending branch). Such data are of value in gauging the need for by-pass surgery, although it should be stressed that the apparent narrowing of a vessel varies with its orientation towards the viewing camera. Reader-to-reader variability in assessment of angiograms also has a standard deviation of 21 per cent (L.M. Zir *et al.*, 1975). Further, exercise-induced vaso-dilatation may modify the extent of obstruction. Finally, since blood flow varies as the fourth power of vessel radius, a small error in the estimate of obstruction can have a large influence upon the presumed adequacy or inadequacy of perfusion; 50 per cent narrowing has little effect upon flow, but 75 per cent narrowing cuts maximum flow by two thirds (K.L. Gould *et al.*, 1974; S.E. Logan, 1975).

The main disadvantages of angiography are the need for cardiac catheterisation, exposure to x irradiation and the injection of a viscous, cardio-toxic contrast medium that can (and sometimes does) provoke ventricular fibrillation.

Alternative procedures

The Fick principle can be applied to the local myocardial uptake of soluble gases such as nitrous oxide (D.E. Gregg *et al.*, 1951; G.G. Rowe, 1959; R.J. Bing *et al.*, 1960; C.R. Jorgensen *et al.*, 1971). It is also possible to measure the uptake of radioactive isotopes (B.L. Zaret *et al.*, 1973) that penetrate the myocardium readily (^{43}K or ^{86}Rb). Such procedures work fairly well in animal experiments, since the radio-isotope can be injected directly into the root of the aorta, and the heart can be excised subsequently for an assessment of its radioactivity. Precordial counters have been used to measure the uptake of radio-isotopes by the human heart, but such techniques lack precision. Furthermore, the myocardial extraction of the radioisotope apparently decreases from 70 to 40 per cent as the rate of coronary blood flow rises, so that accurate measurements demand an assessment of extraction by catheterisation of the coronary sinus (D. Nolting *et al.*, 1958; W.D. Love & Burch, 1959). Even with catheterisation, the value obtained is an average for most of the myocardium, so that local deficiencies of blood flow may pass undetected (F.J. Klocke & Wittenberg, 1969).

Other approaches to the study of myocardial perfusion are currently being developed by the nuclear cardiologists (D.H. Schmidt *et al.*, 1979). To the present, they yield qualitative rather than quantitative results. In addition to technetium pyrophosphate injections and thallium scans, some authors have used radioactive macro-aggregates and microspheres (which become trapped in the finer blood vessels). Others have administered ^{133}Xe (which escapes preferentially into well-perfused regions of the myocardium).

Because of technical difficulties associated with these various approaches, the adequacy of myocardial perfusion is still commonly assessed from the electrocardiographic response to a standard stress test.

Electrocardiogram

Technique

The majority of electrocardiograph machines currently manufactured meet the specifications of the American Heart Association (1967); these requirements — for a 0.05-Hz cut-off and a 6-dB-per-octave roll-off — ensure an error < 0.05 mV in the early part of the ST segment, with a consistent response to high-frequency detail above 100 Hz. Older designs of ECG (Figure 7.1) may respond poorly to both high- and low-frequency signals, obscuring fine details of the record and creating artefactual displacements of the ST segment.

Vectorcardiography continues to be of theoretical interest, although it is now recognised that the hope of representing the entire information content of the electrocardiogram in three 'orthogonal' tracings is unrealistic. Valuable clues to local ischaemia of the myocardium can be obtained by moving a unipolar (exploring) electrode across the praecordium. In the context of physical activity and ischaemic heart disease, the usual requirement is thus for a standard twelve-lead resting ECG, with use of either a single lead (CM_5) or three leads (CM_2, CM_4 and CM_6) during physical activity (Figure 7.2). Because muscle 'noise' is increased by physical activity, the recording

Figure 7.1: To illustrate the influence of a poor low-frequency response on the waveform of a simulated ECG signal.

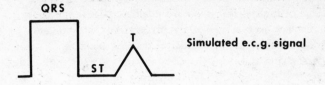

Simulated e.c.g. signal

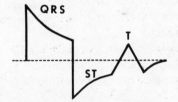

Response of e.c.g. with poor low frequency response. Note artefactual ST segmental depression.

Source: W.E. James & Patnoi (1974).

leads should not be attached to the limbs during exercise. The electrical signal is best measured between the manubrium sterni and the corresponding V position on the praecordium, the neutral electrode being attached to the back of the neck.

It remains quite difficult to obtain high-quality records during vigorous exercise, even if chest leads are used (J. Seymour & Conway, 1969; I. Elgrishi *et al.*, 1970). H. Blackburn *et al.* (1968) asked 14 cardiologists to interpret the same series of tracings. The proportion of abnormal records reported varied from five to 58 per cent, and on different occasions the same physician interpreted the same tracing differently. Reasons for inconsistency included lack of objective criteria, uncertainty about the significance of findings such as junctional depression and the poor technical quality of many records. Interestingly, technical personnel were more consistent readers of the electrocardiogram than were cardiologists. The technicians achieved complete inter-observer agreement in 85 per cent of records, and were also in full agreement as to those patients with clear-cut ischaemia (more than 0.1 mV of ST segmental depression). Keys to the good performance of the paramedical staff were the use of a magnifying lens,

Figure 7.2: To illustrate the recommended placement of electrodes for an exercise electrocardiogram (Lead CM_5). The lead labelled 'right arm' is attached over the upper part of the sternum (manubrium sterni). The lead labelled 'left arm' is attached over the apex beat (in the space between the fifth and sixth ribs, 7-10 cm to the left of the mid-line). The lead marked 'right leg' is attached at the back of the neck. Alternative placements for leads CM_2, CM_4 and CM_6 are also indicated.

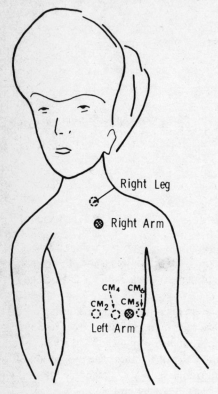

Source: From R.J. Shephard, *Endurance Fitness* (p. 136, second edition, 1977), by permission of the publisher, University of Toronto Press.

simple but standardised measuring techniques and periodic cross-checks of their interpretations against previously evaluated electro-cardiograms.

One of the main technical problems in an exercising subject is a wandering baseline. This reflects a varying electrode impedance. The phenomenon can be minimised by careful skin preparation (removal of the outer layers of the epidermis with a dental burr) and use of an amplifier with a high input impedance (D. Lewes, 1965; R. Tregear, 1965; L.A. Geddes & Baker, 1966). Electrical (60-Hz) 'noise' can be overcome by adequate grounding of the neutral electrode, screening of all cables and use of high-frequency filters with specific ('common-mode') rejection of 60-Hz signals (J. Von der Groeben *et al.*, 1969).

Measurements of the ST segment have been greatly facilitated by the development of analogue and digital averaging techniques (A. Pedersen & Andersen, 1971; P. Rautaharju *et al.*, 1971; W.E. James & Patnoi, 1974; W. Siegel, 1974; L. Jansson *et al.*, 1976; M.L. Simoons, 1976). Analogue equipment gives a visual display of the average tracing derived from 16 or 32 successive heart beats. The usual equipment allows the making up of 1,024 (2^{10}) discreet voltage readings along the length of the QRS-T complex. Noise (Figure 7.3) is thus cancelled out. The quality of the ECG signal improves as the square root of the number of cycles that are averaged; however, if too many complexes are included, a transient ST displacement may be overlooked, while slight asynchrony of the triggering process leads to a progressive rounding of the primary waveform (D.A. Winter, 1969; P. Rautaharju *et al.*, 1971). A single abnormal beat (such as a premature ventricular contraction) also gives a gross distortion of the averaged signal (L.K. Jackson *et al.*, 1969). Some investigators have programmed digital computers to give a more sophisticated solution of the same problem. The 1,024 measurements are made on each of 48 successive heart beats, and the computer program selects for averaging 16 of the 48 QRS complexes that have a mutually similar waveform. Nevertheless, problems still arise. M.L. Simoons (1977) found that in one series of 7,084 tracings incorrect averaging due to excessive drift or noise occurred in 1.8 per cent of subjects. There was also incorrect detection of the QRS complex in 0.04 per cent, P-wave detection errors in 6.5 per cent, and T-wave detection errors in 0.6 per cent. Many of the currently used systems measure ST depression at a fixed time (for example, 80 ms after the ST-T junction, or at a stated interval after the nadir of the R or S waves). Such an approach gives a simple 'packaged' apparatus for clinical purposes, but it does not allow for variations in the duration of the QRS complex and the ST segment. Alternatively, the onset of the T wave can be determined by inspection of the averaged tracing, or by electrical differentiation. Other possibilities are to calculate the slope of the ST segment (F.M. Lester *et al.*, 1967;

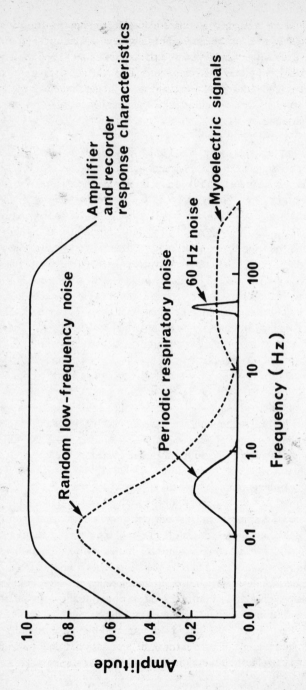

Figure 7.3: Components of noise distorting electrocardiogram.

Source: Based in part on W.E. James & Patnoi (1974).

Figure 7.4: Choice of iso-electric line in assessment of ST displacement. Most authors join successive points of origin of the Q wave, although Lepeschkin has pointed out that P- and U-wave repolarisation may then cause artefactual ST depression. The shaded area is the ST integral. The point (1) is 80 ms after the onset of the ST segment, and the point (2) is the onset of the T wave as determined by inspection.

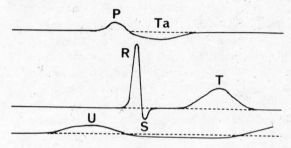

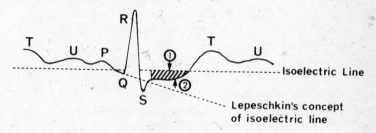

Source: Based on an illustration of E. Lepeschkin (1969).

P.L. McHenry *et al.*, 1968), or the integral of the ST segment below a pre-selected 'iso-electric' baseline (Figure 7.4).

It is not easy to establish the iso-electric ('zero') voltage line during vigorous physical activity, since repolarisation of the U and P waves may extend into the QRS complex and beyond (Figure 7.4). As a matter of convenience, most authors refer measurements to the onset of the Q wave (M. Ellestad, 1975).

Resting electrocardiogram

Many clinicians still search for evidence of myocardial ischaemia in terms of abnormalities of the resting electrocardiogram. However, even if patients have well-marked angina of effort, the resting records commonly remain within normal limits (T.W. Mattingly *et al.*, 1958). Possible clues to ischaemic heart disease include non-specific ST-T wave abnormalities, changes of electrical conduction, dysrhythmias and signs of left-ventricular hypertrophy. Occasionally, there may be ischaemic displacement of the ST segment.

Imminent or recent myocardial infarction is an important contra-indication to exercise. It may be suspected if there are prominent Q waves and elevation of the ST segment, although the latter pheno-menon is sometimes seen also in healthy athletes (S. Zoneraich *et al.*, 1977; J. Morganroth & Maron, 1977; Table 6.9). In doubtful cases, progression of the changes over several days confirms the diagnosis of infarction. If the lesion is on the posterior surface of the heart, the ST segment may be depressed rather than elevated.

Acute myocarditis also causes depression of the ST segment and inversion of the T wave. It is a second important contraindication to exercise.

Exercise should also be avoided if there is a probability of recent *pulmonary embolism*. If the emboli are small, the electrocardiogram may remain normal, but a large embolus is associated with a rapid heart rate and signs of right-heart strain (including inverted T waves over the right ventricle).

Other electrocardiographic indications for caution include dis-orders of cardiac rhythms such as premature ventricular contractions (discussed below), atrial flutter and fibrillation, and the various disturbances of electrical conduction. With *sinu-atrial block*, some of the electrical impulses arising in the sinu-atrial node fail to depolarise the atria; there are thus pauses when an entire ECG complex is missing. When this appearance is seen in athletes, hypertonia of the right vagal nerve is thought to be responsible (F. Plas, 1978; Table 7.3). However, in older adults, coronary vascular disease is often to blame and a 'sick-sinus' syndrome may limit both sinu-atrial conduction and maximum heart rate (M.I. Ferrer, 1973). Blockage of transmission at the *atrio-ventricular node* can also occur. In many athletes, the PR interval is unusually long (> 200 ms, Type I block), and in a proportion of such subjects the PR interval may become progressively extended until a beat is dropped (Wenckeback Type II block; J. Morganroth & Maron, 1977; S. Zoneraich *et al.*, 1977; F. Plas, 1978). More rarely, the PR interval remains constant until a beat is suddenly dropped (Mobitz Type II block). This variety of conduction disturbance is liable to progress to third-degree block, where the atria and ventricles

Table 7.3: Electrocardiographic 'Abnormalities' Observed in 12,000 Athletes

Abnormality	Frequency (%)
Nodal rhythm	0.325
Coronary sinus rhythm	1.15
Atrio-ventricular block	
First degree	6.16
Second degree	0.125
Third degree	0.017
Atrio-ventricular dissociation	0.117
Focal block	3.150
Right bundle-branch block	0.075
Premature ventricular contractions	1.375
Paroxysmal tachycardia	0.067
Ventricular pre-excitation	0.158
Pseudo-ischaemic abnormalities of repolarisation	0.550

Source: Based on data of A. Venerando (1979).

beat independently of each other. Marked atrio-ventricular block usually indicates some disease of the myocardium, and there is a danger of progression to a 'Stokes-Adams' attack, with complete ventricular asystole. *Left bundle-branch block* causes a leftward shift of the QRS vector, with tall and broad R waves in lead I plus deep and broad S waves in lead III. It is usually an indication of cardiac disease. *Right bundle-branch block* causes a rightward shift of the cardiac vector, with broad and late S waves in leads I and II, and a small QRS complex in lead III. It can also be pathological, although a minor degree of right bundle-branch block is a common finding in athletes (N. Hanne-Paparo *et al.*, 1976; W. Kinderman *et al.*, 1978; F. Plas, 1978; B.J.F. de Andrade & Rose, 1979; A. Venco *et al.*, 1980).

Exercise response

The main change in timing of the cardiac cycle during exercise is a shortening of the diastolic phase. However, the P-R interval is also curtailed, often to less than 0.15 seconds, and the Q-T interval is reduced in proportion to the heart rate. There is also an increase in P-wave amplitude, a decrease in T waves during exercise (probably due to sympathetic nerve activity) and an increase in T waves following exercise (possible a response to increased serum potassium concentrations).

The influence of exercise upon premature ventricular contractions and ST segmental voltages is discussed in the following sections.

Premature systoles

Premature beats can arise at any point in the conduction pathway of the electrical impulse. Although sometimes called extra-systoles, they can replace rather than supplement normal cardiac contractions.

A persistent and irregular atrial tachycardia may indicate disease, but it is also compatible with normal health and continued athletic participation (P. Fleischmann & Kellermann, 1969).

Ventricular premature contractions are usually 'ectopic', and in consequence the QRS complex has a broadened and abnormal waveform. Less commonly, a systole may arise within the normal electrical pathway, or impulse conduction may be blocked without the appearance of a visible QRS complex ('concealed conduction'). One factor contributing to premature ventricular contraction is an excessive irritability of the myocardium. This may arise from an accumulation of nicotine or caffeine in the body, or from an excessive sympathetic discharge (as in the chronically anxious person, or the athlete who is competing under intense stress). Some authors have linked emotionally provoked dysrhythmias with an increased frequency of myocardial infarction and sudden death; the effect upon prognosis is probably small (F.D. Fisher & Tyroler, 1963; N. Goldschlager *et al.*, 1973; M. Rodstein *et al.*, 1971), although there is good reason to believe that a sudden outpouring of catecholamines can sometimes contribute to sudden death during intense physical or emotional stress (R.J. Shephard, 1974b).

The premature systoles of an anxious patient usually become less frequent with effort. In other individuals, an abnormality of rhythm appears for the first time during exercise. Overdrive suppression of the abnormal rhythm does not necessarily rule out an ischaemic cause (M.H. Ellestad, 1975; P.L. McHenry & Morris, 1976; G. Koppes *et al.*, 1977). However, appearance of the premature contractions during exercise is generally regarded more seriously (P.L. McHenry *et al.*, 1972; E.F. Beard & Owen, 1973; H. Blackburn *et al.*, 1973). It is clearly associated with an increased probability of cardiac disease (ischaemia and/or scarring) (R.H. Mann & Burchell, 1952; M. Rodstein *et al.*, 1971; J.A. Vedin *et al.*, 1972; M. Ellestad, 1975; B. Surawicz, 1975). The patho-physiology is as follows.

Local hypoxia leads to inhomogeneity of repolarisation, and uni-directional conduction block develops in segments of the myocardium. This facilitates 're-entry' of the electrical impulse into regions of the ventricle that are already repolarised (Figure 1.1; A.M. Katz, 1973; L.S. Gettes, 1975). Circulating catecholamines also lower the threshold of abnormal pace-making foci. These hormones speed both depolarisation and repolarisation of the ventricle (A.M. Katz, 1977), so that non-uniformities of response to the chemical messengers provide a second basis for the 're-entry' phenomenon. The difference of prognosis between resting and exercise-induced premature ventricular contractions is an important issue, for if substantiated it implies that 24-hour tape recordings of the electrocardiogram (L. Mogensen, 1977) have less prognostic value than an exercise ECG.

A polyfocal origin (indicated by differences of QRS waveform between the abnormal beats) is associated with an increased risk of infarction or re-infarction, whereas a unifocal origin (consistent abnormal waveform) is not (T. Kavanagh *et al.*, 1977c). The premature beats are particularly dangerous if they are not only polyfocal, but also occur early in the cardiac cycle (before completion of the T wave). While such premature systoles provide a possible means of diagnosing ischaemic heart disease, it is less clearly established that they add new evidence of risk to that gained from an examination of the ST segment (below).

ST segmental changes

Concept. As the intensity of exercise is increased, the oxygen con-sumed by the ventricles tends to outstrip oxygen delivery via the coronary vessels. Because of differences in work rate and intramural compression of the coronary arteries, the left ventricle is more vulner-able to oxygen lack than the right. Hypoxia alters transmural potentials across individual myocardial cells (W. Trautwein, 1954; W.E. Samson & Scher, 1960) and also changes the pattern of electrical impulse conduc-tion around the two ventricles. In consequence, there is a progressive alteration in the appearance of the ST segment of the electrocardiogram (Figure 7.5), usually seen best in the unipolar chest lead V_4 (H. Feil & Segel, 1928; S. Goldhammer & Schert, 1932; C.C. Wolferth & Wood, 1932). Depression of the S-ST junction is followed by a horizontal or downward sloping depression of the entire ST segment. Unfortun-ately, the phenomenon reflects nonuniform repolarisation of the ventricles rather than ischaemia *per se*, and other possible causes of ST displacement include drug-induced malfunction of the myocardial

Figure 7.5: To illustrate the possible range of appearances of ST segment: (a) normal; (b) junctional depression; (c) horizontal depression; (d) downsloping depression

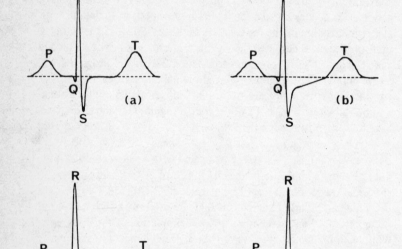

Table 7.4: Factors Influencing ST Segment Displacement during Exercise

False negative results:	Insufficient exercise intensity, resting ST elevation, use of nitroglycerine and other vasodilators, abnormalities of ventricular conduction
False positive results:	Resting ST depression, hyperventilation, cigarette smoking, use of diuretics, potassium loss, glucose and carbohydrate loading, abnormal stress on left ventricle, abnormal conduction (e.g., left-ventricular bundle-branch block), anti-dysrhythmic drugs (e.g., procaine amide, quinidine), digitalis therapy

'sodium pump' and altered concentrations of plasma electrolytes (Table 7.4).

Test format. The exercise format used by many clinicians is still the Master test (A.M. Master & Jaffé, 1941). The patient climbs backwards and forwards over a double nine-inch (22.9 cm) step for 1.5 minutes ('single' test) or three minutes ('double' test), at a rate adjusted somewhat for age, sex and body mass. The main criticisms of the Master test are: (i) reliance on a recovery electrocardiogram; (ii) use of rather mild exercise (the terminal heart rate is typically about 120 beats•min^{-1}); and (iii) a stepping rhythm that imposes a greater strain on elderly than on young subjects.

One possible alternative is to carry all tests to exhaustion, or to a 'symptom-limited' maximum (P.D. Wood *et al.*, 1950; R.A. Bruce *et al.*, 1969). Logic suggests that this will be more risky than a submaximum test, and some (J. McDonough & Bruce, 1969), but not all (P. Rochmis & Blackburn, 1971) of the available data support such a supposition (see below, p. 197). In the clinical setting, one disadvantage of a symptom-linked maximum test is its subjectivity. If the confidence of the patient or his examiner allows a repeat test to be pushed to a higher work rate, a misleading impression of worsening ST depression may be formed. The best approach for the clinician thus seems to record the electrocardiogram when the patient is exercising at a target heart rate corresponding to a fixed percentage, 75 per cent (R.J. Shephard, 1971) or 85 per cent (I. Åstrand, 1967) of maximum oxygen intake (Table 7.5). Some critics of this approach have pointed to the considerable range of maximum heart rates, particularly in older individuals and patients with ischaemic heart disease. However, there is a fairly close relationship between heart rate and myocardial oxygen consumption (Y. Wang, 1972), and the target reading thus provides a reasonable basis for standardising myocardial oxygen demand in patients of a given age.

The observed ST appearance depends also upon the duration of physical activity (R.J. Shephard & Kavanagh, 1978c), since an accumulation of acid metabolites in the myocardium dilates the coronary vessels, relieving the local ischaemia. If comparisons of the ST segment are to be made from one test to another, it is finally important to equate cardiac work rate, whether in terms of heart rate or some more complex measure such as the tension-time index or the triple product (see the discussion of cardiac work rate below, p. 225). It can be quite difficult to calculate the tension element of cardiac work,

Table 7.5: Approximate 'Target' Heart Rates Corresponding to 75 and 85 Per Cent of Maximum Oxygen Intake in Relation to Age

Age (years)	Target heart rate	
	75%	85%
25	160	170
35	150	160
45	140	150
55	130	140

since this depends upon the heart volume and the thickness of the ventricular wall, both factors that can vary from one test to another (K.H. Sidney & Shephard, 1977b).

Interpretation. If the coronary vasculature is healthy, there is normally no more than slight junctional depression, even in maximal exercise (R.A. Bruce *et al.*, 1969). Some authors have attached pathological significance to a marked depression of the S-ST junction (> 0.15 mV) and/or an upward sloping ST segment that remains 0.1 mV below the iso-electric ('zero') potential at the commencement of the T wave (A. Kurita *et al.*, 1977). However, false positive tests are less frequent if attention is directed simply to horizontal and downward sloping ST segments (Table 7.6). Such records are associated with as much as a ten- to 15-fold increase in the risk of future 'coronary events', including premature death from ischaemic heart disease (T.W. Mattingly, 1962; A. Rumball & Acheson, 1963; G.P. Robb & Marks, 1964; I.S. Kasser & Bruce, 1969; W.S. Aronow & Cassidy, 1975; G.P. Robb & Seltzer, 1975; G. Koppes *et al.*, 1977). A combination of ST depression with anginal pain is strong presumptive evidence of significant coronary vascular disease.

For clinical purposes it is necessary to establish an appropriate balance between the sensitivity and the specificity of the ST test criterion (Table 7.6). An increase in sensitivity decreases the number of false negative responses, but also increases the number of false positives. A false positive test may create a cardiac cripple from a healthy middle-aged adult; it may also be followed by an unnecessary angiography (a costly procedure with a significant mortality). On the other hand, a false negative test may encourage a patient to undertake excessively strenuous exertion, with a risk of ventricular fibrillation and sudden

Table 7.6: Critique of Various Procedures for Detecting Myocardial Ischaemia

Test criterion	Sensitivity (%)	Specificity (%)
Junctional depression $\geqslant 0.2$ mV	60	50
Upsloping ST segment	30	93
Horizontal or downsloping ST segment	62	91
Tesr type		
Master test (3-min duration)	33	93
Progressive exercise	59	94

Source: C.A. Ascoop (1977).

Table 7.7: Yield of Exercise Stress Tests in a Low-risk and a High-risk Population

	Ischaemia Present	Absent	Total response
(a) Low risk			
All cases	50	950	1,000
Positive stress test	40	95	135
Negative stress test	10	855	865
(b) High risk			
All cases	425	575	1,000
Positive stress test	340	58	398
Negative stress test	85	517	602

death. When undertaking the routine evaluation of an ostensibly healthy sedentary middle-aged adult, a moderate frequency of false negative tests seems acceptable. Indeed, because the prevalence of disease in the general population is quite low, a fairly high sensitivity is needed to ensure a useful yield of positive tests.

The usual criterion is a horizontal or downward-sloping ST depression of more than 0.1 mV. Given a near-maximum test, with

Table 7.8: Relationship between ECG Abnormalities and Coronary Arterial Disease as Demonstrated at Angiography

Arteriographic status	ECG abnormalities (%)
Normal (n = 370)	8
Single-vessel disease (n = 250)	44
Two-vessel disease (n = 285)	73
Three-vessel disease (n = 367)	88
Left main vessel disease (n = 56)	91

Source: Based on data accumulated by C.G. Blomqvist et al. (1978).

multiple-lead recording both during and following exertion, the sensitivity is then 70–80 per cent, and the specificity is around 90 per cent (Tables 7.6 and 7.7). Statistics depend upon the reference criterion; this may be the angiographic appearance (Table 7.8), which itself is subject to variability, or it may be the subsequent development of manifest ischaemic heart disease (angina, myocardial infarction or death); in the latter case, extended clinical observation can convert a false position to a true positive result, but it also increases the number of false negative findings. The proportion of abnormal records is larger if an exercise electrocardiogram is obtained than if reliance is placed upon the recovery record alone; the latter detects about 60 per cent of abnormalities (G.R. Cumming *et al.*, 1972; K.H. Sidney & Shephard, 1977b), while the exercise record picks out some 87 per cent of the ischaemic tracings encountered in exercise plus recovery.

If a vigorous exercise test is used, some ten per cent of men over the age of 40 years, 20 per cent of men over 60 years and an even higher proportion of women show substantial ST segmental depression (Figure 7.6; Table 7.9). However, not all of these individuals have myocardial ischaemia. Particularly in women (G.R. Cumming *et al.*, 1973; K.H. Sidney & Shephard, 1977b), there is a substantial proportion of false positive results. Taking account also of false negative findings, some authors have maintained that the appearance of angina during exercise provides a better indicator of adverse prognosis than does the interpretation of ST segmental voltages (J.P. Cole & Ellestad, 1978). Nevertheless, the development of exercise-induced ST segmental depression in a person with a previously normal exercise electro-

Figure 7.6: Prevalence of ST segmental depression during maximum or near-maximum exercise, in published reports for middle and old age.

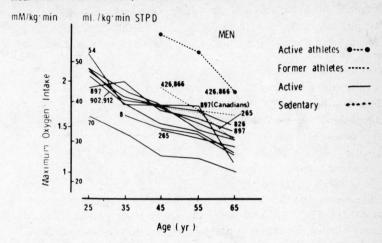

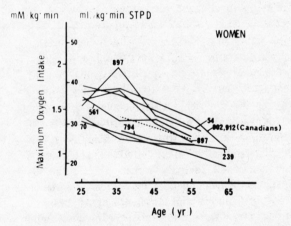

Source: From R.J. Shephard (1978b), by permission of the publishers.

cardiogram is an urgent warning of progressing coronary vascular disease (J.T. Doyle & Kinch, 1970).

Test yield. Mass screening of the general public is sometimes advocated, either in its own right, or as a prelude to the prescription of increased physical activity. However, the wholesale testing of symptomless adults is difficult to justify because of the low yield of useful information.

Table 7.9: Percentage of Elderly Subjects (Usually 60–5 Years Old) showing ECG Evidence of Myocardial Ischaemia (Usually ST Depression > 0.1 mV in Tests at > 75 Per Cent Aerobic Power)

Author*	Percentage of ischaemic records	
	Men	Women
I. Åstrand (1969)	35	55
G.R. Cumming *et al.* (1972, 1973)	37	27
J.R. Brown & Shephard (1967)	—	36
A.E. Doan *et al.* (1965)	46	—
I.S. Kasser & Bruce (1969)	25	—
T. Kavanagh & Shephard (1977a)	17[†]	—
G.R. Profant *et al.* (1972)	—	100
C.P. Riley *et al.* (1970)	32	36
K.H. Sidney & Shephard (1977b)	29	36

* For details of individual references, see Shephard (1978b).
† Masters' Class Athletes.

If 1,000 middle-aged adults are tested, some 135 will show what appears to be an ischaemic stress test, but only 40 of these will be true positive results (Table 7.7). The remainder will receive unnecessary warnings about the dangers of physical activity. A substantial demand will also be created for angiographic tests, the majority of which will prove negative. Of the 40 patients with true positive ischaemic records, perhaps a half will understand and interpret correctly the restrictions that are placed upon their physical activity. Perhaps a half of the 40 true positive tests may also be recommended for coronary by-pass surgery, but since most of them are symptom-free, they will be reluctant to accept this advice. The proportion of the initial screening sample brought to surgical treatment may thus be as low as ten per 1,000, and in the absence of symptoms the usefulness of such surgery will also remain controversial. The remaining 20 true positive patients will probably be recommended for close observation, but again because of the absence of symptoms not all patients will accept this advice. In perhaps ten of the 20, the diagnosis of myocardial ischaemia may reinforce normal medical advice with regard to an improvement of lifestyle. Nevertheless, the total number of individuals helped remains only one person for every fifty tested, so that the cost of such help

Table 7.10: Effective Cost of Helping Patients Through a
Mass-screening Programme for Ischaemic Heart Disease

1,000 stress tests at	$2.43	=	$ 2,430
135 angiographs at	$500 +	=	$67,500
			$69,930
10 patients for surgery 10 patients improve lifestyle		}	cost = $3,497 per person

rises to over $3,000 per patient, a prohibitive figure for a screening programme (Table 7.10).

The yield becomes even smaller, and the cost proportionately higher, if tests are conducted on an annual basis. We are now looking at the incidence rather than the prevalence of disease, in effect progression to the point where ECG changes can be detected. Since subjects usually survive five to ten years after the appearance of ECG changes, incidence is only ten to 20 per cent of prevalence, with a corresponding reduction of yield.

The proportion of positive tests could be increased by augmenting the sensitivity of the test — for example, pushing the patient to a higher intensity of exercise, increasing the number of ECG leads or reducing the amount of ST segmental depression considered as abnormal. However, this would be an unsatisfactory tactic, as it would increase the number of individuals subjected to unnecessary, costly and relatively dangerous angiography.

A more effective approach is to restrict the screening process to individuals with a relatively high risk of coronary arterial disease. R. Paffenbarger (1977) found that the incidence of fatal heart attacks was increased by a factor of 8.5 (from 179 per 100,000 to 1,519 per 100,000) in subjects who combined a low daily energy output with heavy cigarette smoking and a high systolic blood pressure. Assuming that this sub-group had a similarly augmented prevalence of ECG abnormalities, the number of positive tests would rise to 398 per 1,000, more than 85 per cent of these being true positive tests (Table 7.7).

A further factor influencing the practicality of screening procedures is the community participation rate. In Saskatoon, a telephone invitation to attend for a free fitness test and exercise electrocardiogram brought a participation rate of only 35 per cent (D.A. Bailey *et al.*,

1974). In Toronto, establishment of a free clinic in an office building led to participation by about 50 per cent of employees. A half of these went on to join a regular exercise programme that had been organised in the basement of the same building (R.J. Shephard & Cox, in preparation). If the ECG test is to be 'useful', the test result must have a strong impact upon the treatment plan of the physician and/or the health behaviour of the patient. Behavioural scientists have stressed that health behaviour is shaped by health beliefs (M. Becker & Maiman, 1975). In an effective screening programme, the physician or health educator thus takes time to interpret the test result in terms of health outcomes, pointing the path for change (E. Reid, 1979). At a smoking-withdrawal centre where about a third of patients were persuaded to stop smoking for at least one year, many participants commented on the importance of stress-induced ECG abnormalities and dyspnoea as factors contributing to smoking cessation (R.J. Shephard *et al.*, 1972). More recently, paramedical workers have again commented on the value of a simple step test as a motivational tool when seeking lifestyle change (R.J. Shephard, 1980a).

Exercise Stress Tests

General considerations

In the context of ischaemic heart disease, the purposes of an exercise test include: (i) prediction of prognosis; (ii) diagnosis of unusual, exercise induced symptoms; (iii) prescription of an appropriate level of physical activity for both employment and rehabilitation; (iv) monitoring of the response to exercise training; and (v) evaluating the effects of various drugs and of surgical treatment.

Traditionally, observations were confined to the recovery period because of difficulty in counting the pulse and/or recording the electrocardiogram during exercise. However, these difficulties have been overcome by modern ECG technology, and measurements are now routinely made during both exercise and the early recovery period (five to ten minutes post-exercise).

Test protocols

Tests may be made to a target heart rate corresponding to 75 or 85 per cent of maximum oxygen intake. Alternatively, exercise can be continued to a plateau of oxygen consumption (the 'directly measured maximum oxygen intake'), or the test may be 'symptom-limited', activity being halted by the appearance of symptoms such as angina

Figure 7.7: Possible test protocols for carrying a patient to a target heart rate, directly measured maximum oxygen intake or 'symptom-limited' maximum test

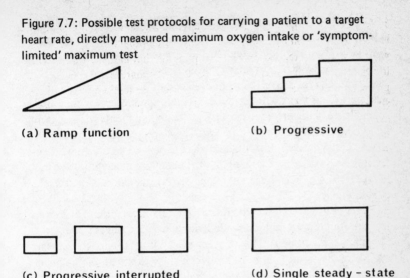

(a) Ramp function   (b) Progressive

(c) Progressive interrupted   (d) Single steady – state

or the appearance of signs (such as an ST segmental depression of more than 0.2 mV).

A variety of test protocols are used to reach these several possible end-points (Figure 7.7). With a *ramp function test*, the loading is increased continuously, or almost continuously, and no steady state is reached. An example of this procedure is the 'Stage One' test of N.L. Jones *et al*. (1975), where the bicycle-ergometer loading is increased by 100 kp·m·min^{-1} at one-minute intervals. The average sedentary subject is carried relatively quickly (within eight or nine minutes) and with little fatigue to a point of voluntary exhaustion. Unfortunately, both heart rate and oxygen consumption lag behind the increase of work rate, so that the subject is incapable of sustaining the 'symptom-limited' power output thus defined. However, the phase lag is relatively similar for heart rate and oxygen intake, so that predictions of maximum oxygen intake based upon the oxygen scale of the Åstrand nomogram do not differ greatly from steady-state values (R.J. Shephard & Kavanagh, 1978c). Perhaps because coronary perfusion improves with a build-up of metabolites in the myocardium, the observed ST segmental depression may be greater with a ramp-function test than with a protocol where a given work rate is sustained for a longer period.

The *progressive sub-maximal test* is the procedure that we have favoured in Toronto. If a cycle ergometer is used, the subject proceeds through three or four stages, each stage augmenting the work rate by 25–50 W; three or at most four minutes are allowed per stage. Normally, this time is sufficient to allow an individual to come very close to a steady-state response of heart rate, blood pressure and oxygen intake for a given work rate, since individual increments of loading are fairly small. Some authors have expressed a fear that longer intervals are necessary to reach a steady state in patients with ischaemic heart disease. This is true of cases with advanced cardiac failure or a 'sick-sinus' syndrome, but in the average patient referred for exercise rehabilitation, the 'on transient' for the exercise-induced increase of heart rate and oxygen intake develops much as in a normal person (Table 7.11).

In the *progressive interrupted test* an interval, sometimes as long as ten minutes, is allowed between individual exercise stages (R.J. Shephard *et al.*, 1968a). The recovery period is short enough that the subject retains some 'warm-up' from one stage to the next. The main advantage of this approach is that it is possible to examine recovery from a given intensity of exercise before proceeding to a higher work rate. This is an important consideration, as dysrhythmias are often concentrated in the recovery phase. Nevertheless, the interrupted protocol is not popular with either physicians or patients, since the total test duration is inevitably extended from a few minutes to almost an hour.

The *single steady-state test* is sometimes used for the direct measurement of maximum oxygen intake. The subject must then return on several occasions to attempt exercise at slightly higher work rates. Now that it is appreciated that a similar result can be obtained by a progressive protocol (R.J. Shephard *et al.*, 1968b), few investigators persist with the single steady-state test.

Choice of ergometer

The most commonly used modes of exercise are a step test, a cycle ergometer and a treadmill (R.J. Shephard, 1977a). The *step test* is simple, inexpensive and needs no calibrating. It is well-suited to mass screening (R.J. Shephard, 1980a). Given careful skin preparation, a good-quality electrocardiogram can be obtained. It is possible to measure the oxygen cost of the activity by the usual open-circuit techniques, and a good estimate of oxygen intake can also be obtained from the rate of working (the product of body mass, step height and the number of ascents per minute). If oxygen intake is estimated rather than measured, it is important that subjects adhere to the required

Table 7.11: Rate of Adjustment to Exercise in Normal Subjects (A), Patients Progressing Well (B), Patients Progressing Poorly (C) and New Entrants to a Post-coronary Rehabilitation Programme (D), Given in the Form of Three-minute Responses to Progressive Exercise Expressed as a Percentage of Five-minute Response

Work rate	Group	Heart rate (%)	Resp. minute volume (%)	Oxygen cons. (%)	Resp. gas exch. ratio (%)	Predicted max O_2 intake
One	A	101.1	92.4	99.7	89.0	—
	B	98.7	98.8	81.2	101.7	—
	C	98.4	101.7	97.7	102.2	—
	D	100.2	103.9	96.2	105.0	—
Two	A	101.1	93.8	100.3	83.9	—
	B	97.6	92.5	88.1	102.9	—
	C	97.5	93.8	95.3	98.9	—
	D	99.0	93.9	93.4	98.7	—
Three	A	101.3	97.8	99.6	103.4	—
	B	96.8	90.0	93.2	99.1	101.9
	C	96.1	88.3	89.1	100.0	96.5
	D	98.1	94.8	97.0	100.0	97.7
Four	A	99.5	96.1	96.8	105.0	—
	B	97.5	99.1	104.5	97.5	108.7
	C	98.0	93.8	98.2	102.0	101.5
	D	95.5	90.1	94.4	100.0	98.7

Source: Based on data of R.J. Shephard & Kavanagh (1978c).

rhythm of stepping, ascending and descending the full height of the step at each cycle. Such exercise is performed with a mechanical efficiency of about 16 per cent (I. Ryhming, 1954; R.J. Shephard, 1967b; Table 7.12). The main disadvantage of a stepping test is that movement of the subject impedes blood sampling, measurements of blood pressure and cardiac-output determinations.

The *cycle ergometer* is quite expensive but, nevertheless, has some attraction for clinical testing. The patient can remain seated

Table 7.12: Estimation of Oxygen Intake from Work Rate during Stepping Exercise

Work rate (kJ•min $^{-1}$)	=	0.00981 × (step height, m) × (Body mass, kg) × (stepping rate per min)
Energy cost (kJ•min $^{-1}$)	=	(100/16) × (work rate)
Oxygen cost (l•min $^{-1}$)	=	(100/16) × (work rate) × (1/21)
Total oxygen intake (l•min $^{-1}$)	=	oxygen cost + resting metabolism
	=	[(100/16) × (work rate) × (1/21)] + [0.3]

Table 7.13: Estimate of Oxygen Intake from Work Rate during Mechanically Braked Cycle Ergometry

Work rate (kJ•min $^{-1}$)	=	(loading, kg) × (flywheel circumference, m) × (gear ratio) × (pedal revs per min)
Energy cost (kJ•min $^{-1}$)	=	(100/23) × (work rate)
Oxygen cost (l•min $^{-1}$)	=	(100/23) × (work rate) × (1/21)
Total oxygen intake (l•min $^{-1}$)	=	oxygen cost + resting metabolism
	=	[(100/23) × (work rate) × (1/21)] + [0.3]

throughout an investigation, and data on blood pressure and cardiac output are readily collected. Unfortunately, the average coronary-prone patient has not used a bicycle for many years. He thus operates the machine in an inefficient manner and this problem can invalidate estimates of oxygen intake that are based upon the mechanical work performed. The standard test format also places a heavy load upon the quadriceps muscle (M. Hoes *et al.*, 1968), and maximum effort is determined by problems in perfusing the active fibres rather than by the performance of the heart (C. Kay & Shephard, 1969). Often, there is a substantial discrepancy between the maximum oxygen intake determined on a cycle ergometer, and that observed during uphill treadmill running (R.J. Shephard *et al.*, 1968b). If oxygen intake is estimated from the work performed (Table 7.13), there are also problems of instrument calibration. Jarring of an electrical ergometer can change dynamo characteristics (N. Jones & Kane, 1979), and supposedly automatic adjustments for variations of pedal speed may also be inappropriate, since efficiency varies with the rate of pedalling

(D. Gueli & Shephard, 1976). In both mechanical and electrical machines, a substantial proportion of unmeasured effort is lost in the pedal bearings and chain mechanism (G.R. Cumming & Alexander, 1968). In some clinical applications, the ergometer is pedalled from the supine or semi-supine position. This allows the use of such techniques as echo-cardiography, nuclear cardiology and cardiac catheterisation, but the activity is then unnatural, and firm shoulder supports are needed to operate the machine. Arm and shoulder ergometers may be used to provide additional information, particularly if a subject's employment calls for vigorous arm exercise. On occasion, a normal electrocardiographic response may be observed during leg ergometry, but during arm exercise ST segmental depression appears as the heart endeavours to pump blood through small but vigorously contracting muscles.

The *treadmill* is bulky, noisy, and expensive. It is sometimes claimed that walking is a very natural form of exercise, but this hardly applies to the task of maintaining a constant position on a narrow and inclined moving belt while breathing through a mouthpiece! Running to exhaustion on a steep and rapidly moving belt is even less natural, and can be quite a frightening experience for the novitiate. One possible advantage of the treadmill when testing a sedentary subject is that exercise is 'machine-paced'. A subject cannot slow down when he becomes tired. This makes it easier to reach the central exhaustion desired in a maximum-oxygen-intake measurement, but at the same time it poses a mechanical danger of stumbling and increases the risk of cardiac problems. Oxygen intake can be measured quite readily while running, but it is difficult to change mouthpieces for a cardiac-output measurement while using the treadmill. Rhythmic vibration of the body may cause a poor-quality electrocardiogram, particularly in a subject who is obese and has pendulous skinfolds. The standard clinical measurement of blood pressure is relatively difficult to obtain while running, and blood sampling is often unsatisfactory unless the subject has an intra-arterial catheter. The oxygen cost of sub-maximal running can be predicted from the speed and slope of the treadmill to about ten per cent (R.J. Shephard, 1968c) and, if the Bruce protocol is followed, the maximum oxygen intake can be estimated (Table 7.14) from the endurance time during a progressive, exhausting test. The treadmill is a particularly valuable tool when it is necessary to obtain a direct measurement of maximum oxygen intake. The results obtained during uphill running to exhaustion are not normally exceeded during any other form of exercise (R.J. Shephard, 1977a).

Table 7.14: Oxygen cost of Treadmill Running

(a)   **Sub-maximal exercise (Shephard, 1968c)**

O_2 intake $(ml \cdot kg^{-1} \cdot min^{-1}) = [V (km \cdot h^{-1}) \times (2.88 + \theta \times 0.23)] + 7.7$
where θ is the treadmill slope in per cent.

(b)   **Maximal oxygen intake**, as predicted from endurance time during
progressive, exhausting exercise (after R.A. Bruce *et al.*, 1973)

Duration (min)	Speed $(km \cdot h^{-1})$	Slope (%)	Approximate O_2 cost $(ml \cdot kg^{-1} \cdot min^{-1})$
3	2.72	10	17.4
4	4.00	12	19.8
5	4.00	12	22.3
6	4.00	12	24.8
7	5.44	14	27.9
8	5.44	14	31.1
9	5.44	14	34.3
10	6.72	16	37.4
11	6.72	16	40.6
12	6.72	16	43.8

Measurements

Aerobic performance. The exercise test is commonly used to assess
aerobic performance. As noted above, the test may be carried to
voluntary or symptom-limited exhaustion. Note can then be kept of the
power output (watts, measured on the cycle ergometer), the treadmill
endurance time (Bruce protocol; Table 7.14), the maximum rate of
climbing of a standard staircase or the distance run in a standard time
(Table 7.15). Alternatively, the oxygen consumption can be measured
at frequent intervals until a plateau is reached despite further increases
of work rate (the 'directly measured maximum oxygen intake'). This is
usually defined as an intensity of exercise where a further five per
cent increase in work rate increases oxygen intake by less than 2
$ml \cdot kg^{-1} \cdot min^{-1}$ (R.J. Shephard *et al.*, 1968b). It is sometimes stated
that it is dangerous to measure the maximum oxygen intake in post-
coronary patients, and that the usually accepted criteria of maximum
effort (R.J. Shephard *et al.*, 1968b) are obscured by such characteristics

Table 7.15: Distance Run over a Twelve-minute Interval and Maximum Oxygen Intake

Distance covered in 12 min* (km)	Maximum oxygen intake $(ml \cdot kg^{-1} \cdot min^{-1})$
< 1.6	< 28.0
1.6–2.0	28.0–34.0
2.0–2.4	34.1–42.0
2.4–2.8	42.1–52.0
> 2.8	> 52.0

* This test requires good cooperation from the subject, a knowledge of pacing and a willingness to undertake twelve minutes of all-out effort. It is thus not suitable for unsupervised testing of newly recruited, sedentary and coronary-prone adults. However, it can be used to monitor progress after rehabilitation has commenced.
Source: Based on the data of K.H. Cooper (1968).

Table 7.16: Characteristics of Maximum Oxygen Intake in Healthy Young Normal Subjects (a), Recently Recruited 'Post-coronary' Patients (b), Successfully Rehabilitated 'Post-coronary' Patients (c), and Patients with a Limited Response to Rehabilitation (d)

Variable	Group (a) Good max.	Group (b) All	Group (b) Good max.[1]	Group (c) All	Group (c) Good max.[1]	Group (d) All	Group (d) Good max.[1]
Age (years)	26.4	45.3		42.2		48.3	
Aerobic power							
($l \cdot min^{-1}$ STPD)	3.81	1.93	—	2.63	—	2.25	—
($ml \cdot kg^{-1} \cdot min^{-1}$ STPD)	49.4	24.6	26.1	36.9	36.9	29.8	29.9
Predicted aerobic power[3]							
($ml \cdot kg^{-1} \cdot min^{-1}$)	45.9	26.1	27.6	35.2	37.7	27.7	29.8
Δ measured	−3.5	−0.5	−1.5	−0.6	−0.8	−2.8	+ 0.1
Max. heart rate							
(beats $\cdot min^{-1}$)	190	161	167	170	170	168	173
Δ predicted[2]	−5	−22	−17	−15	−15	−11	−8
Respiratory gas-exchange ratio	—	—	1.22	—	1.50	—	1.24
Blood lactate ($mmol \cdot l^{-1}$)	13.6	—	11.4	—	13.7	—	11.3

1. Subjects judged from observation to have made a good effort to reach exhaustion.
2. Our prediction is exigent (a linear decline of heart rate from 195 beats $\cdot min^{-1}$ at age 25 to 170 beats $\cdot min^{-1}$ at age 65).
3. Omitting observations where heart rate falls outside range permitted for use of Åstrand nomogram.

Source: Based in part on R.J. Shephard *et al.* (1968b) and T. Kavanagh & Shephard (1976a).

of the disease as a slowing of maximum heart rate, an increase in anaerobic work and a slow approach to an oxygen-intake plateau. T. Kavanagh & Shephard (1976a) examined three groups of post-coronary patients — those recently recruited, those successfully rehabilitated and those responding poorly to rehabilitation (Table 7.16). A total of 36 individuals were tested. One subject developed persistent chest pain, two had transient ventricular tachycardia and one frequent premature ventricular contractions that persisted for about a minute a quarter after exercise. The usual reasons for halting the test were exhaustion, manifested as vertigo, incoordination, a staggering gait, or weakness in the legs. However, two tests were stopped for gross ST depression (> 0.5 mV), and in one patient the limiting factor was back pain. As in normal young subjects, the directly measured maximum oxygen intake on average agreed quite closely with the value predicted from the heart rate response to sub-maximal exercise (Table 7.16). The maximum respiratory gas-exchange ratio exceeded the figure of 1.15 normally anticipated in young and healthy adults, while the terminal blood lactate of those patients who had completed successful rehabilitation was well up to the level required of younger individuals. Heart rates were apparently somewhat less than predicted values, although our predicted figures were based upon a more exigent standard than that used in many reports. These experiments demonstrated that the typical patient referred for 'post-coronary' rehabilitation can perform a directly measured test reasonably well; on the other hand, we observed some potentially dangerous test sequelae, and in view of the correspondence between directly measured and predicted maxima, it seems preferable to base the routine assessment of the post-coronary victim upon a sub-maximum test.

The Åstrand nomogram is one simple approach to sub-maximum assessment. Modifications of the nomogram now permit the prediction of maximum oxygen intake from sex-specific diagrams that need no age correction (Figure 7.8). Alternatively, the equivalent formulae can be used in computer predictions of maximum oxygen intake (R.J. Shephard, 1977a).

A third possibility is to report the heart rate at a fixed oxygen intake or work rate. For example, data from the Southern Ontario multi-centre exercise-heart trial have been interpolated or briefly extrapolated to a common oxygen intake of 1.25 l·min^{-1}, while in the Canadian Home Fitness Test a simple classification of fitness is based upon endurance time and the immediate recovery heart rate when subjects

Figure 7.8: Age- and sex-specific nomogram for the prediction of maximum oxygen intake from heart rate and oxygen intake in sub-maximum effort. In the event that oxygen intake is not measured, it may be estimated as $[0.012W + 0.3]$ l·min^{-1} (where W is the power output in watts, measured on a cycle ergometer), or $[4/3 \times (MN \times 10^{-3}) + 0.3]$ l·min^{-1} (where M is body mass in kg, and N is the number of complete ascents of a 45-cm step per minute).

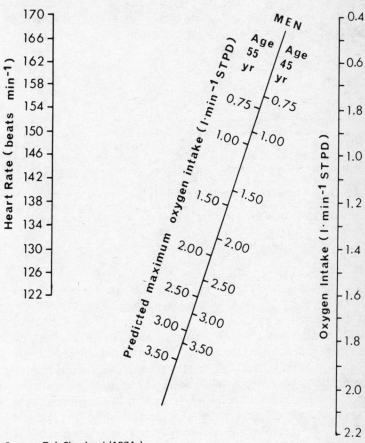

Source: R.J. Shephard (1974c).

Table 7.17: Prediction of Aerobic Fitness from Endurance Time and Immediate Post-exercise Ten-second Pulse Count*

Age (years)	Stepping rate (per min)†	First 3 min (Undesirable fitness level)	Second 3 min	
			(Minimum fitness level)	(Recommended fitness level)
15–19	144	≥ 30	≥ 27	≤ 26
20–9	144	≥ 29	≥ 26	≤ 25
30–9	132	≥ 28	≥ 25	≤ 24
40–9	114	≥ 26	≥ 24	≤ 23
50–9	102	≥ 25	≥ 23	≤ 22
60–9	84	≥ 24	≥ 23	≤ 22
Warm-up for oldest group	66			

* Data for male subjects climbing 40.6-cm double step at age- and sex-specific rhythm set by a long-playing record ('Canadian Home Fitness Test'). Preliminary clearance by a medical screening questionnaire (Par-Q; D. Chisholm *et al.*, 1975) is recommended. Climbing rates are slightly lower for women, to allow for their lower aerobic power per unit of body mass.
† Each subject performs the first three minutes of exercise at a rate appropriate for someone ten years older. Assuming the resultant pulse count is not excessive, he proceeds after a 25-second interval to a rate appropriate for a person of his own age.

Source: D.A. Bailey *et al.* (1974); R.J. Shephard (1980a).

climb a domestic staircase at an age- and sex-specific rate corresponding to an anticipated 70 per cent of maximum oxygen intake (Table 7.17; R.J. Shephard, 1980a).

Difficulties with such sub-maximum assessments include uncertainties about maximum heart rate (a problem with the sick-sinus syndrome and inferior infarcts), inter-individual differences in maximum heart rate, nonlinearity of the oxygen intake/heart rate relationship, drug-induced modifications of the heart-rate response to exercise (for example, β-blocking agents, guanethidine, methyldopa), and possibly activation of ventricular-wall baro-receptors in severely diseased hearts (A.J. Wohl *et al.*, 1977).

Where the test is being conducted for clinical purposes such as exercise prescription, it may suffice to note the heart rate at which electrocardiographic abnormalities appear, setting prescribed activity at a suitable margin below this threshold. One difficulty with this approach is that the increment of blood pressure and thus the cardiac work rate differs when a given heart rate is attained by arm rather than leg exercise. If electrocardiographic abnormalities develop, it is thus preferable to limit effort in terms of some index of cardiac work rate, as discussed below.

Systemic blood pressure. The systemic blood-pressure response to exercise is monitored in order to avoid either an excessive rise or an undue fall in pressure. The pressure recorded by a standard sphygmomanometer cuff may differ from the true intravascular pressure during vigorous exercise (Marx *et al.*, 1967). Nevertheless, cuff recordings are the most practical approach when repeated assessments are required, as in a cardiac-rehabilitation programme. The cuff must be of sufficient size to encircle the arm; if this precaution is neglected, an apparent change of pressure may arise as an obese patient loses sub-cutaneous fat.

Thorough habituation to the investigator and the testing laboratory is also important, otherwise the process of familiarisation may lead to a progressive fall of blood pressure. Of the individuals told that they are hypertensive by a physician, relatively few have a high blood pressure when measurements are made in a relaxed setting (R.J. Shephard *et al.*, 1979b).

Anaerobic threshold. If the work rate is increased progressively, a point is reached where the oxygen delivery to the muscle is no longer sufficient to sustain the activity. Lactic acid begins to accumulate, and there is a disproportionate hyperventilation, with an increase in the respiratory gas-exchange ratio. It has been suggested that this anaerobic threshold bears a consistent relationship to the maximum oxygen intake, thus providing an estimate of endurance fitness that does not require maximal exertion (B. Whipp *et al.*, 1977). In practice, this hope has not been realised. The build-up of lactate varies with the test protocol (for example, step versus ramp function; Figure 7.7); the type of activity (lactate accumulates at a much lower fraction of maximum oxygen intake during cycle ergometry than during step or treadmill tests; R.J. Shephard *et al.*, 1968a); and the level of training (an individual with strongly developed muscles is better able to sustain perfusion during vigorous effort; C. Kay & Shephard, 1969; in contrast, many post-coronary patients have weak muscles, and accumulate lactate at a small fraction of their maximum oxygen intake; S. Degré *et al.*, 1972).

Cardiac work rate. Non-invasive indices of myocardial oxygen consumption include: (i) the heart rate; (ii) the product of systolic pressure and heart rate, sometimes called the tension-time index; (iii) the triple product (systolic pressure × heart rate × duration of systole; G. Blomqvist, 1974); and (iv) multiple regression models based upon systolic pressure and heart rate.

Heart rate is proportional to cardiac work rate only if ventricular pressure, stroke volume, heart size, heart shape and myocardial contractility all remain constant (R.G. Monroe & French, 1961; E.L. Rollett *et al.*, 1965; S. Rodbard *et al.*, 1959; E.H. Sonnenblick *et al.*, 1965; J. Ross, 1972). Despite these limitations, heart rate has proved quite a useful index in some animal experiments (C.R. Jorgensen, 1972; Y. Wang, 1972); this has reflected a close correlation between systemic blood pressure and heart rate in the chosen experimental model (C. Jorgensen *et al.*, 1977), a situation unlikely to prevail in the patient with ischaemic heart disease.

The validity of the systolic pressure-heart rate product and of related multiple-regression equations still depends upon the constancy of stroke volume, heart size and myocardial contractility. The index is said to correlate quite well with more direct measurements of myocardial oxygen consumption (D. Laurent *et al.*, 1956; L.N. Katz & Feinberg, 1958; S.J. Sarnoff *et al.*, 1958; R.G. Monroe & French, 1961; R.J. Ferguson & Gauthier, 1975; E.A. Amsterdam & Mason, 1977; C.R. Jorgensen *et al.*, 1977), although it can be invalidated by drugs that affect ventricular volume and contractility (particularly the β-blocking agents).

The triple product has the soundest theoretical basis, since the only interfering variables are the cardiac stroke volume and heart size. Unfortunately, there is no accurate non-invasive method of measuring systolic contraction time, and for this reason the triple product has no closer correlation with myocardial oxygen consumption than that obtained from the tension-time product (R.G. Monroe, 1964; C.R. Jorgensen *et al.*, 1977).

Test safety. The risks of exercise testing were discussed in the last section of Chapter 6. Given a coronary-prone population, there is a likelihood of one episode of ventricular fibrillation for every 10,000 sub-maximal tests, with as many as one episode for every 3,000 maximal tests. The majority of those affected have a healthier myocardium than patients who develop ventricular fibrillation while at rest. Furthermore, skilled medical attention is at hand, and the myocardium is not subjected to a long period of hypoxia. Resuscitation is thus successful in most instances. Nevertheless, the incidence of cardiac emergencies is sufficient to insist that personnel have recent familiarity with resuscitation procedures, plus the necessary equipment for cardiac massage and/or defibrillation.

Fibrillation is probably provoked by a combination of exercise and fear. Thus, the patient should be reassured before he exercises, and unnecessary frightening apparatus should be removed from view. The test itself should be conducted in a relaxed, informal manner. The safety of informal testing is illustrated by experience with the Canadian Fitness Test. This procedure has now been performed by over 500,000 people of all ages. The required intensity of stepping amounts to 70 per cent of maximum oxygen intake, yet the only known complications have been one ankle injury and a few transient faints following exertion.

How important is the preliminary screening of patients presenting for exercise? Comment has already been made upon the Physical Activity Readiness Questionnaire that is issued with the Canadian Home Fitness Test (PAR-Q; D. Chisholm *et al.*, 1975). This simple screening tool seems to be effective in excluding most of the patients with obvious contraindications to exercise, although it is somewhat over-exigent, since some 20 per cent of office volunteers respond positively to one or more of its seven questions (R.J. Shephard, 1980e). Medical screening is equally unsatisfactory; different physicians prohibit exercise testing in 0.7 to 15.6 per cent of volunteers, and apparently this decision has almost no influence upon the frequency of electrocardiographic abnormalities that develop during exercise (R.J. Shephard, 1980e). Nevertheless, certain well-recognised contra-indications to exercise can be identified at a preliminary medical examination (Table 7.18).

A second safeguard is a careful monitoring of the subject during exercise. Usually accepted indications for halting a test are shown in Table 7.19. Some authors now question the need to abort a test at an ST depression of 0.2 mV. Anginal pain is rarely sensed until there is 0.3–0.4 mV of ST depression, and on occasion subjects have been exercised with impunity to ~ 1 mV of ST depression (G. Cumming, personal communication).

Table 7.18: Contraindications to Exercise Testing

Absolute contraindications

Acute infectious disease

Unstable metabolic disorder

Significant locomotor disturbance

Excessive anxiety

Recent or impending myocardial infarction

Manifest cardiac failure

Acute myocarditis

Aortic stenosis

Probability of recent pulmonary embolism

Special precautions needed

Atrial fibrillation or flutter

Atrio-ventricular block

Left bundle-branch block

Premature ventricular excitation (Wolff-Parkinson-White syndrome)

Table 7.19: Indications for Halting Exercise

Increasing chest pain

Severe dyspnoea or fatigue

Faintness

Claudication

Signs of cerebrovascular insufficiency (pallor, cold moist skin, cyanosis, staggering gait, confusion)

Excessive rise in blood pressure

Sudden fall in systolic pressure

ST segmental depression > 0.2 mV (horizontal or downsloping)

Premature ventricular contractions (more than three in ten seconds, polyfocal, R on T)

Paroxysmal ventricular or supraventricular dysrhythmias

Conduction disturbances other than slight atrio-ventricular block

8 HEART AND CORONARY CIRCULATION IN EXERCISE

In this chapter, we shall take a brief look at normal responses of the heart and coronary circulation to exercise and training. We shall also examine possible modifications of response encountered in patients with ischaemic heart disease.

Heart Rate

Normal values

The 'resting' heart rate is normally 70-80 beats·min $^{-1}$, although much lower values (down to 30 beats·min $^{-1}$) are encountered in highly trained endurance athletes (Chapter 4). Since the resting cardiac output per unit of body surface area is relatively fixed at 3.0-3.5 l·min $^{-1}$·m $^{-2}$, measurement of the resting heart rate provides some guide to resting stroke volume:

Cardiac output = heart rate X stroke volume

In practice, it is difficult to use the resting heart rate in this manner, since the cardiac frequency is increased by anxiety, a high environmental temperature, recent food, drink, drugs such as tobacco and exercise. Two possible approaches are to take the pulse rate immediately on waking, or to measure the sleeping heart rate by means of a portable tape recorder (R.J. Shephard, 1978).

The heart rate increases with exercise, the rate of rise being a linear function of oxygen consumption between 50 and 90-100 per cent of maximum oxygen intake. The linearity of this relationship provides the basis of various procedures for predicting maximum oxygen intake from the heart rate during sub-maximum effort (I. Åstrand, 1960; J.S. Maritz et al., 1961; R. Margaria et al., 1965).

The maximum heart rate of a young man is normally about 195 beats·min $^{-1}$, with an inter-individual variation of some 5-10 beats·min $^{-1}$. Lower maxima (185-195 beats·min $^{-1}$) are sometimes seen in well-trained endurance athletes (C.T.M. Davies, 1967; B. Saltin & Åstrand, 1967; M. Lester et al., 1968) and at high altitudes (threshold for an effect, 2,000 metres, with a decrease to ~ 135 beats•min $^{-1}$ at 6,000 metres; L.G.C.E. Pugh, 1962; E.L. Buskirk *et al.*, 1967).

Aging leads to a progressive reduction in maximum heart rate. At one time it was held that the average value for a 65-year-old man was about 160 beats•min $^{-1}$ (S. Robinson, 1938; E. Asmussen & Molbech, 1959), but more recent observers have set the maximum for a sedentary 65-year old North American at more than 170 beats•min $^{-1}$ (S.M. Fox & Haskell, 1968b; M. Lester *et al.*, 1968; K.H. Sidney & Shephard, 1977c). The reason why aging has this effect is unclear. Unlike the situation at altitude, an old person cannot counteract the slowing of maximum heart rate by the inhalation of oxygen (I. Åstrand *et al.*, 1959). Possibly, the rate of diastolic filling becomes a factor limiting cardiac performance. Greater stiffness of the ventricular wall could increase filling time and modify the feedback of information to the cardio-regulatory centres. Alternatively, the sympathetic drive to the cardiac pacemaker may diminish with age.

Ischaemic heart disease

Several recent reports have suggested a sub-normal response of heart rate to exercise in ischaemic heart disease (L.E. Hinckle *et al.*, 1972; M. Ellestad & Wan, 1975; A.C.P. Powles *et al.*, 1979).

In some cases, there is a simple explanation for this. A stress test may be 'symptom-limited', exercise being halted short of an oxygen consumption plateau on account of concern on the part of the patient or supervising personnel, symptoms such as chest pain, electrocardiographic changes (K.L. Andersen *et al.*, 1971) or an excessive rise in blood pressure. The patient may be receiving β-blocking drugs such as propranolol; he may also have heart failure or an abnormal cardiac rhythm. Because ischaemic heart disease is seen mainly in heavy smokers, there is commonly some associated chronic obstructive lung disease; performance is then limited by respiratory rather than cardiac function (B.W. Armstrong *et al.*, 1967), activity being halted by extreme breathlessness at a relatively low heart rate.

In other instances, the problem lies with test methodology — for instance, maximum exercise may have been attempted on a cycle ergometer rather than a treadmill, with failure to demonstrate an oxygen plateau (A.C.P. Powles *et al.*, 1979); the heart rate is then limited by quadriceps exhaustion rather than the usual ceiling of cardiac performance.

Finally, the proportion of patients rated as having a chronotropic disorder depends markedly upon the placing of the 'normal' age/

maximum heart-rate line (T. Kavanagh & Shephard, 1976). If the data of M. Lester *et al.* (1968) is used as the normal standard, many patients will be rated as abnormal, but if the less rigorous criterion of E. Asmussen & Molbech (1959) is accepted, the proportion so classified will be much smaller. T. Kavanagh & Shephard (1976) asked 36 post-coronary patients to develop a maximum power output by uphill treadmill walking; 20 of the 36 individuals reached a true 'centrally limited' maximum oxygen intake, defined by an oxygen consumption plateau. Maximum heart-rate readings were compared with predicted norms that decreased linearly from a maximum of 195 beats·min^{-1} at age 25 to 170 beats·min^{-1} at age 65. The majority of those tested failed to attain this exacting standard (Table 7.16). Even among the 20 patients who satisfied objective criteria of a centrally limited maximum oxygen intake, the discrepancy between predicted and actual heart rate maxima amounted to about 14 beats·min^{-1}. On the other hand, the observed maxima averaged only 3 beats·min^{-1} less than the earlier age-related standards of E. Asmussen & Molbech (1959).

A.C.P. Powles *et al.* (1979) suggested that 18 of the 39 post-coronary patients that they tested had an abnormal heart-rate maximum. This interpretation was apparently based on an incorrectly plotted line of normality (R.J. Shephard, in preparation) — in fact, only four of the 39 individuals had heart rates more than two standard deviations below the line proposed by E. Asmussen & Molbech (1959). Nevertheless, Powles *et al.* made the interesting observation that the 18 subjects classed as having a low maximum heart rate also tended to show an abnormally slow heart-rate response to sub-maximum effort. Among this sub-group of 18 patients, exercise bradycardia was more marked in those with an inferior than in those with an anterior or an antero-lateral infarct, this difference being increased by vagal blockade. Since there is no great difference in the speed of adaptation to exercise in 'post-coronary' patients (R.J. Shephard & Kavanagh, 1978c; A.C.P. Powles *et al.*, 1979), exercise bradycardia cannot be attributed to a delayed 'on transient'. The most likely explanation is a local ischaemia and/or infarction of the sinu-atrial mode; oxygen lack from any cause impairs the response to both adrenergic and cholinergic stimulation (M.F. Sheets *et al.*, 1975). A further possibility is autonomic imbalance — either failure to withdraw parasympathetic tone during exercise (S. Robinson *et al.*, 1953) or a depletion of myocardial epinephrine stores secondary to cardiac failure (C.A. Chidsey *et al.*, 1965; G.D. Beiser *et al.*, 1968).

Given that at least a small proportion of 'post-coronary' patients show slow heart rates during both sub-maximal and maximal effort, what are the practical implications for exercise testing and prescription? T. Kavanagh & Shephard (1976) tested the accuracy of aerobic power predictions based upon the oxygen consumption at a target heart rate (Table 7.16). The systematic error was smaller than in healthy subjects and the standard deviation of this discrepancy (5-7 ml·kg^{-1}·min^{-1}) was similar to that encountered in normal individuals.

However, in that small sample of subjects with a 'sick-sinus' syndrome, extrapolation to an age-related anticipated maximum heart rate can give a misleading overestimate of maximum oxygen intake and maximum power output (A.C.P. Powles *et al.*, 1979), with a corresponding potential for over-prescription of exercise. There is thus virtue in carrying out at least one simple test to exhaustion on each 'post-coronary' patient; this assesses whether the anticipated age-related maximum heart rate can be reached and, in the event that it cannot, a symptom-limited maximum power output may be established.

Stroke Volume

Normal values

Under normal resting conditions, a standing or a seated subject expels some 80 ml of blood from each ventricle with every heart beat. The diastolic volume of the left ventricle is about 160 ml and around a half of this volume is emptied during systole. Stroke volume is increased with rhythmic exercise, a plateau of some 110-35 ml per beat being reached at 40-50 per cent of maximum oxygen intake. This is achieved by a greater emptying of the heart (increase of contractility and decrease of cardiac reserve). At higher work rates there may also be some increase of end-diastolic volume (L.D. Horwitz *et al.*, 1972) and pressure (J.S. Williamson *et al.*, 1978). Young adults are able to maintain the augmented stroke volume to 100 per cent of maximum oxygen intake, but in older individuals there is a tendency for stroke volume to decrease at the highest work rates (A. Granath *et al.*, 1964; M. Becklake *et al.*, 1965; G. Grimby *et al.*, 1966; J.S. Hanson *et al.*, 1968; V. Niinimaa & Shephard, 1978; Figure 8.1). It is unclear how far this impairment of myocardial performance reflects diminishing myocardial perfusion, lesser cardiac compliance or poorer ventricular contractility; other factors are reduced pre-loading (a failure of venous return) and increased after-loading (a rise in systemic blood pressure).

The maximum stroke volume is influenced by the fitness of an

Figure 8.1: Cardiac response to exercise in normal young adults (solid lines) and elderly subjects (interrupted lines). Subjects walking on treadmill at increasing slopes.

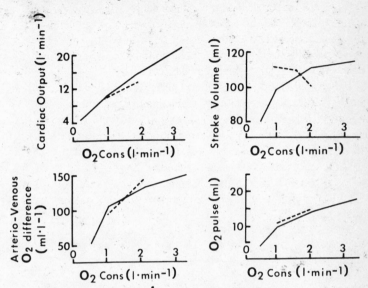

Source: Based on data of V. Niinimaa & Shephard (1978).

individual, being 20–30 ml larger in a well-trained endurance athlete than in a sedentary person. Values obtained on a bicycle ergometer are 10–15 ml lower than those seen on a treadmill (R.J. Shephard, 1977a). If exercise is performed in the supine position, the resting stroke volume is increased to ∼ 110 ml, but little augmentation of output per beat occurs during physical activity.

The largest stroke volume may be seen in the first few seconds after maximum effort, particularly if venous return is sustained by loadless pedalling during the recovery period (D.I. Goldberg & Shephard, 1980). G. Cumming (personal communication) has thus suggested that interval work is the most effective technique for increasing an individual's maximum stroke volume. With static (isometric) exercise, stroke volume shows little change, emptying of the left ventricle against the increased 'after-load' being sustained by an increase in left-ventricular force, with little increase in left-ventricular end-diastolic pressure (R.H. Helfant *et al.*, 1971; C. Kivowitz *et al.*, 1971; C.B. Mullins & Blomqvist, 1973).

Figure 8.2: Relationship between stroke volume and oxygen intake in patients with myocardial infarction alone and in those with infarction plus angina or angina alone. Shading indicates normal response (see D.H. Paterson et al., 1979).

Authors: (1) R. Malmcrona et al. (1963); (2) J.O. Parker et al. (1967); (3) B.E. Higgs et al. (1968); (4) K. Kato & Watanabe (1971); (5) R.A. Bruce et al. (1974a); (6) J. McDonough et al. (1974); (7) N. Rousseau et al. (1973); (8) O. Müller & Rørvik (1958); (9) M. Najmi & Segal (1967); (10) M.H. Frick & Katila (1968); (11) J.P. Clausen et al. (1969); (12) J.V. Messer et al. (1963); (13) R.A. Bruce et al. (1974b); (14) R.P. Malmborg (1964); (15) G.L. Foster & Reeves (1964).

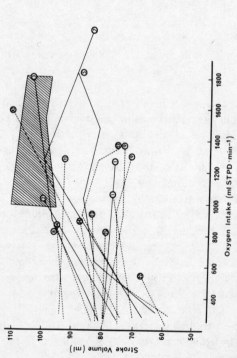

Source: Based on data accumulated by D.H. Paterson.

Figure 8.3: Changes of cardiac function with three weeks of bed rest and seven weeks of subsequent training, for healthy young adults.

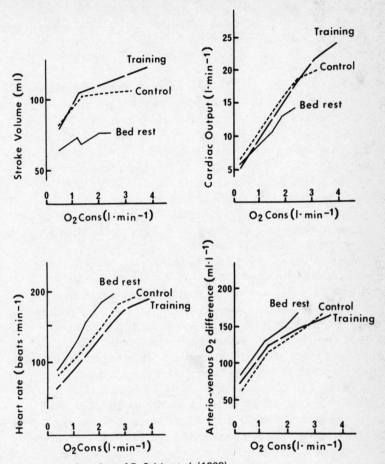

Source: Based on data of B. Saltin *et al.* (1968).

Ischaemic heart disease

Ischaemic heart disease tends to impair stroke volume for several reasons — loss of physical condition during bed rest, abnormal motion of the ventricular wall (Chapter 1) and continuing ischaemia of the myocardium (Figure 8.2).

Two to three weeks of bed rest of itself can cause a 20–30 ml decrease in both resting and exercise cardiac stroke volume (B. Saltin *et al.*, 1968). Thus, a reduced stroke volume is to be anticipated if a 'post-coronary' patient is recruited soon after infarction. In a healthy individual, the normal stroke volume can be restored by a few weeks of training (Figure 8.3; B. Saltin *et al.*, 1968). Following myocardial infarction, the exercise prescription is more cautious, but nevertheless, a gradual reversal of the bed-rest effect occurs (D.H. Paterson *et al.*, 1979).

The pumping function of the ventricular wall may be impaired by electrical-conduction delays, different segments of the wall contracting out of sequence with each other. Severely hypoxic or scarred areas of myocardium may show little or no contractile activity, and occasionally 'paradoxical' bulging of a ventricular aneurysm may occur in phase with cardiac contraction. Finally, hypoxia of the papillary muscles may cause defective functioning of the cardiac valves. Each of these problems inevitably restricts cardiac stroke volume.

More general hypoxia of the myocardium may develop as the cardiac work rate is augmented by an increase in heart rate and systolic blood pressure. There is little scope for anaerobic metabolism in the myocardium. Hence, oxygen lack impairs the regeneration of adenosine triphosphate (ATP) in heart muscle, with a decrease in myocardial contractility (F. Grögler *et al.*, 1973) and a fall in stroke volume; functional impairment can be detected with as little as eight seconds of oxygen lack in the dog heart (H.O. Hirzel *et al.*, 1973).

In practice, the average patient referred for 'post-coronary' rehabilitation has a somewhat lower stroke volume and cardiac output than a normal middle-aged man who is developing a comparable rate of rhythmic work (R.A. Bruce *et al.*, 1974; M. Rousseau *et al.*, 1974; D.H. Paterson *et al.*, 1979). This is due both to impaired contractility and slowed relaxation of the heart (W. Rutihauser *et al.*, 1973). Impaired contractility and a poor stroke volume is particularly likely in the older patient (F. Nager *et al.*, 1967) and the individual with exercise-induced angina (J.V. Messer *et al.*, 1963; G.L. Foster & Reeves, 1964; L.S. Cohen *et al.*, 1965; J.O. Parker *et al.*, 1967; E.A. Amsterdam, 1976). The energy needed for a given bout of dynamic exercise is then obtained by a broadening of arterio-venous oxygen difference and an increase in oxygen debt (Figure 8.4). If ventricular function is impaired, isometric exercise is tolerated particularly poorly, with a decrease in stroke volume and a dramatic rise in left-ventricular end-diastolic pressure.

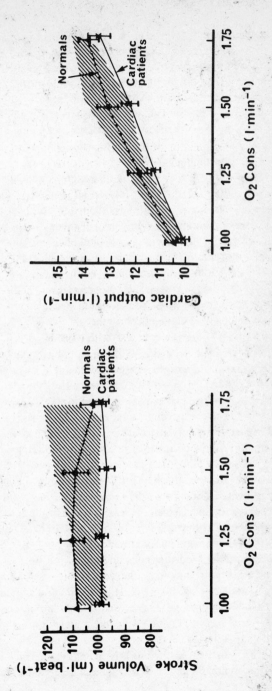

Figure 8.4: Response of 'post-coronary' patients to exercise. Based on cycle-ergometer data for 79 patients with myocardial infarction and nine normal middle-aged men. The shaded area indicates the range of normal values reported in the literature.

Source: Data from Southern Ontario multicentre trial, as repeated by D.H. Paterson et al. (1979).

Training Response

The classical response to training in the healthy person is a decrease in exercise heart rate, associated with an increase in stroke volume (Chapter 4). The maximum heart rate is unchanged, or may show a slight decrease, while the stroke volume is better sustained to maximum effort. This apparently reflects improved coronary blood flow to the active muscles with an increase of actomyosin and myosin ATPase activity (J. Scheuer *et al.*, 1977).

The response of the 'post-coronary' patient is less clear-cut, being influenced by the age of the subject, the severity of the disease process, the time that elapses between infarction and recruitment to the rehabilitation programme, the intensity of the test exercise relative to prescribed training, the rate of progression of the training programme and sometimes changes in medication such as β-blocking drugs. Almost all reports show a moderate increase in heart rate in sub-maximal exercise (Table 8.1), but several studies made over the first six months of rehabilitation show either no increase in stroke volume, or a parallel response of exercised and control subjects (Table 8.2; H. Bergman & Varnauskas, 1970; J.P. Clausen & Trap-Jensen, 1970; J.R. Detry *et al.*, 1971; D.H. Paterson *et al.*, 1979; Figure 8.5). In several of these reports, an increased oxygen delivery is realised by a widening of the maximum systemic arterio-venous oxygen difference.

The reduction in exercise heart rate could reflect: (i) a lessening of drive from the cerebral cortex to the vasomotor centre (E.E. Smith *et al.*, 1976); (ii) lesser activation of the motor cortex secondary to hypertrophy of slow-twitch muscle fibres (H. Roskamm, 1971); (iii) redirection of blood flow from skin to muscle (R.J. Shephard, 1977a); (iv) easier perfusion of the thigh muscles secondary to their hypertrophy (R.J. Shephard, 1977a); and (v) an increased peripheral extraction of oxygen secondary to an increase in the activity of skeletal-muscle enzyme systems (J.P. Clausen, 1976). D.H. Paterson *et al* (1979) found little increase in lean tissue mass over the first six months of training, and thus concluded that factors (ii) and (iv) contributed little to the early conditioning response of post-coronary patients. Blood leaving the active limb muscles also contains very little oxygen (R.J. Shephard, 1977a) so that there is limited scope for factor (v). The early decrease in heart rate with training must thus be attributed to factors (i) and (iii).

The changes of stroke volume arise from the opposing influences of a decreased sympathetic drive (which has a negative inotropic effect

Table 8.1: Effects of Training Programmes in Ischaemic Heart Disease, as Measured by Increase in Maximum Oxygen Intake or Physical Working Capacity and Decrease in Heart Rate during Sub-maximal Working

Patients Total (n)	Myocardial infarction (n)	Angina (n)	Age (years)	Training Frequency (per week)	Training Duration (months)	Response Sub-maximal heart rate (%)	Response Physical working capacity (PWC$_{150}$) (%)	Response Maximum rate of working (%)	Authors
100	92	8	–	3	24	–	–	+17	M. Wassermill & Toor (1966)
12	12	–	48	3	8	–16	–	–	J. Naughton et al. (1966)
254	–	–	–	3–5	33	–	+22 (adherents)	↑ (adherents)	H.K. Hellerstein et al. (1967)
5	5	3	47	2	1–2	–13	–	–	M. Frick et al. (1968)
100	66	47	–	3	33	–13	–	+17	S.H. Saltzman et al. (1969)
11	9	6	–	4	6	–	–	–	F. Kasch & Boyer (1969)
7	6	5	52	5	1	–	+30–40	+33	J.P. Clausen et al. (1969)
9	7	–	53	5	2	–	–	+32	J.P. Clausen & Trap-Jensen (1970)
7	7	6	48	3	4–6	–13	–	–	H. Bergman & Varnauskas (1970)
12	12	–	–	3	6	–	–	–	O. Pedersen-Bjergaard (1971)
14	14	6	47	5	6	–23	+30	–	E.W. Banister & Taunton (1971)
12	12	–	48	3	3	–	–	+23	J.R. Detry et al. (1971)
7	7	6	48	14	1½	–	–	+56	D.R. Redwood et al. (1972)
12	12	7	51	3	2	–7	–	+7	S. Degré et al. (1972)
21	21	3	52	3	3	–9 to –12	+21	+15	A. Biernulf (1973)
28	28	10	50	3	9	–8 to –12	+35	+22	H. Sanne (1973)
16	16	16	50	3	9	–	+33	–	H. Sanne (1973)
16	9	5	51	3	12	–	–	+26	R. Ferguson et al. (1973)
12	12	–	57	3	12	–	–	+17	J.D. Cantwell et al. (1973)
31	31	15	49	5	12	–	–	+35	T. Kavanagh et al. (1973b)
26	26	10	48	3	1½	–11	+24	+24	S. Degré & Denolin (1973)
26	26	13	53	3	3	–	–	–	K. Bergström et al. (1974)
8	8	2	43	5	12–18	–	–	+75	T. Kavanagh et al. (1974b, 1977a)
29	29	15	47	3	3	–13	–	+24	M. Rousseau et al. (1974)
14	7	7	51	3	13	–	+33	+25	R. Ferguson et al. (1974)
12	8	7	50	5	3–24	–	+25	–	D. Cardus et al. (1975)
6	6	3	48	4	6½	–6	–	+41	D.R. McCrimmon et al. (1976)

Source: Based on data collected by D.H. Paterson (1977).

Table 8.2: Changes in Cardiovascular Performance over a 'Post-coronary' Training Programme, as Shown by Data for Exercising Patients

Heart rate Initial (beats/min)	Δ (%)	Stroke volume Initial (ml)	Δ (%)	Cardiac output Initial (l/min)	Δ (%)	Arterio-venous oxygen difference Initial (ml/l)	Δ (%)	Author
133	− 12	110	0	9.5	− 13	101	+ 9	E. Varnauskas (1966)
133	− 8	104	+ 15	14.5	+ 8	107	− 8	M. Frick & Katila (1968)
117	− 8	94	+ 9	13.7	+ 2	96	− 3	M. Frick et al. (1971)
145	− 9	92	+ 6	11.0	− 3	115	+ 1	J.P. Clausen et al. (1969)
131	− 9	93	+ 14	13.0	+ 5	115	− 7	J.P. Clausen & Trap-Jensen (1970)
107	− 14	88	+ 7	12.1	− 9	105	+ 9	J.R. Detry et al. (1971)
119	− 7	81	+ 12	9.4	− 1	108	+ 1	H. Bjernulf (1973)
123	− 13			8.8	+ 2	No data		B. Kirchheiner & Pedersen-Bjergaard (1973)
114	− 7	93	+ 10	11.3	+ 2	101	− 3	S. Degré et al. (1972)
111	− 7	100	+ 2	11.3	0	86	− 1	S. Degré & Denolin (1973)
122	− 8	94	+ 7	10.6	0	93	0	S. Degré & Denolin (1973)
	− 12	86	− 12	10.5	− 2	100	0	M. Rousseau et al. (1974)
Decreased		–		Decreased		Decreased		G.A. Klassen et al. (1972)
Decreased		No change		Decreased		–		P. Gauthier et al. (1973)
		–		No change		–		G. Avon et al. (1973)
Untrained, reference groups of 'post-coronary' patients								
126	− 2	98	+ 8	12.4	+ 6	103	− 4	M. Frick et al. (1971)
107	− 4	85	0	9.0	− 3	99	0	H. Bjernulf (1973)
115	− 3	70	+ 9	7.5	+ 4	No data		B. Kirchheiner & Perdersen-Bjergaard (1973)
111	− 8	91	+ 8	10.0	+ 1	100	− 2	M. Rousseau et al. (1974)

Source: Based on data collected by D.H. Paterson (1977).

upon the myocardium; W.A. Neill, 1977) and an enhancement of intrinsic myocardial contractility (D.A. Cunningham & Rechnitzer, 1974). This may explain why different studies of 'post-coronary' patients have reported training responses ranging from a six per cent decrease to an 18 per cent increase in stroke volume (M.H. Frick & Katila, 1968; H. Bergman & Varnauskas, 1970; J.P. Clausen & Trap-Jensen, 1970; J.R. Detry *et al.*, 1971; A. Bjernulf, 1973; M. Rousseau *et al.*, 1974; S. Degré, *et al.*, 1977; D.H. Paterson *et al.*, 1979).

In the second six months of training, D.H. Paterson *et al.* (1979) saw a six to eleven per cent increase in stroke volume; as in other investigations, this was more marked in heavy than in light work (M.H. Frick & Katila, 1968; J.R. Detry *et al.*, 1971; J.P. Clausen, 1976; S. Degré *et al.*, 1977). It has yet to be resolved why the early training response of a normal person is delayed in the post-coronary patient. Possibly, both the patient and the supervising physician are cautious during the first six months of renewed activity, so that the exercise undertaken at this stage remains insufficient to induce an increase in cardiac stroke volume. J. Scheuer (1973) stressed that increases in myocardial ATPase activity, and thus in intrinsic myocardial contractility, demand a minimum duration and severity of training that is almost certainly lacking in the early coronary rehabilitation programme.

The response from six to twelve months of training (Figure 8.5) cannot be attributed simply to a natural correction of the asynchronous contraction seen immediately after infarction (E. Braunwald *et al.*, 1976); control patients enrolled in a homeopathic exercise programme developed a small *decrease* in stroke volume over the same period of observation. The prime explanation is probably an increase in myocardial contractility due to hypertrophy and/or changes in myocardial metabolism (B. Saltin *et al.*, 1968; J. Scheuer, 1973). However, there may also be some contribution from altered pre- or after-loading of the ventricle. Both J.P. Clausen (1973) and S. Degré *et al.* (1977) have stressed the importance of a decrease in total peripheral resistance. There are several potential mechanisms for producing such a change with training, including: (i) general reduction in sympathetic vasoconstrictor tone; (ii) enzymatic adaptations that allow more muscle fibres to participate in the required activity (thereby increasing the effective vascular bed, and reducing tension per unit of muscle cross section); and (iii) muscle hypertrophy (facilitating perfusion of the thigh muscles, often a limiting factor in cycle-ergometer work; R.J. Shephard, 1977a).

A. Bjernulf (1973) suggested that the response to training was

Figure 8.5: Influence of training upon cardiac stroke volume during exercise, based upon results for 'post-coronary' patients, allocated randomly to 'high-intensity' and 'low-intensity' exercise programmes.

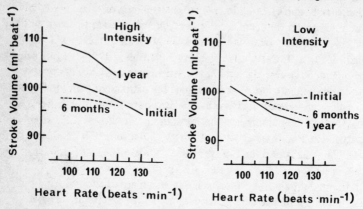

Source: Data from Southern Ontario multicentre trial as reported by D.H. Paterson *et al.* (1979).

influenced by the severity of the disease process, younger and angina-free patients being more likely to show an increase in stroke volume at a given work rate. This seems inherently probable, and indeed absence of the normal augmentation of stroke volume with exercise may be warning of an impending recurrence (R.J. Shephard, 1979a). On the other hand, neither J.R. Detry *et al.* (1971) nor D.H. Paterson *et al.* (1980) found any significant association between the size of the stroke-volume increase with training and the presence or absence of exercise-induced angina. Possibly, future investigators may have more success in relating such changes to objective criteria of hypoxia (such as exercise-induced ST segmental depression).

Cardiac failure

Cardiac failure may be suspected if end-diastolic pressure exceeds 12 mm Hg in the left ventricle or 5 mm Hg in the right ventricle. However, the relationship between diastolic volume and pressure is influenced markedly by: (1) myocardial contractility; (2) myocardial hypertrophy; and (3) fibrosis of the ventricular wall. In a normal subject, the increased stroke volume of exercise is mediated largely by an increase in contractility, with more complete emptying of the ventricle, but in heavy effort some increase in end-diastolic volume may occur (J.H. Mitchell & Wildenthal, 1971).

If the myocardial oxygen supply is inadequate, some degree of cardiac failure is likely during exercise. Initially, stroke output may be maintained at the expense of some increase in diastolic volume (compensated failure), but with a further stretching of the myocardial filaments the force that can be developed by the myosin/actomyosin cross bridges begins to decrease (decompensated failure) (B.M. Lewis *et al.*, 1953; R.M. Harvey *et al.*, 1962; J. Ross *et al.*, 1966). Increases in pulmonary artery, wedge and left ventricular end-diastolic pressures have been linked to exertional angina and low cardiac outputs during exercise (J.O. Parker *et al.*, 1966; L. Wiener *et al.*, 1968; K.P. O'Brien *et al.*, 1969; J. McDonough *et al.*, 1974). In the absence of angina, patients with ischaemic heart disease show a normal left-ventricular end-diastolic pressure during exercise (L.S. Cohen *et al.*, 1965).

Cardiac Output

Normal values

The resting cardiac output is normally $3.0-3.5 \ l \cdot min^{-1} \cdot m^{-2}$, or in a person with a body surface area of $1.8 \ m^2$, $5.4-6.3 \ l \cdot min^{-1}$. During moderate exercise, the oxygen intake increases in close relationship to the increase in cardiac output, although the latter may show a lesser increase from 70 to 100 per cent of maximum oxygen intake (P.O. Åstrand *et al.*, 1964). In our studies of young adults (R. Simmons & Shephard, 1971a, b), the cardiac output at maximum oxygen intake was only marginally less than would be predicted from a linear extrapolation of the cardiac output/oxygen consumption line. Presumably, much depends on the state of training of the subject and his ability to sustain a high stroke volume against the peripheral resistance of strongly contracting leg muscles.

In a well-trained endurance athlete, cardiac output reaches a maximum of $35 \ l \cdot min^{-1}$ or more, but in an older, sedentary individual a peak value of $15-20 \ l \cdot min^{-1}$ is likely.

Ischaemic heart disease

Some authors have found a normal increase in cardiac output when exercise is performed by 'post-coronary' patients (J.A.L. Mathers *et al.*, 1951; C.B. Chapman & Fraser, 1954; J.V. Messer *et al.*, 1963; R.P.A. Malmborg, 1964; R. Malmcrona & Varnauskas, 1964; Figure 8.6). Others have observed a 'hypokinetic' response (K. Kato & Watanabe, 1971; R.A. Bruce *et al.*, 1974; J.S. Forrester *et al.*, 1977; D.H. Paterson *et al.*, 1979), compensated by a broadening of arterio-

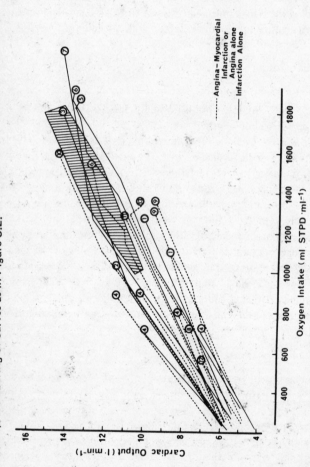

Figure 8.6: Relationship between cardiac output and oxygen intake in patients with myocardial infarction alone and in those with infarction plus angina or angina alone. Shading indicates normal response (see D.H. Paterson *et al.*, 1979). Numbering of curves as in Figure 8.2.

- - - Angina – Myocardial
Infarction or
Angina alone
——— Infarction Alone

Cardiac Output (l·min⁻¹)

Oxygen Intake (ml STPD·ml⁻¹)

Source: Based on data accumulated by D.H. Paterson (1977).

venous oxygen difference in sub-maximal exercise and by an increased proportion of anaerobic metabolism in maximum effort (S. Degré *et al.*, 1972). Among reasons for the discordant reports, we may note the low intensity of exercise used in some early tests, varying intervals between infarction and testing, and varying severity of both infarct and residual coronary vascular disease. Impaired myocardial performance has often been linked with exercise-induced angina (J.V. Messer *et al.*, 1963; L.S. Cohen *et al.*, 1965; G.L. Foster & Reeves, 1964; J. Parker *et al.*, 1966), although the haemodynamic limitation is usually apparent before the onset of clinical symptoms (J.A. Murray *et al.*, 1968).

Slowing of heart rate in the sick-sinus syndrome, hypoxic impairment of myocardial contractility, mechanical problems in the functioning of the ventricular pump, and a delayed 'on transient' at the beginning of exercise are all reasons why the cardiac output of a 'post-coronary' patient would sometimes be less than that of a healthy person with the same power output. However, such problems are by no means universal in ischaemic heart disease. The sick-sinus syndrome is encountered in only about ten per cent of those referred for exercise rehabilitation (A.C.P. Powles *et al.*, 1979; R.J. Shephard, 1980f). Likewise, T. Kavanagh *et al.* (1977c) noted that only 16 of their 610 'post-coronary' patients had radiographic evidence of depression of the ST segment of the electrocardiogram at a target heart rate corresponding to 75 per cent of aerobic power. R.J. Shephard & Kavanagh (1978c) reported a relatively normal exercise 'on transient' in their post-coronary patients (Table 7.11), but A.B. Ford & Hellerstein (1957) observed that an increased fraction of oxygen cost of the 1½-minute Master test was deferred to the recovery period. J.H. Auchincloss *et al.* (1974) tested oxygen consumption one minute after commencing exercise, and found a deficit of ~ 20 per cent in a half of patients with angiographic evidence of coronary arterial disease. Most of the group had severe impairment of myocardial function, with an elevation of diastolic pressure.

Arterio-venous Oxygen Difference

Normal values

The arterio-venous oxygen difference of a normal young adult increases from 40–50 ml·l^{-1} at rest to about 120 ml·l^{-1} at 40 per cent of maximum effort, with a further rise to 130–160 ml·l^{-1} in maximum effort. Higher maxima are seen in endurance athletes and in men generally, while lower maxima are found in the elderly (V. Niinimaa & Shephard, 1978).

Factors influencing the maximum arterio-venous difference include: (i) the haemoglobin level (higher in men than in women); (ii) the extent of the haemoconcentration (between five and ten per cent) induced by exercise; (iii) small effects due to a decrease in arterial pH, an increase in blood temperature and an increase in blood CO_2 content; (iv) the completeness of oxygen extraction in the active muscles (increased by augmentation of the capillary/muscle fibre ratio and by an increase in tissue enzyme concentrations); (v) the redirection of blood from viscera to the active muscles; and (vi) the demand for heat elimination via the cutaneous circulation (increased in obese and poorly trained subjects).

Ischaemic heart disease

Immediately following infarction, the arterial oxygen saturation may be limited by pulmonary oedema, collapse of the lungs (P.A. Valentine *et al.*, 1966) and a hunting of blood through poorly ventilated alveoli (G.J. Mackenzie *et al.*, 1964). This situation is normally corrected within four weeks of the acute episode. Nevertheless, if patients are recruited to an exercise rehabilitation programme some eight weeks after infarction, they may still show a 'hypokinetic' circulation, with an increased arterio-venous oxygen difference at rest and in sub-maximum effort (G.J. Mackenzie *et al.*, 1964; R. Malcroma & Varnauskas, 1964). In contrast, the maximum arterio-venous oxygen difference (130 $ml \cdot l^{-1}$) remains at the lower end of normality (D.H. Paterson *et al.*, 1979).

In the first six months of rehabilitation, the arterio-venous oxygen difference in sub-maximum effort is unchanged (M. Frick & Katila, 1968; J.P. Clausen *et al.*, 1969; S. Degré *et al.*, 1972) or increased somewhat (E. Varnauskas *et al.*, 1966; D.H. Paterson *et al.*, 1979). Any increase may reflect a greater enzyme activity in the working muscles. At a year, the response is much as at the initial testing, with a marginal reduction of the maximum arterio-venous difference to about 127 $ml \cdot l^{-1}$ (D.H. Paterson *et al.*, 1979).

Maximum Oxygen Intake

Normal values

The maximum oxygen intake provides perhaps the best overall estimate of cardio-respiratory performance (R.J. Shephard, 1977a). If data are expressed in units of ml O_2 STPD per kg of body mass per minute, typical values for Canadian city dwellers are as follows:

Age (years)	Men ($ml \cdot kg^{-1} \cdot min^{-1}$)	Women ($ml \cdot kg^{-1} \cdot min^{-1}$)
30-9	39.5	38.6
40-9	34.7	35.1
50-9	33.0	31.6
60-9	26.8	24.1

Rather similar standards have been proposed for the United States (American Heart Association, 1972).

The training response is influenced by the intensity of conditioning in relation to initial fitness, with lesser effects from the frequency and duration of effort and the total quantity of work performed (R.J. Shephard, 1968a, 1977a). If the training intensity is held constant, the half-time of the increase in maximum oxygen intake is about ten days. However, if the training plan is progressive, the increase in condition can extend over many weeks, particularly in older subjects with a poor initial status. The average change is about 20 per cent (R.J. Shephard, 1965, 1977a), but there are occasional reports of much larger gains.

Ischaemic heart disease

Following myocardial infarction, the peak oxygen intake for a man of 45-50 years is reduced to about 25 $ml \cdot kg^{-1} \cdot min^{-1}$ (Table 8.3), about 74 per cent of the Canadian standard, although this deficit can be made good by vigorous training (T. Kavanagh & Shephard, 1976). Angina without infarction is associated with a somewhat lower peak heart rate and peak oxygen intake. In subjects with a combination of angina and infarction, the peak oxygen intake drops to 15–20 $ml \cdot kg^{-1} \cdot min^{-1}$ ($\sim$ 50 per cent of the values encountered in sedentary Torontonians of the same age; C.G. Blomqvist & Mitchell, 1979).

A recent survey of 40 different cardiac rehabilitation experiments (D.H. Paterson, 1977) found a gain in maximum oxygen intake of up to ten per cent in nine studies, ten to 20 per cent in 22 studies, 20–30 per cent in seven studies and more than 30 per cent in the remaining two studies (Table 8.1). The typical response of the 'post-coronary' patient is thus not unlike that seen in a healthy adult. Variations of response reflect programme adherence (H.K. Hellerstein *et al.*, 1967; S.H. Saltzman *et al.*, 1969), fears of over-exertion on the part of patient or physician

Table 8.3: Exercise Tolerance in Patients with Angina Pectoris and/or Previous Myocardial Infarction

N	Age (year)	Peak oxygen intake[†] ($ml \cdot kg^{-1} \cdot min^{-1}$)	Peak heart rate ($beats \cdot min^{-1}$)	Time since infarction (months)	Functional impairment (%)[*]	Author
(a)	Angina pectoris alone					
549	52	22 (approx.)	148		27	R.A. Bruce et al. (1974a)
10	45-69	—	135		—	G.R. Dagenais et al. (1971)
19	40-58	—	119		38	R.P. Malmborg (1964)
(b)	Myocardial infarction alone					
21	50	25.0	150	20	17	A.M. Benestäd (1968)
16	—	26.8	163	3	11	A.M. Benestäd (1972)
249	50	25.0 (approx.)	156	—	17	R.A. Bruce et al. (1974a)
16	48	21.6	150	2-4	28	S. Degré & Denolin (1973)
15	45	24.6	161	3-5 (7-25)	18	T. Kavanagh & Shephard (1976)
(4 with angina pectoris)						
99	<57	24.9	164	3	17	H. Sanne (1973)
25	<57	26.3	169	12	12	H. Sanne (1973)
(c)	Myocardial infarction plus angina pectoris					
497	52	20 (approx.)	145	—	34	R.A. Bruce et al. (1974a)
7	52	—	135	—	53	J.P. Clausen et al. (1969)
10	48	15.6	135	2-4	48	S. Degré et al. (1973)
6	50	19.9	—	24	34	T. Kavanagh & Shephard (1975a)
19	40-58	—	123	—	38	R.P. Malmborg (1964)
71	<57	16.9	133	31	44	H. Sanne (1973)
27	<57	19.6	132	12	35	H. Sanne (1973)

[*] Relative to norms proposed by the American Heart Association (1972).

[†] Values are generally 'symptom-limited' rather than true plateaus of oxygen intake.

(A.J. Barry *et al.*, 1966), age (T. Kavanagh *et al*., 1973b; K. Bergström *et al.*, 1974) and the presence or absence of exercise-induced angina (J.R. Detry *et al.*, 1971; S. Degré *et al.*, 1972; H. Sanne, 1973; M. Rousseau *et al.*, 1974; T. Kavanagh & Shephard, 1975a). In some studies (particularly those over short periods), there has been little change in control subjects (J. Naughton *et al.*, 1966; O. Pedersen-Bjergaard, 1971; T. Kavanagh *et al.*, 1973b; K. Bergström *et al.*, 1974; M. Rousseau *et al.*, 1974). In other, longer programmes, there have been similar gains in control and exercised subjects (Chapter 6; Table 8.4), implying either natural recovery of the oxygen-transport system or a contamination of control subjects by an interest in exercise. The exercised group show fairly rapid early gains, as the effects of bed rest are reversed (H. Sanne, 1973), but given a progressive regimen the response may continue for several years. Indeed, some of our patients who have participated in marathon events have not made dramatic gains of maximum oxygen intake until two or three years after infarction (T. Kavanagh *et al.*, 1977). Possibly, lack of confidence kept them from hard training in the first two years after their acute episode (A.J. Barry *et al.*, 1966). The response to training is less satisfactory in old than in younger patients (T. Kavanagh *et al.*, 1973b; Table 8.5). This is probably an expression of more severe disease and residual myocardial ischaemia in the older individuals. It is also possible that a lessening of financial and family commitments along with reduced physical expectations lessen the drive to vigorous training in an older person. If anginal pain is developed during exercise, training may give a larger than normal increase in symptom-limited performance (M. Rousseau *et al.*, 1974). On the other hand, if the response is assessed from a sub-maximum exercise test (for example, the predicted maximum oxygen intake; Table 8.6), there is plainly a very limited response of anginal patients to continuous endurance training. Nevertheless, such individuals can be treated quite effectively by a programme of modified interval training (H. Sanne, 1973; T. Kavanagh & Shephard, 1965a; Table 8.4). Gains of maximum oxygen intake are accompanied by a lesser reaction to a given intensity of sub-maximum effort (lesser increase in heart rate and respiratory minute volume, lesser increase in blood lactate; Figure 8.7).

Table 8.4: Early Recovery of Maximum Oxygen Intake Following Myocardial Infarction, Presented in the Form of Symptom-limited Maxima Expressed as Percent of Age- and Sex-specific Normal Mean Values

Time post infarction (weeks)		Symptom-limited maximum* (% of normal, mean ± range)	
3	(n = 50)	47	(25–72)
6	(n = 46)	56	(24–92)
13	(n = 38)	56	(31–97)
26	(n = 27)	58	(31–91)

*   First test terminated at a heart rate of 130 beats$\cdot$min^{-1} in the absence of symptoms.

Source: Based on data of A.J. Wohl *et al.* (1977).

Table 8.5: Influence of Patient Age upon Response to Endurance Training

Group	Maximum oxygen intake			
	Initial		After one year	After two years
	l$\cdot$min^{-1} STPD	ml$\cdot$kg$^{-1}\cdot$min^{-1} STPD	l$\cdot$min^{-1} STPD	l$\cdot$min^{-1} STPD
All patients	1.98 ± 0.86	27.0 ± 9.4	+ 0.34 ± 0.69	+ 0.70 ± 0.63
Patients < 50 yrs	2.04 ± 0.65	26.4 ± 6.4	+ 0.32 ± 0.69	+ 0.92 ± 0.76
Patients > 50 yrs	1.89 ± 1.11	27.7 ± 12.6	+ 0.37 ± 0.73	+ 0.51 ± 0.47

Source: T. Kavanagh *et al.* (1973b).

Systemic Blood Pressure

Normal Values

Accurate measurements of systemic blood pressure are important to the assessment of: (i) myocardial performance (a sudden fall in systolic pressure during exercise is of ominous portent); and (ii) cardiac work rate.

Under resting conditions, pressures recorded from a standard sphygmomanometer cuff underestimate the true brachial systolic

Table 8.6: Response of Patients with Exercise-induced Angina to Continuous Endurance Training and Modified Interval Training

Type of patient	Predicted maximum oxygen intake, end year I[1] (ml•kg^{-1}•min^{-1})	Change induced by training year II[2] (ml•kg^{-1}•min^{-1})
Myocardial infarction		
group (a)	25.2	+ 10.7[3]
	± 5.8	± 7.8
group (b)	23.6	+ 6.4[4]
	± 7.0	± 7.3
Myocardial infarction with frequent exercise-induced angina	19.9	+ 9.0[4]
	± 7.4	± 8.1

1. During year I, all subjects attempted a progressive programme of endurance training.
2. During year II, six patients with frequent exercise-induced angina and 20 others were allocated to the interval-training programme.
3. Continuous endurance training.
4. Modified interval training.

Source: T. Kavanagh & Shephard (1975a).

pressure (recorded from in indwelling catheter) by some 10 mm Hg (1.5 kPa; S.N. Hunyor *et al.*, 1978). In contrast, the stethoscopic estimate of diastolic pressure is excessive, even if the point of disappearance of the Korotkov sounds ('fifth phase') rather than muffling ('fourth phase') is noted (J. Fabian *et al.*, 1975). From the viewpoint of cardiac work rate, aortic pressures are more important than peripheral readings, and pulse wave reflections may increase peripheral systolic values.

During exercise, much of the energy in the aorta is in kinetic form. It is important to include this component when examining myocardial performance. Kinetic energy can be detected by a centrally directed catheter and by a sphymomanometer cuff, but not by a laterally tapped or peripherally directed catheter (H.J. Marx *et al.*, 1967). The first two types of measurement indicate a progressive rise of blood pressure during exercise (Table 8.7), the magnitude of this change depending upon the type, intensity and duration of effort and the condition of the myocardium (H. Mellerowicz, 1962; I. Åstrand, 1965; P.O. Åstrand

Figure 8.7: Influence of exercise rehabilitation upon respiratory minute volume and blood lactate during sub-maximal exercise, for 'post-coronary' patients. Authors: (1) E. Varnauskas (1966); (2) J. Naughton *et al.* (1966); (3) M.H. Frick & Katila (1968); (4) J.P. Clausen *et al.* (1970); (5) J.P. Clausen & Trap-Jensen (1970); (6) J.R. Detry *et al.* (1971); (7) S. Degré *et al.* (1972); (8) H. Bjernulf (1973); (9) H. Sanne (1973); (10) S. Degré & Denolin (1973); (11) M. Rousseau *et al.* (1974).

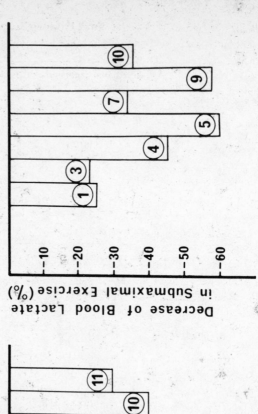

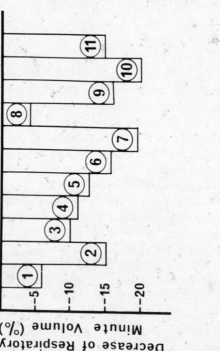

Source: Based on data accumulated by D.H. Paterson (1977).

Table 8.7: Increment in Systolic Blood Pressure (Δ, kPa) in Relation to Age and Work Rate

Age (years)	4 Mets	Work rate and Δ, kPa		
		6 Mets	8 Mets	10 Mets
20-9	3.3	4.8	6.3	7.8
30-9	3.3	5.3	7.2	8.9
40-9	3.5	5.7	6.8	8.1
50-9	3.9	6.4	8.5	10.5

Source: Based on data of S.M. Fox.

et al., 1965; J.S. Hanson *et al.*, 1968). The response to sub-maximal effort varies with the proportion of the maximum oxygen intake that is utilised. Increases of pressure are therefore larger in older subjects (H. Reindell *et al.*, 1960; J.S. Hanson *et al.*, 1968; G. Gerstenblith *et al.*, 1976) and in situations where there is difficulty in perfusing the active tissue (use of small muscles, particularly movements of the arms above the head; P.O. Åstrand *et al.*, 1965; S. Bevegard *et al.*, 1966; I. Åstrand, 1971; J. Schwade *et al.*, 1977; G.E. Adams *et al.*, 1978). Peripheral systolic readings of 180-240 mm Hg (24-32 kPa) may be anticipated with ten to 15 minutes of maximum effort (M. Masuda *et al.*, 1967), although the increase in central arterial pressure is smaller.

Since the maximum stroke volume and cardiac output both decrease with aging, one might have anticipated a lower maximum systemic blood pressure in an old person. However, because of loss of elasticity in the arterial walls, the pressure reached in maximum effort is often higher than in a young adult (A. Granath *et al.*, 1964; I. Åstrand, 1965; S; Julius *et al.*, 1967; I.S. Kasser & Bruce, 1969; L.T. Sheffield & Roitman, 1973). K.H. Sidney & Shephard (unpublished data) found a maximum peripheral systolic pressure of 217 ± 38 mm Hg (28.9 ± 5.1 kPa) in elderly men and 206 ± 32 mm Hg (27.5 ± 4.3 kPa) in elderly women performing maximum aerobic exercise.

Isometric effort gives a large and rapid increase both in systolic and diastolic pressures, with an accompanying tachycardia (A.R. Lind & McNicol, 1967; G.E. Adams *et al.*, 1978). Pressures first rise when the active muscles contract at more than 15 per cent of their maximum voluntary force. At intermediate intensities of effort (20-60 per cent of maximum force), the rate of rise of pressure varies with the intensity

Table 8.8: Systemic Blood Pressure at Rest and During Exercise to 75 Per Cent of Maximum Aerobic Power, Obtained in Patients before and after Three Years of Progressive Endurance Training

	All patients (n = 553)		Hypertensives (n = 141)	
	Initial (mm Hg)	Final (mm Hg)	Initial (mm Hg)	Final (mm Hg)
Resting:				
systolic	133 ± 17	127 ± 15	161 ± 19	154 ± 12
diastolic	85 ± 9	87 ± 11	104 ± 9	103 ± 13
Exercising:				
systolic	169 ± 25	183 ± 29	172 ± 31	188 ± 30
diastolic	96 ± 13	96 ± 12	100 ± 12	99 ± 16
	(kPa)	(kPa)	(kPa)	(kPa)
Resting:				
systolic	17.7	16.9	21.5	20.6
diastolic	11.4	11.6	13.8	13.7
Exercising:				
systolic	22.5	24.5	22.9	25.0
diastolic	12.8	12.8	13.3	13.2

Source: Unpublished data of T. Kavanagh & Shephard.

of contraction, but the pressure at exhaustion is consistent (C.F. Funderburk *et al.*, 1974). A maximum effect is generally attained at 70–80 per cent of maximum voluntary force.

Ischaemic heart disease

Because of associated changes in the peripheral arteries (including the renal artery), many patients with ischaemic heart disease have some resting hypertension. Pulse-wave reflection is also increased, augmenting the central-peripheral pressure gradient.

Hypertension of itself may increase the rise of systemic pressure during sub-maximum exercise (A. Amery *et al.*, 1967). However, increased after-loading of the left ventricle reduces the maximum cardiac response to exercise (R. Sannerstedt, 1966; A. Amery *et al.*, 1967). Theoretically, the patient with coronary vascular disease should withstand such after-loading more poorly than a young person with essential hypertension (H.O. Wong *et al.*, 1969). In practice, the hypertension of ischaemic heart disease is often marginal, with correspondingly smaller haemodynamic consequences. Among one sample of 551 patients referred for exercise rehabilitation, T. Kavanagh & Shephard (Table 8.8) found just over a quarter of the group (141 patients) had a resting peripheral arterial pressure of over 150/100 mm Hg (20.0/13.3 kPa). The initial exercise response of the hypertensive patients was much as in those with a normal resting blood pressure. After an average of three years progressive endurance training, both groups showed a small (6–7 mm Hg) decrease in resting systolic pressure, but an increase in the systolic reading during exercise. The latter presumably reflects an increase of myocardial contractility – an expression of recovery from the acute episode plus a more specific response to prolonged endurance training (D.H. Paterson *et al.*, 1979).

Low maximum systolic pressures are commonly a warning of a deteriorating myocardium (I.S. Kasser & Bruce, 1969; L.T. Sheffield, 1974; M.H. Ellestad, 1975) and are associated with an increased risk of reinfarction (R.J. Shephard, 1979a). However, it remains difficult to disentangle a low maximum pressure due to symptom limitation of effort from a true impairment of myocardial contractility. A sudden drop in systolic pressure during the course of an exercise test is a particularly ominous sign. It suggests circulatory failure, and is an urgent indication to halt exercise while sustaining venous return (R.A. Bruce *et al.*, 1963; K.L. Andersen *et al.*, 1971).

Cardiac Work Rate

Normal values

The elements of cardiac work include 'useful' work carried out in pumping blood around the circulation and 'tension' work performed against intra-ventricular pressure (Chapter 4), plus smaller components due to basal metabolism. electrochemical reactions involved in activation of the heart muscle, the internal work of fibre shortening and energy dissipated in the heart sounds. The last four components normally account for less than two per cent of the total cardiac work, so that they can be ignored in clinical calculations (G. Blomqvist, 1974; E.F. Blick & Stein, 1977; C.R. Jorgensen *et al.*, 1977).

The useful work per heart beat $\dot{W}_a$ is given by the product of intraventricular pressure P_v and volume change ∂V, integrated between the diastolic point V_d and the systolic point V_s:

$$\dot{W}_a = \int_{V_d}^{V_s} P_v \cdot \delta v$$

To a first approximation this expression is equal to the mean ejection pressure times stroke volume. At rest, it amounts to 15 kPa (120 mm Hg) times 80 ml, or 1.2 N-m of useful work per beat. In vigorous exercise, there is an increase to perhaps 22.5 kPa (180 mm Hg) times 110 ml, or 2.5 N-m per beat in a sedentary person and perhaps 22.5 times 140 ml, or 3.2 N-m per beat in an athletic individual.

The tension work per heart beat $\dot{W}_b$ is normally much larger than the useful work. It is calculated from the tension T in the ventricular wall, integrated over the contraction phase of the cardiac cycle. A constant α is introduction into the equation so that units are the same as for useful work:

$$\dot{W}_b = \alpha \int_o^t T \cdot \delta t$$

Wall tension bears a complicated relationship to intraventricular pressure, since the myocardial fibres exhibit both helical and spherical arrangements (Streeter *et al.*, 1969; Jean *et al.*, 1972). One method of calculation modifies the formula of La Place (Chapter 4) to allow for the thickness of the ventricular walls (Mirsky, 1974):

$$T = \frac{P_v}{h} \left[\frac{R_1 \times R_2}{R_1 + R_2} \right]$$

where h is the wall thickness, and R_1 and R_2 are the principal radii of the heart. The efficiency ϵ of the heart is then given by

$$\epsilon = \frac{\dot{W}_a}{\dot{W}_a + \dot{W}_b}$$

An increase in systolic blood pressure (as occurs in prolonged isometric contraction) increases $\dot{W}_b$, thus lowering efficiency and increasing total cardiac work rate. If an increase in cardiac output is required (as in exercise), it is more economical to increase stroke volume (which has its main effect upon $\dot{W}_a$) than heart rate (which influences both $\dot{W}_a$ and $\dot{W}_b$). In practice, the effects of exercise are quite complex. There is usually an increase of myocardial contractility. The direct effect of this, demonstrated in isolated muscle, is to increase oxygen consumption per unit of time, but *in vivo* such an effect is often offset by some shortening of the contraction phase, with a decrease of diastolic volume and thus wall tension (E.H. Sonnenblick, 1971). Endurance training may lead to ventricular hypertrophy (Chapter 4), with a further reduction of tension work per unit of wall cross section.

Since tension work is difficult to measure directly, efficiency is often estimated from the ratio of useful work performed to oxygen consumed by the heart muscle. Useful work increases more than tension work during rhythmic activity. Nevertheless, the efficiency of the heart is no better than 15 per cent, even in maximum exercise (J. Scheuer *et al.*, 1974; A.M. Katz, 1977).

Simple clinical indicators of cardiac work rate were discussed in the previous chapter. Heart rate is an effective index only if work per beat remains constant (no change in stroke volume, blood pressure, contractility or heart size), while the usefulness of the rate-pressure product depends on the constancy of stroke volume, contractility and heart size; the rate-pressure product is normally an acceptable clinical tool, since tension work is the main component of cardiac work.

Attainment of a high rate-pressure product (> 35 m Hg/min) without symptoms or ECG abnormalities is a pointer to a normal coronary circulation. The limiting rate-pressure product is consistent in a given subject (B.F. Robinson, 1967), but unfortunately there is a large overlap of limiting values between subjects with and without angina pectoris (L.T. Sheffield & Roitman, 1973).

Ischaemic heart disease

The resting cardiac work rate is commonly higher in the 'post-coronary' patient than in a normal individual, as deconditioning leads to an increase in heart rate and a diminution in stroke volume. The adverse situation of the 'post-coronary' patient is also apparent during sub-maximum effort, when heart rate continues high and stroke volume low. The work-load of the heart may be further aggravated by cardiac dilatation (whether chronic, due to aneurysmal change, or acute, due to exercise-induced ischaemia of the myocardium).

During vigorous exercise, the coronary vessels of a cardiac patient are less able to dilate than in a normal individual, and there may be various symptoms and signs of local or general ischaemia (anginal pain, dysrhythmias, ST segmental depression and an output of lactate from the ventricles into the coronary circulation). The inner (endocardial) region of the ventricular wall is particularly vulnerable to oxygen lack, since: (i) the complex arrangement of the myocardial fibres creates maximal wall tensions in this zone; and (ii) the coronary arterial supply traverses a substantial thickness of contracting ventricular muscle (I. Mirsky, 1974). In consequence, myocardial infarcts are particularly frequent in the sub-endocardial zone.

At any given intensity of exercise, prolonged and vigorous rehabilitation leads to a reduction of between eight and 33 per cent in such indices of myocardial oxygen consumption as the rate-pressure product, the tension-time index and the triple product (E. Varnauskas, 1966; M.H. Frick & Katila, 1968; J.P. Clausen *et al.*, 1969; F. Kasch & Boyer, 1969; J.P. Clausen & Trap-Jensen, 1970; J.R. Detry *et al.*, 1971; M.H. Frick *et al.*, 1971; S. Degré *et al.*, 1972; B. Kirchheiner & Pedersen-Bjergaard, 1973). This reflects both a relative bradycardia and a lesser rise in blood pressure during exercise, these changes more than outweighing an increased ejection time (S.E. Epstein *et al.*, 1971). Sustained training may also increase the rate-pressure product that can be tolerated before exercise is halted by ischaemic manifestations — indeed, exercise-induced ST segmental depression sometimes disappears completely (T. Kavanagh *et al.*, 1973b).

At one time, it was hoped that a lessening of ST segmental depression might provide evidence of an improved collateral blood flow to hypoxic segments of myocardium. Unfortunately it is now realised that there are other possible explanations of such a change, including a lessening of ventricular dilatation and a reduced wall tension per unit of cross section as the myocardium hypertrophies.

Radiographic estimates of heart volume have shown no significant change with the training of 'post-coronary' patients (E. Varnauskas *et al.*, 1966; P. Rechnitzer *et al.*, 1967; M.H. Frick & Katila, 1968; J.P. Clausen *et al.*, 1969; S. Degré *et al.*, 1972; H. Sanne, 1973). However, an increase in ventricular wall thickness may be inferred from: (i) an increase in left-ventricular end-diastolic pressure measurements (M.H. Frick & Katila, 1968); and (ii) ultrasonic measurements (M.H. Frick, 1969).

Coronary Circulation

Normal values

The resting coronary blood flow of a normal young adult amounts to about five per cent of cardiac output, or $300 \text{ ml} \cdot \text{min}^{-1}$. There is a correspondingly rich capillary supply (2,500–3,000 vessels per mm^2 of fibre section, compared with 200 per mm^2 in resting and 600 per mm^2 in active skeletal muscle).

Oxygen extraction within the heart wall is relatively complete, blood from the coronary sinus having an oxygen content of only 15–50 $\text{ml} \cdot \text{l}^{-1}$, compared with the normal 'mixed' venous oxygen content of $150 \text{ ml} \cdot \text{l}^{-1}$ (E. Varnauskas & Holmberg, 1971). Although haemo-concentration allows a small increase in coronary arterio-venous oxygen difference during exercise (K. Kitamura *et al.*, 1972; R.R. Nelson *et al.*,

1974), the main adaptation to the increased oxygen demand of physical activity comes from an increase in coronary blood flow. The situation of the myocardium is somewhat precarious, since the heart cannot accumulate any significant oxygen debt (A.S. Most *et al.*, 1969; K. Wildenthal *et al.*, 1976). Measurements made upon experimental animals show a three- to six-fold increase in coronary blood flow during vigorous exercise (R. Gorlin, 1971; S.F. Vatner *et al.*, 1972; R.M. Ball *et al.*, 1975; T.M. Sanders *et al.*, 1975). In man, studies have been limited to moderate work rates, but a capacity for a five-fold increase in blood flow may be inferred from responses to vasodilator drugs such as dipyridamole (M. Tauchert *et al.*, 1972). Since the cardiac work rate increases six-fold in maximum effort, a combination of maximum vasodilatation and a small increase in coronary arterio-venous oxygen difference is essential if myocardial hypoxia is not to develop during maximum effort. Nevertheless, there seems a small margin of safety in a healthy person. The maximum heart rate and blood pressure are well sustained even if hypoxic gas mixtures are inspired during vigorous effort (L.E. Lamb *et al.*, 1969), and cardiac performance is also unaffected by the shift of blood flow from sub-endocardial to sub-epicardial tissue during vigorous activity (R.M. Ball *et al.*, 1975; T.M. Sanders *et al.*, 1975).

Ischaemic heart disease

Coronary atherosclerosis limits myocardial perfusion if the lumen of a major vessel is narrowed or blocked by an atheromatous plaque, or fibrosed, calcified vessels fail to undergo the five-fold dilatation seen in a healthy young adult.

Studies correlating coronary angiograms with clinical indices of ischaemia (anginal pain, ST segmental depression and limitations of myocardial performance) suggest that two thirds of a major vessel must be occluded before there is a serious restriction of regional blood flow. Several factors contribute to this finding: (i) obstruction usually develops in the major arteries, but the main resistance to blood flow lies in smaller vessels; (ii) flow resistance is proportional to the fourth power of vessel radius; (iii) apparent narrowing of a main artery can arise from technical problems in the angiogram (filling defects); and (iv) reversible spasm of the coronary vessels (R.C. Schlant, 1974) may develop during angiography.

Methods of evaluating the adequacy of perfusion during exercise include: (i) examination of the ST segment of the electrocardiogram; (ii) various applications of nuclear cardiology; (iii) estimation of lactate levels in coronary sinus blood (F.K. Nakhjavan *et al.*, 1975); and (iv) evaluation of myocardial function during graded exercise. Oxygen lack rapidly leads to a reduction of myocardial contractility and pump failure (A.M. Katz, 1973).

The left-ventricular systolic pressure is usually five to six times larger than that in the right ventricle. The left-ventricular wall is thus much more vulnerable to hypoxia. Its direct blood flow and any collateral supply is delivered almost entirely during diastole (S. Holmberg *et al.*, 1971; B.G. Brown *et al.*, 1972). During exercise, there is a rise in left-ventricular systolic pressure. This facilitates blood flow to the right ventricle, but increases tension in the left-ventricular wall, ensuring that perfusion is restricted to the shortened diastolic phase of the cardiac cycle. Women generally have thinner heart walls than men, but develop a similar maximum systolic pressure; the tension per unit of cross section is thus greater in the female, and this may explain their propensity to 'ischaemic' electrocardiographic appearances (G.R. Cumming *et al.*, 1973; K.H. Sidney & Shephard, 1977b; Figure 7.6; Table 7.9) despite the rarity of vascular narrowing at angiography. Both sexes usually show a sharp fall in diastolic pressure on ceasing exercise, and the resultant decrease in left-ventricular perfusion probably accounts for the frequency of ST depression and dysrhythmias during the early phase of recovery from physical activity.

A combination of exercise and cold exposure is particularly likely to precipitate myocardial ischaemia in a patient with some limitation of coronary blood flow. One possible reason is that the cold air induces a cutaneous vaso-constriction, thus increasing systemic blood pressure and cardiac work load. This general effect is augmented by a more specific cold pressor response (E.M. Glaser, 1966; J. LeBlanc, 1975). Exercise also induces mouth-breathing at a ventilation of 35–40 $l \cdot min^{-1}$ (V. Niinimaa *et al.*, 1980), and it is then possible that a reflex coronary spasm analogous to the Bezold-Jarisch reflex arises from a stimulation of vagal receptors in the air passages (J.G. Widdicombe, 1974). Certainly, the heart has a large autonomic nerve supply, although there is little evidence that sympathetic or parasympathetic nerve fibres contribute to the normal exercise-induced vasodilatation (O. Lundgren & Jodal, 1975). Some authors have thus argued that the angina experienced when jogging on a frosty morning reflects a poor coronary reserve rather than a specific reflex activation of the coronary vasomotor nerves (W.A. Neill *et al.*, 1974).

The immediate treatment of angina is commonly administration of an organic nitrite such as amyl nitrite or the longer acting glyceryl trinitrate. It was once thought that such compounds acted by dilating the coronary vessels (T.V. Brunton, 1871). However, a more important factor is the lowering of systemic pressure. This reduces the work load of the heart, and at the same time facilitates coronary perfusion by easing external compression of the coronary arteries (J.C. Krantz *et al.*, 1962).

Smoking has several adverse effects upon the myocardial oxygen supply (Chapter 2). Heart rate, and thus cardiac work rate, is increased both during rest and exercise (A. Rode *et al.*, 1972). Nicotine is also a coronary vaso-constrictor, so that exercise-induced myocardial ischaemia at a given rate-pressure product tends to be augmented by the smoking of cigarettes with a substantial nicotine delivery (W.S. Aronow *et al.*, 1968; G.R. Wright & Shephard, 1978). The associated dose of carbon monoxide reduces immediate oxygen delivery for a given coronary perfusion and, at least in high doses, a CO-induced shift in the oxyhaemoglobin dissociation curve may facilitate the formation of atherosclerotic plaques (P. Åstrup, 1977).

9 EXERCISE PRESCRIPTION AND ISCHAEMIC HEART DISEASE

We have already noted (Chapter 3) that excessive physical activity can provoke a heart attack. On the other hand, there is a threshold intensity of effort below which no training response occurs. The physician who is prescribing exercise for the 'coronary-prone' individual must thus make a nice judgement between the safety and the therapeutic effectiveness of the regimen he is advocating.

In this chapter, we shall look at appropriate activity prescriptions for the secondary and tertiary prevention of ischaemic heart disease, and will consider the issues of compliance and safety.

Exercise Prescription in Secondary Prevention

Training threshold

Possible mechanisms by which regular exercise could prevent the clinical manifestations of ischaemic heart disease are reviewed in Chapter 4. The most important aspect of training from the viewpoint of prevention and therapy seems to be the development of endurance fitness (as indicated by an increase in maximum oxygen intake). It is in this context that we shall discuss the 'training threshold'.

Many authors cite the classical experiments of M.J. Karvonen *et al.* (1957), inferring from these observations that the minimum intensity of physical activity needed to induce conditioning is that associated with a heart rate of 140 beats·min^{-1}, or an oxygen consumption that is 60 per cent of maximum. In fact, Karvonen examined one specific situation (young men running upon a treadmill for 30 minutes, four or five times per week); training was observed at a terminal heart rate of 160–180 beats·min^{-1}, but not at 135 beats·min^{-1}.

When applying such observations to a middle-aged, coronary-prone population, we must note that maximum heart rate decreases with age. A 45-year-old man thus reaches 60 per cent of maximum oxygen intake at a lower heart rate than his 25-year-old counterpart. Furthermore, initial fitness is often poor in a middle-aged person, and this probably lowers the training threshold (R.J. Shephard, 1968a). It seems logical that if exercise is rarely undertaken at 50 per cent of maximum oxygen

232

intake, this can become an effective training stimulus (R.J. Shephard, 1967a).

The nature of the interaction between the duration of activity and the training threshold is also poorly understood. P.O. Åstrand (1967) suggested that 30 minutes of activity, five times per week, was necessary to initiate training. Others have claimed that, if the intensity of exercise is substantially greater than 60 per cent of maximum oxygen intake, then the minimum period of training can be shortened, possibly to as little as five minutes per day (C. Bouchard *et al.*, 1966; K.H. Cooper, 1968; R.J. Shephard, 1968a). A brief training session is of interest to the over-worked businessman, but from the viewpoint of safety there are attractions to a more extended, low-intensity programme. Physiologists commonly examine training responses after a fixed time interval such as twelve weeks, but there is evidence that, ultimately, equal gains of physical condition can be achieved by less frequent and/or less intense activity sessions (K.H. Sidney & Shephard, 1978).

Optimum prescription

Given current ignorance about training thresholds, any exercise prescription is at best an educated guess, and it scarcely merits the mystery with which it has sometimes been surrounded.

The aim should be a gradual but steady progression of endurance activity to the point where at least 60 per cent of maximum oxygen intake is being developed for 30 minutes, four or five times per week. A simple guide to a suitable starting point for a given subject can be obtained by using the self-administered version of the Canadian Home Fitness Kit (R.J. Shephard, 1980a). The time (T, min) to cover one mile (1.6 km) is given by the formula:

$$T = 44.7 - 0.45 \, V_{O_2} - 12.3H + 0.015M$$

where $\dot{V}_{O_2}$ is 60 per cent of the maximum oxygen intake as predicted from the Canadian Home Fitness Test score; H is the standing height in metres: and M is the body mass in kg. Thus, a man with a $\dot{V}_{O_2 \, (max)}$ of 40 ml·kg^{-1}·min^{-1}, a height of 1.7 m and a mass of 70 kg would be required to cover 1.6 km in 14.0 min, while an older subject of the same size but with a $\dot{V}_{O_2 \, (max)}$ of 20 ml·kg^{-1}·min^{-1} would be allowed 19.4 min to complete the same prescription.

Fast walking is a safe and effective method of accomplishing the required effort in an older person. It has some advantages over jogging. The dangers of slipping and ankle injury are smaller when walking, while the forces transmitted from the ground to the ankle, knee and spine are only a third or a half of those developed in jogging and running.

Other activities that involve a large proportion of the body musculature such as swimming, cross-country skiing and cycling provide useful alternative forms of exercise. However, regulation of the intensity of activity is more difficult than for walking or jogging. K.H. Cooper (1968) attempted to equate various sports in terms of their training effects, using a 'points' scheme. His system can give some guidance to the layman who is planning his own programme; nevertheless, there remains considerable uncertainty as to the relative value of brief intense activity versus more sustained but leisurely pastimes, and participants seem to earn their 'points' more easily in some sports than in others (Massie *et al.*, 1970). Other texts provide tables showing the average energy cost of various sports (Table 9.1), but again such figures can be rather misleading, since: (i) energy costs increase exponentially with the speed of movement; and (ii) there are large inter-individual differences in mechanical efficiency and thus the energy costs of most sports. Light palpation of the carotid artery during or immediately following a burst of movement provides a fair check that the intensity of activity lies in the prescriptive zone, although due note must be taken of the effects upon the exercise heart rate of: (i) isometric contractions; (ii) excitement; (iii) heat; and (iv) recent smoking. I say 'light palpation' because it has been suggested that over-vigorous palpation of the carotid artery can cause: (i) slowing of the heart rate; and (ii) loss of consciousness through compression of the carotid sinus (J.R. White, 1977). Recent reports indicate that such risks are small and outweighed by the ease of counting the carotid pulse rate during exercise (G.W. Gardner *et al.*, 1979).

Other factors to be considered in recommending activity to a patient include: (i) his skills and interests; (ii) his personality (group versus solitary pursuits); (iii) available local facilities; and (iv) possibilities for pursuit of the prescription as a family. Where possible, a substantial part of the activity should be built into the normal day — for instance, a fast 2-km walk to the subway is less easily forgotten than is the requirement to cover an equivalent distance at a gymnasium. Electrical equipment such as lawn mowers and snow-blowers can be replaced by muscle power, and stairs can be used in place of an elevator. Fardy & Ilmarinen (1975) showed that a man could increase his aerobic power substantially by deliberate climbing of at least 25 flights of stairs per

Table 9.1: Classification of Various Recreational Activities

Light activity (12–20 kJ•min^{-1})*	Moderate activity (20–40 kJ•min^{-1})*	Heavy activity (40–80 kJ•min^{-1})*
Archery	Badminton	Athletics
Billiards	Canoeing	Basketball
Bowls	Recreational cycling	Boxing
Cricket	Dancing	Climbing
Golf	Gardening	Competitive running
Table tennis	Gymnastics	Association football
Recreational volleyball	Field hockey	Rowing
Walking	Horse riding	Squash rackets
	Jogging	
	Recreational cross-country skiing	
	Downhill skiing	
	Recreational swimming	
	Tennis	

* The energy cost depends greatly on the pace of performance, and the skill of the participant and of other players. In most activities, energy expenditures also vary almost linearly with body mass. The figures cited are for a young adult, but a lower energy expenditure may be heavy effort for an older person.

Source: Based in part on data of J.V.G. Durnin & Passmore (1967).

day. A London bus conductor ascends up to 60 flights of stairs per day (J.N. Morris, personal communication), and this may be one reason why he develops less heart attacks than the driver of the same vehicle.

The average middle-aged exerciser does not normally need specific routines to develop his muscle strength. Sufficient training of the body musculature is obtained from aerobic activity. Sustained isometric effort is indeed best avoided by the middle-aged adult. Isometrics induce an undesirable immediate increase in systemic blood pressure, and may add to the long-term work of the heart by encouraging an unnecessary development of the chest and shoulder muscles.

The total exercise prescription should include a brief (between five and ten minutes) warm-up and warm-down, plus advice on other changes of lifestyle. The warm-up is intended to minimise the risk of cardiac dysrhythmia (R.J. Barnard *et al.*, 1973) and skeletal injury; it usually takes the form of progressive calisthenics, including gentle stretching exercises that improve flexibility. The warm-down sustains venous return during the early recovery period. Fluid is returned from the muscles to the central circulation, avoiding a precipitous fall in blood pressure and minimising post-exercise stiffness. Slow walking is suitable for this purpose.

Whatever form of activity is prescribed, the patient should feel no more than pleasantly tired on the following day. If there are severe residual symptoms, then the training plan is too vigorous. The coronary-prone individual with an aggressive ('Type A') personality may need strong warnings to compete only against himself, not exceeding the stipulated dose of physical activity. Because a 2-km walk is good for his health, he must not assume that a 4-km run is even better! On the other hand, the training plan must show progression, the duration and/or the intensity of exercise being increased every few weeks as the patient adapts to his current prescription. Regular assessment of fitness, whether by a paramedical professional or by the Canadian Home Fitness Test (R.J. Shephard, 1980a), provides an objective indication of the progress that has been realised. Such 'feedback' is important to motivation of the subject and gives appropriate guidance for upward adjustment of the prescription.

Specific prescriptions

The general pattern of training discussed above should induce a substantial increase in aerobic power — at least 20 per cent in an average adult (R.J. Shephard, 1965), with larger gains in those who train exceedingly hard or who have previously lived very sedentary lives. Individual modification of the basic prescription may be needed to correct particular risk factors such as obesity, and to induce the development of specific muscle groups.

An obese patient may initially be incapable of sustaining high-intensity activity. Nevertheless, an extended programme of moderate activity (for example, progression to one hour of deliberate walking per day) may achieve a small negative energy balance, with gradual correction of the obesity. In a typical older person, an hour of deliberate fast walking four days per week for a year is sufficient to eliminate three quarters of the body fat accumulated between the ages of 25 and 65 years (K.H. Sidney & Shephard, 1978).

Deliberate muscular development is normally unnecessary for a middle-aged adult. However, if a person's work calls for the occasional performance of very heavy work by the arms and shoulder girdle, specific training of the muscles concerned will minimise the resultant rise in systemic blood pressure and thus in cardiac work rate during the activity. Specific development of the knee or the back muscles may also be helpful if there is a previous history that regular exercise was hampered by musculo-skeletal problems in these areas. The maximum isometric force of a muscle can apparently be increased by contractions lasting no longer than six seconds (T. Hettinger, 1961) and, if adequate rest intervals are allowed, isometric training can be performed without either skeletal injury or an excessive rise in systemic blood pressure.

Pulse-rate palpation

The accuracy of self-determined Canadian Home Fitness Test scores and the subsequent regulation of training intensity depend upon the ability of the ordinary middle-aged adult to count his pulse rate with reasonable accuracy (R.J. Shephard, 1980a).

In the original Saskatoon trial of the Canadian Home Fitness Test, subjects were given no specific instruction in pulse counting, and relatively large errors occurred; the coefficient of correlation between cardiotachometer readings and palpated rates was only 0.50. M. Jetté *et al.* (1976) taught their subjects to count the pulse 'until they could do this accurately'. Average readings immediately following vigorous exercise were 154 ± 22 as measured from the ECG and 147 ± 23 as obtained by palpation (difference = 7.0 ± 5.6). D. Bailey & Mirwald (1975) found a similar discrepancy (average of ECG readings, 135, average of palpated values 127 beats·min^{-1}) when they tested children aged between eleven and 14 who were used to counting their pulse (track and speed-skating contestants). In the latter experiments, the coefficient of correlation between measured and palpated readings was 0.94 for the athletes, but only 0.37 for children with no previous experience in pulse counting. We have recently observed similar results when testing office workers in Toronto (Table 9.2).

Although it is undoubtedly possible to find subjects who are inept at pulse counting (G.R. Cumming & Glenn, 1977; A. Bonen *et al.*, 1977), the majority of adults make a reasonable estimate of their heart rate. Accuracy is improved by use of the carotid rather than the radial pulse and by a modest amount of practice. Perhaps because of greater motivation, and perhaps because they have received more careful instruction, 'post-coronary' patients make a particularly valid assessment of their heart rates (W.R. Duncan *et al.*, 1968); T. Kavanagh & Shephard, unpublished data).

Table 9.2: Relationship between Heart Rate as Measured by ECG and Palpated Pulse Rate for Office Workers Carrying Out Canadian Home Fitness Test with Only the Instructions Provided on the Jacket of the Record

	ECG-measured heart rate (beats•min^{-1})*	Palpated pulse rate (beats•min^{-1})	Difference (beats•min^{-1})	Coefficient of correlation (r)
Rest	75.8 ± 10.6	75.8 ± 12.9	0.1 ± 11.3	0.55
Test stage I	125.6 ± 18.4	119.6 ± 25.8	5.9 ± 20.1	0.63
Test stage II	142.8 ± 17.2	138.8 ± 24.8	4.0 ± 18.1	0.68
Test stage III	148.7 ± 16.1	141.8 ± 19.1	6.9 ± 20.6	0.33

* The time was measured for the ECG complexes presented during the ten-second counting interval.

Source: Shephard, Cox, Corey & Smyth (in preparation).

Exercise Prescription in Tertiary Prevention

Hospital phase

At one time, coronary patients followed a regimen of strict bed rest while in hospital. It was feared that the slightest physical activity might precipitate rupture of the weakened segment of ventricular wall. However, it is now realised that such a 'cardiac tamponade' is a rare complication of myocardial infarction. The majority of deaths occur in the first 24 hours after the acute episode, the usual cause being a dysrhythmia of sudden onset, or the progressive development of left-ventricular failure. If cardiac rhythm is normal and there is an adequate systemic blood pressure, the prognosis improves rapidly thereafter.

Exercise is best begun early, when the patient is most amenable to recommendations for a change of lifestyle. This allows hospital staff to supervise the early phases of rehabilitation. Treatment should commence within 24 hours of infarction, assuming there are no signs of heart failure, shock, intractable pain or persistent dysrhythmias (J. Acker, 1973; L.L. Brook, 1973; N.K. Wenger, 1973; L.R. Zohman, 1973).

Over the first week, activity is limited to an intensity of about 10 kJ•min^{-1}. The patient commences by sitting at 45° in his bed, feeding himself, and carrying out light exercises for individual muscle groups. By the end of the week, he is able to sit in a chair for three one-hour periods per day.

During the second and third weeks, activity is gradually increased, with occasional peaks to 16 kJ·min⁻¹. The patient attends to his personal toilet and carries out light craftwork. Walking begins, and by the third week he is covering 30 metres per trip. Each new stage of activity is initiated before rather than after a meal, and where possible it is monitored by ECG.

In the fourth week, the patient walks 0.8–1.0 km at a stretch, and returns to his home or a convalescent facility (O.A. Brusis, 1977). If progress is maintained, the pre-infarction level of activity should be reached at about eight weeks. The patient is then qualified to resume most types of daily work, and can also contemplate further training through a specific out-patient rehabilitation programme.

Outpatient phase

On recruitment to an outpatient programme, the average patient has recovered sufficient physical condition to allow performance of a standard sub-maximal laboratory stress test. This is usually carried to a target heart rate (75 or 85 per cent of maximum oxygen intake), although most patients can continue activity to a symptom-limited maximum without excessive risk (R.A. Bruce *et al.*, 1973; T. Kavanagh & Shephard, 1976). Laboratory evaluation allows the supervising physician: (i) to define an intensity of activity that is tolerated without excessive ST segmental depression or dysrhythmias; (ii) to prescribe a dose of endurance exercise appropriate for further conditioning; and (iii) to establish a 'bench-mark' for subsequent monitoring of progress.

In the first six to eight weeks of outpatient therapy, the patient should attend two or three closely monitored exercise class sessions per week. He should also exercise himself to a total of five sessions per week. In the supervised sessions, he learns the theory of walking and jogging, including such matters as an appropriate choice of clothing and footwear. The technique of pulse counting is demonstrated, and an assistant checks that the subject is recording an accurate estimate of his heart rate. If abnormal rhythms or deep ST segmental depression develop during exercise, the patient is taught to recognise the corresponding sensations, and he is counselled to halt exercise briefly until such symptoms pass. As in a healthy adult, the endurance prescription is based on both general condition and the maximum oxygen intake as determined during laboratory testing. A typical recommendation for a patient with obesity, low back-pain, osteoarthritis of the knees or moderately impaired oxygen transport (maximum oxygen intake of less than 16 ml·kg⁻¹·min⁻¹) calls for a progressive extension of the required walking distance over the eight weeks (T. Kavanagh, 1976):

Weeks 1–2	1.6 km in 30 minutes
Weeks 3–4	2.4 km in 42 minutes
Weeks 5–6	3.2 km in 50 minutes
Weeks 7–8	4.0 km in 57.5 minutes

If the initial maximum oxygen intake is greater than 16 ml·kg^{-1}·min^{-1}, the preliminary period can be shortened to six weeks. For example, with a maximum oxygen intake of 21.4–22.7 ml·kg^{-1}·min^{-1}, a patient aged 42 might commence by covering 1.6 km in 17 minutes; he would progress to 3.2 km in 34 minutes for weeks 3–4, and 4.8 km in 51 minutes for weeks 5–6. Starting levels for other degrees of disability are shown in Table 9.3.

The patient may move to a higher intensity of training when his existing prescription has been well tolerated for at least two weeks. Requirements include: (i) an exercise heart rate consistently below the target value (equivalent to 60 per cent of maximum oxygen intake; Table 9.4); and (ii) no signs of over-training such as muscular aches and pains, excessive tiredness or premature ventricular contractions. If maximum effort is 'symptom-limited' (anginal pain, premature ventricular contractions or deep ST segmental depression) the target heart rate is proportionately reduced (to a figure equivalent to 60 per cent of the symptom-limited maximum oxygen intake; Table 9.4) and progression to a higher intensity of effort is not attempted until the exercise heart rate has fallen at least 10 beats·min^{-1} below the modified target value.

When the patient has reached the fastest walking time of Table 9.3, he is ready to progress to Table 9.5. He now follows the training pattern adopted by long-distance runners — firstly a quickening of pace with some shortening of the running time, and then a lengthening of the training session at a constant running speed (9.6 km·h^{-1} if under age 45 years, and 8.0 km·h^{-1} if over the age of 45 years). Criteria for progression follow the pattern already discussed. At a speed between 6.4 and 7.2 km·h^{-1} (depending on height and leg length) most patients find it convenient to pass from fast walking to jogging. Since the latter activity involves a rather different group of leg muscles to those used in walking, the change is introduced gradually at an appropriate point in the prescription. The patient begins by jogging 15 seconds out of each minute in order to make his required

Table 9.3: Relationship between Initial Maximum Oxygen Intake and Exercise Prescription for 'Post-coronary' Patients

Maximum oxygen intake (ml kg^{-1}•min^{-1} STPD)	Walking time (min)*
16.1–17.5	60
17.6–18.4	57
18.5–21.3	54
21.4–22.7	51
22.8–25.6	48
25.7–28.5	45
> 28.6	42

* All times are for a walking distance of 4.8 km; however, for weeks 1–2, 1.6 km and for weeks 3–4, 3.2 km should be covered at the same pace. An additional three minutes should be allowed if the patient is more than 45 years old.

Source: T. Kavanagh (1976).

Table 9.4: Target Heart Rate for Training of the Post-coronary Patient

Age (years)	Maximum heart rate (beats•min^{-1})	Target heart rate* (beats•min^{-1})
25	195	147
30	190	144
35	185	141
40	180	138
45	175	135
50	170	132
55	165	129
60	160	126
65	155	123

* The target is equivalent to 60 per cent of maximum oxygen intake, based on a conservative estimate of maximum heart rate (220 − age, years) and a resting heart rate of 75 beats•min^{-1}. If the resting heart rate deviates by 10 beats•min^{-1} from this standard, the target heart rate must be correspondingly adjusted upwards or downwards by 6 beats•min^{-1}. If the maximum heart rate is limited by symptoms such as angina, frequent premature ventricular contractions, or deep downward sloping ST segmental depression, the target heart rate is set at 60 per cent of this symptom-limited maximum oxygen intake. For example, if the symptom-limited heart rate at age 45 years is reduced by 15 beats•min^{-1} (160 instead of 175 beats•min^{-1}), the target heart rate is reduced by 60 per cent of 15, i.e., 9 beats•min^{-1}.

Table 9.5: Further Stages in the Training of the 'Post-coronary' Patient

Age < 45 years			Age > 45 years		
Distance (km)	Time (min)	Speed (km·h^{-1})	Distance (km)	Time (min)	Speed (km·h^{-1})
4.4	36.5	7.2	4.4	41	6.4
4.4	35	7.5	4.4	39	6.7
4.4	34	7.8	4.4	37.5	7.0
4.4	33	8.0	4.4	36.5	7.2
4.4	31	8.5	4.4	35	7.5
4.0	27	8.9	4.0	31	7.7
4.0	26	9.2	3.2	24	8.0
3.2	20	9.6	4.0	30	8.0
4.0	25	9.6	4.4	33	8.0
4.4	27.5	9.6	4.8	36	8.0
4.8	30	9.6	4.8	36	8.0
5.2	32.5	9.6	5.2	39	8.0
5.6	35	9.6	5.6	42	8.0
6.0	37.5	9.6	6.0	45	8.0
6.4	40	9.6	6.4	48	8.0
6.8	42.5	9.6	6.8	51	8.0
7.2	45	9.6	7.2	54	8.0
7.6	47.5	9.6	7.6	57	8.0
8.0	50	9.6	8.0	60	8.0

Source: T. Kavanagh (1976).

average speed. He then progresses to 30 seconds jogging and 30 seconds walking before attempting to cover all of the required distance at a jog.

Other activities may be substituted for jogging, particularly if this is made necessary by musculo-skeletal problems or by an adverse outdoor climate. An equivalent intensity of activity may be established with the guidance of data such as Table 9.1 and the resultant heart rate. If a different set of muscles are to be used (for example, a transition from outdoor jogging to indoor rope skipping), some temporary moderation of the prescription is desirable.

Class organisation

The general pattern of the 'post-coronary' exercise class is much as in a programme for a healthy person — a typical routine including five or ten minutes of calisthenics for 'warm-up' and flexibility, the prescribed endurance exercise, a 'fun' activity such as a game of recreational volleyball in order to increase motivation and a gentle warm-down. Each class is preceded by a short discussion period, when patients can review problems of training and lifestyle that are of interest to the group. Those with unusual symptoms are asked to report this to the supervising physician; they may undergo a full clinical examination and even laboratory testing before admission to the class session. One important function of the supervised class is to evaluate how the patient is reacting to his prescribed exercise. Where necessary, obscure symptoms can be evaluated by telemetry; for example, it may be necessary to distinguish the arm pain of angina from that due to osteo-arthritis. The patient must be kept under close observation not only while exercising, but also during the recovery period. Two of our patients developed ventricular fibrillation shortly after exercise, one whole standing in a hot and rather humid shower area, and the other sitting awaiting a taxi to return home. Finally, discussion periods should be arranged for the patients' wives — often spouses become more tense and anxious than the patients themselves, and they will pose many questions at such sessions, ranging from problems of dietary modification to appropriate modes of sexual expression (T. Kavanagh & Shephard, 1977b; Table 9.6).

We advise a patient who has graduated from the preparatory class to attend the Toronto Rehabilitation Centre once a week, carrying out a further four sessions of prescribed exercise on his own. This pattern of conditioning strikes a reasonable balance between the need for careful supervision of the patient and the physical problems of driving to and from an outpatient centre in a large city. Adherence to the home prescription is checked by having the patient bring an 'exercise-log' to the Centre at each visit. The log lists the walking or jogging distances actually covered each day, times, pulse rates before and after exercise and any unusual circumstances (Figure 9.1).

After a year of weekly attendance at the Rehabilitation Centre, we promote the patient to an eight-week inter-class interval. This is made necessary by problems of logistics. A visit to the Centre every two months provides an opportunity to review progress and discuss symptoms. In general, it also gives sufficient motivation to sustain the initial gains of training, although there is relatively little further progress after transfer to this type of regimen (Table 9.7). Indeed, in some patients ST segment depression is increased.

Table 9.6: Wives' Appraisal of Patients' Attitudes to Sexual Activity and to Other Socio-economic Problems

Characteristic	Normal or increased sexual activity, $n = 51$ (% showing characteristic)	Decreased sexual activity, $n = 49$ (% showing characteristic)
Patient takes less responsibility in marriage	52.9	79.5
Decrease in living standards (social, domestic or financial)	39.2	59.1
Prone to symptom claiming	27.4	57.1
Insecure in employment	15.6	38.7
Depressed	7.9	26.2

Source: T. Kavanagh & Shephard (1977b).

Table 9.7: Response of Post-coronary Patients to Infrequently Supervised Exercise

Variable	Group A (training already plateaued)		Group B (condition still improving)	
	Initial value	Change over one year[1]	Initial value	Change over one year[3]
Maximum oxygen intake:				
($l \cdot min^{-1}$)	2.02 ± 0.66	0.00 ± 0.45	2.02 ± 0.42	+ 0.12 ± 0.46
($ml \cdot kg^{-1} \cdot min^{-1}$)	27.5 ± 8.2	−0.7 ± 6.2	25.7 ± 4.5	+ 1.4 ± 5.5
ST depression (mV at comparable heart rate)	−0.03 ± 0.15[2]	0.07 ± 0.13[2]	0.01 ± 0.12	0.10 ± 0.12

1. Training sustained in 23 of 30 patients.
2. Sample initially showed small elevation of ST segment on average; positive change indicates worsening of condition.
3. Training sustained in 16 of 19 patients.

Source: Based on data of T. Kavanagh & Shephard (1980).

Figure 9.1: An example of an 'exercise-log' for monitoring prescribed exercise.

Day	Type of exercise	Distance (km)	Time (min, s)	10-second pulse count (before exercise)	(after exercise)	Symptoms and comments
Sunday	Jogging	5.6	40.10	11	21	–
Monday	Jogging	5.6	40.15	12	22	Slight tightness in chest
Tuesday	Jogging	5.6	40.00	10	20	Had a good day
Wednesday	Jogging	5.6	40.04	11	21	–
Thursday	Rest day	–	–	–	–	–
Friday	Jogging	5.6	40.10	11	21	–
Saturday	Rest day	–	–	–	–	–

S.M. Fox (1979) has advocated a similar pattern of tapering super-vision following infarction. His plan envisions twelve weeks at three sessions per week, twelve weeks at two sessions per week, twelve weeks at one session per week and twelve weeks at one session alternate weeks. The patient himself is encouraged to exercise at least three times per week throughout, either on his own or at some community facility. S.M. Fox has proposed that supervised training be terminated when the patient attains a reasonable level of physical working capacity, the required standard decreasing from 10 Mets in men and 8 Mets in women aged less than 49 years to 7 Mets in men and 6.5 Mets in women over 70 years of age.

Jogging technique

Although it is sometimes shrouded in mystery, the technique of jogging is simple. Basic needs are a good pair of shoes, clothes that are permeable to sweat, and (possibly) a cheap wallet-style-computer with timing and pacing options. The patient should run with short steps, landing in a flat-footed manner. The body is held erect, with the shoulders and neck relaxed. Running on the toes or an exaggerated heel roll are liable to cause various orthopaedic injuries. The shoes that are chosen should not be too light – the aim is comfort rather than a racing performance. The sole should be thick and resilient enough to absorb some of the shock of ground impact. Arch and ankle support should be provided, and the heel should not be too low. Padding around the instep and at the back of the heel will minimise chafing. Hard running surfaces (concrete or tiled floors and sidewalks) are best avoided. Natural turf should also be well-groomed, without pot-holes or obstacles.

Hot climates

Sustained jogging produces an increase in core temperature in 'post-coronary' patients, much as in normal individuals (R.J. Shephard & Kavanagh, 1975; T. Kavanagh & Shephard, 1975b; T. Kavanagh *et al.*, 1975a; T. Kavanagh *et al.*, 1977a; R.J. Shephard *et al.*, 1978a). Indeed, since the rise of core temperature is a function of the percentage of maximum oxygen intake that is exerted (B. Nielsen, 1969), a cardiac patient is more vulnerable to hyperthermia than a fit young man at any given speed of running. Limiting temperatures for the runner are summarised in Table 9.8. These values should be approached with caution if the patient is obese, or is not yet acclimatised to summer heat. The best remedy for a prolonged hot spell

Table 9.8: Limiting Environmental Temperatures for Outdoor Running and Jogging, as Specified by US National Road Running Club

Temperature		Relative
Dry bulb ($^\circ$C)	Wet bulb ($^\circ$C)	humidity (%)
35.0		
29.4	24.3	60
26.7	23.3	75

Table 9.9: Some Changes Induced by Running over a Marathon Distance, Shown by Data for Post-coronary Patients Participating in 1975 Boston Marathon Run

Decrease in body mass	2.8 ± 0.5 kg	(4.1 ± 0.8%)
Sweat loss	3.6 ± 0.5 l	
Estimated dehydration*	0.7 ± 0.5 l	(1.8 ± 1.5%)
Rectal temperature	1.6 ± 0.5 $^\circ$C	
Plasma		
$\quad$ Na$^+$	+ 4 ± 3 $\quad$ mmol•l^{-1}	
$\quad$ K$^+$	0 ± 0.2 mmol•l^{-1}	
$\quad$ HCO$'_3$	− 1.5 ± 0.8 mmol•l^{-1}	
$\quad$ urea	+ 5.8 ± 1.7 mg•dg^{-1}	

* Dehydration is less than sweat loss as a result of: (i) fluid ingestion; (ii) metabolic production of water; and (iii) (probably) liberation of water from glycogen.

Source: R.J. Shephard *et al.* (1978a).

may be a temporary replacement of jogging by swimming.

A group of post-coronary patients who ran the Boston marathon in 1975 averaged a 2.9 kg decrease in body mass and a 1.6°C increase in rectal temperature, despite copious use of fluids (Table 9.9). If the weather is warm, it is important to choose clothes that allow a ready evaporation of sweat, and to insist upon an adequate fluid intake. A jogger should be 'pre-loaded' with 500 ml of fluid a few minutes before running begins, and should ingest a further 150 ml every 15 minutes while he is running. During exercise, this type of intake is not easily achieved, since it is much larger than dictated by the sensation of thirst. During exercise, the sodium and potassium ion content of the plasma either rise or remain constant (R.J. Shephard & Kavanagh, 1975; R.J. Shephard *et al.*, 1978a; Table 9.9). There is thus little point in spending money on expensive replacement fluids — indeed, by causing an unnecessary rise in serum potassium, certain proprietary fluids may increase the danger of a dysrhythmia. The best drink for the runner is probably water or an isotonic solution of glucose. Following exercise, the potassium and sodium lost in the sweat should be replaced. Normally, this is accomplished by increased salting of food, but during a prolonged spell of hot weather, a cumulative mineral ion deficit can develop (C.H. Wyndham & Strydom, 1972). The affected patient becomes irritable and loses 'weight'. The blood volume and thus the stroke volume are reduced, so that a given rate of work induces a higher heart rate and a higher cardiac work rate. This may lead to a worsening of angina and/or an increased frequency of abnormal heart rhythms. The remedy is to maintain salt intake, and to moderate training temporarily if symptoms of mineral deficiency develop.

Cold weather

Very cold weather also restricts outdoor activity. Cold air causes cutaneous vasoconstriction, with an increase in central blood volume and a rise in systemic blood pressure. Inspiration of cold, dry air may also induce bronchospasm in an individual with sensitive airways (R.J. Shephard, 1977b), and it is reputed to provoke angina through a reflex narrowing of the coronary arteries. Substantial adaptation to cold is possible through an appropriate choice of clothing and the adoption of a brisk movement pattern. Cross-country skiing, for example, is an enjoyable sport on a sunny afternoon even when the temperature is as low as −15°C. Much depends on the wind chill factor (Table 9.10) and the extent of radiant heating from the sun; the comfort of a given environment may decrease rapidly once the sun sets, a point to be noted by those exercising in the evening. If inspiration of cold air is inducing symptoms, a patient may find it helpful to use a jogging mask (T. Kavanagh, 1970). This device allows the inspiration of air that has been warmed and humidified within the patient's own sweat suit.

It is important to note that the 'warm-up' must be extended if injuries are to be avoided in cold weather. Sudden chilling during the warm-down phase can be a danger if too much clothing has been worn, and garments have become saturated with sweat. Another danger, most marked in late February, is that of slipping on patches of ice. Freezing

Table 9.10: Thermal Comfort in Relation to Air Speed

Thermal comfort*	Air speed (m•sec^{-1})			
	0	5	10	20
Pleasant	10	26	27	28
Cool	0	19	21	21.5
Very cold	−14	11	14	16
Bitterly cold	−50	−11	−4	0

* All temperatures refer to dry air, and are expressed in degrees Celsius.

rain is an obvious hazard, but greater danger comes from small ice patches formed by alternate melting and freezing of the winter snows. Finally, the dirty windshields of the winter season put the night-time jogger at considerable danger from passing motorists.

Slowing of training

Many factors necessitate a temporary reduction of the training prescription for a 'post-coronary' patient. In place of pleasant tiredness, there may be persistent muscle soreness; if ignored, this could progress to a frank musculo-skeletal injury. The systemic blood pressure, both in rest and in exercise, may be increased by a period of domestic or business anxiety. Myocardial irritability may be augmented by a viral infection. Finally, the patient may complain of increased chest pain, an abnormal heart rhythm or a vague malaise suggesting an extension of the disease process. All of these items should be referred to the supervising physician as soon as possible; he will then decide whether a more formal reduction of prescription is necessary and, if so, for how long this should be enforced.

Recruitment and Compliance

The major challenges to exercise prescription are patient recruitment and compliance. The statistics are discouraging. Even if an exercise programme is established on company premises, the proportion of staff recruited to such a programme is unlikely to exceed 20 per cent (M. Collis, 1975; R.J. Shephard *et al.*, 1980a). Many participants will be people who were previously taking exercise in some other facility. Finally, as many as 50 per cent of 'high-risk' recruits may drop out of

Table 9.11: Drop-out Rate Observed in 'Post-coronary' Exercise Rehabilitation Programmes

Period of rehabilitation (months)	Drop-out rate (cumulative % of initial sample)	Drop-out rate plus poor attendance (cumulative % of initial sample)	Percentage of drop-outs due to medical problems	Authors
36	40	–	–	V. Gottheiner (1968)
36	25	–	–	H.K. Hellerstein (1968)
60	52	–	–	E.R. Nye & Poulsen (1974)
22	56	–	–	E.H. Bruce et al. (1976)
2–5	36	57	36.4	E. Kentala (1972)
6–12	52	78*	32.3	
12	40	61*	7.1	L. Wilhelmsen et al. (1975)
48	70	87*	–	
12	23	–	–	
24	38	–	–	
36	50	–	11.9	P. Rechnitzer et al. (in preparation)
36	4.4	17.2†	17.4	R.J. Shephard & Kavanagh (in preparation)

* Some of subjects reported exercising on their own.

† A further 12.7 per cent of subjects had moved to other cities, but were continuing to exercise three or more times per week.

Source: Based in part on data accumulated by N.R. Oldridge (1979).

an exercise class over a six-month period.

In patients who have already sustained a myocardial infarction, losses are not quite so severe (Table 9.11). The Southern Ontario multicentre exercise-heart trial lost about ten per cent of its residual sample every six months (R.J. Shephard, 1979b). The Toronto Rehabilitation Centre has fared even better, a total of 17.2 per cent of initial recruits having poor or zero attendance at the exercise class over an average of three years (R.J. Shephard, 1979b).

Recruitment

Factors influencing middle-aged adults to join a fitness programme differ from those that sustain their interest (Stiles, 1967; Heinzelman & Baggley, 1970). In a 'representative' group of US men, Stiles (1967) concluded that fear of incapacitation and a desire for buoyant health were frequent reasons for beginning to exercise. Less common initial motivations were a desire to compete and a history of family involvement in a specific sport. Heinzelmann & Baggley (1970) noted that workers joined their employee-fitness programme in order: (i) to feel healthier; (ii) to reduces chances of a heart attack; and (iii) to help research. The President's Council on Fitness (1973) cited as common reasons for regular physical activity: (i) a desire for good health (23 per cent); (ii) a belief that exercise was 'a good thing'; and (iii) a wish to lose 'weight' (13 per cent). Non-participants blamed their inactivity upon (i) lack of time (13 per cent); (ii) the amount of exercise taken at work (11 per cent); (iii) medical reasons (8 per cent); and (iv) age (5 per cent); they were the older, less well-educated and less affluent members of the sample, and were less likely to have participated in exercise programmes at school. D.V. Harris (1970) commented that middle-aged men who were physically active had a history of participation in athletic camps, school and university sports teams. Typically, they enjoyed both competition and the resultant fatigue, and their parents had encouraged them to participate in sports from an early age. B.C. Brunner (1969) also observed that middle-aged men joined a fitness programme to keep fit and develop a sense of well-being, while non-participants complained of lack of time.

Recruitment apparently occurs for similar reasons in other parts of the world. P. Teraslinna *et al.* (1970) listed improvement of health (63 per cent), improvement of fitness (19 per cent) and control of body 'weight' (7 per cent) as the perceived motives of Finnish executives who joined an exercise programme. The men recruited lived near the exercise facility, had an above average initial level of activity

Table 9.12: Reasons for Participation in an Industrial Fitness Programme

Variable	Always or frequently a motivation		Rarely or never a motivation	
	Men (%)	Women (%)	Men (%)	Women (%)
Health and fitness	83.2	91.2	16.8	8.9
Release of tension	58.5	57.5	41.5	42.5
Games and competition	70.0	38.3	30.0	61.7
Fun and enjoyment	90.4	92.5	9.6	7.5
Socialising, making friends	37.9	56.0	62.1	43.9
Self-discipline	50.0	52.5	50.0	46.5
Appearance	51.2	88.3	48.8	16.7

Source: Based on data of R.J. Shephard *et al.* (1980a).

and, contrary to many studies, were likely to be cigarette smokers.

R.J. Shephard *et al.* (1980a) studied US office staff who joined an employee fitness programme at the Westchester (NY) head offices of General Foods. They noted that male recruits had an above average maximum oxygen intake and muscle strength, but were also somewhat overweight and fat. Women participants were closer to the actuarial 'ideal' body mass, but had lower levels of cardio-respiratory and muscular fitness than the men. Factors of programme acceptability such as travelling time from the employee's home, hours worked in the office and the cost of an annual membership ($48) had little impact upon participation. Perceived attractions of the increased activity (Table 9.12) included health, fitness, competition (particularly in the men) and appearance (particularly in the women). General and specific health beliefs of employees were well developed, but contrary to the arguments advanced by Marshall Becker and his associates (M. Becker & Maiman, 1975; M. Fishbein & Ajzen, 1975; M. Becker *et al.*, 1977), the relationship between health beliefs, health practices and health outcomes was limited (Table 9.13). Our findings thus suggest that personal trial of an exercise programme may be a more effective technique of recruitment than a campaign intended to induce a more general change of attitudes and values.

In older adults (K.H. Sidney & Shephard, 1977a), findings are similar; reasons why men joined an experimental pre-retirement

Table 9.13: A Comparison of Health Beliefs between Participants in an Employee Fitness Programme and Control Workers from the Same Company (Scores Expressed in Arbitrary Units)

Variable	Men		Women	
	Members (*n* = 256)	Non-members (*n* = 217)	Members (*n* = 153)	Non-members (*n* = 151)
General health beliefs				
Current health	4.58	4.46†	4.59*	4.29
Possibility of improvement	1.41*	1.67	1.55	1.66
Heart-attack beliefs				
Smoking a risk factor	4.06	4.14	3.86*	4.16
Beliefs about exercise				
Prevents heart attacks	1.85*	2.21†	1.91*	2.19†
Spouse believes in it	1.57*	1.28	1.46	1.23
Friends believe in it	1.83*	1.46	1.71*	1.36
Reasons for exercise				
Health	1.92*	2.23†	1.63*	2.05†
Fun	1.84	1.81	1.66*	1.88
Socialising	2.69	2.83	2.48*	2.85
Self-discipline	2.50*	2.69†	2.49	2.67†
Personal appearance	2.51*	2.78†	1.85*	2.20†

* Significantly better score than corresponding sub-group (*P* < 0.01).
† Subjects in non-member sample exercising away from the facility show favourable scores relative to those not taking any exercise.

Source: Based on data of R.J. Shephard *et al.* (1980a).

exercise class included (in order of perceived importance) the improvement of health and/or fitness, opportunity for exercise instruction and testing, altruism ('to help science') and hedonistic ('fun', 'curiosity'). Women recruits again cited improvement of health and fitness, opportunities for instruction and testing, altruism and hedonism, but they also remarked upon anticipated gains of mental vigour and alertness, along with opportunities to socialise and pressure exerted by their friends. Other factors important to the motivation of this age group were the provision of appropriate facilities, instructions on how to exercise safely and opportunities for regular supervised activity. Not one of our elderly recruits had received any advice on the merits of increased physical activity from their personal physicians (R.J. Shephard, 1978b).

The situation is a little different after myocardial infarction. Many doctors have now accepted the value of progressive exercise in the treatment of younger 'post-coronary' patients, and recruits to such programmes are commonly received on the basis of medical referral. Given an incidence of three heart attacks per 1,000 men aged 35-65 years, and an average survival of ten years, the total patient base in a metropolitan area such as Toronto (population 2.5 million) is about 15,000. Relating these statistics to our actual enrolment of about 1,250, we would judge that one male patient in twelve is now being referred for exercise. Presumably, at least a proportion of such men have relatively small infarcts; this suggestion is strongly supported by: (i) the short average duration of ischaemic pain in the Toronto series (Table 9.14); and (ii) the low rates of recurrence and mortality seen in those patients recruited to a control programme of homeopathic exercise (1.5 and 0.4 events per 100 person-years respectively).

Compliance

Knowledge of factors influencing compliance with exercise programmes is in its infancy. Plainly, much depends upon the characteristics of the individual and our success in matching the prescribed programme to his temperament and abilities.

Drop-out rates among apparently healthy subjects depend greatly upon the basis of initial recruitment and screening, the type of programme that is offered and criteria of non-compliance. Thus, Teräslinna *et al.* (1969) had only one of 89 subjects defect over nine months of exercise. On the other hand, losses from a jogging programme amount to 35 per cent at ten weeks (J.H. Wilmore *et al.*, 1970), 41 per cent at six months (G.V. Mann *et al.*, 1969) and 53 per cent at seven months (J. Massie & Shephard, 1971; H.L. Taylor *et al.*, 1973). Typical figures for a gymnasium-based exercise programme are a 17 per cent sample attrition at three months (H.P. Elder, 1969) and an 18 per cent loss at seven months (J. Massie & Shephard, 1971). N. Oldridge (1977) noted that 50 per cent of his sample had defected at 18 months, 60 per cent at 48 months and 70 per cent at 84 months.

The gregarious middle-aged adult responds better to a group programme than to solitary jogging (J. Massie & Shephard, 1971), whereas the reverse is often true of the introvert. Among the Toronto

Table 9.14: Characteristics of Myocardial Infarction among Patients Referred to the Toronto Rehabilitation Centre

Duration of pain (min)	Proportion of sample (%)	Severity of pain	Proportion of sample (%)
Nil	4.2	Nil	4.1
0–2	11.7	Mild	29.6
2–10	22.3	Severe	29.6
10–20	3.2	Very severe*	25.5
20–30*	14.9	Unbearable*	11.2
30–60*	43.7		

* Typical of a classical myocardial infarction.

Source: Based on data of T. Kavanagh & Shephard (1973a).

sample of 'post-coronary' patients, a surprisingly large 45 per cent said that they were happiest when exercising on their own (R.J. Shephard & Kavanagh, 1978d). Possible attractions of solitary exercise for the cardiac patient are an absence of 'competition' and avoidance of comparisons with others who may be progressing faster in their prescribed activity.

Reactions to an industrial fitness programme depend upon the overall attitude of the employee (favourable or otherwise) towards his company (R.J. Shephard & Cox, 1980). In vigorous programmes, it is the heavy subjects with a large excess body mass, a high percentage of body fat and a low maximum oxygen intake who are the commonest defectors (Table 9.15). Presumably, the physical demands made upon them are excessive relative to either their physiological ability or their perceived needs. In some instances, a failure to fulfil the expectations of the instructor leads to a deterioration of self-image. In programmes where a more gradual progression of exercise intensity has been adopted, the interaction between initial fitness and compliance is less obvious (R.J. Shephard & Cox, 1980); however, a light, rhythmic gymnastics class selectively attracts the shorter members of an office population (mean height of participating men 173.5 ± 0.7 cm and of women, 160.3 ± 0.6 compared with values of 175.0 ± 1.5 and 162.3 ± 1.1 cm for 'drop-outs', and of 178.4 ± 0.9 and 161.9 ± 0.8 cm for non-participants). Other features of the 'drop-out' include extroversion, persistent cigarette smoking, a poor credit-rating (J. Massie & Shephard,

Table 9.15: Three Comparisons between Good Participants (P) and Drop-outs (D) from Exercise Programmes

Variable	Middle-aged volunteers Men		Middle-aged office workers				Elderly subjects Men and women	
			Men		Women			
	P	D	P	D	P	D	P	D
Body mass (kg)	76.9	84.8[2]	76.4	75.4	57.2	59.3	64.1	70.8
	±7.8	±11.6	±1.3	±2.7	±0.9	±1.8	±10.2	±12.2
Excess mass (kg)	9.6	16.1[2]	5.1	4.2	6.0	6.7	3.6	13.3[3]
	±6.9	±9.4					±6.0	±6.9
Body fat (%)	23.0	26.2[1]	21.1	19.9	27.9	28.5	22.2	28.6
	±4.0	±4.2	±0.7	±1.5	±0.7	±0.8	±5.6	±6.3
Maximum oxygen intake ($ml \cdot kg^{-1} \cdot min^{-1}$ STPD)	36.5	33.2	36.6	38.6	32.0	31.1	29.8	24.0[1]
	±10.2	±5.6	±0.8	±1.6	±0.5	±0.8	±1.4	±4.1
Percentage of smokers	25	55[1]						

1. $P < 0.05$.
2. $P < 0.01$.
3. $P < 0.001$.

Source: Data of J. Massie & Shephard (1971) for middle-aged volunteers, of R.J. Shephard & Cox (1980) for middle-aged office workers and of K.H. Sidney & Shephard (1978) for elderly subjects.

1971) and (at least in 'post-coronary' patients; Table 9.16) a 'Type A' personality, a 'blue-collar' job, light occupational activity and an inactive leisure (N. Oldridge, 1979b).

Among 'post-coronary' patients, some defections are attributed to severe disease (for example, worsening angina, or the onset of cardiac failure), but most authors agree that medical problems are a fairly infrequent cause of poor compliance (R.A. Bruce *et al.*, 1974b; T. Kavanagh *et al.*, 1979; R.J. Shephard *et al.*, 1979a). In the Southern Ontario multicentre exercise-heart trial, 22 percent of sample attrition was due to medical causes (13.2 per cent cardiac, 8.8 per cent non-cardiac; N. Oldridge & Andrew, 1979); 25 per cent of losses were regarded as unavoidable (factors such as a change of work shift or removal to another city) and 42 per cent were blamed on psycho-social causes. In Göteborg (L. Wilhelmsen *et al.*, 1975), drop-outs were

Table 9.16: Identification of the Exercise 'Drop-out', Based on a Multiple-regression Analysis

Characteristic	Cumulative likelihood of dropping out of programme in 2 years* (%)
Average patient	45
Cigarette smoker	58
Smoker + blue-collar worker	69
Smoker + blue-collar worker + inactive leisure	80
Smoker + blue-collar worker + inactive leisure + light activity at work	95

* For the purpose of the Southern Ontario multicentre exercise-heart trial, a 'drop-out' was defined as a person who failed to attend class sessions for eight consecutive weeks.

Source: Data from Southern Ontario multicentre trial, as reported by N. Oldridge (1979b).

Table 9.17: A Comparison of Drop-out Rates and Reinfarction Rates for the Southern Ontario Multicentre Exercise-heart Trial

	Cumulative drop-outs	Reinfarction rate (per 100 person-years)
Centres recruiting from hospitals (n = 367)	52.6%	5.1
Centres where physician referred (n = 384)	38.5%	2.7

Source: Based on preliminary analysis of data from Southern Ontario multicentre trial, as reported by R.J. Shephard (1979c).

blamed upon lack of transportation (34 per cent), poor motivation (24 per cent), cardiac problems (25 per cent) and other medical problems (17 per cent).

One striking feature of the Southern Ontario trial analysed to date has been a two-fold difference of compliance between cooperating centres. This reflects in part varying patterns of recruitment (physician referral versus the 'scouring' of intensive-care hospital wards; Table 9.17) — and in part differences in the personality of the individuals leading the exercise classes. The class leader must plainly be enthusiastic, but not to the point of making excessive demands upon his patients. There is a need for a regular feedback of test scores and interpretation of current symptoms, and in this connection the personal involvement of the medical director is very important. In such a setting, a relatively close linkage can be established between physical activity and health. Thus the perceived benefits reported by our 'post-coronary' patients (R.J. Shephard and Kavanagh, 1978d) have included advice on fitness, health and heart problems, regular testing, safe supervised exercise, encouragement and camaraderie. Many patients have also valued our associated programme of psychological rehabilitation, making a plea for its wider availability.

Some authors have found that the drop-out rate is highest in the first three months after recruitment (N.B. Oldridge, 1979). If this were generally true, it would have important implications for both the design of experiments and the use of scarce resources in the rehabilitation of 'post-coronary' patients. In fact, if the annual loss from the Southern Ontario multicentre exercise-heart trial is expressed as a percentage of the residual sample, overall defections amount to about 20 per cent in the fourth as in the first year of recruitment (R.J. Shephard, 1979c).

Techniques of sustaining exercise compliance become of particular importance one to two years after recruitment, when the average 'post-coronary' patient must be weaned from one supervised class per week to one class in eight weeks. As might be predicted, the transition is harder for extroverts than for introverts (R.J. Shephard & Kavanagh, 1978d). T. Kavanagh & Shephard (1979) noted that 67 per cent of patients who had reached a plateau of training and 63 per cent of patients who were still progressing found it 'no problem' or 'relatively easy' to continue with their prescribed activity while making only one visit to the Centre every eight weeks. The remainder of the sample missed the encouragement they had drawn from other members of the class and the discipline of regular observation, complaining that 'suitable' exercise facilities were lacking in their area of residence. Nevertheless, attendance at the eight-weekly classes was good. After allowing for an average of one legitimate absence per year (due to an acute infection, or a journey out of town), the attendance averaged more than 90 per cent of potential. It may be that the patient accepts the reduced class frequency as a practicable commitment, and is thus willing to reschedule conflicting engagements, avoiding the establishment of a pattern of chronic non-attendance.

Safety of Prescribed Exercise

The safe operation of an exercise class is essential not only in its own right, but also in terms of sustaining compliance and avoiding expensive litigation.

Cardiac problems

The cardiac problems that may arise from injudicious exercise have already been discussed in Chapter 3. Current estimates of risk run from one in 100,000 to one in 300,000 man-hours of exercise, figures varying with the precise status of the 'post-coronary' patients that are included in a class. A cardiac facility operating five one-hour classes per week, each with 50 members, might thus encounter one episode of ventricular fibrillation in eight years. This is a sufficiently likely event that staff should have the training to administer prompt and effective resuscitation.

Many patients experience some warning of impending reinfarction (symptoms such as increasing anginal pain, premature beats or general malaise). Prompt reporting of such problems prior to a class can allow a careful clinical and physiological re-evaluation of the individual, thereby minimising the chances of an emergency during the exercise session (H. Pyfer, 1979). Sometimes pride or worsening cerebral perfusion may cause a class member to ignore exercise-induced symptoms, and class members should thus learn to watch not only themselves but also their colleagues. The prescribed intensity of activity should be reduced for any adverse circumstance (environmental or personal) and should be halted for any acute infection. Subjects with deep exercise-induced ST segmental depression and/or dysrhythmias must be observed with particular care, the prescribed activity being kept to a cardiac frequency at least 10 beats$\cdot$min^{-1} below that causing symptoms and signs. Both the warm-up and the warm-down should be carefully carried out, and patients should sit when changing. Showers should be locked to prevent use of excessively hot or cold water, and ventilation should be adequate to prevent a build-up of humidity in the locker room.

The relatives of the patient and other class members should be taught the principles of cardiac resuscitation, and where possible exercise should be carried out in pairs.

Musculo-skeletal problems

In some exercise programmes for middle-aged adults, as many as a half of the group have had to stop exercising within six months due to musculo-skeletal problems (such as ankle and knee injuries, prolapsed intervertebral discs, stress fractures of the metatarsals and 'shin-splints'; Å. Kilbom *et al.*, 1969; G.V. Mann *et al.*, 1969). T. Kavanagh & Shephard (1977a) found that among participants in the 1975 World Masters' competition, 57.2 per cent had suffered an injury of sufficient severity to interrupt training during the previous year. Of those injured, 39.6 per cent had experienced at least one week of disability, 26.7 per cent had been incapacitated for between one and four weeks, and 33.7 per cent had been affected for more than four weeks.

This alarming toll of injuries is not necessary in a well-designed and carefully graded recreational or therapeutic programme. K.H. Sidney & Shephard (1977a) prescribed a regimen of increased activity for 42 men and women aged 60–83 years, encountering only one or two minor tendon pulls requiring no more than one or two weeks of reduced activity.

The risk of such problems apparently increases with age, as a result of: (i) greater muscle stiffness secondary to greater fatigue; (ii) less rapid relaxation of antagonist muscles; (iii) loss of elastic tissue, shortening of tendons and alterations in structure of the collagen molecule; (iv) loss of flexibility and degeneration of the joints; (v) a decreased blood supply to the tendons; (vi) loss of both organic matter and minerals from bone; (vii) clumsiness due to lack of recent exercise and impairment of special senses, balance and reflexes; and (viii) obesity.

Keys to the minimisation of musculo-skeletal problems include: (i) a thorough initial medical examination, with avoidance of stress upon vulnerable joints; (ii) adequate warm-up at each session of activity; (iii) gradual progression of the required training; (iv) the use of appropriate footwear and soft running surfaces such as well-groomed natural or artificial turf; (v) emphasis upon walking rather than jogging in the early phases of conditioning; (vi) a temporary reduction of the prescription if the pattern of activity is changed; and (vii) avoidance of violent calisthenics (especially rapid twisting movements and excessive stretching).

10 ADJUVANTS TO EXERCISE

It is not the purpose of this book to provide detailed instructions regarding such aspects of 'prudent living' as the reduction in body fat, adoption of special diets, cessation of smoking, relaxation and the use of various drugs.

Nevertheless, an exercise programme may involve several years of regular contact between class leader and participant, and many opportunities arise to offer advice on these issues. Furthermore, prudent living can itself have a beneficial effect upon prognosis. Indeed, some authors have gone so far as to claim that the benefits of regular exercise are brought about simply by reductions in body mass and systemic blood pressure (Chapter 8). A few comments will thus be made on possible adjuvants to exercise.

Reduction in Body Mass

Tables of 'ideal' body mass (Table 10.1) have been developed by the Society of Actuaries (1959). Their suggested classification of subjects by body frame (light, medium or heavy) is very subjective, and the present author has therefore proposed using as a reference criterion the average ideal mass for a given standing height, irrespective of body frame (R.J. Shephard, 1974d). The figures thus derived provide simple target 'weights' from the viewpoint of minimising cardiovascular mortality, but they must be interpreted with discretion. A very muscular individual may exceed the 'ideal' mass by 10 kg and yet have little body fat. At the other extreme, a woman may be 5 kg below the ideal mass, while combining an excess of fat with very poor muscular development. A low body mass was once linked to a poor prognosis, since it often heralded either tuberculosis or carcinoma. With current advances in medical treatment, there is no longer any obvious prognostic penalty in subjects who fall a little under the ideal mass; indeed, many people have a more pleasing appearance when their mass is a little less than the quoted figure.

The majority of sedentary, middle-aged North-Americans exceed the target figures. Typically, 5–10 kg of tissue is added between late adolescence and the age of 45 years (R.J. Shephard, 1977a).

Table 10.1: 'Ideal' Body Mass, Derived from Data of the Society of Actuaries (1959)

Standing height, for subjects wearing no shoes (cm)	Ideal mass,* for subjects wearing indoor clothing	
	Men (kg)	Women (kg)
147.3	–	48.5
149.9	–	49.9
152.4	–	51.2
155.0	–	52.6
157.5	57.6	54.2
160.0	58.9	55.8
162.6	60.3	57.8
165.1	61.9	60.0
167.6	63.7	61.7
170.2	65.7	63.5
172.7	67.6	65.3
175.3	69.4	66.8
177.8	71.4	68.5
180.3	73.5	–
182.9	75.5	–
185.4	77.5	–
188.0	79.8	–
190.5	82.1	–
193.0	84.3	–

*   For discussion, see R.J. Shephard (1974d).

In older age groups, fat persists but some lean tissue is lost, so that the total body mass of a senior citizen gradually reverts towards the supposed target.

Since obesity is well recognised as a cardiovascular 'risk factor' (Table 10.2), one might anticipate substantial numbers of very heavy patients in a 'post-coronary' exercise programme. In practice, this does not seem to be the case. The number of very obese subjects reporting to a coronary rehabilitation class is quite small, and changes in body fat over the course of training are also quite limited (Table 10.3). One reason for this anomalous finding is that body fat has already been reduced during the hospital phase of treatment. It may also be that

Table 10.2: Mortality of Grossly Obese Men and Women from Selected Causes in Relation to Excess Body Mass for Subjects Aged 15-69 Years

Disease	Men*		Women*	
	+ 24 kg	+ 42 kg	+ 28 kg	+ 37 kg
Heart and circulation	131	185	175	178
Renal	146	298	93	122
Vascular diseases of brain	136	215	143	142
All causes	123	168	130	138

* Data expressed as a percentage of standard values for subjects of same sex. Excess mass associated with a given mortality ratio varies slightly with stature.

Source: Based on data of *Build and Blood Pressure Study*, Society of Actuaries (1959).

Table 10.3: Initial Body Composition of Patients Referred to a 'Post-coronary' Programme, and Changes Observed over One Year of either Vigorous or Homeopathic Exercise

	Vigorous exercise		Homeopathic exercise	
	Initial	One year	Initial	One year
Body mass (kg)	74.6	+0.1	75.6	+1.5
	±10.5	±1.8	±11.0	±3.4
Skinfold thicknesses:				
triceps (mm)	10.9	−0.1	10.1	+1.2
	±4.3	±2.5	±2.5	±1.6
subscapular (mm)	20.2	−1.1	19.6	+3.3
	±6.1	±5.4	±3.8	±6.9
suprailiac (mm)	18.3	−1.8	18.9	+0.2
	±8.7	±5.8	±8.2	±6.7
Estimated body fat (%)	27.3	−0.4	26.2	+1.2
	±5.7	±3.0	±3.8	±1.9

Source: Based on Toronto segment of Southern Ontario multicentre trial, to be reported by R.J. Shephard, Cox & Kavanagh.

those with persistent obesity seek some alternative form of treatment, or indeed reject medical advice concerning lifestyle.

Patients who are above the ideal mass often claim that they are carrying muscle rather than fat. Some bias towards a well-muscled

Table 10.4: The Average Thickness of Eight Skinfolds in Subjects
Approximating the 'Ideal' Body Mass of Table 10.1

Skinfold site	Skinfold thickness (mm)	
	Men	Women
Chin	5.8	7.1
Triceps	7.8	15.6
Chest	12.0	8.6
Subscapular	11.9	11.3
Suprailiac	12.7	14.6
Waist	14.3	15.3
Suprapubic	11.0	20.5
Knee (medial aspect)	8.6	11.8
Average, eight folds	10.4	13.9

Source: R.J. Shephard (1977a).

sample is indeed possible among recruits to an exercise class.
However, there are several simple methods of checking this potential
alibi. An increase in body mass after the age of 25 is more likely to
be fat than muscle. The amount of fat can be estimated by caliper
measurements of skinfold thickness (Table 10.4). More direct
assessments of the percentage body fat are also possible by such
techniques as water displacement, underwater weighing, isotopic
determinations of body water and determinations of lean body mass
from ^{40}K counts.

On a warm day, elimination of body heat is impeded in a fat person.
Heat energy can be transferred through the insulating layer of
subcutaneous adipose tissue only at the expense of an increased skin
blood flow. The associated increase in body mass boosts the oxygen
cost of most physical tasks (G. Godin & Shephard, 1973b). This in turn
throws a greater strain on both the heart and the musculo-skeletal
system. When planning a training programme for an obese subject,
gentle progression is thus important in avoidance of cardiac and
musculo-skeletal problems and an associated high drop-out rate.

The desired result of an activity programme is loss of fat rather than
a loss of 'weight'. In a woman who has taken too little activity and too
little food for many years, an increase in total body mass through
some muscular development may be a healthy development. The

method of reducing body fat is simply to create a negative energy balance. If the body consumes less food energy than the combined costs of lean tissue synthesis and external work, the body fat content must diminish (W. O'Hara *et al.*, 1979). Drastic or even complete starvation is sometimes proposed for the obese individual, but this is dangerous unless conducted in a hospital setting; risks are particularly grave in the coronary-prone patient, where potassium ions liberated by tissue breakdown could provoke a fatal dysrhythmia. Since the original gain in body mass in a middle-aged adult has typically occurred over a span of ten to 20 years, it is usually better to aim at a relatively slow correction of the problem, with the intention of creating a new lifestyle that will persist once the target body mass has been reached. Starvation diets occasionally achieve dramatic initial reductions in excess mass, but the fat is commonly replaced once dietary restrictions are lifted (E. Sohar & Sneh, 1973; J.A. Innes *et al.*, 1974).

Body mass can undoubtedly be reduced by a modest restriction of diet, even in the absence of deliberate physical activity, but this has the major disadvantage that tissue protein is sacrificed along with the unwanted fat. A combination of increased activity (500–1,000 $kJ \cdot day^{-1}$, as developed through a typical exercise prescription), and a normal or slightly reduced energy intake (e.g., 500 $kJ \cdot day^{-1}$ diminution of food supply) provides the most effective 'reducing' regimen. Regularly spaced meals help to avoid the peaks and troughs of blood sugar that favour overeating, but snacks, alcohol and sweetened soft drinks must be held to a minimum. A daily energy deficit of 1,000 kJ will reduce body mass by at least 1 kg per month, more if energy loss is accelerated by an increased protein turnover. This is a satisfactory regimen for the average 'coronary-prone' patient who is 10–15 kg overweight, although more drastic measures may be needed for the occasional individual who presents with 50–100 kg of excess fat.

Although the necessary increase in physical activity was once regarded as impracticable by some nutritionists, simple calculations show that the exercise prescription of Chapter 9 readily meets the requirements of fat loss. The prescribed energy expenditure (60 per cent of maximum oxygen intake) amounts to an added 20–2 $kJ \cdot min^{-1}$, or 600–60 kJ over a 30-minute exercise class. If two flights of stairs are also climbed only three times during the day, a further 100 kJ are added, for a total of 700–60 $kJ \cdot day^{-1}$. A negative energy balance may give rise to a rapid early decrease in body mass. This reflects a loss of tissue fluids, probably including water 'coupled' to food stores such as glycogen (R.J. Shephard, 1980c). Although the phenomenon is sometimes exploited by those marketing dubious methods of 'instantaneous weight reduction', any such fluid loss is replaced within a few days, to the great discouragement of the 'weight watcher'. The early loss of fluid is often accompanied by disturbances of mineral balance, and this problem must be carefully watched in an individual with ischaemic heart disease.

The response of the post-coronary patients to a year of exercise rehabilitation (Table 10.3) is a little disappointing in terms of further changes in body fat content. Nevertheless, if the required activity does no more than maintain the fat loss achieved in hospital, this is in itself a major accomplishment relative to the known failure rate of traditional 'weight-loss' programmes.

Special Diets

Saturated fat

A number of trials are currently evaluating the preventive and thera-peutic value of diets low in saturated (animal) fat (Chapter 5). In general, it seems that the patient with a risk of ischaemic heart disease gains a marginal advantage of prognosis if he switches to a vegetable-oil diet that has a low cholesterol content (Dayton *et al.*, 1969). However, dramatic benefits cannot be expected from a sudden change of feeding patterns in late life. A high proportion of the undesired serum cholesterol comes not from the diet (500–600 mg·day^{-1}), but rather from hepatic and intestinal synthesis (about 1,000 mg·day^{-1}). If energy intake is excessive relative to physical activity and other sources of energy expenditure, cholesterol formation will occur whether fat or sugar is ingested (K.J. Ho *et al.*, 1970). Since atherosclerotic changes begin in childhood (Chapter 1), dietary manipulations in adult life are unlikely to resolve existing vascular disease such as advanced plaque formation with thrombosis and calcification. While a high serum cholesterol remains a risk factor for the patient who has already sustained a myocardial infarction (Table 10.5), there is no guarantee that prognosis can be improved by dietary attempts (J. Stamler, 1971) to reduce serum cholesterol. Furthermore, critics of low-animal-fat diets have pointed to several risks of alternative eating patterns, including: (i) a build-up of the wax-like vegetable fat ceroid (which is not attacked by body enzymes; A.N. Howard, 1970); (ii) an accumula-tion of straight-chain (trans-) unsaturated fatty acids, with possible damage to cell membranes (M.G. Enig, 1979); and an increased intake of refined sugar (which may favour both cholesterol formation and

Table 10.5: Classification of Blood Lipid Abnormalities with Main Basis of Treatment

Type of abnormality	Characteristics	Treatment Drug	Diet and Exercise
I	Increased low-density lipoproteins, lack of enzymes to break down chylomicrons, xanthomata	Thyroid hormone	Medium-length tri-glycerides
II	Increased low-density lipoproteins, lack of serum bile acids — inherited	Clofibrate and/or cholestyr-amine	Unsaturated fat
III	Increased very-low-density lipoproteins, xanthomata	Clofibrate	Exercise, negative energy balance
IV	Increased very-low-density lipoproteins, reduced low-density, increased cholesterol synthesis		Exercise, negative energy balance
V	Increased high- and low-density lipoproteins	Thyroxine + clofibrate	Exercise, negative energy balance, high-protein diet

Source: D.S. Fredrickson (1974).

damage to the pancreatic islets).

The first practical step in the dietary treatment of a coronary-prone individual is to obtain a lipid profile. Certain specific abnormalities of cholesterol and triglyceride metabolism can be corrected by use of drugs and dietary modification (Table 10.5). Some post-coronary patients with less clear-cut lipid disorders may still seek possible prognostic gains from a restricted diet and a low fat intake, but others may decide that the purchase and preparation of special food for one member of the family would cause a domestic upheaval that is unwarranted by present scientific evidence.

Increased physical activity modifies serum cholesterol only if there is an associated negative energy balance. However, vigorous endurance exercise induces favourable changes in the ratio of high-density to low-density lipoproteins, with some reduction in serum triglyceride readings (Chapter 4).

Vitamins

While large quantities of vitamins are consumed by the public, there is little evidence that such materials are deficient in a normal well-balanced western diet. Indeed, in war-time experiments, volunteers survived for several months on a vitamin-free-diet before symptoms occurred.

Exercisers are particularly prone to ingest large quantities of vitamins and other dietary supplements (T. Kavanagh & Shephard, 1977a). There seem several reasons for this. Successful competitors from Eastern Europe follow this practice, partly because the food in many communist states is less varied than in North America and partly because Eastern physiologists argue that for optimum performance the body must be 'saturated' to the point that the excretion of a given vitamin exactly matches the amount ingested. In North America, the more active members of the total population are often 'health-conscious' individuals and this causes them to explore possible methods of improving physique, including the use of dietary supplements.

A number of vitamins, particularly members of the B complex, are involved in carbohydrate metabolism, and the need for such compounds may thus rise with an increase in daily energy expenditure. However, if the diet remains well balanced, the added demand for vitamins is balanced by the added intake of food. One possible minor exception is the small loss of water-soluble vitamins that occurs in an individual who sweats heavily (R.J. Shephard, 1980c). Massive doses of vitamin C are sometimes taken by athletes in an attempt to ward off upper respiratory infections, and speed recovery following musculo-skeletal injuries (T. Kavanagh & Shephard, 1977a), although there is little hard evidence that the supplement is of benefit in either situation. Among 'post-coronary' patients, there is also a vogue for ingestion of vitamin E, although there is no objective evidence that this affects prognosis (R.E. Olson, 1973; T.W. Anderson, 1974).

Smoking Withdrawal

Cigarette-smoking is a clearly-identified 'risk factor' for the development of clinically manifest ischaemic heart disease (Chapter 2).

Table 10.6: Some Adverse Effects of Smoking upon Oxygen Transport
and the Cardiovascular System

Decreased maximum oxygen intake:
    combination of CO with haemoglobin
    displacement of oxygen dissociation curve for haemoglobin
    combination with myoglobin
    ? effects on tissue enzymes
Increased work of breathing:
    bronchospasm
    chronic bronchitis
Increased cardiac work rate:
    increase in heart rate
    increase in systemic blood pressure
    increased velocity of myocardial contraction
    increased stroke volume and cardiac output
Decreased coronary blood flow
Decreased flow to skeletal muscles
Increased risk of abnormal cardiac rhythm
Increased platelet adhesiveness
Increased serum free fatty acids

Source: A. Rode & Shephard (1971b); A. Rode *et al*. (1972); Wright & Shephard
(1979).

Several constituents of cigarette smoke (including carbon monoxide
and nicotine) have adverse effects upon oxygen transport and the
cardiovascular system (Table 10.6). Among ostensibly healthy middle-
aged adults who smoke, the reduction in 'coronary risk' associated with
regular exercise habits is also less than that seen in non-smokers (Table
10.6). Further, continued smoking increases the risk of recurrent
infarction for patients who are already enrolled in a rehabilitation
programme. It is thus logical to commend smoking withdrawal as an
important adjuvant to an increase of physical activity in both secondary
and tertiary preventive programme.

It is not our intention to discuss here the various possible techniques
of smoking withdrawal, although a few practical points deserve
emphasis. Firstly, an initial exercise test and/or participation in a
regular training programme may provide motivation to quit smoking,
particularly if clinically significant findings are carefully interpreted to

Table 10.7: Effects of Smoking Habits and of Physical Activity upon Total Mortality (47 Per cent due to Ischaemic Heart Disease)

Habitual level of activity	Total mortality (relative to corresponding sedentary group)	
	Never smoked regularly	Smoked > 20 cigarettes•day^{-1}
Sedentary	1.00	1.00
Light	0.69	0.95
Moderate	0.58	0.75
Heavy	0.57	0.70

Source: Based on data of E.C. Hammond (1964).

Table 10.8: Smoking Status of Distance Runners by Age at Which They Began Running

Smoking status	Began running	
	Before age 21	After age 21
Never smoked (%)	56	36
Former smoker (%)	36	60
Current smoker (%)	8	4

Source: Based on data of P. Morgan *et al.* (1976).

the patient (Table 10.8). The cigarette habit leads to various respiratory symptoms such as cough, sputum and breathlessness, with a substantial associated increase in the work of breathing (A. Rode & Shephard, 1971b). However, the severity of the respiratory disorder does not become obvious to a sedentary middle-aged adult until he tries to exercise. Equally, the initial stress test may provide the first warning of myocardial ischaemia. Personal experience of a smoking-withdrawal clinic has shown that exercise-induced dyspnoea and ST segmental depression are both strong factors influencing the decision of an individual to stop smoking (R.J. Shephard *et al.*, 1972).

The percentage of continuing smokers among men attending the Toronto 'post-coronary' rehabilitation programme is about 35 per cent (T. Kavanagh *et al.*, 1977c). A large proportion of our group stopped smoking soon after infarction. There is little evidence that the remaining subjects followed this example with continued rehabilitation. Nevertheless, the combined effects of regular exercise and contact with Centre staff probably played a useful role in avoiding the recidivism that normally afflicts ex-smokers.

Relatively few middle-aged adults who engage in distance running are smokers. Some authors have argued that this reflects the attraction of health conscious non-smokers to active pursuits. P. Morgan *et al.* (1976) presented statistics for Masters' Athletes. The initial percentage of smokers was much the same as in the general population (64 per cent in men who began distance running after age 21 years), but at the time of examination (after many years of running) it was only four to eight per cent. In this group, it is thus likely that running caused smoking cessation. However, the required weekly mileage (40–50 km) falls outside the scope of most recreational programmes.

It is important to persuade patients to quit smoking and not merely to switch from cigarettes to a cigar or pipe. Although the latter two forms of tobacco usage are normally associated with a lower primary risk of ischaemic heart disease than cigarette smoking, this is mainly because the smoke is not inhaled, with a correspondingly smaller absorption of carbon monoxide. Unfortunately, many cigarette smokers continue to inhale the more pungent smoke if they switch to a cigar or a pipe, so that their final health status may actually be worsened by this change of behaviour (C.M. Castleden & Cole, 1973).

Any decision to stop smoking should be linked with a total appraisal of health attitudes; otherwise, the potential gain in life expectancy may be whittled away by adverse changes such as an increase in mental tension, or a large increase in body fat. The ideal goal is to change attitudes in at least four areas of health behaviour, smoking cessation being linked to an increase in physical activity, control of food intake and adoption of a more relaxed attitude to life. In many patients, the well-disciplined atmosphere of the regular exercise class provides a format that is helpful in realising these objectives. But even if the patient shows a transient period of tension, or a small gain in body mass following smoking withdrawal, this should not be regarded as an indication to resume the cigarette habit; the accumulation of one or two kilograms of additional body mass is a negligible risk factor relative to the continued inhalation of tobacco smoke.

Relaxation

In the view of many authors, typical coronary-prone individuals are
tense, restless, time-oriented individuals, with what M. Friedman and
Rosenman (1974) would class as 'Type A' behaviour (Chapter 11). Of
the 751 patients referred to the Southern Ontario multicentre exercise
heart trial, 489 cases (65.1 per cent) were placed in this category.

Participation in an exercise programme sometimes has a relaxing
effect, with a reduction of state anxiety (W.P. Morgan, 1979), cardiac
frequency (J.F. Patton *et al.*, 1977), blood pressure (H.J. Montoye,
1975), lactate production (J.O. Holloszy *et al.*, 1971), catecholamine
output (L. Hartley *et al.*, 1972) and rating of perceived exertion
(J.F. Patton *et al.*, 1977). However, the response depends very much
upon the manner in which physical activity is pursued. Despite advice
to the contrary, many patients with ischaemic heart disease choose
to participate in a tense, competitive manner. They arrive at the
rehabilitation class begrudging the time that must be devoted to
physical activity, their minds seething with other plans and problems.
The prescribed exercise is performed in a rigid, obsessional manner,
with the hope not only of improving physical condition, but of out-
performing other class members. If business or social commitments
prevent the daily dose of exercise, such individuals may show a substantial increase in tension and anxiety.

In these circumstances, real benefit may be gained from various
types of relaxation therapy — deep-breathing exercises, yoga and even
hypnosis. At the Toronto Rehabilitation Centre, instruction in
hypnosis is arranged for many of the 'post-coronary' patients. The
rudiments of the necessary procedures are taught to individuals by a
physician with special experience in this art, and then regular weekly
practice classes are scheduled for groups of between eight and ten
men. Over the course of a year or so, the majority of patients reach the
point where they can induce deep relaxation on their own and, by
daily practice of hypnosis, many of these individuals apparently
develop a healthier attitude to life. While this is difficult to quantify,
T. Kavanagh *et al.* (1973b) found that over the first year of rehabilitation, the improvements in exercise-test responses in patients receiving
hypnosis almost matched the gains of those enrolled in the exercise
class!

Drugs

Space does not permit a detailed discussion of the place of drugs in the treatment of ischaemic heart disease. However, comment will be made on interactions between physical activity and some of the more commonly used pharmaceutical agents.

Nitroglycerin

Patients with exercise-induced angina may find a need to take trinitrin, isosorbide dinitrate or a related drug immediately before or during prescribed activity. The implication is that in addition to the primary myocardial infarction, other areas of the heart muscle are becoming perilously short of oxygen. Such a patient is at a greater risk of recurrence than the individual with an uncomplicated infarct and, accordingly, training must proceed more cautiously. In particular, activity must be kept below an intensity that would provoke cardiac failure (J.O. Parker *et al.*, 1966), and a close watch must be kept for any worsening of angina that would herald a potential reinfarction.

Nitroglycerin substantially augments the amount of work that can be performed by symptom-limited patients (Table 10.9). Some (R.E. Goldstein *et al.*, 1971; J.P. Bronstet *et al.*, 1978) but not all (A.N. Goldbarg, 1973) authors have also found gains from the administration of longer-acting nitrates. Failure to respond to these compounds may reflect either a non-ischaemic cause for the supposed anginal pain, or advanced coronary disease (L.D . Horwitz *et al.*, 1972).

The nitrates as a class were originally thought to be coronary vasodilator agents, although it would be surprising if much dilatation could occur in the hardened vessels of a typical anginal patient. Such drugs may have some effect upon coronary collateral vessels (W. Ganz *et al.*, 1978). Amyl nitrate also causes a general arteriolar dilatation (D.T. Mason *et al.*, 1972), while nitroglycerin is reputed to have a positive inotropic action that shortens the duration of systole (B.E. Strauer, 1973). Nevertheless, it is now widely accepted that most nitrates act primarily through an increase in venous pooling (H. Westling, 1971). Cardiac filling pressure is reduced, with a reduction in the systemic blood pressure and thus the work rate of the heart (B.F. Robinson, 1968; R.E. Goldstein *et al.*, 1971; V. Kötter *et al.*, 1978). A small reduction in pressure can be beneficial to a heart that is failing from oxygen lack, but an excessive fall in diastolic filling pressure reduces cardiac output and thus physical performance. It is still hotly debated whether the response can be improved by using a

Table 10.9: Changes in Response to Progressive Cycle-ergometer Test with Sublingual Nitroglycerine, a Long-acting Nitrate (Nifedipine) and Placebo in Patients with Angina

Drug	Max. heart rate	Max. systolic blood pressure	Max. work performed	Final ST depression
	(beats·min^{-1})	(mm Hg)	(kp-m)	(mV)
Control	122	170	3,015	0.38
Placebo (30 min)	125	168	3,220	0.39
(180 min)	127	174	3,313	0.39
Nitroglycerine (immediate)	140	183	4,861	0.33
Nifedipine (30 min)	143	164	4,254	0.40
(180 min)	146	171	4,947	0.34

Source: Based on data of J.P. Bronstet *et al.* (1978).

combination of nitrates with β-blocking drugs that counter coronary vascular spasm (H.I. Russek, 1968; W.S. Aronow & Kaplan, 1969; D.J. Battock *et al.*, 1969; J.P. Bronstet *et al.*, 1978; C. De Ponti *et al.*, 1978). Presumably, much depends upon the extent of coronary calcification. Some authors also advocate combining nitrates with calcium inhibitors; the latter modulate the breakdown of adenosine triphosphate and thus affect the development of tension by the myocardium (I.P. Clements *et al.*, 1978; B. Niehnes *et al.*, 1978).

Since nitroglycerin reduces cardiac stroke volume, the heart rate for a given power output is increased after administration of this drug. The assessment of responses to sub-maximal exercise then becomes complicated, particularly if reliance is placed upon heart-rate measurements at a given work load. However, to the extent that patients with angina take nitroglycerin as a normal prelude to exercise, it can be argued that the observed performance scores are realistic.

The response of anginal patients to regular, slow, long-distance exercise is often disappointing, and such individuals fare much better if transferred to a modified interval training programme (T. Kavanagh & Shephard, 1975a). The rest intervals apparently allow opportunity for re-oxygenation of poorly vascularised areas of the myocardium. The need for nitroglycerin can be reduced by a thorough warm-up and (in cold weather) the use of a jogging mask (T. Kavanagh, 1970).

Fortunately, the modification of the exercise/heart-rate relationship by nitroglycerin does not seem to prevent some training from occurring, provided that the patient is made sufficiently comfortable that he can increase his activity by a significant amount.

β-Blocking agents

Agents that block β-receptors of the sympathetic nervous system (for example, propranolol) are given to an ever-increasing proportion of 'post-coronary' patients. One common reason for such therapy is to decrease the frequency of premature ventricular contractions and other abnormal cardiac rhythms. Catecholamines provoke such disturbances by causing a patchy disturbance of ventricular function; there is an increase in calcium conductance across the cell membrane which increases contractility and shortens the refractory period, while at the same time an increase in potassium conductance accelerates repolarization (A.M. Katz, 1977). Both of these changes favour re-entry of the electrical signal into a part of the myocardium that has already undergone contraction. β-Blocking agents counter this trend by making the myocardial membrane less sensitive to catecholamines (P. Kühn, 1977).

Abnormalities of ventricular rhythm such as premature ventricular contractions and tachycardia are of particular importance as possible precursors of ventricular fibrillation. The need for β-blocking drugs is thus a warning that exercise testing and prescription must proceed with caution.

A.N. Goldbarg *et al.* (1971) found that after administration of propranolol the heart rate of healthy adults was reduced at rest (9 beats·min^{-1}), in light activity (17 beats·min^{-1}) and during maximal effort (36 beats·min^{-1}). However, there was considerable compensation for this bradycardia through an increase in the end-diastolic volume, with a resultant increase in stroke volume and a widening of arterio-venous oxygen difference. Maximum oxygen intake was unchanged, but the period for which maximum power output could be sustained was shortened by 25 per cent. Other suggested effects of propranolol have included a favourable distribution of coronary blood flow within the myocardium (L.C. Becker *et al.*, 1971) and an enhanced release of oxygen from the red cells (F.A. Oski *et al.*, 1972).

It is uncertain how far these various patterns of adaptation operate when β-blocking drugs are administered to patients with advanced coronary vascular disease. If a reduction in heart rate, systemic blood pressure and myocardial contractility occur, this should reduce the oxygen demand of the myocardium (C.R. Jorgensen *et al.*, 1977).

Propranolol is thus commended by most authors (H.I. Russek, 1968; D.J. Battock *et al.*, 1969; G.R. Dagenais *et al.*, 1971; A.N. Goldbarg, 1973) for the relief of pain in anginal patients. Most but not all (W.S. Aronow & Kaplan, 1969; A.N. Goldbarg, 1973) investigators find that the exercise tolerance of the anginal victim is improved by β-blockade. Much probably depends upon the cause of his disability. If the angina is arising from an excessive myocardial oxygen demand, then propranolol will help performance. However, if activity is limited by poor myocardial pumping, a further reduction in contractility will have a deleterious effect upon effort tolerance (D.T. Mason *et al.*, 1972); indeed, it may even precipitate cardiac failure. There may thus be advantages in the use of newer and more selective drugs such as practolol and oxprenolol, which produce cardiac β-blockade with less depression of myocardial contractility (E.A. Amsterdam *et al.*, 1971).

The slow heart rate of the patient treated by β-blockade complicates the normal process of stress testing and exercise prescription. The ideal arrangement would be to halt administration of the drug a few days prior to laboratory evaluation. However, withdrawal must be arranged with the concurrence of the supervising clinician, and a gradual tapering of dosage over a week or longer is necessary to avoid provoking a 'rebound' dysrhythmia. If, for any reason, the drug cannot be withdrawn, exercise tolerance cannot be judged from observations of heart rate; exercise prescription must be based on the power output as measured on a cycle ergometer, or the oxygen intake attained during treadmill walking. Any attempt to push such a patient to a normal target heart rate would of course be fraught with disaster.

A slowing of the heart-rate response to exercise is not necessarily an indication of improved physical condition in this class of person. It is equally conceivable that the clinical status has worsened, and the supervising physician has found it necessary to increase the dose of β-blocking agent. If the exercise prescription has previously been based upon heart rate, the first administration of β-blocking drugs is an urgent indication to re-evaluate the permitted work rate.

α-Blocking agents

α-Blocking agents such as phentolamine are occasionally administered to improve myocardial contractility. Such drugs are helpful to the patient whose performance is limited by function of the cardiac pump (H. Zebe *et al.*, 1978). α-Blockade leads to a substantial drop of end-diastolic pressure, with an increase in stroke volume and exercise tolerance.

Calcium antagonists

Drugs such as Verapamil and Nifedipine inhibit calcium transport. In consequence, myocardial-tension development is reduced, heart rate is slowed and blood pressure falls, all of these changes being helpful to the patient with exercise-induced angina (J.P. Bronstet *et al.*, 1978; I.P. Clements *et al.*, 1978; B. Niehnes *et al.*, 1978). The delay in calcium transport at the myocardial membrane also decreases the likelihood of developing a ventricular dysrhythmia (P. Kühn, 1977). Indications for the use of these compounds are much as for β-blocking agents; they should be avoided if there is any suspicion of cardiac failure.

Cardiac glycosides

Cardiac glycosides such as digoxin may be administered to treat residual heart failure following myocardial infarction, and/or to lower ventricular rate in the presence of an abnormal atrial rhythm. In either case, recovery of myocardial function is less than complete, and the exercise prescription must be correspondingly cautious.

Unfortunately, it is particular difficult to interpret behaviour of the exercise electrocardiogram after administration of digoxin, since this drug can of itself delay repolarisation, giving rise to ST segmental depression (L. Zwillinger, 1935; A.M. Katz, 1977). The slow resting heart rate of over-digitalisation must also be distinguished clearly from a training bradycardia.

Functional effects upon the myocardium are complex. Contractility and the velocity of cardiac contraction are increased (E.H. Sonnenblick *et al.*, 1965). At the same time, end-diastolic pressure and ventricular dimensions are diminished (J.O. Parker *et al.*, 1969; R.O. Malmborg, 1965). It is thus difficult to predict whether the cardiac glycosides will increase or decrease myocardial oxygen consumption, angina and symptom-limited effort tolerance.

Diuretics

Diuretics are commonly administered to 'post-coronary' patients who show a tendency to cardiac failure. They are an indicator of an adverse prognosis (T. Kavanagh *et al.*, 1977c).

Such drugs lower blood pressure, and thus the rate-pressure product. They also reduce ventricular volume and cardiac output, and thus have a beneficial effect upon those patients whose effort tolerance is impaired by angina. If there is depletion of body potassium stores, the ECG may show a falsely positive ST depression during exercise (A.J. Georgopoulos *et al.*, 1961).

Hypotensive agents

Hypotensive agents such as the Raowolfia alkaloids may be administered to patients with ischaemic heart disease in order to control an associated hypertension. Heart rate, cardiac output and myocardial contractility may all be reduced (R.L. Kahler *et al.*, 1962; S.I. Cohen *et al.*, 1968). However, the potential reduction in cardiac work rate is offset by an increase in ventricular volume.

Again, there is a likely implication of advanced atherosclerotic disease, with an impaired exercise response. In the early stages of therapy, control of blood pressure may be less than perfect, the patient swinging from hypertension to hypotension. Allowance must be made for this when monitoring the blood-pressure response to exercise. If the patient is in the hypotensive phase, particular care must be taken to ensure a slow warm-down, with avoidance of hot showers. Carelessness in this respect could cause hypotensive collapse or ventricular fibrillation.

Sedatives and relaxants

In view of the personality disorders encountered in many patients with ischaemic heart disease (Chapter 11), a case could be made for the pre-scription of sedative and/or relaxant drugs. However, the problem of impaired myocardial function can be life-long, and the danger of addic-tion to a 'remedy' such as Valium or Librium is then very real.

Endurance exercise has an immediate arousing effect, but if it is timed to take place two to three hours prior to the patient's bed-time, it has an effective secondary sedative action. The degree of relaxation that results from exercise depends upon the spirit in which it is pursued (see the comments on relaxation above).

Insulin

Maturity-onset diabetes is frequently associated with ischaemic heart disease. Before acceptance into an exercise programme, the blood sugar should be well controlled. Care should also be taken to have a sweetened drink before commencing an extended bout of exercise.

The long-term prognosis of the diabetic is improved by an increase in physical activity, and in many cases the need for insulin is diminished or abolished (J. Devlin, 1963; G.M. Grodsky & Benoit, 1967).

11 PSYCHO-SOCIAL CONSIDERATIONS

Although physicians place great emphasis upon statistics for mortality and recurrence rates in ischaemic heart disease, a more important aspect of therapy in many respects is the success of psycho-social readaptation. This chapter will look briefly at the issues of employment, resumption of normal sexual activity and adjustments of mood state.

Employment

We have already noted (Table 2.2) that premature death from ischaemic heart disease leads to a substantial economic loss. The typical cardiac victim is a successful, well-trained executive at the peak of his career. Sudden death robs society of a potential ten or 20 years of benefit from accumulated skills and experience. One estimate calculated the cost to the US economy at $19.4 billion per year (H.E. Klarman, 1964). The same author estimated the additional costs of caring for cardiac cripples at $3.0 billion per year. At the time of Klarman's report, the emphasis was upon work classification (L.H. Bronstein, 1959; R.J. Clark, 1959; D. Gelfand, 1959; T.V. Parran et al., 1959), with cardiologists making maximum use of residual function in the light of physiological, psycho-social and occupational evaluation (Table 11.1; N.K. Weaver, 1959; H.K. Hellerstein, 1979). It was soon found that the great majority of cardiac patients could return to gainful employment without risk to themselves or their employers (D.J. Turell & Hellerstein, 1958). More recently, the process of re-integration into society has been aided by active rehabilitation. S.R. Doehrman (1977) found that 60 per cent of one sample had resumed work after three to four months, 79 per cent at six months and 81 per cent at one year. N.K. Weaver (1959) had an even better experience (Table 11.2).

Those who remain unemployed after six months seem unlikely to change their status. Age is the main determinant of successful re-adaptation, the percentage returning to work being 88 per cent at 45–60 years, 85 per cent at 60–5 years, and 67 per cent in those over 65 years (E. Weinblatt et al., 1966; B.M. Groden, 1967; S. Fisher, 1970;

Table 11.1: Apparent Needs of Patients with Ischaemic Heart Disease Attending the Cleveland Work Classification Unit

Reassurance	73%
Intellectual interpretation	60
Vocational guidance	41
Emotional rehabilitation	28
More medical treatment	15
Vocational rehabilitation	8
Physical rehabilitation	6
Diagnosis	3
Avocational guidance	2

Source: T.V. Parran *et al.* (1959).

Table 11.2: Cumulative Percentage of Patients Resuming Work at an Oil Refinery

Number of months post-infarction	Percentage of patients returned to work
0	5.2
1	17.7
2	34.4
3	63.5
4	75.0
5	87.5
6	93.8

Source: Based on data of N.K. Weaver (1959).

S. Hinohara, 1970; R. Nagle *et al.*, 1971). A second important variable is the severity of infarction. One year after the acute episode, E. Weinblatt *et al.* (1966) found 86 per cent employment in those who were not severely disabled, compared with 54 per cent in those who had severe disability. A history of vigorous physical activity prior to infarction doubles the chances of a return to full-time work (E. Weinblatt *et al.*, 1966). Other important variables include motivation, skills and experience (R.J. Clark, 1959; D. Gelfand, 1959; A. Morgan Jones, 1959; T.V. Parran *et al.*, 1959), financial status (R. Nagle *et al.*, 1971), the attitude of relatives (R. Mulcahy *et al.*, 1972), the physical demands of the job (B.M. Groden, 1967; N.K. Wenger *et al.*, 1973) and the presence of associated diseases such as diabetes (B.M. Groden, 1967; S. Hinohara, 1970; N.K. Wenger *et al.*, 1973).

The anxiety that follows infarction (T. Hackett & Cassem, 1973) may delay a return to work (S. Hinohara, 1970), but it does not seem to be a major determinant of ultimate employability. S. Fisher (1970a) found no greater anxiety levels among the unemployed than in those who resumed their job, while H.A. Wishnie *et al.* (1971) and N.K. Wenger *et al.* (1973) considered anxiety and depression were limiting factors in no more than a quarter of chronically unemployed cardiac patients.

A proportion of more severely disabled patients benefit from coronary by-pass surgery (Chapter 12). G.K. Barnes *et al.* (1977) found that after such treatment 19 per cent of those previously unemployed returned to full-time work, and a further 35 per cent accepted part-time employment.

Given that most patients do resume regular work, should any restriction be placed on such activity? If the job involves occasional heavy tasks such as lifting, these should be simulated in the laboratory under telemetric control. If severe ST depression or dysrhythmias develop during this testing, the two possible options are: (i) to proscribe those duties that provoke undesirable signs; or (ii) to prescribe local muscular training until the heaviest physical demands are better tolerated. Attention must also be directed to the psychological demands of the job; while argument continues over 'stress' and infarction (L.E. Hinckle, 1972), a surprisingly large percentage of patients note business problems in the period immediately preceding a coronary attack (Chapter 3). The typical history is of a man who is spending long hours at each of two jobs. It is thus discouraging to find that after their 'heart attack' many patients remain fiercely competitive, still working 44–72 hours per week (D.E. Sharland, 1964). A. Jezer & Warshaw (1960) suggested that before returning to work employees should undergo a 'stress interview', with simultaneous recording of the electrocardiogram and blood pressure. L. Zohman & Tobis (1970) added a galvanic skin response measurement to the protocol in order to quantify the stress imposed.

Some employers have feared the legal implications of employing 'post-coronary' patients (L. Price, 1959; Ungerleider & Gubner, 1959). The number of cases where employment has been judged a primary or a contributing cause of myocardial infarction has increased dramatically in recent years. An early study from New York State set the annual total of Compensation Board payments for heart disease at $2 million (L.J. Goldwater & Weiss, 1951). In contrast, the US Disability Insurance Program received 43,979 claims for arteriosclerotic and degenerative heart disease between July 1955 and August 1956; furthermore, 64.2 per cent of these claims were allowed (A.B. Price, 1959). A cause-and-effect relationship may be postulated if the 'heart attack' begins less than six hours following performance of some unusual task; the case for compensation is naturally strengthened if there is a history of bridging symptoms (M. Texon, 1959).

The employment record of the cardiac patient is usually well up to average. W.E.R. Greer (1959) examined the experience of the Gillette razor company. Some 23.5 per cent of employees with ischaemic heart disease were premium workers (expected figure 20 per cent), while 8.8 per cent were base or unsatisfactory employees (expected figure 8 per cent). Absenteeism averaged 13.3 days per year (expected figure 11.3 days per year), and there were no major accidents among the cardiac group (expected figure 2.6 per cent of employees losing two or more weeks' work per year from major accidents). We may conclude that, given adequate rehabilitation and proper placement, the 'post-coronary' patient can become a safe and effective member of the labour force.

Resumption of Sexual Activity

Relatively little is known about the sexual behaviour of the older person (A.C. Kinsey, 1948; W.R. Stokes, 1951; A.L. Finkle, 1959; G. Newman & Nichols, 1960; R.J. Shephard, 1978b), and information regarding the 'post-coronary' patient is even more sketchy. A major textbook on ischaemic heart disease (T.R. Harrison & Reeves, 1968) makes no mention of sexual activity, while an otherwise excellent monograph from the International Society of Cardiology (T. Semple, 1973) contents itself with the delicate comment: 'family relationships may so deteriorate that resumption of normal married life becomes very difficult'. Nevertheless, sexual relations are an important aspect of healthy living at all ages, and the physician who is guiding a patient's recovery from myocardial infarction should be able to offer competent advice on the resumption of normal sexual activity.

There is both subjective and physiological evidence that exercise helps the process of readaptation (H.K. Hellerstein, 1970; R.A. Stein,

1977). Certainly, the physical demands of sexual activity can be substantial in a young person. There are reports of heart rates rising to 170 beats•min^{-1} and systemic blood pressures reaching levels as high as 250/120 mm Hg (G. Klumbies & Kleinsorge, 1930; E.P. Boas & Goldschmidt, 1932; R.G. Bartlett & Bohr, 1956). Such figures would place an undesirable load upon the heart after infarction, particularly if due account is taken of: (i) the absence of a steady state; (ii) the contraction of small muscles; (iii) the combination of isometric and isotonic work, often with a need for postural support; and (iv) associated autonomic reactions (J.S. Skinner, 1979). However, the typical 'post-coronary' patient has been married for many years, and his response to normal intercourse is much less dramatic than that of a young student. A peak pulse rate averaging 117 beats•min^{-1} (range 90–144 beats•min^{-1}) is sustained for only ten to 15 seconds, and the resultant cardiac stress can be compared with the ascent of a couple of flights of stairs (an oxygen consumption of 4.5 Mets; L. Zohman & Tobis, 1970; H.K. Hellerstein & Friedman, 1973).

Many patients harbour the myth that repeat infarctions tend to occur at orgasm, so that sexual intercourse should never again be attempted (T.P. Hackett & Cassem, 1973). A number of authors have documented the decreased frequency of intercourse following infarction, although a part of this change could be a normal con-comitant of aging (R.J. Shephard, 1978b). H.K. Hellerstein & Friedman (1970) noted a drop from 2.1 to 1.6 orgasms per week in 49-year-old men, and A. Bloch *et al.* (1975) a decrease from 1.2 to 0.6 per week. Others (W.B. Tuttle *et al.*, 1964; R.F. Klein *et al.*, 1965; D. Dorossiev *et al.*, 1976) report similar findings. The altered behaviour apparently bears more relationship to pscyhological factors including the sexual drive prior to infarction (Table 11.3) than to age, working capacity or disease severity.

A study from the Toronto Rehabilitation Centre (T. Kavanagh & Shephard, 1977b) noted that while 80 of 161 patients showed either no change or an increase in sexual activity, in the remaining 81 patients the frequency of intercourse was reduced. Reasons cited for the diminished frequency included the patient's apprehension (21 per cent), the wife's apprehension (23 per cent), loss of desire (37 per cent) and a combination of these factors (19 per cent). Of the patients with reduced frequency, 20 were encountering anginal pain and six were developing premature ventricular beats during intercourse. These 26 individuals noted that sexual activity was less enjoyable than before infarction. Eight of their number feared that intercourse would provoke

Table 11.3: Cited Reasons for Reduction in Sexual Activity

Reason	Author
Loss of desire	A. Bloch *et al.* (1975)
	H.K. Hellerstein & Friedman (1970)
	T. Kavanagh & Shephard (1977b)
Depression	A. Bloch *et al.* (1975)
Apprehension	A. Bloch *et al.* (1975)
	H.K. Hellerstein & Friedman (1970)
	T. Kavanagh & Shephard (1977b)
Wife's apprehension	A. Bloch *et al.* (1975)
	H.K. Hellerstein & Friedman (1970)
	T. Kavanagh & Shephard (1977b)
Symptoms and fatigue	A. Bloch *et al.* (1975)
	H.K. Hellerstein & Friedman (1970)
Impotence*	A. Bloch *et al.* (1975)
	H.K. Hellerstein & Friedman (1970)
	E. Weiss & English (1957)
	W.B. Tuttle *et al.* (1964)

* Many North American patients appear to deny impotence (J.S. Skinner, 1979).

Source: Based in part on reports collected by J.S. Skinner (1979).

another infarct, and in a further eight cases their wives had similar fears. The remainder of the 26 men were apathetic because of symptoms that arose during intercourse.

Formal tests of personality disclosed no clear relationship between reduced sexual activity and post-infarct depression. However, discussion with the wives revealed certain differences of behaviour relative to those with normal or increased sexual activity (Table 9.6). The gain in maximum oxygen intake with training (19.1 versus 11.6 per cent) also favoured the group who resumed normal sexual activity, an observation confirmed by R.A. Stein (1977). It is less clear whether the difference in training response is the cause or an effect of sexual problems. Certainly, self-esteem is important to successful completion of an exercise rehabilitation programme. T.H. Hackett & Cassem (1973) have commented on the decreased ego strength and sense of emasculation that exacerbate feelings of fatigue and weakness in the 'post-coronary' patient, and it is highly probable that the resumption of normal sexual activity plays an important role in restoring self-esteem.

Some authors (for example, M. Brenton, 1968; J.F. Briggs, 1972) have suggested that the cardiac patients should adopt a physically less demanding position such as side-lying when sexual activity is resumed. In the Toronto study, only 18 per cent of patients elected a more passive position and, whether cause or effect, all 18 per cent showed a decline in sexual activity. L. Zohman & Tobis (1970) also found that a change of technique hampered a return of normal sexual response. Passive positions are now largely discredited, since E.D. Nemec *et al.* (1964) have found that such changes yield no advantage in terms of lowering the heart rate or blood pressure at orgasm.

The relative risks of intercourse and normal rhythmic exercise can be judged from the respective incidence of symptoms; 12.4 per cent of the Toronto patients developed angina during intercourse, compared with 36.0 per cent during a standard laboratory stress test to 75 per cent of maximum oxygen intake (T. Kavanagh & Shephard, 1977b). Likewise, the percentage of patients experiencing ventricular premature beats was 3.7 per cent, compared with 4.6 per cent during the stress test. Nevertheless, in one series of just over 200 primary non-fatal infarctions, two patients admitted that their cardiac episodes had arisen during normal sexual activity (R.J. Shephard, 1974b). M. Ueno (1963) found 34 of 5,559 sudden deaths (0.6 per cent) were related to coitus, 0.3 per cent being attributable to cardiovascular disease, while H.K. Hellerstein & Friedman (1970) estimated sexually related cardiac fatalities at 0.6 per cent of deaths in the Cleveland area. Some 80 per cent of the Japanese incidents occurred during extra-marital affairs, many being associated with overeating and overdrinking. Given that the average frequency of intercourse in a coronary-prone man is about once in five days (H.K. Hellerstein & Friedman, 1970; A. Bloch *et al.*, 1975; T. Kavanagh & Shephard, 1977b), and allowing between ten and 15 minutes for the discharge of marital responsibilities (R.G. Bartlett, 1956; H.K. Hellerstein & Friedman, 1970; W.A. Littler *et al.*, 1974), it can be estimated that the risk of a first heart attack is increased at least two- to three-fold during the period of sexual activity (E. Massie, 1969; R.J. Shephard, 1974b).

It has been recommended that patients who are liable to angina take nitroglycerin, standard cardiac drugs and possibly tranquillisers prior to the sex act (J.F. Briggs, 1972; Q.R. Regestein & Horn, 1978; W.S. Aronow, 1979). Unfortunately, many of the medications commonly prescribed for the cardiac patient (digoxin, β-blockers, antidepressants, alcohol and tranquillisers, anti-hypertensive drugs) are liable to reduce libido, impair ejaculation and cause impotence (F.O. Simpson, 1974; R.S. Eliot & Miles, 1975). Because of the greater heart rate and blood pressure response evoked in such circumstances, there are strong medical arguments against marital adventures with an unfamiliar partner (L.D. Scheingold & Wagner, 1974). Coitus should also be avoided after a heavy meal, particularly if the subject is fatigued, anxious or emotionally upset. Reassurance may be necessary if the first few attempts at intercourse are unsuccessful following a prolonged period of abstinence; in this regard, advice from a general practitioner who is familiar with both the topic and the patient may be as effective as more specialised sexual counselling (B. Kushnir *et al.*, 1976).

In women who have sustained infarction, sexual frigidity and dissatisfaction are common, although such problems are almost always blamed upon the male partner rather than the disease process (L. Abramov, 1976). It may be wise to recommend some method of contraception other than the 'pill' to female cardiac patients (Chapter 12).

Adjustment of Mood State

Patients participating in a 'post-coronary' exercise rehabilitation programme often show serious disturbances of mood (J. Bendien & Groen, 1963; D.L. Keegan, 1973; T. Kavanagh *et al.*, 1977a), but it is less clear how far such disturbances are a reflection of the original personality (C.D. Jenkins, 1971; M.J. Segers & Mertens, 1974; B. Lebovits *et al.*, 1975; P. Siltanen *et al.*, 1975), and how far they reflect a reaction to the loss of financial, social and emotional security that accompanies a heart attack. The Napoleonic physician Corvisart (1806) wrote: 'repeated depressing emotions . . . may be the origin of refractory disorders of the heart'. More recently, M. Friedman & Rosenman (1974) described an association between a specific personality ('Type A') and heart disease, but others (E.H. Friedman, 1974; J.L. Marx, 1977; H. Selye, 1978) have argued that this thesis has been exaggerated, thereby causing unnecessary anxiety to patients fitting the 'Type A' description. D. Eden *et al.* (1977) went further, finding in a group of kibbutzim workers a negative correlation of overload, conflict and social pressure with conventional cardiac risk factors such as serum cholesterol. They concluded that the managers under study thrived in stressful situations.

Nevertheless, it seems likely that problems of personality and attitude can not only contribute to the critical 'coronary' incident (R.A. Keith, 1966; J.R.P. French & Caplan, 1970; M. Friedman & Rosenman, 1974), but also can influence the timing of the decision to call a physician, and the subsequent response to rehabilitation (D. Gelfand, 1959; B.D. McPherson *et al.*, 1967; M. Dobson *et al.*, 1971; T. Kavanagh *et al.*, 1973b). Clinicians also have the impression that there is an increased incidence of depression in the months immediately following myocardial infarction (A. Verwoerdt & Dovenmuehle, 1964; C.K. Miller, 1965; H.P. Klein & Parsons, 1968; D.L. Keegan, 1973). The question thus arises whether 'post-infarction' patients are individuals with a particular liability to depression (J. Brozek *et al.*, 1966), the 'heart attack' merely serving as a trigger that reveals an underlying personality defect.

T. Kavanagh *et al.* (1975b) applied the Minnesota Multiphasic Personality Inventory (MMPI) to a sample of 96 patients after between twelve and 15 months of rehabilitation. Almost all patients exceeded the theoretical D (depression) score of 50 (Figure 11.1), which may reflect in part the normal effect of age upon D scores, but about a third of the sample (34/96) had very high D scores (> 70 units, two standard deviations greater than normal). Individuals with the pathological increase in D score also showed high values for the 'neurotic triad' (hysteria, hypochrondriasis and psychasthenia; Table 11.4). Other authors (H.D. Ruskin *et al.*, 1970) have reported similar findings. It is popularly held that the MMPI is a measure of 'trait' rather than 'state', and in support of this view J. Brozek *et al.* (1966) found pre-existing high hypochondriasis scores in men who later sustained a 'heart attack'. On the other hand, A.M. Ostfeld *et al.* (1964) found no initial difference in MMPI scores between normal subjects and those individuals who subsequently developed myocardial infarction. A further possible complication is that individuals with an unusual personality tend to volunteer for physiological and psychological testing (R.J. Shephard & Kemp, unpublished data). Thus J. Naughton *et al.* (1968) recorded high D, Hy and Hs scores for a group of sedentary control subjects who agreed to complete the MMPI. However, depression inhibits physical activity (particularly in a post-coronary patient; D. Gelfand, 1959), and it is thus unlikely that a rehabilitation programme will selectively attract patients with a high D score. It could be argued that depression is a side-effect of the medication used to treat hypertension (rauwolfia and guanethidine) and dysrhythmia (β-blockers). Some 30 per cent of the depressed patients in the Toronto series were receiving propranolol, but scores

Figure 11.1: Distribution of depression (D) scores on the Minnesota Multiphasic Personality Inventory (MMPI). The solid line shows the anticipated distribution of normalised D scores and the broken line the distribution for a unimodal sample of patients with mild depression. The shaded area indicates the proportion of the sample with gross depression.

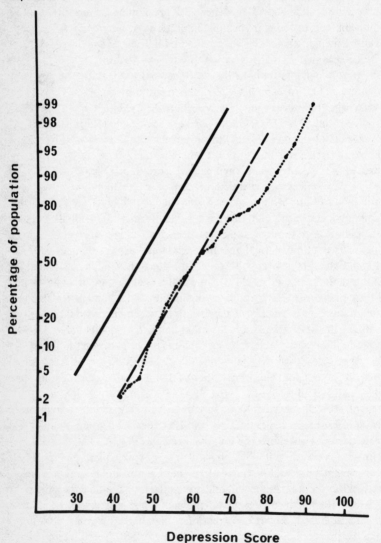

Source: T. Kavanagh *et al*. (1975b).

Table 11.4: Normalised Scores from Minnesota Multiphasic Personality Inventory Data for Post-coronary Patients, a Score of 50 on Each Measure Being Expected for a Normal Healthy Subject

Psychological characteristic	H.D. Ruskin *et al.* (1970)	T. Kavanagh *et al.* (1975b)	
		Entire sample (n = 96)	Grossly depressed patients (n = 34)
Depression	70.1	63.3	79.2
Hysteria	63.1	54.2	66.3
Hypochondriasis	63.7	55.4	64.2
Psychasthenia	59.2	55.5	65.2

for this sub-group did not differ from those for patients who were not receiving drugs. Possibly, the direct mood-depressing effect of β-blocking agents is outweighed by the resultant relief of symptoms.

We may conclude that a proportion of patients became severely depressed as a reaction to their infarction. T.H. Hackett & Cassem (1973) estimated that during the acute episode, 75 of 100 patients admitted to the coronary care unit became depressed. The peak effect was seen on the third day post-infarction. The abnormality of mood persists with the return home, as the patient senses the threat of invalidism, loss of autonomy and independence. Contributory factors include weakness resulting from the heart attack and subsequent bed rest, sexual problems (T.H. Hackett & Cassem, 1973), inappropriate and inadequate explanation from the attending physician (S. Hinohara, 1970), interaction with an over-anxious wife (H.D. Ruskin *et al.*, 1970; M. Dobson *et al.*, 1971; M. Skelton & Dominian, 1973), frequent hospital admissions (A. Verwoerdt & Dovenmuehle, 1964) and the patient's own anxiety, lack of confidence and fear of sudden death (V.B.O. Hammett, 1963; S. Fisher, 1970). In the Toronto series (T. Kavanagh *et al.*, 1975b), the depressed group were older than those with normal D scores (average age 51 as opposed to 45 years). A higher proportion of the depressed group also suffered from angina and hypertension. Prior to infarction, a higher percentage reported facing major worries, both in business (74.1 per cent of sample versus 60.6 per cent) and at home (32.2 versus 20.0 per cent). However, the information was collected retrospectively, and it could thus reflect either a true difference in exogenous pressure (C.M. Parkes *et al.*, 1969; C.D. Jenkins, 1971), or a magnified perception of difficulties secondary to depression. As previously noted by M. Dobson *et al.* (1971), the depression was also related to physical disability, affecting subjects that showed a poorer than average training response. It could be argued that depression weakened motivation, leading to exaggeration of symptoms and inadequate training (R.R.H. Lovell & Verghese, 1967). On the other hand, in the Toronto experiments, depressed and non-depressed subjects attained an almost equal walking distance and speed. Despite equal effort, the training response was poorer in the depressed subjects. The most reasonable explanation of our findings is thus that difficulties encountered in training contributed to their depression, and indeed it is arguable that some cases might have responded more favourably to a less vigorous programme.

Many patients deny their depression (A.D. Weisman & Hackett, 1961), to the point where it may be overlooked (J.G. Bruhn, 1973; T. Kavanagh *et al.*, 1975b; M. Dobson *et al.*, 1971). However, the psychological profile has important implications when planning a rehabilitation programme. The non-depressed hypomanic patient is a driving, ambitious individual, eager to excel in his prescribed exercise, and he must be cautioned against training in too aggressive and competitive a manner. Such an individual may use the mechanism of denying symptoms to enable him to cope with heavy business commitments or strenuous physical exertion in the face of niggling pains. To a point, this is a useful mechanism, and it accounts for his favourable progress after infarction. On the other hand, it can lead to a dangerous delay in seeking medical advice when symptoms warn that a recurrence of the infarction is imminent (V.B.O. Hammett, 1963).

The depressed patient, in contrast, may need much encouragement in order to undertake the rehabilitation needed for a return to work (D. Gelfand, 1959). Nevertheless, the Toronto Rehabilitation Centre team ultimately persuaded 95 per cent of their depressed patients to resume full-time employment. Depressed patients are likely to benefit from psychotherapy (C.A. Adsett & Bruhn, 1968), hypnosis (T. Kavanagh *et al.*, 1974a) or a combination of these two types of treatment. Small-group sessions allow covert problems to be revealed and discussed, with substantial therapeutic benefit. Some psychiatrists have regarded depression as a functionally useful withdrawal from a noxious situation, but in the context of ischaemic heart disease there is a good deal of evidence that hope and optimism are necessary to a favourable prognosis (W.A. Greene, 1954; B.Z. Lebovits *et al.*, 1967;

A.H. Schmale & Engel, 1967; J.G. Bruhn *et al.*, 1971).

Patients frequently comment on the improvement of mood that follows participation in a regular exercise programme (W.P. Morgan *et al.*, 1970, 1971). This thus seems an important reason for recommending an increase in physical activity. Amidst a list of medical prohibitions (food, cigarettes, alcohol, sex, . . .) exercise stands out as both a positive recommendation and a means of reducing the dependency of the cardiac victim. Nevertheless, it is not easy to document large changes of mood by objective tests. In one group of 'post-coronary' patients who progressed to marathon running (T. Kavanagh *et al.*, 1977a), D scores were lower than in the average cardiac patients, but were still substantially greater than for the general population. T. Kavanagh *et al.* (1977b) carried out a longitudinal 'follow-up' on 44 patients with high initial scores for depression and the 'neurotic triad'. Four years later, there was a substantial reversion towards normal scores (Table 11.5). Likewise, J.G. Bruhn (1973) found that relative to an inactive group, post-coronary patients who increased their physical activity had lower scores for depression and hypochrondriasis, with higher scores for ego strength. H.K. Hellerstein (1965) also showed decreases in depression and psychasthenia scores among patients enrolled in his cardiac reconditioning programme. It is arguable that at least a part of these various changes reflects an inevitable adaptation of the patient and his spouse to the problems created by the infarct (A. Verwoerdt & Dovenmuehle, 1964; M. Skelton & Dominian, 1973). Furthermore, in the Toronto study, the sample was initially selected on the basis of a high D score, thus increasing the likelihood that scores would revert towards the mean (B.D. McPherson *et al.*, 1967; C.O. Dotson, 1973). Several other groups of investigators have described a reduction in depression coincident with exercise participation (A. Verwoerdt & Dovenmuehle, 1964; J. Naughton *et al.*, 1968; B.M. Groden & Brown, 1970; W.P. Morgan *et al.*, 1970; J.G. Bruhn, 1973; E.H. Friedman & Hellerstein, 1973) but, in the one controlled trial (J. Naughton *et al.*, 1968), the decrease in depression was not significantly enhanced by training. B.D. McPherson *et al.* (1967) suggested that much of the observed improvement might be a result of group support rather than exercise *per se*, since some changes occurred when patients carried out homoeopathic doses of exercise. Certainly, in the Toronto series, gains of aerobic power were as great in those who did not improve their D score as in those who did; however, persistently high D scores were linked to a lability of resting systemic blood pressure and a worsening

Table 11.5: Changes of Minnesota Multiphasic Personality Inventory Score over Four Years of Exercise Rehabilitation for Subjects with High Initial D

Variable	Initial score	Final score	Δ	P	Normal score
Depression (D)	29.0	25.9	−3.1 ± 6.0	< 0.05	16.7
Hysteria (Hy)	25.1	22.5	−2.6 ± 4.9	< 0.05	16.5
Hypochondriasis (Hs)	18.2	16.0	−2.2 ± 4.9	< 0.05	11.3
Psychasthenia (Pt)	30.6	28.6	−2.1 ± 5.7	< 0.05	23.0

* Data are here presented as 'raw' scores.

Source: T. Kavanagh *et al.* (1977b).

of exercise-induced ST segmental depression (T. Kavanagh *et al.*, 1977b).

W.P. Morgan (1979) has emphasised that excessive training can have an adverse effect upon mood, with associated physiological disturbances (heart rate, blood pressure, catecholamine output and — in women — menstrual disorders). This picture of 'overtraining' is well recognised among athletes, but it can also develop in a post-coronary patient who is exercising too hard.

One last personality characteristic that deserves comment is the MF (masculinity/femininity) scale of the MMPI. 'Post-coronary' patients have a high score on this variable (T. Kavanagh *et al.*, 1977b). One may link this observation to the feminine characteristics of heavy smokers (A. Rode *et al.*, 1972). It is conceivable that stress may arise because of a conflict between the individual's personality and the perceived demands of a traditional male sex role (H.I. Russek, 1966), with both recourse to cigarettes and development of a heart attack. Alternatively, the MF score could be increased as a consequence of emasculating changes forced upon the patient by his heart attack. The lack of change in MF scores over four years of rehabilitation seems rather against the latter explanation. Finally, since most of the Toronto sample were well-educated 'white-collar' workers, it is possible that a high level of education affected the choice of cultural vocational and avocational attitudes (ballet, poetry, art, . . .) in a manner leading to a 'feminine' score.

12 MISCELLANEOUS TOPICS

This chapter will examine briefly a miscellany of topics relating to exercise and ischaemic heart disease, including problems of the female patient, anginal pain, by-pass operations and peripheral vascular disease.

The Female Patient

Until recently, the loss of productive years from ischaemic heart disease in women amounted to only a small fraction of the male total. In a classical study of 100 coronary heart disease patients under the age of 40 years, only four cases were women (R.E. Glendy *et al.*, 1937). More recent Canadian statistics (Table 2.2) put female deaths between one quarter and one fifth of the male total. Since the relative immunity of women to heart attacks is particularly noticeable in the younger age groups, it has been argued that women gain an advantage from their characteristic pattern of hormone secretions. In support of this view, animals gain some protection from oestrogen-feeding, and men who have undergone bilateral orchidectomy in early life are also less liable to heart attacks (J.B. Hamilton, 1948; M.M. Gertler & White, 1976). On the other hand, several recent observations have tended to discredit the hormonal hypothesis, as follows:

(1) Men suffering myocardial infarctions have a personality that is rated as feminine rather than masculine on traditional assessments such as the Terman-Miles test (Chapter 11); they are less aggressive, less adventurous, less enterprising and less self-assertive than controls, being 'actively sympathetic and concerned with domestic affairs, art and literature' (M.M. Gertler & White, 1976).
(2) 'Post-coronary' men have above average serum levels of oestradiol, with possible adverse effects upon the metabolism of sugar and fat.
(3) Women taking female sex hormones for purposes of contraception apparently have an increased risk of 'heart attacks' (W.H.W. Inman & Vessey, 1968; J.E. Wood, 1972; L.D. Ostrander & Lamphiear, 1978), with a reduction in hepatic triglyceride lipase

(D. Applebaum-Bowden & Hazzard, 1979).
(4)   Finally, the incidence of 'heart attacks' in women has increased
       progressively as they have adopted a more 'masculine' lifestyle.

Current thinking is thus that women gained a substantial part of their
historic immunity to myocardial infarction through such characteristics
as a low average consumption of cigarettes. Furthermore, this advantage
is now being dissipated through heavy smoking and the adoption of
aggressive 'Type A' behaviour in occupational and leisure activity.

Relatively few authors have compared the circumstances of heart
attacks in men and women (B. Wikland, 1971; M. Romo, 1972; G.
Bentsson, 1973). M. Romo (1972) found that 15 per cent of men were
physically active during or immediately prior to infarction, whereas
only one per cent of women were active at the time of attack (Chapter
3). This may reflect a lack of heavy physical activity among middle-
aged European women prior to 1970. If so, the statistics that are now
being collected will probably show a higher proportion of incidents in
women who are exercising.

The paradoxical behaviour of the ST segment in women has already
been discussed (G. Cumming *et al.*, 1973b; K.H. Sidney & Shephard,
1977b; Chapter 7). 'Abnormal' electrocardiograms are as frequent
in elderly women as in men. However, female subjects show less
evidence of coronary atherosclerosis at angiography, and they sustain less heart attacks than the men. One possible explanation of the
paradox (K.H. Sidney & Shephard, 1977b) is that the ventricular wall
has a lesser cross section in women than in men. Attempts to develop
a similar systemic pressure thus place the myocardial fibres under
greater tension, and ischaemia occurs during vigorous exercise, even
if the coronary vasculature is relatively normal. If this explanation is
correct, it is then necessary to explain why ischaemia does not provoke
fibrillation in the women. Possibly, the intensity of effort needed to
reveal ischaemia (75–100 per cent of maximum oxygen intake) is not
normally attained by a middle-aged lady.

There have been several comparisons of prognosis between men and
women. One early report found that the five-year survival after myocardial infarction was only 39 per cent in women, compared with 60
per cent in men (J.L. Juergens *et al.*, 1960). However, a part of this
difference was due to the greater average age of the females (67.5 as
opposed to 60.0 years). More recent studies have found either no
difference in prognosis (G.E. Honey & Truelove, 1957), or a slight
advantage to female patients compatible with the normal difference of

Table 12.1: Probability of Death within First 4.5 Years of Diagnosis of Angina or Myocardial Infarction — a Comparison of Statistics for Women and Men, Based on Abnormality of Four Variables

| Variable | Probability of cardiac death | | | |
| | Women | | Men | |
	Normal	Abnormal	Normal	Abnormal
Electrocardiogram	0.047	0.149	0.062	0.190
Systemic blood pressure	0.102	0.093	0.101	0.227
Serum cholesterol	0.048	0.163	0.137	0.122
Blood-sugar regulation	0.071	0.278	0.133	0.197

Source: E. Weinblatt *et al*. (1973).

Table 12.2: Perceived Reasons for Joining a Physical-activity Programme — a Comparison of Ranked Data for Elderly Men and Women

Men	Women
1. Physical health	1. Physical health
2. Programme and facilities	2. Programme and facilities
3. Altruism	3. Psychological well-being
4. Recreational/hedonistic	4. Altruism
	5. Recreational/hedonistic
	6. Socialising

Source: K.H. Sidney & Shephard (1977a).

longevity between older men and women (E. Weinblatt *et al*., 1973; A. Vedin *et al*., 1975). Diabetes has a greater adverse effect on post-infarction prognosis in women, while angina has less impact in a woman than in a man. The last finding may reflect the fact that a larger proportion of women have vague symptoms that prove not to be true angina (E. Weinblatt *et al*., 1973). Likewise, a much higher proportion of women than men are diagnosed as hypertensive, but many have labile hypertension. The recorded pressure therefore has less influence on prognosis in women than in men. On the other hand, a high serum cholesterol has a greater adverse effect in women (Table 12.1).

Attitudes to an increase in physical activity differ substantially

Table 12.3: Attitudes towards Physical Activity as Assessed by the Kenyon Inventory — a Comparison of Data for Elderly Men and Women

Concept of physical activity	Arbitrary score	
	Men	Women
Aesthetic experience	49.2	51.0
Health and fitness	48.2	49.2
Catharsis of tension	45.9	48.0
Social experience	46.9	46.1
Ascetic experience	34.2	33.8
Pursuit of vertigo	38.6	30.9
Game of chance	29.7	29.7

Source: K.H. Sidney & Shephard (1977a).

between men and women (M. Dosch *et al.*, 1975). Women are less attracted to physical development than men, but are more interested in psychological well-being and a reduction in body fat, with improvements of posture and carriage (R.J. Shephard, 1977a). Appealing items of programme content for the female include health and fitness, relief of tension, plus the social and aesthetic aspects of activity; however, there is less appreciation of the vertiginous component than in men (Tables 12.2 and 12.3).

Track events are well accepted by young women, but older females still resist a programme that places a heavy emphasis upon jogging, particularly if they are somewhat obese. At the Toronto Rehabilitation Centre, a battery of cycle ergometers has provided a satisfactory basis for regular exercise. These machines allow the women to undertake a graded activity programme while conversing with their friends. Swimming and aquabatics (underwater gymnastics) are other forms of exercise suitable for an older woman who is somewhat obese; during such activities, excess body fat provides a useful bonus of both buoyancy and insulation against cool water.

Anginal Pain

Anginal pain arises from myocardial ischaemia (L. Katz & Landt, 1935; Chapter 1). The chain of events leading to this symptom often

includes a rise in peripheral venous tone and thus in cardiac work-
load (H. Westling, 1971). The tissue malfunction is reversible, in
contrast with infarction (where the myocardial cells die and are
replaced by scar tissue). It might therefore be inferred that angina
is an earlier manifestation of ischaemic heart disease than is an
infarct. However, in practice, this is not the case. Angiograms often
show extensive disease in the patient with angina. The cumulative
likelihood of death in the first five years after diagnosis is very similar
for angina and for myocardial infarction (E. Weinblatt *et al.*, 1973),
while disability prior to death is typically greater among those
with angina. Furthermore, the prognosis of the post-infarction patient
is substantially worsened by concurrent angina (R.J. Shephard, 1979a),
while the development of an infarct may cure angina, at least
temporarily.

Angina usually has a precipitating cause (such as exposure to cold,
physical activity or emotional excitement), and recovery is relatively
rapid as soon as the provoking agent is withdrawn. A proportion of
patients can 'walk through' an exercise-induced anginal attack.
Possibly, continued exercise leads to dilatation of either the normal or
the collateral blood supply to the affected segment of myocardium,
or possibly a progressive increase in systemic blood pressure improves
myocardial flow. In any event, 'walking through' an attack is not a
technique to recommend to angina patients. Careful measurements
usually show impaired cardiac contractility (decrease of $\dot{V}_{max}$, dP/dt
and circumferential fibre shortening; M.H. Ellestad, 1975) with a stiff-
ening of the ventricular wall (A.M. Fogelman *et al.*, 1972) during an
attack. If affected individuals persist with physical activity in the face
of anginal pain, they can precipitate a situation where stroke output
diminishes, end-diastolic volume increases and cardiac failure develops
(J.O. Parker *et al.*, 1966; T.W. Moir & Debra, 1967). The astute clinician
will infer impairment of myocardial function from an atrial or ventricular
'gallop' rhythm, heard immediately following an exercise bout.

There is a general relationship between exercise-induced
ST-segmental depression and angina, but many patients can develop
several millimetres of ST displacement and a rise in end-diastolic
pressure without symptoms (M. Ellestad, 1975). Again, some women
show both retrosternal discomfort and ST changes without angio-
graphically demonstrable narrowing of the coronary vessels (R. Gorlin,
1967; T.N. James, 1970; W. Likoff, 1972). Despite these anomalies,
ECG telemetry during exercise provides an objective basis for
distinguishing angina from musculo-skeletal pains and symptom-

claiming associated with a secondary cardiac neurosis.

Patients who show a deep ST-segmental depression or true angina following infarction have an adverse prognosis. Training is contra-indicated for the individual who develops angina or cardiac failure at rest. In other anginal patients, activity must be prescribed with caution. If there is ECG evidence of exercise-induced ischaemia, the maximum permissible level of training should be defined by a laboratory stress test (R.E. Goldstein & Epstein, 1973; L.T. Sheffield & Roitman, 1973), and the individual should be taught the symptom pattern of angina as a further safeguard in regulating his habitual activity. Some authors (for example, J.J. Kellermann *et al.*, 1977) have observed a substantial improvement in effort tolerance when anginal patients undertake regular bouts of vigorous continuous training. Others have found a poor response to continuous activity, possibly because the patients were unable to reach a training threshold (T. Kavanagh & Shephard, 1975a); nevertheless, when the individuals concerned were transferred to a modified interval training plan, gains in maximum oxygen intake were almost as large as those seen in asymptomatic 'post-coronary' patients.

The optimum regimen for the person with angina seems to be about a minute of exercise, followed by a slow-walking recovery interval of sufficient duration to allow oxidation of accumulated metabolites (typically 1–1½ minutes). Sudden bursts of activity without a warm-up must be avoided, as must sustained isometric contractions. Exercise is also contraindicated for this class of patient if there has been recent emotional excitement, a heavy meal or exposure to extreme heat or cold.

If a patient is severely disabled by chest pain, preliminary medication with trinitrin and/or the administration of oxygen may help to raise confidence sufficiently so that a significant volume of training can be undertaken. Trinitrin affords relief to about 90 per cent of anginal victims, usually within five minutes of sub-lingual administration. If relief is not obtained, one must suspect either a loss of potency in the drug or a non-anginal explanation of the discomfort. Other drugs used in the relief of angina are discussed in Chapter 11. The angina threshold is lowered by exposure to carbon monoxide, whether from cigarette smoking (W.S. Aronow, 1976) or freeway travel (W.S. Aronow *et al.*, 1972). Regular ingestion of alcohol may also have an adverse effect (J. Orlando *et al.*, 1976).

The frequency of exercise-induced ST segmental depression and angina diminishes with conditioning (A. Kattus, 1970; J. Detry &

Bruce, 1971; D.R. Redwood *et al.*, 1972; T. Kavanagh *et al.*, 1973b).
Possible explanations include: (i) a lesser emotional reaction to a given
exercise task; (ii) a decrease in cardiac work rate for a given intensity of
exercise (D.R. Redwood *et al.*, 1972; D.N. Sim & Neill, 1974; C.K.
Kennedy *et al.*, 1976); and (iii) a true increase in myocardial blood
supply. Often, the first of these mechanisms is the most important.
Angina arises because a patient fears he will be unable to complete a
task or senses that he is being hurried (W.A. Aronow, 1979).
Substantial benefit is then derived from reassurance, judicious use of
tranquillisers and sedatives and simple psychotherapy. L. Zohman &
Tobis (1967) provided an interesting demonstration of the importance
of psychological factors in an experiment where patients were
supplied with compressed air via a mask; this led to a 50 per cent
increase in effort tolerance and a 20 per cent decrease in ECG changes
at a given work rate, changes comparable with those observed after a
short period of training. With regard to the third mechanism, A.A.
Kattus & Grollman (1972) found little relationship between development of the coronary collateral circulation and relief of angina.
However, more recent observations (G. Kober *et al.*, 1978) have noted
a better recovery of left ventricular function in patients with well-
developed collateral vessels.

By-pass Operations

There remain substantial differences of opinion concerning the indications for and the benefit to be anticipated from coronary by-pass
operations in ischaemic heart disease. The goals of surgery are similar
to those of exercise rehabilitation — extension of longevity,
restoration of function and an improvement in the quality of life.
There is good evidence that a by-pass may provide six to twelve
months of relief from disabling angina (W.C. Sheldon *et al.*, 1969;
E.L. Alderman *et al.*, 1973). In some instances, this may reflect an
increase in blood flow to ischaemic areas of the myocardium (J.A.
Walker *et al.*, 1971; D.G. Greene *et al.*, 1972; P. Lichtlen *et al.*, 1973).
However, in other patients, the mechanism of pain relief seems to be
the provocation of a perioperational infarct (H.I. Russek, 1970; R.E
Goldstein & Epstein, 1973; R.S. Ross, 1975; G.A. Guinn & Mathur,
1976; G.M. Lawrie *et al.*, 1977; H.D. McIntosh & Garcia, 1978).
   There are reports that surgery has improved longevity in patients
with significant disease of the left main coronary artery (T. Takaro

et al., 1976; R.C. Read *et al.*, 1978), isolated disease of the anterior descending artery (W.C. Sheldon *et al.*, 1975), two-vessel disease (K.E. Hammermeister *et al.*, 1977), severe three-vessel disease (J.F. McNeer *et al.*, 1974; R.C. Read *et al.*, 1978) and anginal pain with minimal laboratory exercise (J.R. Margolis, 1975). Proponents of medical treatment suggest that there is no sound theoretical reason for such claims, since the majority of coronary veins grafts do not remain patent for more than one to two years (M.L. Murphy *et al.*, 1979). They argue that surgeons have generally compared their data with inappropriate controls — a medically treated group reported by the Cleveland Clinic (A.V.G. Bruschke *et al.*, 1973), or other non-concurrent data drawn from the literature (A. Oberman *et al.*, 1972; J.O. Humphries *et al.*, 1974). Randomised controlled trials fail to support the claims made for surgical treatment (V.S. Mathur & Guinn, 1975; M.L. Murphy *et al.*, 1979). Some surgeons have in turn retorted that this reflects the unexpectedly poor experience of the surgically treated patients. If the controlled series had received the best possible standard of surgery, benefit would have been observed. Thus W.D. Johnson (1979) claimed that in patients without significant irreversible myocardial damage, surgery should yield a 95 per cent five-year survival rate, irrespective of the number of diseased vessels, 90 per cent of patients getting partial relief and up to 70 per cent total relief from angina (Table 12.4). However, cynics have replied that part of the apparent improvement in surgical statistics reflects the extension of operative treatment to patients with less severe disease. The debate continues, but for the present we must conclude that the superiority of surgical treatment has only been established for patients with left main coronary artery disease (F. Kloster *et al.*, 1975; M.H. Frick *et al.*, 1976; T. Takaro *et al.*, 1976; Table 12.5).

Functional tests have shown little difference in the incidence of dysrhythmia during normal daily activity between surgically and medically treated patients (N. de Soyza *et al.*, 1976). There have been reports of augmented tolerance to exercise, with a higher limiting rate-pressure product (W.D. Johnson *et al.*, 1970; E.A. Amsterdam *et al.*, 1973), a decrease in left-ventricular end-diastolic pressure (W.D. Johnson *et al.*, 1970; K. Chatterjee *et al.*, 1972), a gain in cardiac index (K. Chatterjee *et al.*, 1972) and an increased ventricular ejection fraction after surgery (G. Rees *et al.*, 1971; M.G. Bourassa *et al.*, 1972), but other investigators have found no greater improvements than would be expected during conservative treatment (A.G. Tilkian *et al.*, 1976). The quantitation of left-ventricular function after a by-pass operation

Table 12.4: Relief of Angina with Coronary By-pass Surgery, Based on Data for 1,150 Unselected Patients

Angina status	Ventricular function		
	Normal (47% of sample) (%)	Mild impairment (34% of sample) (%)	Severe impairment (19% of sample) (%)
Total relief*	66	66	63
Improved	25	23	24
No change	6	7	6
Worsened	3	4	7

* Figures for 1975–6 show 68.5 per cent of patients with total relief of angina.

Source: W.D. Johnson (1979).

Table 12.5: Long-term Results of Coronary By-pass Surgery

Type of vessel	Post-operative period (yr)	Progression of stenosis (%)
Vessels with patent grafts	1	57
	6	66
Vessels with occluded grafts	1	53
	6	57
Non-grafted vessels	1	9.5
	6	46

Source: Based on data of M.G. Bourassa *et al.* (1978).

is complicated by changes in both ventricular volume and compliance (J.H. Caldwell *et al.*, 1975; U. Sigwart *et al.*, 1975; B. Sharma *et al.*, 1976). Nevertheless, a disappointingly small percentage of subjects show improved left-ventricular performance (R. Balcon & Rickards, 1973; K.E. Hammermeister *et al.*, 1974; P. Steele *et al.*, 1977).

J.C. Manley (1979) has suggested that the response to surgery depends on both pre-operative left-ventricular impairment (which reflects the size of the scar) and the patency of the graft (Table 12.6). If initial function is relatively normal, substantial gains in performance

Table 12.6: Improvement of Left-ventricular Function in Relation to Extent of Scarring and Success of Revascularisation

Extent of myocardial scar	Improvement of left-ventricular function	
	Good revascularisation (%)	Poor revascularisation (%)
Small	94	73
Moderate	75	56
Large	20	25

Source: Based on data of J.C. Manley (1979).

appear soon after surgery, and persist as long as the graft remains patent. However, gains are less likely if there is initially a moderate or a severe impairment of function and, in patients who have suffered a post-operative infarction, a deterioration in ventricular performance is likely. While revascularisation can improve the function of a hypokinetic segment of the ventricular wall, it is unlikely to restore the contraction of akinetic tissue (J.C. Manley & Johnson, 1972; W.P. Geis *et al.*, 1975). A combination of persistent angina, a low resting cardiac index, a poor ejection fraction and an elevated left-ventricular end-diastolic pressure points to a large infarct and a poor response to surgery (P.E. Cohn *et al.*, 1975). On the other hand, the patient who has normal resting function but develops angina and a rising left-ventricular end-diastolic pressure during exercise may well benefit from a by-pass operation. If there is a clear-cut aneurysm with paradoxical motion of the ventricular wall, function may be improved by excision of the affected segment (D.E. Harken, 1972; W. Delius *et al.*, 1973; R.W. Hacker, 1973; M. Rothlin *et al.*, 1973).

Peripheral Vascular Disease

Many patients with ischaemic heart disease also have atherosclerotic lesions in their peripheral vasculature (L.K. Widmer *et al.*, 1969). Such lesions worsen prognosis for several reasons, as follows:

(1)   They generally lead to an increase in systolic blood pressure and thus in cardiac work-load.

(2)   They hamper peripheral perfusion, compounding problems that

arise from poor maintenance of the cardiac stroke volume during vigorous exercise.

(3) Peripheral ischaemia may limit participation in a training programme (as a result of the development of intermittent claudicant pain when the patient walks a short distance).

(4) A combination of diabetes and peripheral ischaemia may progress to gangrene, with a need to amputate one or both lower limbs. The diseased heart must then sustain the heavy demands of locomotion in a wheel chair, on crutches or on a prosthesis (T. Kavanagh *et al.*, 1973a).

The pain of intermittent claudication is typically felt in the calf muscles (J.A. Gillespie, 1960). It is brought about by moderate exercise (such as walking 200 metres) and is relieved by rest. S.O. Isacsson (1972) observed symptoms of this type in 2.8 per cent of a random sample of 55-year-old men living in Malmo, Sweden. While the main risk factor is cigarette smoking, Isacsson also noted a significant correlation between calf blood flow and reported leisure activity.

The traditional treatment of claudicant pain has been surgical (excision of the thrombus, vascular graft or lumbar sympathectomy). However, A. Singer & Rob (1960) commented that the condition of 20 out of 22 patients receiving conservative treatment remained unchanged or improved, and a more recent review estimated that surgery was necessary in only 20 per cent of patients (British Medical Journal, 1976).

The walking distance to the onset of claudicant pain can be extended by a programme of regular exercise (S. Hedlund & Porjé, 1964; O.A. Larsen & Lassen, 1968; B. Ericsson *et al.*, 1971; Table 12.7), although the mechanism leading to the improvement of function remains unclear. H. Sanne & Sivertsson (1968) noted a development of collateral vessels in the cat when experimental occlusion of the femoral artery was followed by five weeks of treadmill training. On the other hand, O.A. Larsen & Lassen (1968) did not see any increase in limb flow when men with peripheral vascular disease underwent a training programme. Other possible mechanisms for improvement of peripheral oxygen supply include: (i) a recanalisation of existing vessels; (ii) a strengthening of the active muscles; and (iii) an increased peripheral oxygen extraction related to a redistribution of blood flow between skin and muscle, a redistribution of flow between active and inactive fibres and possibly an increased oxygen extraction within a given fibre through an increase in enzyme activity

Table 12.7: The Influence of Endurance Training upon Patients with Intermittent Claudication, Based on Data for Eleven Months of Training

Variable	Exercise group (n = 7)		Control group (n = 6)	
	Initial status	Change (%)	Initial status	Change (%)
Walking distance	273 m	+ 95	298 m	+ 17
Painless distance	186 m	+ 104	184 m	− 22
Maximum flow	15.7 ml/dl	+ 41	17.5 ml/dl	+ 6

Source: B. Ericsson *et al.* (1971).

(S. Zetterquist, 1971). It is also conceivable that psychological support allows a patient to perform more work before activity is halted by symptoms.

Practical suggestions for the claudicant subject include: (i) the wearing of well-insulated footwear in cold weather; (ii) correction of any anaemia; (iii) cessation of smoking; and (iv) the taking of a peripheral vasodilator drug prior to vigorous exercise. The traditional Buerger's exercises involve elevating the legs at 45-90° for three minutes, three or four times per day. Such therapy is supposed to improve collateral flow by inducing a reactive vasodilatation. However, if the exercises have more than a psychological effect, it is likely that this arises through a strengthening of the leg muscles, with a resultant facilitation of perfusion of the active fibres (J.P. Clausen & Larsen, 1971; M. Hirai, 1974).

13 EPILOGUE: THE BOTTOM LINE

While commercial organisations increasingly keep their focus upon the 'bottom line', there remains resistance to a cost-benefit analysis of health care. Somehow, it seems distasteful to set a dollar value on an individual human life. Nevertheless, how available health care resources should be deployed is becoming an important ethical decision. For example, is it appropriate to spend money on the primary and secondary prevention of heart disease, or should it be diverted to modern marvels of treatment such as by-pass surgery and cardiac transplants? Accordingly, this final chapter will attempt a brief review of cost-benefit issues from the standpoint of the patient, the physician and the community as a whole.

Cost-benefit Considerations for the Patient

Heart disease and health insurance costs

Strident argument continues between the proponents and antagonists of 'socialised' medicine, but prepaid health care by government and/or private insurance carriers is becoming a fact of life in almost all nations. Even in New York, the last bastion of free-enterprise medicine, L.R. Zohman (1973) found that a third of patients attending her exercise test and rehabilitation facility received 50 per cent or more reimbursement from Health Insurance carriers. Furthermore, social provision for the disabled and their dependants has become a responsibility of the state. Thus, fatal and non-fatal episodes of ischaemic heart disease impose a substantial financial burden upon the community (Table 13.1). Measured in current (1981) dollars, this amounts to at least $900 per wage-earner (R.J. Shephard, 1977a).

Since many of the causes of ischaemic heart disease reflect personal lifestyle (including items such as cigarette consumption, physical inactivity, overeating, and 'Type-A' behaviour, it becomes an important question of public policy how firm a government should be in moulding individual behaviour patterns.

One possible way of encouraging a favourable lifestyle is to develop a system of differential health-insurance premiums, based upon the risk-taking behaviour of the insured person. This approach has been adopted successfully with automobile insurance (reduced premiums for teetotallers), fire insurance (reduced premiums for non-smokers) and some forms of life assurance (increased premiums if overweight, reduced premiums for non-smokers). The concept would be more difficult to apply and to police if a total allowance were to be made for 'diseases of choice' when calculating annual insurance premiums. For example, it could be argued that a small proportion of those who are obese have an intractable metabolic disorder; this is not their choice, and it would be unfair to penalise such individuals. Nevertheless, a potential instrument for measuring overall risk-taking behaviour has now been developed by the Canadian Federal Government — a health-hazard-appraisal questionnaire. A simple computer programme calculates the difference between the individual's calendar age and an appraised age based upon personal lifestyle (cigarette smoking habits, physical inactivity, excessive consumption of alcohol, failure to use a seat belt, etc.). At present, the score from this instrument is being used as a motivational tool, and there is now evidence that a favourable change of appraised age can result from participation in an employee fitness programme (Table 13.2).

A second possible tactic for discouraging poor health behaviour is to charge the resultant health cost at source, imposing a heavy tax on items such as cigarettes and alcohol. For some reason, this expedient is politically more acceptable than the use of differential health-insurance premiums. Nevertheless, it remains difficult to attribute an appropriate cost to any given risk factor and, to avoid the wrath of powerful lobbies maintained by the industries concerned, the tax that is levied rarely covers the full health cost of the adverse behaviour. Furthermore, there is a danger that a government may perceive the tax as a source of revenue rather than as a partial payment of health costs already incurred. It is then but a short step to accept and even tacitly to encourage the risk-taking behaviour. Physical inactivity is particularly difficult to tax, except indirectly through such items as petrol for cars and electricity for power appliances. A possible alternative is to offer tax relief to corporations that introduce low-cost employee-fitness programmes. The self-employed could receive similar encouragement through tax deductions for membership in approved health clubs.

A third method of health promotion is a massive advertising campaign. There seems sufficient evidence to warrant persuading people to become physically more active. In the past, it has been argued that advertising is singularly ineffective in changing personal habits. While commercial Fitness Spas often spend a substantial proportion of their

Table 13.1: Estimated Impact of Cardiovascular Disease upon the US Economy, Measured in 1962 Dollars

	Annual cost (billion dollars)
Direct costs:	
personal services and supplies (hospital care, services of physicians and nurses, provision of drugs)	2.6
non-personal items (research, training, public-health services, capital construction and insurance schemes)	0.5
Indirect costs:	
premature death (see Table 2.2)	19.4
loss of output from illness	3.0
intangibles (e.g. pain, suffering, orphanhood)	5.2
Total	30.7

Source: H.E. Klarman (1964).

Table 13.2: Appraised Age, as Determined by the Canadian Health Hazard Appraisal, Showing the Change of Score among Men and Women Participating Regularly in an Industrial Fitness Programme

	Change of appraised age over 6 months	
Nature of participation	Men	Women
Control subject	−0.42	1.37
Non-participant	0.25	1.87
Drop-out	−0.24	−0.27
Low adherent	−0.44	0.53
High adherent	−1.91	0.39

Source: R.J. Shephard, Corey & Cox (in preparation).

income on recruitment, it is possible that the individuals thus attracted have already been active elsewhere. Again, the short-term results of massive 'lifestyle' documents such as the US Surgeon General's reports on 'Smoking and Health' have been disappointing. On the other hand, the funds allocated to smoking-withdrawal programmes have remained only a small fraction of those expended by cigarette manufacturers in promoting their sales. More encouragement can be drawn from long-term changes in the cardiac epidemic (Chapter 2). The most reasonable explanation of the downturn in cardiac deaths is that there has been a slow but progressive improvement in lifestyle in response to 15 years of well-coordinated health education.

Techniques of mass stress-testing

Some authors have advocated mass stress-testing, both as a means of detecting individuals who are vulnerable to a 'heart attack' and as a prelude to an increase in physical activity. In the United States, it is current wisdom that an exercise ECG should be obtained prior to the prescription of physical activity for any patient over 35 years of age (K.H. Cooper, 1970; American College of Sports Medicine, 1975). This is largely an example of the practice of 'defensive medicine'. Physicians fear to use less than the maximum available diagnostic aids in case a cardiac emergency should occur, with a subsequent claim of professional negligence (G.H. Siegel, 1973). However, we have already seen that an exercise stress-test is a relatively ineffective screening procedure when dealing with apparently healthy 35-year-old subjects. In Canada, the option of universal physician-supervised stress-tests was reviewed at a National Conference on Fitness and Health (W.R. Orban, 1974); delegates concluded that such a policy would generate unwarranted expense. A simple, three-tiered test structure was proposed as a workable alternative. At the lowest level of sophistication would be a self-administered test, the Canadian Home Fitness Test (R.J. Shephard, 1980a). This would cost from $5-7, the charge being borne by the individual himself. The relative safety of the procedure would be assured by details of test design (R.J. Shephard, 1980a), and by completion of an initial health questionnaire (PAR-Q, the physical activity readiness questionnaire; D. Chisholm *et al.*, 1975). The score from the Home Fitness Test was intended to motivate patients to an increase in physical activity, while providing them with an approximate guide to a suitable exercise prescription.

At the second level of sophistication, the Canadian National Conference proposed a more comprehensive fitness test, supervised by paramedical personnel, and costing about $15. In some instances, this cost might be borne by the individual, and in other instances it might be arranged as an employee benefit. A prototype of this system can be seen in seven 'fitness vans' currently operated by the Province of Ontario. These are staffed by five paramedical workers, and they offer simple assessments of lung function, muscle strength, body fat and flexibility in addition to an ECG-monitored version of the Canadian Home Fitness Test. The ECG is used primarily to obtain an accurate heart-rate count, although the paramedical staff of the vans have had instruction in ECG interpretation, and are thus able to refer suspicious-looking records to a physician for expert appraisal. At the third level of investigation is a full physician-supervised laboratory stress-test. Many clinics in the United States charge $ 150–200 (L.R. Zohman, 1973) for this service.

It is obviously much cheaper to leave the great mass of routine exercise testing to paramedical personnel, but questions may be asked concerning the safety of such an approach. In practice, the risks are remarkably small. The Canadian Home Fitness Test has now been carried out by upwards of 500,000 people, with no serious complications (R.J. Shephard, 1980a). A typical experience from a series of 15,000 supervised tests is a transient loss of consciousness in three subjects and one minor ankle strain (R.J. Shephard, 1980a). Many would maintain that the involvement of a physician helps to avoid a heart attack during testing or subsequent prescribed exercise. However, we found that different physicians advised anywhere from 0.7 to 15.0 per cent of ostensibly healthy patients against performance of the Canadian Home Fitness Test. Furthermore, the proportion of ECG abnormalities observed during testing was unrelated to the proportion of subjects that had been excluded. On the basis that prolonged exercise such as a marathon ski event increased the risk of a heart attack by a factor of only three or four (R.J. Shephard, 1976), we calculated that if five million middle-aged Canadian men and women performed the Canadian Home Fitness Test once every year, 16 to 33 years would elapse before there was a single fatality attributable to the test. On the reasonable assumption that the PAR-Q test would exclude at least a half of the 'high-risk' patients, the time to a cardiac emergency would increase to 33–66 years. The advantage of having a physician present to administer resuscitation during the 66th year seems indisputable. However, if his cardiac resuscitation had a success rate of 80 per cent, the cost would exceed $ 25 billion dollars per resuscitation measured in 1981 currency. While the physician might be successful in his treatment of the emergency, it is further quite unlikely that he would have averted the incident, since there are few clear guidelines as to precipitating factors. Permissible test limits for the three most promising indicators (excessive ST depression, excessive dysrhythmias and excessive rise in systemic blood pressure) are all hotly debated between different laboratories. Plainly, there are more economic strategies than physician supervision for combating one emergency in 330 million man-years; one obvious possibility is the training of the general population in techniques of cardiac resuscitation (L.A. Cobb *et al.*, 1975).

If tests are conducted in their entirety by paramedical workers, the disposition of the exercise electrocardiogram becomes an important consideration. Some physicians have argued that paramedical personnel should be required to use a device other than an ECG for accurate heart-rate counting. The main basis for this suggestion is that patients may believe they have received ECG clearance for exercise, when in fact they have not. There are two simple remedies: (i) the patient can be given a written statement that the ECG is used only to count the heart rate; or (ii) the paramedical worker can be taught to interpret the ECG. The latter approach seems the more sensible, and indeed H. Blackburn (1968) has shown that a competent technician can provide more accurate routine screening than a physician (Chapter 7). Test records that appear to be abnormal can be referred to a resident cardiologist for evaluation, and where necessary the patient can then be referred for a full medically supervised stress-test. If a large population is to be screened, another possible option is to group subjects by age, sex and fitness level, carrying out the stress-tests 16 at a time. A bank of 16 ECGs can then be monitored by an intensive-care nurse and a cardiology resident on a highly cost-effective basis; indeed, with careful scheduling, two individuals can carry out at least 100 stress tests per hour (R.J. Shephard, 1980a).

Value of screening

Using this last approach, the cost of a medically supervised ECG stress-test can be brought under $2.50 per individual (Table 13.3). The examination takes a little over the optimal time for a screening procedure, but nevertheless it is well accepted by most patients. The main argument against its general application is a low effectiveness in detecting ischaemic heart disease (Table 7.1; Chapter 7). Furthermore, there are inevitably many false positive diagnoses, a situation that creates both cardiac cripples and an unnecessary demand for the potentially dangerous procedure of coronary angiography. Taking account of the costs of angiography, the total expense involved in bringing ten of 1,000 screened individuals to by-pass sugery and a further ten patients to a test-reinforced improvement in lifestyle exceeds $60,000, more than $3,000 for every individual that is helped (Table 7.3). Moreover, the value of such help is doubtful. The usefulness of coronary by-pass

Table 13.3: Cost of Mass Stress-testing with Medically Supervised ECG Recording

Test time =	10 min	
Staff	one salaried physician at $42 \cdot h^{-1}$	= $ 7.00
	one coronary care nurse at $21 \cdot h^{-1}$	= $ 3.50
	ten junior assistants at $6 \cdot h^{-1}$	= $10.00
Equipment	depreciation at $20,000 \cdot yr^{-1}$	= $ 2.38
Supplies		= $16.00
Total for 16 patients		= $38.00
	Cost per patient = $2.43	

Source: Based on calculations of R.J. Shephard (1980a).

surgery in the absence of cardiac symptoms remains highly debatable (Chapter 12), and there are cheaper and possibly more certain means of reinforcing behavioural change than mass screening.

Cost-effectiveness is substantially improved (Table 7.3) if exercise testing is limited to candidates identified as having a high risk of ischaemic heart disease on the basis of simple clinical questioning (family history, smoking habits, excess body mass, etc.).

Medical supervision of exercise programmes

Similar questions of cost-effectiveness may be posed concerning the medical supervision of exercise programmes. To reach informed and ethical decisions, it is necessary to set a dollar value upon the life that is being protected. For example, an apparently healthy 40-year-old man has the potential to earn for 25 years and collect a pension for a further ten years. Given a current annual income of $30,000, his total financial worth is thus $900,000, measured in 1981 dollars. In contrast, a post-coronary patient aged 50 may have the prospect of survival for only ten years. Assuming the same annual salary, his total worth would be about $300,000. How do these figures compare with the cost of providing a medically supervised exercise programme?

Let us suppose that a middle-aged population of five million adults are each performing five hours of exercise per week. The total number of exercise-related cardiac emergencies will then be about 910 per year (R.J. Shephard, 1976). This estimate is admittedly based on many assumptions, but it is partially corroborated by an alternative figure of

1,900 incidents per year, derived from the experience of *males* with an above-average cardiac risk (individuals who have already survived a non-fatal heart attack). Grouping the population of five million adults into 100,000 exercise classes, each with 50 members, the risk that an emergency will arise in any given class is about one in 110 per year. By using a simple self-administered health questionnaire, the risk is reduced, probably to one in 220 class-years or lower. Let us assume that medical cover is to be provided, and that 100,000 physicians are persuaded to undertake regular supervisory duties for an honorarium of $50 per class. The cost of such supervision is $12,500 per class-year, $2,750,000 per emergency or about $3.5 million per successful resuscitation; unfortunately, this cost is almost four times the worth of the person whose life has been saved.

The risk of a cardiac emergency is greater when dealing with 'post-coronary' patients. W. Haskell (1978) has estimated that in recently designed 'cardiac' rehabilitation programmes there is one cardiac emergency in 1,000 man-years. Given a class size of 50 patients, the risk is one in 20 class-years, $250,000 per emergency or about $300,000 per successful resuscitation. Although the financial worth of the 'post-coronary' patient is lower than that of his healthy counterpart, there is plainly more economic justification for medical supervision of a 'cardiac' exercise programme.

Assuming a class size of 40–50 patients, and allowing one hour of physician time, one hour of gym time and 2½ hours of physical activity supervisor time per session, H. Pyfer & Doane (1973) calculated a total operating cost of $4.50 per person-session over the first three months of post-coronary rehabilitation, $4.00 per person-session for the remainder of the first year, and $25 per person-month (three sessions per week) thereafter. L.R. Zohman cited a similar figure ($5 per session for supervised cycle-ergometer exercise). In Toronto, we have used one physician and four supervisors for a group of 50 'cardiac' patients (R.J. Shephard, 1976); the cost is about $90 per session, excluding gymnasium rental (R.J. Shephard, 1976).

It is also instructive to calculate the economic cost of insuring against a cardiac emergency. One recent discussion recommended a minimum personal protection of $500,000 per incident (R.B. Parr & Kerr, 1975), with additional coverage for the responsible hospital or university. Let us suppose an apparently healthy 40-year-old man with a net worth of $900,000, and a risk of one in 220 class-years. Simple calculation suggests that an appropriate charge for insurance would be $82 per person-year. A class of 50 members could thus be insured

for an annual premium of $4,100; if resuscitation were 80 per cent
successful, the cost would drop further to $820 per class-year. Parallel
calculations can be carried out for 50-year-old post-coronary patients
with a worth of $300,000 and a risk of one cardiac emergency in 20
class-years. An appropriate insurance cost is then $300 per participant-
year, or $15,000 per class-year ($3,000 per class-year, given 80 per
cent success of resuscitation). However, these relatively low figures are
based on well-designed medically supervised programmes. A cost at
least ten times greater would be anticipated for less satisfactory classes
(W. Haskell, 1978).

Few people would seriously argue against medical supervision of
exercise in the early stages of post-coronary rehabilitation (B. Erb,
1969; J.K. Cooper & Willig, 1971). On the other hand, the possibility
of arranging long-term medically supervised rehabilitation may be
limited by the willingness of physicians to undertake this type of duty.
The annual incidence of non-fatal infarcts is about 250 per 100,000
population, and about a half of these are suitable candidates for
exercise rehabilitation (L.L. Brock, 1974). Thus, the total number of
recruits to a Canada-wide cardiac rehabilitation programme might be
30,000 patients per year. Assuming an average survival of ten years, the
size of the post-coronary exercise class would soon grow to 300,000
members. Maintaining a 1:50 physician/patient ratio there would be a
need for 6,000 suitably trained physicians (cost $75 million per year)
and 6,000 gymnasia equipped for cardiac resuscitation.

It is hardly surprising that both Canadian and US experts have
recommended a progressive 'tapering' of medically supervised exercise
programmes (Chapter 9) over a period of between one and two years
following infarction. There is pragmatic justification for such a plan,
since the mortality of patients who remain enrolled in an exercise
programme drops progressively in the second and subsequent years of
activity (Chapter 6).

Cost-benefit Considerations for the Physician

Traditionally, the Hippocratic oath has kept physicians from crass
cost-benefit analyses in the operation of their practices. Such a view of
medicine was appropriate when the main diagnostic tool was a $2
stethoscope, office costs were limited to the occasional re-upholstering
of a living-room chair and secretarial help could be obtained by buying
an occasional bouquet for one's wife. However, current patterns of

practice demand the use of expensive diagnostic equipment, salaried paramedical assistants and costly office suites, and in this situation a careful cost-benefit analysis is necessary to economic survival (H. Pyfer & Doane, 1973).

Primary and secondary prevention

Many physicians believe that lifestyle counselling is too expensive to be undertaken within the fee schedules offered by insurance carriers. If such a viewpoint were correct, this would present a major obstacle to the development of practical programmes for the prevention of ischaemic heart disease. However, there has been a rapid growth in commercial lifestyle counselling services such as 'weight-watchers' and 'smoke-enders', suggesting that the medical community has a false perception of the economics of health promotion.

There is some virtue in offering incidental counsel on exercise, obesity and smoking habits during the course of a general medical examination, but the keys to a successful preventive programme include: (i) automation; (ii) gathering of a sufficient audience; and (iii) delegation of attitude changing to well-trained professionals. Many patients spend at least 15 minutes in the doctor's waiting room, and a good tape/slide presentation on a healthy lifestyle could be offered at this time for a capital investment of perhaps $ 1,000. The cost could be reduced proportionately if several doctors shared a common waiting room.

One-to-one lifestyle counselling is uneconomic, but an instructor with appropriate group skills can sustain the effective involvement of up to 30 patients. The role of the physician should be to supervise such programmes, monitoring the medical information that is transmitted, but leaving to behavioural experts the detailed organisation of a given class-session. Often, a meeting place such as a church hall can be reserved for a nominal fee, so that a nightly payment of $ 2–3 per patient is enough to meet the costs of therapy. Pre-paid insurance does not always cover charges for lifestyle counselling. Nevertheless small payments often serve a useful function, encouraging the patient to adhere to the proposed lifestyle.

Exercise testing and prescription

Many practices are sorely underequipped for purposes of exercise testing and prescription. Other physicians are dazzled by promotional literature, and make excessive purchases of electronic gadgetry that are hard to justify. The most economical arrangement is to ensure that

Table 13.4: Costs of Maintaining a Simple Exercise Test Facility

		$	Per year $
Office space, 20 square metres			2,000
Paramedical professional			20,000
Equipment:	defibrillator	1,000	
	electrocardiogram	500	
	cycle ergometer	200	
	sphygmomanometer	200	
	skinfold calipers	200	
	handgrip dynamometer	200	
	flexibility test	200	
	spirometer	400	
	timing device	25	
	oxygen and medical supplies	200	
		$4,125	
	amortized over five years:		825
Supplies and repairs			1,000
	Total:		$23,825

Capacity 20 patients per day, 4,600 patients per year

Cost per patient: $ 5.20*

* This estimate does not include allowance for medical consultation, initial training costs, delays in response to billings or administration. In the first year of operation, these factors could increase costs by up to 50 per cent (H. Pyfer & Doane, 1973). H. Pyfer & Doane have calculated the much higher cost of $ 48 per maximum exercise-tolerance test. However, this is based on a much smaller-scale operation (40 cardiac patients), with incomplete usage of facilities. They also make the generous allowance of half an hour of physician time and one hour of paramedical time for each stress test. L.R. Zohman (1973) presents calculations based upon $ 155 per stress test; again this higher figure reflects underutilisation of the facility (50 patients per month) and a generous allowance for medical consultation.

one set of equipment is shared by a group of at least three to four physicians. Given a case load of 20 patients per day, the approximate cost per patient (exclusive of medical consultation and billing charges) can be as low as $ 5.20 (Table 13.4). The main expense is the salary of a well-trained paramedical professional. Given an adequate case load, a simple facility such as that outlined in Table 13.4 should not impose a severe financial burden upon a group medical practice.

Malpractice insurance

Theoretically, the physician who performs or supervises an exercise test at a level of care commensurate with his training should be immune from malpractice suits. Unfortunately, much effort has been expended by personal-injury lawyers in recent years, and in some cases substantial damages have been awarded against physicians on account of problems arising from exercise testing, exercise prescription and authorisation of a return to normal employment (E.L. Sagall, 1979). Successful suits have been based on professional negligence (harm resulting from acts of commision or omission), failure to obtain 'informed consent' for the test or exercise programme, and a combination of these factors. The present author has personal recollection of one patient, an apparently healthy middle-aged shop assistant, who performed a brief sub-maximal step test on company premises. She had been given a careful preliminary medical examination, and the step test was performed under medical supervision, without apparent mishap. Nevertheless, the following day, she complained of a swollen, painful ankle, and was unable to stand at work for about three months. She presented a claim for damages, although it was difficult to determine whether her tendonitis had been provoked by the step test or had arisen elsewhere. Certainly, there was no evidence that the condition was caused directly by a deviation from normal standards of care, and the patient could not prove that her own actions in the 24 hours following the test had not contributed to her condition. On the advice of her lawyer, she was thus persuaded to accept normal occupational-disability payments for the period that she was absent from work.

The appropriate level of medical care for exercise testing and prescription is now clearly documented in numerous publications. Defence against malpractice must thus be based on testimony and records showing that such norms of clinical expertise were met.

E.L. Sagall (1979) noted common basis for legal claims as follows:

(1)   Failure to detect pre-existing medical abnormalities contra-indicating a proposed stress test or conditioning programme;
(2)   Failure to monitor the patient adequately before, during and after exercise;
(3)   Lack of skill or delay in the handling of an emergency;
(4)   Lack of equipment, drugs and trained personnel necessary for effective resuscitation;
(5)   Lack of informed consent;
(6)   Inadequate documentation of the procedures followed;

(7) Inappropriate clearance for return to work with subsequent
     reinfarction.

E.L. Sagall suggested that the consent form should list specifically all
hazards of exercise, including death, myocardial infarction, acute
congestive heart failure and cerebrovascular accident. It should also
explain appropriate alternative procedures with their risks. He
commented that the signing of a printed consent form (G.H.
Siegel, 1973; American College of Sports Medicine, 1975) might not
be enough to establish informed consent. The physician should
therefore note in his records at the time of testing that a verbal
explanation had been fully understood by the patient.

Given that fatalities occur almost exclusively among 'cardiac'
patients, and that resuscitation is about 80 per cent successful, the risk
of death is approximately one in 50,000 patients. Assuming the net
worth of a 'post-coronary' patient is $300,000, an appropriate
insurance allowance would be $6 per test, more than 100 per cent of
the basic cost of the examination.

In contrast, when a sub-maximal test is performed on a 'normal'
adult, the risk of a cardiac emergency is about one in 80 million;
assuming an 80 per cent chance of successful resuscitation, the cost of
providing $1,000,000 insurance would then be no more than 0.25 ¢
per test. Given the total annual test population of 4,600 patients
postulated in Table 13.4, insurance against possible fatalities in healthy
subjects would not add more than five per cent to operating costs.

Cost-benefit Considerations for the Community

Physical activity has potential benefits for the community in terms of
the prevention of ischaemic heart disease, plus a more general impact
on other health problems (smoking, obesity, diabetes, etc.), productivity
and the costs of self-care during old age (Table 13.5). Against these
possible gains must be set the costs of promoting physical activity and
of providing the necessary facilities.

Costs of ischaemic heart disease

In discussing cost-benefit considerations for the patient, we estimated
the probable cost of ischaemic heart disease at $900 per wage-earner
per year. The community would not recover all of this money if there
were a mass increase in physical activity. The most optimistic forecasts

Table 13.5: Potential Annual Savings from an Increase in Physical Activity, Calculated per Wage-earner, Assuming 20 Per cent Participation in the Exercise Programme

	$ per annum
Ischaemic heart disease	90
Chronic chest disease	?
Improved lifestyle	150
Absenteeism	37
Employee turnover	216
Geriatric care	17
	—
	510*

*   In estimating this figure, note that: (1) not all savings are necessarily mutually exclusive; (2) ischaemic heart disease patients may live to collect longer pensions; (3) geriatric savings have been adjusted downwards by 25 per cent to allow for the cost of specific exercise classes for the elderly.

(Chapter 5) point to an immediate halving of cardiac deaths ($900/5 × 2 = $90 p.a.). However, cynics have suggested that the resultant survivors might live to collect a substantial old-age pension, eventually requiring several years of expensive geriatric care that would have been avoided by a heart attack. From the purely economic point of view, savings to the community are most likely if exercise postpones death from 40 to no later than 65 years of age.

Costs of other health problems

A stronger economic case can be made for the savings that result from avoidance of other health problems, particularly the chronic chest disease that is linked to cigarette smoking (C.M. Fletcher, 1959). It is uncertain how far physical activity checks the cigarette habit, but there is some evidence that the commencement of long-distance running can have this type of effect (P. Morgan *et al.*, 1976).

In our employee fitness programme, 'high adherents' showed a gain of 1.5-2 years appraised age relative to 'non-participants' and 'drop-outs' over a six-month study (R.J. Shephard & Cox, in preparation). Assuming an income of $30,000 per year, this is equivalent to a total of between $45,000 and $60,000 per individual, or $650-850 per participant per year of life. At present, sustained participation in employee fitness programmes does not exceed 20 per cent of company staff, so the community saving is the smaller sum of $130–70 per individual per year.

Industrial productivity

Important practical effects of an employee fitness programme are a decrease of absenteeism and a reduced employee turnover (M. Cox & Shephard, 1979). In our study, 'high adherents' showed a drop in in absenteeism relative to other employees. The resultant saving averaged 1.4 days per employee per year. Assuming 230 days were spent earning $30,000, the annual saving per employee would average $183, or 0.61 per cent of salary. Given a company of 1,400 employees, with 20 per cent of high adherents, the total payroll saving would be a useful $51,000 per annum (0.12 per cent).

An even bigger cost factor is the employee turnover rate. In the company that we examined (M. Cox & Shephard, 1979) there was an average turnover rate of 20 per cent per annum. The cost was $6,000 per individual, $1,200 per employee per year (or four per cent of payroll). However, 'high adherents' to the industrial fitness programme had a turnover rate of only two per cent per annum (some 0.4 per cent of payroll). Given 20 per cent participation in the employee fitness programme, the overall turnover should thus drop from 20 to 16.4 per cent, with a payroll saving of 0.72 per cent. In a company of 1,400 employees, this could yield a total dividend of just over $300,000 per annum.

Costs of geriatric care

In 1975, the annual cost of institutional care for the elderly citizens of Canada amounted to $1,897 million, about $82 per citizen and $200 per wage-earner (R.J. Shephard, 1978b). Measured in 1981 dollars, the cost would be at least $250 per wage-earner.

Much of this expense is incurred simply because senior citizens become too weak to look after themselves. If increased physical activity were to push back the age of dependency by eight or nine years without altering the age at death, this would reduce the number of dependent patients by a factor of two thirds. Given also some impact on acute and chronic care (particularly for cardiorespiratory diseases) and a small reduction in mental illness, 1975 geriatric costs for Canada would have shown a 44 per cent reduction, as follows:

Active and chronic care = $\$1,169 \text{ M} \times 1/3 = \$386 \text{ M}$
Mental care   = $\$\ \ \ 60 \text{ M} \times 1/10 = \$\ \ 6 \text{ M}$
Extended care   = $\$\ \ 668 \text{ M} \times 2/3 = \$445 \text{ M}$

  Total saving = $\$837 \text{ M}$

Against this saving, it would be necessary to set the costs of suitable exercise classes for the elderly. The true financial benefit to the community would thus be about $\$633$ million per year, or 34 per cent of geriatric-care costs. Assuming a participation rate of 20 per cent, the annual savings from a geriatric exercise programme would be $\$17$ per wage-earner per year ($\$250 \times 34\% \times 20\%$).

Costs of promoting physical activity

There are few reliable guides to the costs of promoting physical activity. One may presume that at one extreme there is a potentially active minority of adults who are easily persuaded to undertake regular exercise, but at the other extreme there are very inactive individuals who would be recruited only with extreme difficulty.

One possible indicator of the expenditure needed to influence life-style is the budget for advertising cigarettes (about $\$300$ M per year in the US). Much of this money maintains the cigarette habit rather than recruits new smokers. Nevertheless, the annual cost is approximately $\$3$ per wage-earner, with a 40–50 per cent adult participation rate.

A second statistic is the advertising budget for commercial health spas. One popular chain of health clubs in Southern Ontario boasts about 130,000 members, and it is reputed to spend $\$1,500,000$ per year on advertising. Since the majority of those recruited sign an initial three-year contract, and some subsequently renew their membership, it costs this company about $\$50$ for every contract that is completed. The club membership accounts for less than five per cent of the adults in Ontario, and it is thus difficult to be certain that the advertising programme has achieved any large-scale conversion to the habit of regular exercise. Many of the people who join both private and industrial fitness clubs have previously been active elsewhere (R.J. Shephard *et al.*, 1980a).

In Canada, governmental expenditures on the promotion of fitness are made through agencies such as the Canadian crown corporation 'Participaction', the Federal Department of Health and Welfare, and corresponding Provincial and municipal departments. The overall Federal expenditure on 'lifestyle' programmes was estimated at $\$45$

million for the fiscal year 1973/4 (M. Lalonde, 1974). However, this total covered a wide range of public-health programmes, and even in 1981 it is unlikely that governmental allocations for the promotion of physical activity exceed $10 million per year (about 80 ¢ per wage-earner). Some ten years of expenditure at this rate has undoubtedly increased Canadian awareness of a need for voluntary activity, but changes in behaviour have been quite small. Particular effort has been concentrated on Saskatoon, and in that city as many as 50 per cent of adults have been persuaded to participate in specific projects such as a communal 'walk around the block'.

Costs of facilities

Many forms of physical activity involve substantial expense in terms of equipment, facilities and land usage (R.J. Shephard, 1977a; Tables 13.6 and 13.7). Indeed, at a first glance, the potential health savings seem eclipsed by the costs of the increased activity. However, if due allowance is made for economies from careful scheduling and incomplete participation, the cost-benefit ratio becomes more favourable.

Jogging is often regarded as the 'poor-man's sport', but a realistic appraisal of costs would amount to $200-300 per individual per year, at least $100 of this being attributable to clothing and equipment. Cross-country skiing (minimal equipment about $20 per year, amortized over five years) appears to be cheaper than jogging, although account must also be taken of the short 'season' (typically, two months of the year). While these costs do not deter an executive, many blue-collar workers perceive fitness as an expensive luxury. Thus, when a Hamilton hospital arranged 'post-coronary' exercise classes for employees at a steel mill, they found that in order to ensure regular attendance it was necessary to offer not only a free programme but free parking facilities.

Capital costs of physical facilities include construction and the land that is used by both the playing area and parked vehicles. The total expense would be much lower if the provision of recreational lands became a firmer condition of permission for residential developments. The costs cited in Table 13.7 exceed the basic fees charged by many commercial fitness clubs; for instance, a new and lavishly equipped YMCA in North Toronto is offering membership for $500 per year. This discrepancy arises partly because the costs of Table 13.7 are calculated per wage-earner rather than per participant, and partly because the space allocated is sufficient to allow all of the population

Table 13.6: Costs of One-year Jogging Programme

	$
Two pairs of good-quality running shoes	80
Two pairs of socks	10
Sweat suit (five-year depreciation)	5
Rain gear (five-year depreciation)	5
Stop watch (five-year depreciation)	5
Shorts (five-year depreciation)	2
Winter track admission ($ 1 per night)	90
Total*	197

* No allowance has been made for added food consumption. Depending on the distance covered and the type of food eaten, this could range from $ 25 to $ 100 per year.

Table 13.7: Estimated Capital Cost of Providing Facilities for Selected Types of Exercise in a Metropolitan Population of 2.4 Million, Measured in 1981 Dollars

Sport	Construction ($ billion)	Costs[2] Land ($ billion)	Total ($ billion)	Annual cost per wage-earner if loan at 15% interest ($)	Ratio to health savings of Table 13.5[3]
Football/soccer	1.4	14.0	15.4	2,310	0.076
Tennis (doubles, three shifts)[1]	2.0	1.8	3.8	570	0.057
Conservation park (swimming)	—	0.45	0.45	68	0.023[4]
Urban swimming (360 per pool):					
indoor	5.2	8.4	13.6	2,040	0.067
outdoor	1.7	8.4	10.1	1,515	0.050
Urban skating (1,000 per rink):					
indoor	2.1	4.2	6.3	945	0.031
outdoor	1.1	4.2	6.3	795	0.026

1. It is assumed that the tennis courts are distributed on a neighbourhood basis, with no specific need for parking facilities.
2. Costs are calculated on the basis that all of the 2.4-million population will wish to use the facilities at peak hours. The values cited would drop proportionately if: (a) usage could be scheduled in one hour segments of a 12-hour day; and (b) participation rates were only 20 per cent of the total population.
3. Assuming usage scheduled over twelve-hour day with 20 per cent participation, at 1 hour per participant; eg. (2310/12)/5 $\times$ 510.
4. Assuming occupancy by 20 per cent of population throughout twelve-hour day.

to participate at peak hours. Commercial fitness organisations are profitable because: (i) scheduling allows distribution of member usage over at least twelve hours per day; (ii) only a small segment (commonly less than ten per cent of members) make full use of their privileges; and (iii) supplements are usually charged for popular activities such as tennis and squash.

Even a humble walk to the station is surprisingly expensive if careful accounting is made. Let us suppose than an 8-km walk is introduced into the normal working day. Although there is no charge for facilities (since sidewalks are probably available), a good pair of shoes may cost $50 per year, and a further expense arises from the food energy consumed — about 1.3 MJ per day, equal to four or five slices of bread per day, or about $25 of bakery products per year. On the credit side, we may note that maintenance costs are lower for a sidewalk than for a road, and the non-pedestrian will use gasoline ($270\,1 \cdot yr^{-1}$, $65 at 24 ¢ per litre) and parking facilities or will pay bus fares ($230 per year). The calculation is interesting in showing the problem of present-day society. Given the fact of universal car ownership, the cost of operating a vehicle over a short-haul journey that can and should be walked is remarkably low — indeed, for a family of four it is only about 22 per cent of self-propulsion! Plainly, it is desirable to modify our economic structure to correct this situation, conserving both our health and non-renewable resources such as gasoline in the process.

The next decade will undoubtedly see a trend towards demechanisation. Rising energy costs will encourage use of our muscles for performing more everyday activities. It may become economically advantageous to walk to the station and to use a handmower to cut the lawn. But even if this change is not realised, it would be wrong to conceive our cost-benefit analysis rigidly in terms of dollars and cents. Good health and an ability to live life to the full are priceless commodities. Those who have personal experience of a healthy life-style do not need strong economic incentives to persist in an active way of life — indeed, many are prepared to make considerable financial investments to enhance their newly discovered happiness.

BIBLIOGRAPHY

Abramov, L. Sexual life and sexual frigidity among women developing acute myocardial infarction. *Psychosom. Med., 38*, 418–25 (1976)

Acker, J. Early activity after myocardial infarction. In: *Exercise Testing and Exercise Training in Coronary Heart Disease*, ed. J.P. Naughton, H.K. Hellerstein & I.C. Mohler (Academic Press, New York, 1973) pp. 311–14

Adams, G.E., Bonner, E.A., Ribisl, P.M. & Miller, H.S. Blood pressure during heavy work on the treadmill and bicycle ergometer. *Med. Sci. Sports, 10*, 50 (1978)

Adelson, L. Sudden death from coronary disease — the cardiac conundrum. *Postgrad. Med., 30*, 139–47 (1961)

Adsett, C.A. & Bruhn, J.G. Short-term group psychotherapy for post-myocardial infarction patients and their wives. *Canad. Med. Assoc. J., 99*, 577–84 (1968)

Alderman, E.L., Matlof, H.J., Wexler, L., Shunway, N.E. & Harrison, D.C. Results of direct coronary artery surgery for treatment of angina pectoris. *New Engl. J. Med., 288*, 535–9 (1973)

Aldinger, E.E. & Sohal, R.S. Effects of digitoxin on the ultrastructural myocardial changes in the rat subjected to chronic exercise. *Amer. J. Cardiol., 26*, 369–74 (1970)

Allan, T.M. & Dawson, A.A. ABO blood groups and ischaemic heart disease in man. *Br. Heart J., 30*, 377-82 (1968)

Allen, J.G. Aerobic capacity and physiological fitness of Australian men. *Ergonomics, 9*, 485–94 (1966)

Altekruse, E.B. & Wilmore, J.H. Changes in blood chemistry following a controlled exercise program. *J. Occup. Med., 15*, 110–13 (1973)

American College of Sports Medicine. Guidelines for graded exercise testing and exercise prescription and behavioural objectives for physicians, program directors, exercise leaders and exercise technicians (Amer. Coll. Sports Med., Madison, Wisc., 1975)

American Heart Association. Report of committee on electro-cardiography (Chairman C.E. Kossmann). Recommendations for standardization of leads and specifications for instruments in electrocardiography and vectorcardiography. *Circulation 35*, 583–602 (1967)

American Heart Association, Committee on Exercise. *Exercise Testing and Training of Apparently Healthy Individuals. A Handbook for Physicians* (American Heart Association, New York, 1972)

Amery, A., Billiet, L., Conway, J. & Reybrouck, T. Comparison of cardiac output determined by a CO_2 rebreathing method at rest and during graded sub-maximal exercise. *J. Physiol.*, *267*, 34–5p (1977)

Amery, A., Julius, S., Whitlock, L.S. & Conway, J. Influence of hypertension on the hemodynamic response to exercise. *Circulation 36*, 231–7 (1967)

Amsterdam, E.A. Function of the hypoxic myocardium. In: *Congestive Heart Failure*, ed. D.T. Mason (Yorke Medical Books, New York, 1976) pp. 147–58

Amsterdam, E.A., Hughes, J.L., Mansour, E., Salel, A.F., Bonnano, J.A., Zelis, R. & Mason, D.T. Circulatory effects of practolol: selective cardiac beta adrenergic blockade in arrythmias and angina pectoris. *Clin. Res.*, *19*, 109 (abstr.) (1971)

Amsterdam, E.A., Hughes, J.L., Miller, R.R., Massumi, R.A., Zelis, R. & Mason, D.T. Physiologic approach to the medical and surgical treatment of angina pectoris. In: *Exercise Testing and Exercise Training in Coronary Heart Disease*, ed. J.P. Naughton, H.K. Hellerstein & I.C. Mohler (Academic Press, New York, 1973) pp. 103–17

Amsterdam, E.A. & Mason, D.T. Exercise testing and indirect assessment of myocardial oxygen consumption in evaluation of angina pectoris. *Cardiology 62*, 174–89 (1977)

Andersen, K.L., Shephard, R.J., Denolin, H., Varnauskas, E. & Masironi, R. *Fundamentals of Exercise Testing* (World Health Organization, Geneva, 1971)

Anderson, T.W. Double blind trial of vitamin E in angina pectoris. *Amer. J. Chem. Nutr.*, *27*, 1174–8 (1974)

Anderson, T.W. The myocardium in coronary heart disease. In: *Proceedings of International Symposium on Exercise and Coronary Artery Disease*, ed. T. Kavanagh (Toronto Rehabilitation Centre, Toronto, 1976) pp. 32–44

Anderson, T.W. A new view of heart disease. *New Scientist 77*,

374–6 (1978a)

Anderson, T.W. *Comments to Conference on Decline in CHD Mortality* (National Institutes of Health, Bethesda, Md., 1978b)

Anderson, T.W, & Halliday, M.L. The male epidemic: 50 years of ischaemic heart disease. *Publ. Hlth. (Lond.)*, *93*, 163–72 (1979)

Anderson, T.W. & Le Riche, W.H. Ischaemic heart disease and sudden death, 1901–1961. *Brit. J. Prev. Soc. Med.*, *24*, 1–9 (1970)

Applebaum-Bowden, D. & Hazzard, W.R. Ethinyl estradiol lowers liver levels of triglyceride lipase. *Circulation 59/60*, Suppl. II–186 (abstr.) (1979)

Arcos, J.C., Sohal, R.S., Sun, S.C. & Burch, G.E. Changes in ultra structure and respiratory control in mitochondria of rat heart hypertrophied by exercise. *Exp. Molec. Pathol.*, *8*, 49–65 (1968)

Arlow, J.A. Identification mechanisms in coronary occlusion. *Psychosom. Med.*, *7*, 195–209 (1945)

Armstrong, A., Duncan, B., Oliver, M.F., Julian, D.G., Donald, K.W., Fulton, M., Lutz, W. & Morrison, S.L. Natural history of acute coronary heart attacks. A community study. *Brit. Heart J.*, *34*, 67–80 (1972)

Armstrong, B.W., Workman, J.M., Hurt, H.H. & Roemich, W.R. Clinico-physiologic evaluation of physical working capacity in persons with pulmonary disease; rationale and application of a method based on estimating maximal oxygen consuming capacity from MBC and O_2V_e. *Amer. Rev. Resp. Dis.*, *93*, 223–33 (1967)

Armstrong, M.L. Regression of atherosclerosis. *Atheroscler. Rev.*, *1*, 137–82 (1976)

Aronow, W.S. Effect of cigarette smoking and of carbon monoxide on coronary heart disease. *Chest 70*, 514–18 (1976)

Aronow, W.S. Medical management of stable angina pectoris. In: *Heart Disease and Rehabilitation*, ed. M.L. Pollock & D.H. Schmidt (Houghton Mifflin, Boston, 1979) pp. 212–27

Aronow, W.S. & Cassidy, J. Five years follow-up of double Master's Test, maximal treadmill stress test and resting and post-exercise apexcardiogram in asymptomatic persons. *Circulation 52*, 616–18 (1975)

Aronow, W.S., Harris, C.N., Isbell, M.W. *et al.* Effect of freeway travel on angina pectoris. *Ann. Intern. Med.*, *77*, 669–76 (1972)

Aronow, W.S. & Kaplan, M.A. Propranolol combined with isosorbide dinitrate versus placebo in angina pectoris. *New Engl.*

J. Med., *280*, 847–50 (1969)

Aronow, W.S., Kaplan, M.A. & Jacob, D. Tobacco: a precipitating factor in angina pectoris. *Ann. Intern. Med.*, *69*, 529–36 (1968)

Asano, K., Ogawa, S. & Furuta, T. Aerobic work capacity in middle- and old-aged runners. In: *Exercise Physiology*, ed. F. Landry & W.A.R. Orban (Symposia Specialists, Miami, Fla., 1978) pp. 465–71

Ascoop, C.A. What is an abnormal ischemic ECG response to exercise? In: *Coronary Heart Disease, Exercise Testing and Cardiac Rehabilitation*, ed. W.E. James & E.A. Amsterdam (Symposia Specialists, Miami, 1977) pp. 145–54

Ashley, F.W., & Kannel, W.B. Relation of weight change to changes in atherogenic traits: the Framingham study. *J. Chr. Dis.*, *27*, 103–4 (1974)

Asmussen, E. & Molbech, S.V. Methods and standards for evaluation of the physiological working capacity of patients. *Comm. Test. Obs. Inst.*, No. 4 (Hellerup, Denmark, 1959)

Åstrand, I. Aerobic work capacity in men and women with special reference to age. *Acta Physiol. Scand.*, *49*, suppl. 169, 1–92 (1960)

Åstrand, I. Blood pressure during physical work in a group of 221 women and men 48–63 years old. *Acta Med. Scand.*, *178*, 41–6 (1965)

Åstrand, I. The Scandinavian Committee on ECG classification. The 'Minnesota Code' for ECG classification. Adaptation to CR leads and modification of the code for ECGs recorded during and after exercise. *Acta Med. Scand.*, suppl. 481 (1967)

Åstrand, I. Electrocardiographic changes in relation to the type of exercise, the work load, age and sex. In: *Measurement in Exercise Electrocardiography*, ed. H. Blackburn (C.C. Thomas, Springfield, Ill., 1969) pp. 309–21

Åstrand, I. Circulatory responses to arm exercise in different work positions. *Scand. J. Clin. Lab. Invest.*, 27, 293–7 (1971)

Astrand, I., Åstrand, P.O. & Rodahl, K. Maximal heart rate during work in older men. *J. Appl. Physiol.*, *14*, 562–6 (1959)

Åstrand, P.O. Concluding remarks. *Canad. Med. Assoc. J.*, *96*, 907–11 (1967)

Åstrand, P.O., Cuddy, T.E., Saltin, B. & Stenberg, J. Cardiac output during submaximal and maximal work. *J. Appl. Physiol.*, *19*, 268–74 (1964)

Åstrand, P.O., Ekblom, B., Messin, R., Saltin, B. & Stenberg, J. Intra-arterial blood pressure during exercise with different muscle groups. *J. Appl. Physiol.*, *20*, 253–6 (1965)

Åstrand, P.O., Engström, L., Eriksson, B., Karlberg, P., Nylander, I., Saltin, B. & Thorén, C. Girl swimmers. *Acta Paed. Scand.*, *147*, supp., 1–75 (1963)

Åstrand, P.O. & Rodahl, K. *Textbook of Work Physiology* (McGraw Hill, New York, 1977)

Åstrup, P. Atherogenic compounds of tobacco smoke. In: *Atherosclerosis IV*, ed. G. Schettler, Y. Goto, Y. Hata & G. Close (Springer Verlag, Berlin, 1977) pp. 156–61

Åstrup, P., Hellung-Larsen, P., Kjeldsen, K. & Mellemgaard, K. The effect of tobacco smoking on the dissociation curve of oxhaemoglobin. *Scand. J. Clin. Lab. Invest.*, *18*, 450–7 (1966)

Åstrup, T. The effects of physical activity on blood coagulation and fibrinolysis. In: *Exercise Testing and Exercise Training in Coronary Heart Disease*, ed. J.P. Naughton, H.K. Hellerstein & I.C. Mohler (Academic Press, New York, 1973) pp. 169–92

Atkins, J.M., Matthews, O.A., Blomqvist, C.G. & Mullins, C.B. Incidence of arrhythmias induced by isometric and dynamic exercise. *Brit. Heart J.*, *38*, 465–71 (1976)

Auchincloss, J.H., Gilbert, R.G. & Bowman, J.L. Response of oxygen uptake to exercise in coronary artery disease. *Chest 65*, 500–6 (1974)

Avon, G., Ferguson, R.J., Chaniotis, L., Choquette, G. & Gauthier, P. *Estimation du Débit Cardiaque par 'CO₂ Rebreathing' avant et après l'Entrainement Physique chez le Coronarien. Anstract* (First Canadian Congress of Sport and Physical Activity, Montreal, 1973)

Ayotte, B., Seymour, J. & McIlroy, M. A new method for measurement of cardiac output with nitrous oxide. *J. Appl. Physiol.*, *28*, 863–6 (1970)

Bailey, D.A. & Mirwald, R.L. *A Children's Test of Fitness* (Action British Columbia, June, 1975)

Bailey, D.A., Shephard, R.J., Mirwald, R.L. & McBride, G.A. Current levels of Canadian cardio-respiratory fitness. *Canad. Med. Assoc. J.*, *111*, 25–30 (1974)

Balcon, R., Jewitt, D.E., Davies, J.P.H. & Oram, S. A controlled trial of propranolol in acute myocardial infarction. *Lancet* (ii), 917–20 (1966)

Balcon, R. & Rickards, A. Evaluation of results after aorto-

coronary bypass. In: *Coronary Heart Disease*, ed. M.
Kaltenbach, P. Lichten & G.C. Friesinger (G. Thieme, Stuttgart, 1973) pp. 296–300

Ball, R.M., Bache, R.J., Cobb, F.R. & Greenfield, J.C. Regional
myocardial blood flow during graded treadmill exercise in the
dog. *J. Clin. Invest.*, *55*, 43–9 (1975)

Bang, H.O., Dyerberg, J. & Hjørne, N. Investigations of blood
lipids and food composition of Greenlandic Eskimos. In:
Circumpolar Health, ed. R.J. Shephard & S. Itoh (University of
Toronto Press, Toronto, 1976) pp. 141–5

Banister, E.W. & Griffiths, J. Blood levels of adrenergic amines
during exercise. *J. Appl. Physiol.*, *33*, 674–6 (1972)

Banister, E.W. & Taunton, J.E. A rehabilitation program after
myocardial infarction. *Brit. Col. Med. J.*, 1–4 (October, 1971)

Banister, E.W., Tomanek, R.J. & Cvorkov, N. Ultrastructural
modifications in rat heart-responses to exercise and training.
Amer. J. Physiol., *220*, 1935–40 (1971)

Barnard, R.J. Long-term effects of exercise on cardiac function.
Exercise Sports Sci. Rev., *3*, 113–33 (1975)

Barnard, R.J., MacAlpin, R.N., Kattus, A.A. & Buckberg, G.D.
Ischemic response to sudden strenuous exercise in healthy men.
Circulation 48, 936–42 (1973)

Barnes, G.K., Ray, M.J., Oberman, A., *et al*. Changes in working
status of patients following coronary bypass surgery. *J. Amer.
Med. Assoc.*, *238*, 1259–62 (1977)

Barry, A.J., Daly, J.W., Pruett, E.D.R., Steinmetz, J.R.,
Birkhead, N.C. & Rodahl, K. Effects of physical training in
patients who have had myocardial infarction. *Amer. J. Cardiol.*,
17, 1–7 (1966)

Bartle, S.H. & Sanmarco, M.E. Comparison of angiographic and
thermal washout techniques for left ventricular volume
measurement. *Amer. J. Cardiol.*, *18*, 235–52 (1966)

Bartlett, R.G. Physiologic responses during coitus. *J. Appl.
Physiol.*, *9*, 469–72 (1956)

Bartlett, R.G. & Bohr, V.C. Physiologic responses during coitus in
the human. *Fed. Proc.*, *15*, 10 (abstr.) (1956)

Bassett, D.R., Rosenblatt, G., Moellering, R.C. & Hartwell, A.S.
Cardiovascular disease, diabetes mellitus and anthropometric
evaluation in Polynesian males on the Island of Nichau, 1963.
Circulation 34, 1088–97 (1966)

Bassler, T.J. Marathon running and immunity to atherosclerosis.

Ann. N.Y. Acad. Sci., 301, 579–92 (1977)

Battock, D.J., Alvarez, H. & Chidsey, C.A. Effects of propranolol and isosorbide dinitrate on exercise performance and adrenergic activity in patients with angina pectoris. *Circulation 39*, 157–69 (1969)

Bauss, R. & Roth, K. *Motorisch Entwicklung. Probleme und Ergebnisse von Längsschnittuntersuchungen* (Institut für Sportwissenschaft, Darmstadt, 1977)

Beard, O.W., Hipp, H.R., Robins, M., Taylor, J.S., Ebert, R.V & Bevan, L.G. Initial myocardial infarction among 503 veterans — 5 year survival. *Amer. J. Med., 28*, 871–83 (1960)

Beard, E.F. & Owen, C.A. Cardiac arrhythmias during exercise testing in healthy men. *Aerospace Med., 44*, 286–9 (1973)

Becker, L.C., Fortuin, N.J. & Pitt, B. Effect of ischemia and antianginal drugs on the distribution of radioactive microspheres in the canine left ventricle. *Circ. Res., 28*, 263–9 (1971)

Becker, M., Haefner, D.P., Kasl, S.V., Kirscht, J.P., Maiman, L.A. & Rosenstock, I.M. Selected psychosocial models and correlates of individual health-related behaviours. *Medical Care 15* (5) (suppl.), 27–46 (1977)

Becker, M. & Maiman, L.A. Socio-behavioural determinants of compliance with health and medical care recommendations. *Medical Care 13* 10–24 (1975)

Becklake, M.R., Frank, H., Dagenais, G.R., Ostiguy, G.L. & Guzman, G.A. Influence of age and sex on exercise cardiac output. *J. Appl. Physiol., 20*, 938–47 (1965)

Becklake, M., Varvis, C.J., Pengelly, L.D., Kenning, S., McGregor, M. & Bates, D.V. Measurement of pulmonary blood flow during exercise using nitrous oxide. *J. Appl. Physiol., 17*, 579–86 (1962)

Beiser, G.D., Epstein, S.E. & Goldstein, R.E. Impaired heart rate response to sympathetic nerve stimulation in patients with cardiac decompensation. *Circulation 37*, Suppl VI, 40 (1968)

Bendien, J. & Groen, J. A psychological statistical study of neuroticism and extroversion in patients with myocardial infarction. *J. Psychosomat. Res., 7*, 11–14 (1963)

Benditt, E.P. The origin of atherosclerosis. *Sci. Amer., 236* (2), 74–85 (1977)

Benestad, A.M. Determination of PWC and exercise tolerance in cardiac patients. *Acta Med. Scand., 183*, 521–9 (1968)

Benestad, A.M. The deteriorative effect of myocardial infarction upon physiological indices of work capacity. *Acta Med. Scand.,* *191*, 67–75 (1972)

Benfari, R.C. Lifestyle alteration and the primary prevention of CHD: the Multiple Risk Factor Intervention Trial (MRFIT). In: *Heart Disease and Rehabilitation*, ed. M.L. Pollock & D.H. Schmidt (Houghton Mifflin, Boston, Mass., 1979) pp. 341–51

Bengtsson, C. Ischaemic heart disease in women. *Acta Med. Scand., 549*, suppl., 1–128 (1973)

Bennett, D.H. & Evans, D.W. Correlation of left ventricular mass determined by echocardiography with vectorcardiographic and electrocardiographic voltage measurements. *Brit. Heart J., 36*, 981–7 (1974)

Berenson, G.S. & Burch, G.E. The response of patients with congestive heart failure to a rapid elevation in atmospheric temperature and humidity. *Amer. J. Med. Sci., 223*, 45–53 (1952)

Bergman, H. & Varnauskas, E. The haemodynamic effects of physical training in coronary patients. *Medicine and Sport 4*, 138–47 (Karger, Basel, 1970)

Bergström, K., Bjernulf, A. & Erikson, U. Work capacity, heart and blood volume, before and after physical training in male patients after myocardial infarction. *Scand. J. Rehabil. Med., 6*, 51–64 (1974)

Berkada, B., Akokan, G. & Derman, V. Fibrinolytic response to physical exercise in males. *Atherosclerosis 13*, 85–91 (1971)

Bevegard, S., Freyschuss, H. & Strandell, T. Circulatory adaptations to arm and leg exercise in supine and sitting positions. *J. Appl. Physiol., 21*, 37–46 (1966)

Bing, R.J., Hellems, H.K. & Regan, T.J. Measurement of . coronary blood flow in man. *Circulation 22*, 1–3 (1960)

Biorck, G., Blomqvist, G. & Sievers, J. Studies on myocardial infarction in Malmo, 1935 to 1954. 1. Morbidity and mortality in hospital material. *Acta Med. Scand., 159*, 253–74 (1957)

Biss, K., Ho, K.J., Mikkelson, B., Lewis, L. & Taylor, C.B. Some unique biologic characteristics of the Masai of East Africa. *New Engl. J. Med., 284*, 694–9 (1971)

Bjernulf, A. Haemodynamic aspects of physical training after myocardial infarction. *Acta Med. Scand., 548*, suppl., 1–50 (1973)

Björntrop, B.P., Fahlen, M., Grimby, G., Gustafson, A., Holm, J., Renström, P. & Schersten, T. Carbohydrate and lipid metabolism in middle-aged physically well-trained men. *Metabolism 21*, 1037–44 (1972)

Blackburn, H. The exercise electrocardiogram. Technological, procedural and conceptual developments. In: *Measurement in Exercise Electrocardiography. The Ernst Simonsen Conference*, ed. H. Blackburn (C.C. Thomas, Springfield, Ill., 1968), pp. 220–58

Blackburn, H. Multifactor preventive trials in coronary heart disease. In: *Trends in Epidemiology*, ed. G.T. Stewart (C.C. Thomas, Springfield, Ill., 1972)

Blackburn, H. Disadvantages of intensive exercise therapy after myocardial infarction. In: *Controversy in Internal Medicine*, ed. F. Ingelfinger (W.B. Saunders, Philadelphia, 1974) p. 162

Blackburn, H. Preventive cardiology in practice: Minnesota studies on risk factor reduction. In: *Heart Disease and Rehabilitation*, ed. M.L. Pollock & D.H. Schmidt (Houghton Mifflin, Boston, Mass., 1979) pp. 245–75

Blackburn, H., Blomqvist, G., Freiman, A., Freisinger, G.C., *et al.* The exercise electrocardiogram: differences in interpretation. *Amer. J. Cardiol., 21*, 871–80 (1968)

Blackburn, H., Debacker, G. & Crow, R. Epidemiology and prevention of ventricular ectopic rhythms. *Adv. Cardiol., 18*, 208–16 (1976)

Blackburn, H., Taylor, H.L., Hamrell, B., Buskirk, E., Nicholas, W.C. & Thorsen, R.D. Premature ventricular complexes induced by stress testing, their frequency and response to physical conditioning. *Amer. J. Cardiol., 31*, 441–9 (1973)

Blake, H.A., Manion, W.C., Mattingly, T.W., *et al.* Coronary artery anomalies. *Circulation 30*, 927–40 (1964)

Blick, E.F. & Stein, P.D. *Work of the Heart: a General Thermodynamic Analysis* (Pergamon Press, New York, 1977)

Bloch, A., Maeder, J.P. & Haissly, J.C. Sexual problems after myocardial infarction. *Amer. Heart J., 90*, 536–7 (1975)

Blomqvist, C.G., Gaffney, F.A., Atkins, J.M. *et al.* The exercise ECG and related physiological data as markers of critical coronary artery lesions. *Acta Med. Scand., 615*, suppl., 51–62 (1978)

Blomqvist, C.G. & Mitchell, J.H. Exercise testing and electrocardiographic interpretation. In: *Heart Disease and Rehabilitation*, ed. M.L. Pollock & D.H. Schmidt (Houghton-Mifflin, Boston, 1979)

Blomqvist, G. Exercise physiology related to diagnosis of coronary artery disease. In: *Coronary Heart Disease: Prevention, Detection, Rehabilitation with Emphasis on Exercise Testing*, ed. S.M. Fox (Internationl Medical Corporation, Denver, Colorado, 1974) pp. (2-1)–(2-26)

Bloom, D.S. & Vecht, R.H. Circulatory changes during isometric exercise measured by transcutaneous aortovelography. *J. Physiol., 281*, 21–2p (1978)

Boas, E.P. & Goldschmidt, E.F. *The Heart Rate* (C.C. Thomas, Springfield, Ill., 1932)

Bonen, A., Gardner, J., Primrose, J., Quigley, R. & Smith, D. An evaluation of the Canadian Home Fitness Test. *Canad. J. Appl. Sports. Sci., 2*, 133–6 (1977)

Borer, J.S., Bacharach, S.L., Green, M.V., *et al.* Real-time radionuclide cineangiography in the non-invasive evaluation of global and regional left ventricular function at rest and during exercise in patients with coronary artery disease. *New Engl. J. Med., 296*, 839–44 (1977)

Boshoff, W.H. Ergonomic aspects of traditional and modern cultivation tasks in Uganda. In: *Proceedings of the Fourth International Congress on Rural Medicine* (Usada, Japan, 1965)

Bouchard, C., Hollmann, W., Venrath, H., Herkenrath, G. & Schlüssel, H. Minimalbelastungen zur Prävention kardiovaskularer Erkrankungen. *Sportarzt und Sportmedizin 7*, 348–57 (1966)

Bourassa, M.G. Corbara, F., Lésperance, J. & Campeau, L. Progression of coronary disease five to seven years after aortocoronary bypass surgery. In: *Coronary Heart Disease*, ed. M. Kaltenbach, P. Lichtlen, R. Balcon & W.D. Bussmann (G. Thieme, Stuttgart, 1978) pp. 139–44

Bourassa, M.G., Lésperance, J., Campeau, L. & Saltiel, J. Fate of left ventricular contraction following aortocoronary venous grafts. *Ciculation 46*, 724–30 (1972)

Bourne, G. An attempt at the clinical classification of premature ventricular beats. *Quart. J. Med., 20*, 219–43 (1927)

Braunwald, E., Ross, J. & Sonnenblick, E.H. *Mechanisms of Contraction of the Normal and Failing Heart*, 2nd edn (Little, Brown, Boston, Mass., 1976)

Brenton, M. *Sex and Your Heart* (Coward, New York, 1968)

Briggs, J.F. The role of emotions in the rehabilitation of the cardiac patient. In: *Changing Concepts in Cardiovascular Disease*, ed. H.I. Russek & B.L. Zohman (Williams & Wilkins, Baltimore,

1972) pp. 393–7

British Medical Journal. Intermittent claudication. *Brit. Med. J.*, *6019*, 1165–6 (1976)

Brock, L.L. Stress testing in work evaluation units. In: *Work Evaluation Units Sub-committee Newsletter* (American Heart Association, New York, 1967)

Brock, L. Early reconditioning for post-myocardial infarction patients: Spalding Rehabilitation Center. In: *Exercise Testing and Exercise Training in Coronary Heart Disease*, ed. J.P. Naughton, H.K. Hellerstein and I.C. Mohler (Academic Press, New York, 1973) pp. 315–23

Brock, L.L. Administrative considerations. In: *Coronary Disease, Exercise Testing, Rehabilitation Therapy*, ed. S. Fox (International Medical Corporation, Denver, Col., 1974) pp. (10-1)–(10-8)

Brodsky, M., Wu, D., Denes, P., Kanakis, C. & Rosen, K.M. Arrhythmias documented by 24 hour continuous electrocardiographic monitoring in 50 male medical students without apparent heart disease. *Amer. J. Cardiol., 39*, 390–5 (1977)

Brody, A.J. Master two-step test in clinically unselected patients. *J. Amer. Med. Assoc., 171*, 1195–8 (1959)

Bronstein, L.H. Experience of the work classification unit at BelleVue Hospital. In: *Work and the Heart*, ed. F.F. Rosenbaum & E.L. Belknap (P.B. Hoeber, New York, 1959)

Bronstet, J.P., Series, E., Guern, P., Vallot, F. & Pic, A. Matching Nifedipine and Nitroglycerine in the prevention of exercise-induced angina. In: *Coronary Heart Disease*, ed. M. Kaltenbach, P. Lichtlen, R. Balcon & W.D. Bussmann (G. Thieme, Stuttgart, 1978) pp. 309–16

Brown, B.G., Gundel, W.D., Gott, V.L. & Covell, J.W. Hemodynamic determinants of retrograde arterial coronary flow following acute coronary occlusion. *Circulation 46*, suppl. 2, 100 (Abstr.) (1972)

Brown, J.R. & Shephard, R.J. Some measurements of fitness in older female employees of a Toronto department store. *Canad. Med. Assoc. J., 97*, 1208–13 (1967)

Brozek, J., Keys, A. & Blackburn, H. Personality differences between potential coronary and non-coronary subjects. *Ann. N.Y. Acad. Sci., 134*, 1056–64 (1966)

Bruce, E.H., Frederick, R., Bruce, R.A. *et al.* Comparison of active participants and drop-outs in CAPRI cardiopulmonary rehabilitation programs. *Amer. J. Cardiol, 37*, 53–60 (1976)

Bruce, R.A. Atherosclerosis. In: *Coronary Heart Disease: Prevention, Detection, Rehabilitation with Emphasis on Exercise Testing*, ed. S.M. Fox (International Medical Corp., Denver, Col., 1974) chap. 1, pp. 1–16

Bruce, R.A, Alexander, E.R., Li, Y.B., Chiang, B.N., Ting, N. & Hornsten, T.R. Electrocardiographic responses to maximal exercise in American and Chinese population samples. In: *Measurement in Exercise Electrocardiography*, ed. H. Blackburn (C.C. Thomas, Springfield, Ill., 1969) pp. 413–44

Bruce, R.A., Blackmon, J.R., Jones, J.W. & Strait, G. Exercise testing in adult normal subjects and cardiac patients. *Pediatrics 32*, suppl., 742–56 (1963)

Bruce, R.A., Fisher, L.D., Cooper, M.N. & Gey, G.O. Separation of effects of cardiovascular disease and age on ventricular function with maximal exercise. *Amer. J. Cardiol., 34*, 757–63 (1974a)

Bruce, R.A., Hornsten, T.R. & Blackmon, J.R. Myocardial infarction after normal responses to maximal exercise. *Circulation 38*, 552–8 (1968)

Bruce, R.A., Kusumi, F., Culver, B.H. & Butler, J. Cardiac limitation to maximal oxygen transport and changes in components after jogging across the U.S. *J. Appl. Physiol., 39*, 958–64 (1975)

Bruce, R.A., Kusumi, F. & Hosmer, D. Maximal oxygen intake and nomographic assessment of functional aerobic impairment in cardiovascular disease. *Amer. Heart J., 85*, 546–62 (1973)

Bruce, R.A., Kusumi, F., Niederberger, M. & Peterson, J.L. Cardiovascular mechanisms of functional aerobic impairment in patients with coronary heart disease. *Circulation 49*, 696–702 (1974b)

Bruhn, J.G. Obtaining and interpreting psychosocial data in studies of coronary heart disease. In: *Exercise Testing and Exercise Training in Coronary Heart Disease*, ed. J.P. Naughton & H.K. Hellerstein (Academic Press, New York, 1973)

Bruhn, J.G., Wolf, S. & Philips, B.V. Depression and death in myocardial infarction: a psychosocial study of screening male coronary patients over nine years. *Psychosom. Res., 15*, 305–13 (1971)

Brunner, B.C. Personality and motivating factors influencing adult participation in vigorous physical activity. *Res. Quart.*, *40*, 464–8 (1969)

Brunner, D. Active exercise for coronary patients. *Rehab. Rec.*, *9*, 29–31 (1968)

Brunner, D. *Studies in Preventive Cardiology. Coronary Heart Disease — Epidemiology and Rehabilitation* (Government Hospital, Donolo, Jaffa, 1973)

Brunner, D. & Manelis, G. Physical activity at work and ischemic heart disease. In: *Coronary Heart Disease and Physical Fitness*, ed. O.A. Larsen and R.O. Malmborg (University Park Press, Baltimore, Md., 1971)

Brunton, T.L. On the action of nitrite of amyl on the circulation. *J. Anat. Physiol.*, *5*, 92–101 (1871)

Bruschke, A.V.G. Management of the patient with severe symptoms of coronary artery disease. In: *Coronary Heart Disease, Exercise Testing and Cardiac Rehabilitation*, ed. W.E. James & E.A. Amsterdam (Symposia Specialists, Miami, Fla., 1977) pp. 37–45

Bruschke, A.V.G., Proudfit, W.L. & Sones, F.M. Progress study of 590 consecutive nonsurgical cases of coronary disease followed 5–9 years. I. Arteriographic correlations. *Circulation* *47*, 1147–53 (1973)

Bruschke, A.V.G., Proudfit, W.L. & Sones, F.M. Progress study of 590 consecutive nonsurgical cases of coronary disease followed 5–9 years. II. Ventriculographic and other correlations. *Circulation 47*, 1154–63 (1973)

Brusis, O.A. Guidelines for supervised and non-supervised cardiac rehabilitation programs. In: *Coronary Heart Disease, Exercise Testing and Cardiac Rehabilitation*, ed. W.E. James and E.A. Amsterdam (Symposia Specialists, Miami, Fla., 1977) pp. 233–45

Bubenheimer, P., Samek, L., Schmeisser, H.J. & Roskamm, H. Echocardiographic evaluation of left ventricular function during exercise in untrained young men and athletes. In: *International Conference on Sports Cardiology*, ed. T. Lubich & A. Venerando (1980) pp. 787–92

Burch, G.E. & De Pasquale, N.P. Sudden, unexpected natural death. *Amer. J. Med. Sci.*, *249*, 86–97 (1965)

Burrow, R.D., Strauss, H.W., Singleton, R., *et al.* Analysis of left ventricular function from multiple gated acquisition cardiac blood pool imaging: comparison to contrast angiography.

Circulation 56, 1024–8 (1977)

Burt, J.J. & Jackson, R. The effects of physical exercise on the coronary collateral circulation of dogs. *J. Sports Med. Phys. Fitness 5*, 203–6 (1965)

Burton, A.C. *Physiology and Biophysics of the Circulation* (Year Book Publishers, Chicago, Ill., 1965)

Buskirk, E.R., Kollias, J., Piconreatigue, E., Akers, R., Prokop, E. & Baker, P. In: *International Symposium on the Effects of Altitude on Physical Performance*, ed. R. Goddard (Athletic Institute, Chicago, 1967)

Cadlwell, J.H., Stewart, D.K., Frimer, M., *et al.* Left ventricular volume during maximal supine exercise. *Circulation 51/52*, suppl. II, 140 (1975)

Cander, L. & Forster, R.E. Determination of pulmonary parenchymal tissue volume and pulmonary capillary blood flow in man. *J. Appl. Physiol., 14*, 541–51 (1959)

Cantwell, J.D., Walter, J.B., Watt, E.W. & Fletcher, G.F. Dynamic exercise training in post-myocardial infarction patients. *Med. Sci. Sports 5*, 66–7 (1973)

Cardus, D., Fluentes, F. & Srinivasan, R. Cardiac evaluation of a physical rehabilitation program for patients with ischemic heart disease. *Arch. Phys. Med. Rehabil., 56*, 419–25 (1975)

Carlson, L.A. Plasma lipids and lipoproteins and tissue lipids during exercise. In: *Nutrition and Physical Activity*, ed. G. Blix (Almqvist & Wiksell, Uppsala, 1967) p. 16

Carrier, R., Landry, F., Potvin, R., *et al.* Comparisons between athletes, normal and Eskimo subjects from the view of selected biochemical parameters. In: *Training: Scientific Basis and Application*, ed. A.W. Taylor (C.C. Thomas, Springfield, Ill., 1972)

Carrow, R.E., Brown, R.E. & Van Huss, W.D. Fiber sizes and capillary to fiber ratios in skeletal muscle of exercised rats. *Anat. Record 159*, 33–40 (1967)

Cash, J.D. & McGill, R.C. Fibrinolytic response to moderate exercise in young male diabetics and non-diabetics. *J. Clin. Pathol., 22*, 32–5 (1969)

Casssel, J., Heyden, S., Bartel, A.G., Kaplan, B.H., Tyroler, H.A, Cornoni, J.C. & Hames, C.G. Occupation and physical activity and coronary heart disease. *Arch. Int. Med., 128*, 920–8 (1971)

Castelli, W.P., Doyle, J.T., Gordon, T., Hames, C.G., Hjortland,

M.C., Hulley, S.B., Kagan, A. & Zukel, W.J. HDL cholesterol and other lipids in coronary heart disease — the cooperative lipoprotein phenotyping study. *Circulation 55*, 767–72 (1977)

Castleden, C.M. & Cole, P.V. Inhalation of tobacco smoke by pipe and cigar smokers. *Lancet* (2), 21–2 (July, 1973)

Cederlöf, R., Friberg, L. & Jonsson, E. Hereditary factors and 'angina pectoris'. A study of 5,877 twin-pairs with the aid of mailed questionnaires. *Arch. Env. Health 14*, 397–400 (1967)

Cermak, J. Changes of the heart volume and of the basic somatometric indices in 12–15 years old boys with an intense exercise regime. A long term study. *Brit. J. Sports Med., 7*, 241–4 (1973)

Chamberlain, D.A. Role of coronary ambulances in reduction of sudden coronary death. In: *Sudden Coronary Death*, ed. V. Manninen & P.I. Halonen (Karger, Basel, 1978a) pp. 191–2

Chamberlain, D.A. Beta-adrenergic blocking agents in prevention of sudden death. In: *Sudden Coronary Death*, ed. V. Manninen & P.I. Halonen (Karger, Basel, 1978b) pp. 196–205

Chapman, C.B. & Fraser, R.S. Studies on the effect of exercise on cardio-vascular function. III. Cardiovascular response to exercise in patients with healed myocardial infarction. *Circulation 9*, 347–51 (1954)

Chapman, J.M. & Massey, F.J. The interrelationship of serum cholesterol, hypertension, body weight, and risk of coronary disease. Results of the first ten years' follow up in the Los Angeles Heart Study. *J. Chron. Dis., 17*, 933–49 (1964)

Chatterjee, K., Swan, H.J.C., Parmley, W.W., Sustaita, H., Marcus, H. & Matloff, J. Depression of left ventricular function due to acute myocardial ischemia and its reversal after aortocoronary saphenous-vein bypass. *New Engl. J. Med., 286*, 1117–22 (1972)

Chiang, B., Perlman, L.V., Ostrander, L.D., *et al.* Relationship of premature systoles to coronary heart disease and sudden death in the Tecumseh epidemiological study. *Ann. Intern. Med., 70*, 1159–66 (1969)

Chidsey, C.A, Braunwald, E. & Morrow, A.G. Catecholamine excretion and cardiac stores of norepinephrine in congestive heart failure. *Amer. J. Med., 39*, 442–51 (1965)

Chisholm, D.M., Collis, M.L., Kulak, L.L., Davenport, W. & Gruber, N. Physical activity readiness. *Brit. Col. Med. J., 17*, 375–8 (1975)

Choquette, G. & Ferguson, R. Blood pressure reduction in 'borderline' hypertensives following physical training. *Canad. Med. Assoc. J., 108*, 699–703 (1973)

Chrastek, J. & Adimirova, J. Höher Blütdruck und körperliche Übungen. *Sportarzt und Sportmedizin 21* (3), 61–6 (1970)

Clark, R.J. Experience of the cardiac work classification unit in Boston, Massachusetts. In: *Work and the Heart*, ed. F.F. Rosenbaum & E.L. Belknap (P.B. Hoeber, New York, 1959) pp. 311–21

Clarke, H.H. *Physical and Motor Tests in the Medford Boy's Growth Study* (Prentice Hall, Englewood Cliffs, N.J., 1971)

Clarke, H.J. Physical activity and coronary heart disease. Washington, D.C. — President's Council on Physical Fitness and Sports. *Physical Fitness Research Digest 2* (2), 1–13 (1972)

Clarke, H.H. Update: physical activity and coronary heart disease. *Physical Fitness Research Digest 9* (2), 1–25 (1979)

Clarke, J.M., Shelton, J.R., Hamer, J., Taylor, S. & Venning, G.R. The rhythm of the normal human heart. *Lancet* (ii), 508–12 (1976)

Clausen, J.P. Circulatory adjustments to dynamic exercise and effect of physical training in normal subjects and patients with coronary artery disease. *Progr. Cardiovasc. Dis., 18*, 459–95 (1976)

Clausen, J., Felsby, M., Schønau-Jørgensen, F., Lyager-Nielsen, B., Roin, J. & Strange, B. Absence of prophylactic effect of propranolol in myocardial infarction. *Lancet* (ii) 920–4 (1966)

Clausen, J.P., Klausen, K., Rasmussen, B. & Trap-Jensen, J. Central and peripheral circulatory changes after training of the arms and legs. *Amer. J. Physiol., 225*, 675–82 (1973)

Clausen, J.P. & Larsen, N.A. Muscle blood flow during exercise in normal men studied by the Xe^{133} clearance method. *Cardiovasc. Res., , 245–54 (1971)

Clausen, J.P., Larsen, O.A. & Trap-Jensen, J. Physical training in the management of coronary artery disease. *Circulation 40*, 143–54 (1969)

Clausen, J.P. & Trap-Jensen, J. Effects of training on the distribution of cardiac output in patients with coronary artery disease. *Circulation 42*, 611–24 (1970)

Clausen, J.P., Trap-Jensen, J. & Lassen, N.A. The effects of training on the heart rate during arm and leg exercise. *Scand. J. Clin. Lab. Invest., 26*, 295–301 (1970)

Clausen, J.P., Trap-Jensen, J. & Lassen, N.A. Evidence that the relative exercise-bradycardia induced by training can be caused by extra-cardiac factors. In: *Coronary Heart Disease and Physical Fitness*, ed. O.A. Larsen & R.O. Malmborg (University Park Press, Baltimore, Md., 1971) pp. 27–8

Clements, I.P., Vliestra, R.E., Dewey, J.D. & Harrison, C.E. Protective effect of verpamil infusion on mitochondrial respiratory function in ischemic myocardium. In: *Coronary Heart Disease*, ed. M. Kaltenbach, P. Lichtlen, R. Balcon & W.D. Bussman (G. Thieme, Stuttgart, 1978) pp. 284–96

Cobb, F.R., Ruby, R.L. & Fariss, B.L. Effects of exercise on acute coronary occlusion in dogs with prior partial occlusion (abstr.) *Circulation 37/38*, 104 (1968)

Cobb, L.A., Baum, R.S., Alvarez, H. & Schaffer, W.A. Resuscitation from out-of-hospital ventricular fibrillation: 4 years follow up. *Circulation 52*, suppl. III, 223–8 (1975)

Cohen, L. Contributions of serum enzymes and isoenzymes to the diagnosis of myocardial injury. I. *Mod. Concepts Cardiovasc. Dis., 36*, 43–7 (1967)

Cohen, L.S., Elliott, W.C., Rolett, E.L. & Gorlin, R. Haemodynamic studies during angina pectoris. *Circulation 31*, 409–16 (1965)

Cohen, S.I., Young, M.W., Lau, S.H., Haft, J.I. & Damato, A.N. Effects of reserpine on cardiac output and A-V conduction at rest and controlled heart rates in patients with essential hypertension. *Circulation 37*, 738–46 (1968)

Cohn, P.F., Gorlin, R., Herman, M.V. *et al*. Relation between contractile reserve and prognosis in patients with coronary artery disease and a depressed ejection fraction. *Circulation 51*, 414–20 (1975)

Cole, J.P. & Ellestad, M.H. Significance of chest pain during treadmill exercise: correlation with coronary events. *Amer. J. Cardiol., 41*, 227–32 (1978)

Cole, D.R., Singian, E.B. & Katz, L.N. Long-term prognosis following myocardial infarction, and some factors which affect it. *Circulation 9*, 321–34 (1954)

Collis, M. *Employee Fitness* (Minister of State for Fitness and Amateur Sport, Ottawa, 1975)

Cooksey, W.B. Letter to the Editor. *J. Amer. Med. Assoc., 113*, 351–2 (1939)

Cooper, J.K. & Willig, S.H. Nonphysicians for coronary care

delivery: Are they legal? *Amer. J. Cardiol.*, *28*, 363–5 (1971)

Cooper, K.H. *Aerobics* (Evans, New York, 1968)

Cooper, K.H. Guidelines in the management of the exercising patient. *J. Amer. Med. Assoc.*, *211*, 1663–7 (1970)

Cooper, K.H., Meyer, B.U., Blide, R., Pollock, M. & Gibbons, L. The important role of fitness determination and stress testing in predicting coronary incidence. *Ann. N.Y. Acad. Sci.*, *301*, 642–52 (1977)

Corliss, R.J. Cardiac catheterization. In: *Heart Disease and Rehabilitation*, ed. M. Pollock & D.H. Schmidt (Houghton Mifflin, Boston, 1979) pp. 140–56

Coronary Drug Project Research Group. Clofibrate and niacin in coronary heart disease. *J. Amer. Med. Assoc.*, *231*, 360–81 (1975)

Corvisart. *Essai sur les Maladies du Coeur et des Gros Vaisseaux* (Paris, 1806). Cited by L.F. Bishop & P. Reichart, *Psychosomatics 12*, 412–15 (1971)

Council on Rehabilitation. International Society of Cardiology. *Myocardial Infarction. How to Prevent. How to Rehabilitate*. Ed. T. Semple (Brussels, 1973)

Cox, M.H. & Shephard, R.J. Employee fitness, absenteeism, and job satisfaction. *Med. Sci. Sports 11*, 105 (abstr.) (1979)

Crews, J. & Aldinger, E.E. Effect of chronic exercise on myocardial function. *Amer. Heart. J.*, *74*, 536–42 (1967)

Criterion Committee of New York Heart Association. *Diseases of the Heart and Blood Vessels. Nomenclature and Criteria for Diagnosis* (Little, Brown, Boston, 1964)

Cumming, G.R. & Alexander, W.D. The calibration of bicycle ergometers. *Canad. J. Physiol. Pharm.*, *46*, 917–19 (1968)

Cumming, G.R., Borysyk, L.M. & Dufresne, C. The maximal exercise ECG in asymptomatic men. *Canad. Med. Assoc. J.*, *106*, 649–53 (1972)

Cumming, G.R., Dufresne, C., Kich, L. & Samm, J. Exercise electrocardiogram patterns in normal women. *Brit. Heart J.*, *35*, 1055–61 (1973a)

Cumming, G.R., Dufresne, C. & Samm, J. Exercise ECG changes in normal women. *Canad. Med. Assoc. J.*, *109*, 108–11 (1973b)

Cumming, G.R. & Edwards, A.H. Indirect measurement of left ventricular function during exercise. *Canad. Med. Assoc., J.*, *89*, 219–21 (1963)

Cumming, G.R., & Glenn, J. Evaluation of the Canadian Home

Fitness Test in middle-aged men. *Canad. Med. Assoc. J.*, *117*, 346–9 (1977)

Cunningham, D.A., Ingram, K.J. & Rechnitzer, P.A. The effect of training: physiological responses. *Med. Sci. Sports 11*, 379–81 (1979)

Cunningham, D.A., Ingram, K.J., Rechnitzer, P.A., Jones, N.L., Shephard, R.J., Sangal, S., Andrew, G., Buck, C., Kavanagh, T., Parker, J.O. & Yuhasz, M.S. Effect of a 2-year program of exercise training on cardiovascular fitness and recurrence rates in post-myocardial infarction patients. *Cardiology 62*, 136–7 (1977)

Cunningham, D.A. & Rechnitzer, P.A. Exercise prescription and the post-coronary patient. *Arch. Phys. Med. Rehab.*, *55*, 296–300 (1974)

Cureton, T.K. Improving the physical fitness of youth. A report of research in the sports-fitness school of the University of Illinois. *Monographs of Society for Research in Child Development 29* (4), 1–221 (1964)

Dagenais, G.R., Pitt, B. & Ross, R.S. Exercise tolerance in patients with angina pectoris. *Amer. J. Cardiol.*, *28*, 10–16 (1971)

Daoud, A.S., Fritz, K.E., Jarmolych, J., Augustyn, J.M., Lee, K.T. & Thomas, W.A. Regression of complicated atherosclerotic lesions in the abdominal aortas of swine. *Adv. Exp. Med. Biol.*, *82*, 447–52 (1977)

Davies, C.T.M. Submaximal tests for estimating maximum oxygen intake. Commentary. In: *Proceedings of an International Symposium on Physical Activity and Cardiovascular Health. Canad. Med. Assoc. J.*, *96*, 743–4 (1967)

Dayton, S., Hashimoto, S.D., Dixon, W.J. & Tomiyasu, W. A controlled clinical trial of a diet high in unsaturated fat in preventing complications of atherosclerosis. *Circulation 40*, Suppl. II, 1–63 (1969)

d'Andrade, B.J.F. & Rose, E.H. Study of the rest e.c.g. of marathon runners. In: *Proceedings of the International Conference on Sports Cardiology*, ed. A. Venerando (A. Gaggi, Bologna, 1979)

Defares, J.G. *A Study of the Carbon Dioxide Time Course during Rebreathing*. Ph.D. Thesis (University of Utrecht, 1956)

Degré, S., Degré-Coustry, C., Hoylaerts, M., Grevisse, M. & Denolin, H. Therapeutic effects of physical training in coronary heart disease. *Cardiology 62*, 206–17 (1977)

Degré, S. & Denolin, H. Bases physiologiques de l'entrainement musculaire chez les patients atteints d'infarctus du myocarde et premiers resultats d'un programme de réadaptation physqiue. *Médicine et Hygiene 31*, 978–80 (1973)

Degré, S., Messin, R., Vandermoten, P., Bemaret, B., Haissly, J.C., Salhadin, P.H. & Denolin, H. Aspects physio-pathologiques de l'entrainement musculaire chez des patients atteinte d'infarctus du myocarde. *Acta Cardiol.*, *27*, 445–62 (1972)

Delhez, L., Bottin, R., Thonon, A. & Petit, J.M. Influence de l'entrainment sur la force maximum des muscles repiratoires. *Soc. Med. Belg. Ed. Phys.*, *20*, 52–63 (1967–8)

Delius, W., Cullhed, I., Björk, L. & Hallen, A. Left ventricular aneurysmectomy. Clinical, haemodynamic and angiographic results. In: *Coronary Heart Disease*, ed. M. Kaltenbach, P. Lichtlen & G.C. Friesinger. (G. Thieme, Stuttgart, 1973) pp. 223–8

de Marées, H. & Barbey, K. Änderung der peripheren Durchblutung durch Ausdauertraining. *Z. f. Kardiol.*, *62*, 653–63 (1973)

De Palma, R.G., Bellon, E.M., Klein, L., Koletsky, S. & Insull, W. Approaches to evaluating regression of experimental atherosclerosis. *Adv. Exp. Med. Biol.*, *82*, 459–70 (1977)

De Ponti, C., Galli, M.A., Mauri, F., Salvadé, P. & Caru, B. Effects of association of calcium antagonists with nitro-derivatives or beta-blocking drugs in effort angina. In: *Coronary Heart Disease*, ed. M. Kaltenbach, P. Lichtlen, R. Balcon & W.D. Bussmann (G. Thieme, Stuttgart, 1978) pp. 316–21

de Soyza, N., Murphy, M.L., Bissett, H.K. *et al.* A comparison of ventricular arrhythmia in coronary artery disease patients randomized to surgical and medical therapy. *Clin. Res.*, *24*, 2A (abstr.) (1976)

Detry, J. & Bruce, R.A. Effects of physical training on exertional ST segment depression in coronary heart disease. *Circulation 44*, 390–6 (1971)

Detry, J.R., Rousseau, M., Vanden Broucke, G., Kusumi, L., Brausseur, A. & Bruce, R.A. Increased arterio-venous oxygen difference after physical training in coronary heart disease. *Circulation 44*, 109–18 (1971)

Devlin, J. The effect of training and acute physical exercise on plasma-insulin like activity. *Irish J. Med. Sci., 6*, 423–5 (1963)

de Vries, H.A. Physiological effects of an exercise training regimen upon men aged 52 to 88. *J. Gerontol., 25*, 325–36 (1970)

de Wijn, J.F., de Jongste, J.L., Mosterd, W. & Willebrand, D. Haemoglobin, packed cell volume, serum iron-binding capacity of selected athletes during training. *J. Sports Med. Phys. Fitness 11*, 42–51 (1971)

Dimond, G.E. Prognosis of men returning to work after first myocardial infarction. *Circulation 23*, 881–5 (1961)

Doan, A.E., Peterson, D.R., Blackmon, J.R. & Bruce, R.A. Myocardial ischemia after maximal exercise in healthy men. *Amer. Heart. J., 69*, 11–21 (1965)

Dobson, M., Tattersfield, A.E., Adler, M.W. and McNicol, M.W. Attitudes and long-term adjustment of patients surviving cardiac arrest. *Brit. Med. J., 3*, 207–12 (1971)

Doehrman, S.R. Psycho-social aspects of recovery from coronary heart disease: a review. *Soc. Sci. Med., 11*, 199–218 (1977)

Dohm, G.L., Huston, R.L., Askew, H.N. & Weiser, P.C. Effects of exercise on activity of heart and muscle mitochondria. *Amer. J. Physiol., 223*, 783–7 (1972)

Doll, E., Keul, J. & Maiwald, C. Oxygen tension and acid-base equilibria in venous blood of working muscle. *Amer. J. Physiol., 215*, 23–9 (1968)

Dorossiev, D., Paskova, V. & Zachariev, Z. Psychological problems of cardiac rehabilitation. In: *Psychological Approach to the Rehabilitation of Coronary Patients*, ed. U. Stocksmeier (Springer Verlag, Berlin, 1976) pp. 26–31

Dosch, M., Ozburn, D. & Stephens, M. Motivating the female to exercise. In: *Adult Fitness and Cardiac Rehabilitation*, ed. P.K. Wilson (University Park Press, Baltimore, Md., 1975) pp. 275–9

Dotson, C.O. Analysis of change. *Ex. Sports. Sci. Rev., 1*, 393–420 (1973)

Douglas, F.G.V. & Becklake, M.R. Effect of seasonal training on maximal cardiac output. *J. Appl. Physiol., 25*, 600–5 (1968)

Doyle, J.T. & Kinch, S.H. The prognosis of an abnormal electrocardiographic stress test. *Circulation 41*, 545–53 (1970)

Draper, H.H. A review of recent nutritional research in the arctic. In: *Circumpolar Health*, ed. R.J. Shephard & S. Itoh (University of Toronto Press, Toronto, 1976) pp. 120–9

Drinkwater, B. & Horvath, S.M. Detraining effects on young women. *Med. Sci. Sports 4*, 91–5 (1972)

Dublin, L.I. Longevity of college athletes. *Harper's Monthly Mag.*, *157*, 229–38 (1928)

Duncan, W.R., Ross, W.D. & Banister, E.W. Heart rate monitoring as a guide to the intensity of an exercise programme. *Brit. Col. Med. J.*, *10* (8), 219–20 (1968)

Dunkman, W.B., Perloff, J.K., Kastor, J.A. *et al.* Medical perspectives in coronary artery surgery — a caveat. *Ann. Intern. Med.*, *81*, 817–37 (1974)

Durnin, J.V.G. & Passmore, R. *Energy, Work and Leisure* (Heinemann, London, 1967)

Durrer, D., Janse, M.J. & Lie, K.I. Electrophysiological mechanisms for sudden coronary death. In: *Sudden Coronary Death*, ed. V. Manninen & P.I. Halonen (Karger, Basel, 1978)

Eckstein, R.W. Effect of exercise and coronary artery narrowing on coronary collateral circulation. *Circ. Res.*, *5*, 230–5 (1957)

Eden, D., Shiron, A., Kellerman, J.J., *et al.* Stress, anxiety, and coronary risk in a supportive society. In: *Stress and Anxiety*, ed. C.D. Spielberger & I.G. Sarason (Hemisphere Publishing, New York, 1977)

Edholm, O.G. The changing pattern of human activity. *Ergonomics 13*, 625–43 (1970)

Edholm, O.G., Humphrey, S., Lourie, J.A., *et al.* Energy expenditure and climatic exposure of Yemenite and Kurdish Jews in Israel. *Philos. Trans. R. Soc. Lond. (Biol. Sci.) 266B*, 127–40 (1973)

Edington, D.W., Cosmas, A.C. & McCaffery, W.B. Exercise and longevity: evidence for a threshold age. *J. Gerontol.*, *27*, 341–3 (1972)

Edler, E.I. The diagnostic use of ultrasound in heart disease. In: *Ultrasonic Energy*, ed. E. Kelly (Univ. of Illinois Press, Urbana, Ill., 1965)

Ekblom, B., Åstrand, P.O., Saltin, B., Stenberg, J. & Wallstrom, B. Effect of training on circulatory response to exercise. *J. Appl. Physiol.*, *24*, 518–28 (1968)

Elder, H.P. The effects of training on middle-aged men. In: *Exercise and Fitness*, ed. D.P. Franks (Athletic Institute, Chicago, 1969)

Elgrishi, I., Ducimetière, P. & Richard, J.L. Reproducibility of analysis of the electrocardiogram in epidemiology using the 'Minnesota Code'. *Brit. J. Prev. Soc. Med.*, *24*, 197–200 (1970)

Eliot, R.S. *Stress and the Heart* (Futura Publishing, Mount Kisko,

N.Y., 1974)

Eliot, R.S. & Miles, R.R. Advising the cardiac patient about sexual intercourse. *Med. Asp. Hum. Sex., 9*, 49–50 (1975)

Ellestad, M.H. *Stress Testing. Principles and Practice* (F.A. Davis, Philadelphia, 1975)

Ellestad, M., Allen, W., Wan, M.K.C. & Kemp, G.L. Maximal treadmill stress testing for cardiovascular evaluation. *Circulation 39*, 517–22 (1969)

Ellestad, M.H. & Wan, M.K.C. Predictive implications of stress testing: follow-up of 2,700 subjects after maximum treadmill stress testing. *Circulation 51*, 363–9 (1975)

Elmfeldt, D., Wilhelmsson, C., Vedin, A., Tibblin, G. & Wilhelmsen, L. Characteristics of representative male survivors of myocardial infarction compared with representative population samples. *Acta Med. Scand., 199*, 387–98 (1976)

Enig, M.G. The problem of trans-fatty acids in modern diet. In: *Topics in Ischaemic Heart Disease — An International Symposium* (Toronto Rehabilitation Centre, Toronto, 1979)

Enos, W.F., Bayer, J.C. & Holmes, R.H. Pathogenesis of coronary disease in American soldiers killed in Korea. *J. Amer. Med. Assoc., 158*, 912–14 (1955)

Enos, W.F., Holmes, R.H. & Bayer, J.C. Coronary artery sclerosis in American soldiers killed during the Korean war. *J. Amer. Med. Assoc., 152*, 1090–3 (1953)

Epstein, F.H. Glucose intolerance and coronary heart disease incidence — recent observations. In: *Lipid Metabolism, Obesity and Diabetes Mellitus: Impact upon Atherosclerosis*, ed. H. Greten, R. Levine, E.F. Pfeiffer & A.E. Renold (G. Thieme, Stuttgart, 1974) pp. 174–9

Epstein, L., Miller, G.J., Stitt, F.W. & Morris, J.N. Vigorous exercise in leisure time, coronary risk factors, and resting electrocardiogram in middle-aged male civil servants. *Brit. Heart J., 38*, 403–9 (1976)

Epstein, S.E., Redwood, D.R., Goldstein, R.E., Beiser, G.D., Rosing, D.R., Glancy, D.L., Reis, R.L. & Stinson, E.B. Angina pectoris — pathophysiology, evaluation and treatment. *Ann. Int. Med., 75*, 263–96 (1971)

Erb, B. *Proceedings, National Conference on Exercise in Prevention, Evaluation, and Treatment of Heart Disease, S. Carol. Med. Assoc. J., 65* suppl. I, 73–85 (1969)

Ericsson, B. Haeger, K. & Lindell, S. Maximal flow capacity before and after training. In: *Coronary Heart Disease and Physical Fitness*, ed. O.A. Lassen & R.O. Malborg (University Park Press, Baltimore, 1971) pp. 155–7

Estes, E.H. Electrocardiography and vectorcardiography. In: *The Heart*, 3rd edn, ed. J.W. Hurst, R.B. Logue, R.C. Schlant & N.K. Wenger (McGraw Hill, New York, 1974) pp. 267–85

Fabian, J., Stolz, I., Janota, M., *et al*. Reproducibility of exercise tests in patients with symptomatic ischaemic heart disease. *Brit. Heart. J., 37*, 785–9 (1975)

Fardy, P.S. Effects of soccer training and detraining upon selected cardiac and metabolic measures. *Res. Quart., 40*, 502–8 (1969)

Fardy, P.S. & Ilmarinen, J. Evaluating the effects and feasibility of an at work stairclimbing intervention program for men. *Med. Sci. Sports 7*, 91–3 (1975)

Fardy, P., Maresh, C.M. & Abbott, R.D. A comparison of myocardial function in former athletes and non-athletes. *Med. Sci. Sports 8*, 26–30 (1976)

Feigenbaum, H. Use of echocardiography to evaluate cardiac performance. In: *Cardiac Mechanics: Physiological, Clinical and Mathematical Considerations*, ed. I. Mirsky, D. Ghista & H. Sandler (Wiley, New York, 1974) pp. 203–31

Feil, H. & Siegel, M.L. Electrocardiographic changes during attacks of angina pectoris. *Amer. J. Med. Sci., 175*, 255–60 (1928)

Feldman, S.A., Ho, K.J., Lewis, L.A., Mikkelson, B. & Taylor, C.B. Lipid and cholesterol metabolism in Alaskan Arctic Eskimos. *Arch. Pathol., 94*, 43–58 (1972)

Ferguson, R.J., Choquette, G., Chanioto, L., Jankowski, L.W. & Huot, E. Role de la marche dans la réadaptation des patients coronariens. *Arch. Mal. Coeur 66* (8), 995–1001 (1973)

Ferguson, R.J., Gauthier, P., Coté, P. & Bourassa, M.G. Coronary hemodynamics during upright exercise in patients with angina pectoris. *Circulation 52*, suppl. II, 115 (abstr.) (1975)

Ferguson, R.J., Petitclerc, R., Choquette, G., *et al*. Effect of physical training on treadmill exercise capacity, collateral circulation and progression of coronary disease. *Amer. J. Cardiol., 34*, 764–9 (1974)

Ferrer, M.I. The sick sinus syndrome. *Circulation 47*, 635–41 (1973)

Finkle, A.L. Sexual potency in aging males. Part I. Frequency of coitus among clinical patients. *J. Amer. Med. Assoc., 170*, 1391–

3 (1959)

Fishbein, M. & Ajzen, J. *Belief, Attitude, Intention and Behavior* (Addison Wesley, Reading, Mass., 1975)

Fisher, F.D. & Tyroler, H.A. Relationship between ventricular premature contractions in routine electrocardiograms and subsequent death from coronary heart disease. *Circulation 47*, 712–19 (1963)

Fisher, S. Impact of physical disability on vocational activity: work status following myocardial infarction. *Scand. J. Rehabil. Med., 3*, 65–70 (1970a)

Fisher, S. International survey on the psychological aspects of cardiac rehabilitation. *Scand. J. Rehab. Med., 2–3*, 71–7 (1970b)

Fitzhugh, G. & Hamilton, B.E. Coronary occlusion and fatal angina pectoris. *J. Amer. Med. Assoc., 100*, 475–80 (1933)

Flaherty, J.T., Ferans, V.J., Pierce, J.E., Carew, T.E. & Fry, D.L. Localizing factors in experimental atherosclerosis. In: *Atherosclerosis and Coronary Heart Disease*, ed. W. Likoff, B.L. Segal & W. Insull (Grune & Stratton, New York, 1972) pp. 40–83

Fleischmann, P. & Kellermann, J.J. Persistent irregular tachycardia in a successful athlete without impairment of performance. *Israeli J. Med. Sci., 5*, 950–2 (1969)

Fletcher, C.M. Chronic bronchitis. Its prevalence, nature and pathogenesis. *Amer. Rev. Resp. Dis., 80*, 483–94 (1959)

Fletcher, G.F. & Cantwell, J.D. *Exercise in the Management of Coronary Heart Disease. A Guide for the Practicing Physician* (C.C. Thomas, Springfield, Ill., 1971)

Fletcher, G.F. & Cantwell, J.D. *Exercise and Coronary Heart Disease. Role in Prevention, Diagnosis, Treatment* (C.C. Thomas, Springfield, Ill., 1974)

Florey, Du V.C., Melia, R.J.W. & Darby, S.C. Changing mortality from ischaemic heart disease in Great Britain 1966–76. *Brit. Med. J., 1*, 635–7 (1978)

Fogelman, M., Abbasi, A.S., Pearce, M.L. & Kattus, A.A. Echocardiographic study of the abnormal motion of the posterior left ventricular wall during angina pectoris. *Circulation 46*, 905–13 (1972)

Ford, A.B. & Hellerstein, H.K. Energy cost of the Master two-step test. *J. Amer. Med. Assoc., 164*, 1868–74 (1957)

Forrester, J.S., Diamond, G.A. & Swan, H.J.C. Correlation classification of clinical and hemodynamic function after acute myocardial infarction. *Amer. J. Cardiol., 39*, 137–45 (1977)

Foster, G.L. & Reeves, T.J. Haemodynamic response to exercise in clinically normal middle-aged men and those with angina pectoris. *J. Clin. Invest., 43*, 1758–68 (1964)

Fox, S.M. Heart disease and rehabilitation: scope of the problem. In: *Heart Disease and Rehabilitation*, ed. M.L. Pollock & D.H. Schmidt. (Houghton Mifflin, Boston, 1979) pp. 3–12

Fox, S.M. & Haskell, W.L. Population studies. *Canad. Med. Assoc. J., 96*, 808–11 (1967)

Fox, S.M. & Haskell, W.L. Physical activity and the prevention of coronary heart disease. *Bull. N.Y. Acad. Sci., 44*, 950–65 (1968a)

Fox, S.M. & Haskell, W.L. The exercise stress test: needs for standardisation. Presented at the Fourth Asian/Pacific Congress of Cardiology, Tel Aviv. Cited by S. Fox, Exercise and stress testing workshop report. National Conference on Exercise in the Prevention, in the Evaluation and in the Treatment of Heart Disease. *J. S. Carol. Med. Assoc., 65*, suppl. 1, 77 (1968b)

Fox, S.M., Naughton, J.P. & Gorman, P.A. Physical activity and cardiovascular health. *Mod. Concepts Cardiovasc. Dis., 41*, 17–30 (1972)

Fox, S.M. Skinner, J.S. Physical activity and cardiovascular health. *Amer. J. Cardiol., 14*, 731–46 (1964)

Framingham Heart Study. *Habits and Coronary Heart Disease*. US National Heart Institute Public Health Service Publication 1515 (US Government Printing Office, Washington, D.C., 1966) pp. 1–13

Franks, B.D. & Cureton, T.K. Effects of training on time components of the left ventricle. *J. Sports. Med. Phys. Fitness 9*, 80–8 (1969)

Fredrickson, D.S. Function and structure of plasma lipoproteins. In: *Lipid Metabolism, Obesity and Diabetes Mellitus: Impact upon Atherosclerosis*, ed. H. Greten, R. Levine, E.F. Pfeiffer & A.E. Renold (G. Thieme, Stuttgart, 1974)

French, A.J. & Dock, W. Fatal coronary arteriosclerosis in young soldiers. *J. Amer. Med. Assoc., 124*, 1233–7 (1944)

French, J.R.P. & Caplan, R.D. *Psychosocial Factors in Coronary Heart Disease* (US National Air & Space Administration, 1970)

Frick, M.H. The response of heart volume and ventricular functions to physical training in coronary heart disease. *Mal. Cardiovasc., 10*, 331–9 (1969)

Frick, M.H., Harjola, P.T. & Valle, M. The prognostic impact of coronary by-pass surgery. In:' *Internal Medicine: 1976 Topics* (Karger, Basel, 1976) pp. 287–92

Frick, M.H., Harjola, P.T. & Valle, M. Influence of coronary bypass surgery on sudden death in chronic artery disease. In: *Sudden Coronary Death*, ed. V. Manninen & P.I. Halonen (Karger, Basel, 1978) pp. 229–31

Frick, M.H. & Katila, M. Hemodynamic consequences of physical training after myocardial infarction. *Circulation 37*, 192–202 (1968)

Frick, M.H., Katila, M. & Sjörgen, A.L. Cardiac function and physical training after myocardial infarction. In: *Coronary Heart Disease and Physical Fitness*, ed. O.A. Larsen & R.O. Malmborg (University Park Press, Baltimore, Md., 1971) pp. 44–7

Frick, M.H., Konttinen, A. & Sarajas, S.H.S. Effects of physical training on circulation at rest and during exercise. *Amer. J. Cardiol., 12*, 142–7 (1963)

Fried, T. & Shephard, R.J. Deterioration and restoration of physical fitness after training. *Canad. Med. Assoc. J., 100*, 831–7 (1969)

Friedberg, C.K. *Diseases of the Heart* (W.B. Saunders, Philadelphia, 1966)

Friedberg, C.K. & Unger, A.H. The natural history of coronary heart disease. In: *Atherosclerotic Vascular Disease*, ed. A.N. Brest & G.H. Moyer (Appleton Century Crofts, New York, 1967) pp. 300–8

Friedman, E.H. Type A or B behavior. *J. Amer. Med. Assoc., 228*, 1369 (1974)

Friedman, E.H. & Hellerstein, H.K. Influence of psychosocial factors on coronary risk and adaptation to a physical fitness evaluation programme. In: *Exercise Testing and Exercise Training in Coronary Heart Disease*, ed. J.P. Naughton & H.K. Hellerstein (Academic Press, New York, 1973)

Friedman, M., Manwaring, J.H., Rosenman, R.H., Donion, G. & Ortega, P. Instantaneous and sudden deaths. *J. Amer. Med. Assoc., 225*, 1319–28 (1973)

Friedman, M. & Rosenman, R.H. Type A behavior and your heart (Fawcett, Greenwich, Conn., 1974)

Friedman, R.J., More, S., Singal., D.P. & Gent, M. Regression of injury-induced atheromatous lesions in rabbits. *Arch. Pathol.*

Lab. Med., *100*, 189–95 (1976)

Friend, B., Page, L. & Marston, R. Food consumption patterns in the United States: 1909–13 to 1976. In: *Nutrition, Lipids and Coronary Heart Disease*, ed. R. Levy, B. Rifkind, B. Dennis & N. Ernst (Raven Press, New York, 1979) pp. 489–522

Froehlicher, V.F. Animal studies of the effect of chronic exercise on the heart and atherosclerosis. A review. *Amer. Heart. J.*, *84*, 496–506 (1972)

Froehlicher, V.F. *The Effect of Chronic Exercise on the Heart and on Coronary Atherosclerotic Heart Disease. A Literature Survey.* US Airforce, Brooks Air Force Base Report SAM-TR-76-69 (1976)

Froehlicher, V.F. & Oberman, A. Analysis of epidemiologic studies of physical inactivity as risk factor for coronary artery disease. *Progr. Cardiovasc. Dis.*, *15*, 41–65 (1972)

Funderburk, C.F., Hipskind, S.G., Welton, R.C. & Lind, A.R. Development of and recovery from fatigue induced by static effort at various tensions. *J. Appl. Physiol.*, *37*, 392–6 (1974)

Galbo, H., Hoist, J.J. & Christensen, N.J. Glucagon and plasma catecholamine responses to graded and prolonged exercise in man. *J. Appl. Physiol.*, *38*, 70–6 (1975)

Ganz, W., Cribier, A., Chew, C., Kanmatsuse, K., Tzivoni, D., Nair, R. & Swan, H.J.C. Effect of nitroglycerin on the acutely ischemic myocardium. In: *Coronary Heart Disease*, ed. M. Kaltenbach, P. Lichtlen, R. Balcon & W.D. Bussmann (G. Thieme, Stuttgart, 1978) pp. 256–61

Gardner, G.W., Danks, D.L. & Scharfstein, L. Use of carotid pulse for heart rate monitoring. *Med. Sci. Sports 11* (1), 111 (abstr.) (1979)

Gauthier, P., Ferguson, R.J., Chaniotis, L., Avon, G. & Choquette, G. Evaluation hémodynamique en position couchée et assise avant et après l'entrainement chez le coronarien. In: *Abstracts from First Canadian Congress of Sport and Physical Activity* (Montreal, 1973) p. 13

Geddes, L.A. & Baker, L.E. The relationship between input impedance and electrode area in recording the ECG. *Med. Biol. Eng.*, *4*, 439–50 (1966)

Geer, J.C. & McGill, H.C. The evolution of the fatty streak. In: *Atherosclerotic Vascular Disease*, ed. A.N. Brest & J.H. Moyer (Appleton Century Crofts, New York, 1967) pp. 8–22

Geis, W.P., Ardekani, R.G., Rahimtoola, S.H., *et al.* Delineation

of improved ventricular wall motion after coronary
revascularization. In: *Coronary Artery Surgery*, ed. J.C.
Norman. (Appleton Century Crofts, New York, 1975) pp.
846–55

Gelfand, D. Experience at the cardiac work classification unit of the
heart association of southeastern Pennsylvania (Philadelphia).
In: *Work and the Heart*, ed. F.F. Rosenbaum & E.L. Belknap
(P.B. Hoeber, New York, 1959) pp. 322–9

Gentry, W.D. Psychosocial concerns and benefits in cardiac
rehabilitation. In: *Heart Disease and Rehabilitation*, ed. M.L.
Pollock & D.H. Schmidt (Houghton Mifflin, Boston, 1979)

Georgopoulos, A.J., Proudfit, W.L. & Page, I.H. Effect of exercise
on electrocardiograms of patients with low serum potassium.
Circulation 23, 567–72 (1961)

Gerstenblith, G., Lakatta, E.G. & Weisfeldt, M.L. Age changes in
myocardial function and exercise response. *Progr. Cardiovasc.
Dis., 19*, 1–21 (1976)

Gertler, M.M. & White, P.D. *Coronary Artery Disease in Young
Adults* (Harvard University Printer, Cambridge, Mass., 1954)

Gertler, M.M. & White, P.D. *Coronary Heart Disease. A 25-year
Study in Retrospect* (Medical Economics, Oradell, N.J., 1976)

Gettes, L.S. Electrophysiologic basis of arrhythmias and acute
myocardial ischemia. In: *Modern trends in Cardiology*, vol. 3, ed.
M.F. Olives (Butterworths, London, 1975) pp. 218–46

Gillespie, J.A. Future place of lumbar sympathectomy in
obliterative vascular disease of lower limbs. *Brit. Med. J.* (ii),
1640–42 (1960)

Gilson, J.C. & Hugh-Jones, P. *Lung Function in Coalworkers'
Pneumoconiosis*. Special Report Series 290 (UK Medical
Research Council, 1955) pp. 1–226

Glaser, E.M. *The Physiological Basis of Habituation* (Oxford
University Press, London, 1966) pp. 1–102

Glendy, R.E., Levine, S.A. & White, P.D. Coronary disease in
youth. Comparison of 100 patients under 40 with 300 persons
past 80. *JAMA, 109*, 1775–81 (1937)

Gluckman, M. Sport and conflict. In: *Sport in the Modern World —
Chances and Problems*, ed. O. Grupe, D. Kurz & J.M. Teipel
(Springer Verlag, New York, 1973) pp. 48–54

Godin, G. & Shephard, R.J. Activity patterns of the Canadian
Eskimo. In: *Polar Human Biology*, ed. O.G. Edholm & E.K.E.
Gunderson (Heineman, Cambridge, 1973a)

Godin, G. & Shephard, R.J. Body weight and the energy cost of activity. *Arch. Env. Health 27*, 289–93 (1973b)

Goldbarg, A.N. The effects of pharmacological agents on human performance. In: *Exercise Testing and Exercise Training in Coronary Heart Disease*, ed. J.P. Naughton, H.K. Hellerstein & I.C. Mohler (Academic Press, New York, 1973)

Goldbarg, A.N., Ekblom,. B. & Åstrand, P.O. Effects of blocking the autonomic nervous system during exercise. *Circulation 44*, suppl. II, 118 (abstr.) (1971)

Goldberg, D.I. & Shephard, R.J. Stroke volume during recovery from upright bicycle exercise. *J. Appl. Physiol., 48*, 833–7 (1980)

Goldhammer, S. & Schert, D. Elektrokardiographische untersuchungen bei Kranken mit Angina Pectoris ('ambulatorischer' Typus). *Z. f. Klin. Med., 122*, 134–51 (1932)

Goldschlager, N., Cake, D. & Cohn, K. Exercise-induced ventricular arrhythmias in patients with coronary artery disease. Their relation to angiographic findings. *Amer. J. Cardiol., 31*, 434–40 (1973)

Goldstein, R.E. & Epstein, S.E. The use of indirect indices of myocardial oxygen consumption in evaluating angina pectoris. *Chest 63*, 302–6 (1973)

Goldstein, R.E., Rosing, D.R., Redwood, D.R., Beiser, G.D. & Epstein, S.E. Clinical and circulatory effects of isosorbide dinitrate. Comparisons with nitroglycerine. *Circulation 43*, 629–40 (1971)

Goldwater, L.J. & Weiss, N.M. Study of workmen's compensation and heart disease in New York City. *New York J. Med., 51*, 2754–8 (1951)

Gollnick, P. & Hermansen, L. Biochemical adaptations to exercise anaerobic metabolism. *Exercise Sport Sci. Rev., 1*, 1–43 (1973)

Gollnick, P.D. & Ianuzzo, C.D. Hormonal deficiencies and the metabolic adaptations of rats to training. *Amer. J. Physiol., 223*, 278–82 (1972)

Goode, R.C., Firstbrook, J. & Shephard, R.J. Effects of exercise and a cholesterol-free diet on human serum lipids. *Canad. J. Physiol. Pharm., 44*, 575–80 (1966)

Gordon, T., Castelli, W.P., Hjortland, M.C., Kannel, W.B. & Dawber. T.R. High density lipoprotein as a protective factor against coronary heart disease. The Framingham study. *Amer. J. Med., 62*, 707–14 (1977)

Gordon, T., Sorlie, P. & McNamara, P. Physical activity and

coronary vulnerability. The Framingham study. *Cardiol. Digest* 6, 28 (1971)

Gorlin, R. Anginal pain without atherosclerosis. *JAMA, 201* (9), 27–8 (1967)

Gorlin, R. Myocardial blood flow and metabolism in coronary disease. In: *Coronary Heart Disease and Physical Fitness*, ed. O.A. Larsen & R.O. Malmborg (University Park Press, Baltimore, 1971) pp. 97–101

Gorlin, R. *Coronary Artery Disease* (W.B. Saunders, Philadelphia, 1976)

Gottheiner, V. Herzinfarkt und sport. In: *Proceedings of Sports Medical Symposium of Seventeenth Olympic Games* (Rome, 1960)

Gottheiner, V. Long range strenuous sports training for cardiac reconditioning and rehabilitation. *Amer. J. Cardiol., 22*, 426–35 (1968)

Gould, K.L. & Lipscomb, K. Effects of coronary stenoses on coronary flow reserve and resistance. *Amer. J. Cardiol., 34*, 48–55 (1974)

Graievskaia, N.D. & Markov, L.N. Post-mortem anatomical and histological findings in sudden death in sport. *Brit. J. Sports Med., 7*, 159–61 (1973)

Granath, A., Johnson, B. & Strandell, T. Circulation in healthy old men studied by right heart catheterization at rest during exercise in supine and sitting position. *Acta Med. Scand., 1976*, 425–46 (1964)

Greene, D.G, Klocke, F.J., Schimert, G.L., Bunnell, I.L., Wittemberg, S.M. & Lajos, T. Evaluation of venous bypass grafts from aorta to coronary artery by inert gas desaturation and direct flowmeter techniques. *J. Clin. Invest., 51*, 191–6 (1972)

Greene, W.A. Psychological factors and reticuloendothelial disease. *Psychosom. Med., 16*, 220–30 (1954)

Greer, W.E.R. Experience in selective placement and follow-up on cardiacs. In: *Work and the Heart*, ed. F.F. Rosenbaum & E.L. Belknap (P.B. Hoeber, New York, 1959) pp. 383–6

Gregg, D.E. & Fisher, L.C. Blood supply to the heart. In: *Handbook of Physiology. Section 2. Circulation*, vol. II (American Physiological Society, Washington, D.C., 1963) pp. 1517–84

Gregg, D.E., Longino, F.H., Green, P.A. & Czerwonka, L.J. A comparison of coronary flow determined by the nitrous oxide method and by a direct method using the rotameter. *Circulation* *3*, 89–94 (1951)

Grendahl, H. Early death in acute myocardial infarction. A retrospective study of 302 cases. *Acta Med. Scand., 181*, 655–62 (1967)

Grimby, G., Nilsson, N.J. & Saltin, B. Cardiac output during sub-maximal and maximal exercise in active middle-aged athletes. *J. Appl. Physiol., 21*, 1150–6 (1966)

Groden, B.M. Return to work after myocardial infarction. *Scott. Med. J., 12*, 297–301 (1967)

Groden, B.M. & Brown, R.I.F. Differential psychological effects of early and late mobilization after myocardial infarction. *Scand. J. Rehab. Med., 2–3*, 60–4 (1970)

Grodsky, G.M. & Benoit, F. Effect of massive weight reduction on insulin secretion in obese subjects. *International Diabetes Symposium* (Stockholm, 1967)

Groen, J.J., Tijong, B.K., Willebrandt, A.F. & Kamminga, C.J. Influence of nutrition, individuality and different forms of stress on blood cholesterol. Results of an experiment of 9 months duration in 60 normal volunters. In: *Proceedings of an International Congress of Dieticians* (1959) p. 19

Grögler, F., Beddermann, C., Frank, G. & Borst, H.G. Myocardial contraction and hemodynamics before, during and after coronary occlusion in the pig. In: *Coronary Heart Disease*, ed. M. Kaltenbach, P. Lichtlen & G.C. Friesinger (G. Thieme, Stuttgart, 1973) pp. 162–6

Grollman, A. The determination of cardiac output of man by the use of acetylene. *Amer. J. Physiol., 88*, 432–45 (1929)

Groom, D. Cardiovascular observations on Tarahumara Indian runners — the modern Spartans. *Amer. Heart J., 81*, 304–14 (1971)

Gueli, D. & Shephard, R.J. Pedal frequency in bicycle ergometry. *Canad. J. Appl. Sports Sci., 1*, 137–42 (1976)

Guinn, G.A. & Mathur, V.S. Surgical versus medical treatment of stable angina pectoris: prospective randomized study with 1- to 4-year follow up. *Ann. Thor. Surg., 22*, 524–7 (1976)

Gwinup, G. Effect of exercise alone on the weight of obese women. *Arch. Int. Med., 135*, 676–80 (1975)

Hacker, R.W. Resection of aneurysms, akinetic areas and infarctions in coronary heart disease. In: *Coronary Heart Disease*, ed. M. Kaltenbach, P. Lichtlen & G.C. Friesinger (G.

Thieme, Stuttgart, 1973) pp. 207–16

Hackett, T.P. & Cassem, N.H. Psychological adaptation to convalescence in myocardial infarction patients. In: *Exercise Testing and Exercise Training in Coronary Heart Disease*, ed. J.P. Naughton & H.K. Hellerstein (Academic Press, New York, 1973) pp. 253–62

Hakkila, J. Studies of the myocardial capillary concentration in cardiac hypertrophy due to training. *Ann. Med. Exp. Biol. Fenn., 33*, suppl. 10, 1–82 (1955)

Halliday, M. & Anderson, T.W. The sex differential in ischaemic heart disease: trends by social class 1931 to 1971. *Epidemiol. & Comm. Health 33*, 74–7 (1979)

Halter, J., Moccetti, T., Gattiker, K. & Lichtlen, P. Left ventricular dynamics before and after aneurysmectomy. In: *Coronary Heart Disease*, ed. M. Kaltenbach, P. Lichtlen & G.C. Friesinger (G. Thieme, Stuttgart, 1973) pp. 228–38

Hames, C. 'Most likely to succeed' as a candidate for a coronary attack. In: *New Horizons in Cardiovasculuar Practice*, ed. H.I. Russek (University Park Press, Baltimore, Md., 1975)

Hamilton, J.B. The role of testicular secretions as indicated by the effects of castration in men and by studies of pathological conditions and the short life-span associated with maleness. *Recent Prog. in Hormone Res., 3*, 257–322 (1948)

Hamilton, M.J. & Ferguson, J.H. Effects of exercise and cold acclimation on the ventricular and skeletal muscles of white mice (*Mus. musculus*). I. Succinic dehydrogenase activity. *Comp. Biochem. Physiol., A43*, 815–24 (1972)

Hamilton, W.F. Measurement of cardiac output. In: *Handbook of Physiology*. Section 2. *Circulation*, vol. I, ed. W.F. Hamilton (American Physiological Society, Washington, D.C., 1962) pp. 551–84

Hammermeister, K.E., DeRouen, T.A., Murray, J.A., *et al*. Effect of aortocoronary saphenous vein by-pass grafting on death and sudden death: comparison of non-randomized medically and surgically treated cohorts with comparable coronary disease and left ventricular function. *Amer. J. Cardiol., 39*, 925–34 (1977)

Hammermeister, K.E., Kennedy, J.W., Hamilton, G.W., *et al*. Aortocoronary saphenous vein bypass: failure of successful grafting to improve resting left ventricular function in chronic angina. *New Engl. J. Med., 290*, 196–92 (1974)

Hammett, V.B.O. Recognition and management of abnormal

psychological reactions to coronary heart disease. In: *Coronary Heart Disease*, ed. W. Likoff & J.H. Moyer (Grune & Stratton, New York, 1963) pp. 459–63

Hammond, E.C. Smoking in relation to mortality and morbidity. Findings in first thirty-four months of follow-up in a prospective study started in 1959. *J. Nat. Cancer Inst., 32*, 1161–88 (1964)

Hampton, J.R. & Nicholas, C. Randomized trial of a mobile coronary care unit for emergency calls. *Brit. Med. J.* (i), 1118–21 (1978)

Hanne-Paparo, N., Drory, Y., Schoenfeld, Y., Shapira, Y. & Kellermann, J.J. Common ECG changes in athletes. *Cardiology 61*, 267–78 (1976)

Hanson, J.S. & Nedde, W.H. Preliminary observations on physical training for hypertensive males. *Circ. Research 36/37*, suppl. I, 49–53 (1970)

Hanson, J.S., Tabakin, B.S. & Levy, A.M. Comparative exercise cardio-respiratory performance of normal men in the third, fourth and fifth decades of life. *Circulation 37*, 345–60 (1968)

Harken, D.E. Changing concepts in mechanical assistance and surgical excision. In: *Changing Concepts in Cardiovascular Disease*, ed. H.I. Russek & B.L. Zohman (Williams & Wilkins, Baltimore, 1972) pp. 281–7

Harris, D.V. Physical activity history and attitudes of middle-aged men. *Med. Sci. Sports 2*, 203–8 (1970)

Harris, W.S. Systolic time intervals in the non-invasive assessment of left ventricular performance in man. In: *Cardiac Mechanics: Physiological, Clinical and Mathematical Considerations*, ed. I. Mirsky, D. Ghista & H. Sandler (Wiley, New York, 1974) pp. 233–92

Harrison, T.R. & Reeves, T.J. *Principles and Problems of Ischemic Heart Disease* (Year Book Publishers, Chicago, 1968)

Hartley, L.H. Growth hormone and catecholamine response to exercise in relation to physical training. *Med. Sci. Sports 7*, 34–6 (1975)

Hartley, L.H., Grimby, G., Kilbom, A., Nilsson, N.J., Åstrand, I., Bjure, J., Ekblom, B. & Saltin, B. Physical training in sedentary middle-aged and older men. III. Cardiac output and gas exchange at submaximal and maximal exercise. *Scand. J. Clin. Lab. Invest., 24*, 335–44 (1969)

Hartley, L.H., Mason, J.W., Hogan, R.P., Jones, L.G., Kotchen, T.A., Mougey, E.H., Wherry, F.E., Pennington, L.L. &

Ricketts, P.T. Multiple hormone responses to graded exercise in relation to physical training. *J. Appl. Physiol.*, *33*, 602–6 (1972)

Hartley, L.H. & Saltin, B. Blood gas tensions and pH in brachial artery, femoral vein and brachial vein during maximal exercise. *Med. Sci. Sports 3*, 66–72 (1969)

Hartung, G.H. Physical activity and coronary heart disease risk: a review. *Amer. Corr. Therap. J.*, *31* (4), 110–15 (1977)

Hartung, G.H., Smith, L.C., Foreyt, J., Gorry, A.G. & Gotto, A.M. Plasma lipid levels in middle-aged runners, joggers, and sedentary men. *International Conference on Sports Cardiology* (Rome, 1978)

Harvey, R.M., Smith, W.M., Parker, J.O. & Ferrer, M.I. The response of the abnormal heart to exercise. *Circulation 26*, 341–62 (1962)

Haskell, W.L. Cardiovascular complications during exercise training of cardiac patients. *Circulation 57*, 920–4 (1978)

Haskell, W.L. Mechanisms by which physical activity may enhance the clinical status of cardiac patients. In: *Heart Disease and Rehabilitation*, ed. M.L. Pollock & D.H. Schmidt (Houghton Mifflin, Boston, Mass., 1979) pp. 276–96

Haskell, W.L. & Fox, S.N. Physical activity in the prevention and therapy of cardiovascular disease. In: *Science and Medicine of Exercise and Sport*, 2nd edn, ed. W.R. Johnson & E.R. Burkirk (Harper & Row, New York, 1974) pp. 455–68

Hatch, T. & Cook, K.M. Partitional respirometry. *AMA Arch. Industr. Health 11*, 142–58 (1955)

Haust, M.D. Injury and repair in the pathogenesis of atherosclerotic lesions. In: *Atherosclerosis*, ed. R.J. Jones (Springer Verlag, Berlin, 1970) pp. 12–20

Heberden, W. Some account of a disorder of the breast. *Med. Trans. Roy. Coll. Phys.*, *2*, 59 (1772)

Hedley, O.F. Analysis of 5,116 deaths reported as due to coronary occlusion in Philadelphia. *US Weekly Public Health Rep.*, *54*, 972 (1959)

Hedlund, S. & Porjé, J.B. Cirkulationstörningar hos äldre. Synpunkter på fysiologi och fysisk träning som terapiform. *Svenska Läk-Tidn 61*, 2970–85 (1964)

Heintzen, P.H., Moldenhauer, K. & Lange, P.E. Three dimensional computerized contraction pattern analysis: description of methodology and its validation. *Europ. J. Cardiol.*, *1*, 229–39 (1974)

Heinzelmann, F. & Baggley, R. Response to physical activity programs and their effects on health behavior. *Publ. Health Rep.*, *85*, 905–11 (1970)

Helander, S. & Levander, M. Primary mortality and 5-year prognosis of cardiac infarction. Study which considers in particular how prognosis is affected by composition of materials as regards age and sex of patients and severity of infarction. *Acta Med. Scand.*, *163*, 289–304 (1959)

Helfant, R.H., deVilla, M.A. & Meister, S.G. Effect of sustained isometric handgrip exercise on left ventricular performance. *Circulation 44*, 982–93 (1971)

Heller, E.M. Four year practical experience with a graded exercise program for myocardial infarction patients. Paper presented to Ontario Medical Association Annual Meeting (Toronto, May, 1968)

Heller, E.M. A practical graded exercise program for post-coronary patients — five year review. *Modern Medicine of Canada 27* (7), 529–42 (1972)

Hellerstein, H.K. Active physical reconditioning of coronary patients. *Circulation 32*, suppl. II, 110 (abstr.) (1965)

Hellerstein, H.K. Exercise therapy in coronary disease. *Bull. N.Y. Acad. Med.*, *44*, 1208–47 (1968)

Hellerstein, H.K. Exercise therapy in coronary heart disease. In: *Ischaemic Heart Disease*, ed. J.H. De Haas *et al.* (Williams & Wilkins, Baltimore, 1970) pp. 406–29

Hellerstein, H.K. A misguided goal or unrealized objective? In: *Critical Evaluation of Cardiac Rehabilitation*, ed. J.J. Kellermann & H. Denolin (Karger, Basel, 1977) pp. 125–35

Hellerstein, H.K. Cardiac rehabilitation: a retrospective view. In: *Heart Disease and Rehabilitation*, ed. M.L. Pollock & D.H. Schmidt (Houghton-Mifflin, Boston, 1979) pp. 509–20

Hellerstein, H.K. & Friedman, E.H. Sexual activity and the post-coronary patient. *Arch. Int. Med.*, *125*, 987–99 (1970)

Hellerstein, H.K. & Friedman, E.H. Sexual activity and the post-coronary patient. *Med. Aspects Hum. Sex.*, *3*, 70 (1973)

Hellerstein, H.K., Hornsten, T.R., Goldberg, A., Burlando, A.G., Friedman, E.H., Hirsch, E.Z. & Marik, S. The influence of active conditioning upon subjects with coronary artery disease. Cardio-respiratory changes during training in 67 patients. *Canad. Med. Assoc. J.*, *96*, 758–9, 901–3 (1967)

Hellerstein, H.K. & Turrell, D.J. The mode of death in coronary artery disease. An electrocardiograophic and clinicopathological correlation. In: *Sudden Cardiac Death*, ed. B. Surawicz & E.E. Pellegrino (Grune & Stratton, New York, 1964)

Herman, M.V., Heinle, R.A., Klein, M.D. & Gorlin, R. Localized disorders in myocardial contraction: asynergy and its role in congestive heart failure. *N. Engl. J. Med., 277*, 222–32 (1967)

Hermansen, L. & Ekblom, B. Physical fitness of an arctic and a tropical population. In: *Physical Activity in Health and Disease*, ed. E. Evang & K.L. Andersen (Williams & Wilkins, Baltimore, 1966)

Hermansen, L. & Wachtlová, M. Capillary density of skeletal muscle in well-trained and untrained men. *J. Appl. Physiol., 30*, 860–3 (1971)

Herrick, J.B. Clinical features of sudden obstruction of the coronary arteries. *JAMA, 59*, 2015–20 (1912)

Hettinger, T. *Physiology of Strength* (C.C. Thomas, Springfield, Ill., 1961)

Hickey, N., Mulcahy, R., Bourke, G.J., Graham, I. & Wilson-Davis, K. Study of coronary risk factors related to physical activity in 15,171 men. *Brit. Med. J.* (3), 507–9 (1975)

Higgs, B.E., Clode, M. & Campbell, E.J.M. Changes in ventilation, gas exchange and circulation during exercise after recovery from myocardial infarction. *Lancet* (ii), 793–5 (1968)

Hill, A. Bradford. *Principles of Medical Statistics*, 9th edn. (University Press, New York, 1971)

Hill, J.D., Hampton, J.R. & Mitchell, J.R.A. A randomized trial of home versus hospital management for patients with suspected myocardial infarction. *Lancet* (i), 837–41 (1978)

Hinckle, L.E. An estimate of the effects of 'stress' on the incidence and prevalence of coronary heart disease in a large industrial population in the United States. *Thromb. Diath. Haemorrh., 51*, suppl., 15–65 (1972)

Hinckle, L.E., Carver, S.T. & Plakun, A. Slow heart rate and increased risk of cardiac death in middle-aged men. *Arch. Int. Med., 129*, 732–48 (1972)

Hinckle, L.E., Carver, S.T. & Stevens, M. The frequency of asymptomatic disturbances of cardiac rhythm and conduction in middle-aged men. *Amer. J. Cardiol., 24*, 629–50 (1969)

Hinckle, L.E, Whitney, L.A., Lehman, E.W., Dunn, J. & Benjamin, B. Occupation, education and coronary heart disease. *Science 161*, 238–46 (1968)

Hinckle, L.E. & Wolff, H.G. The role of emotional and environmental factors in essential hypertension. In: *The Pathology of Essential Hypertension*, ed. J.H. Cort, V. Fencl, Z. Hejl & J. Jirka (State Medical Publishing House, Prague, 1962)

Hinohara, S. Psychological aspects in rehabilitation of coronary heart disease. *Scand. J. Rehabil. Med., 2*, 53–9 (1970)

Hirai, M. Muscle blood flow measured by Xe^{133} clearance method and peripheral vascular diseases. Part I. Standard exercise method — with special reference to work load and volume injected. *Jap. Circ. J., 38*, 655–9 (1974)

Hirzel, H.O., Meier, W., Mehmel, H. & Krayenbühl, H.P. Left ventricular dynamics during acute ischemia in the dog. In: *Coronary Heart Disease*, ed. M. Kaltenbach, P. Lichtlen & G.C. Friesinger (G. Thieme, Stuttgart, 1973) pp. 156–61

Hiss, R.G. & Lamb, L.E. Electrocardiographic findings in 122,043 individuals. *Circulation 25*, 947–61 (1962)

Ho, K., Mikkelson, B., Lewis, L.A., Feldman, S.A. & Taylor, C.B. Alaskan Arctic eskimo: responses to a customary high fat diet. *Amer. J. Clin. Nutr., 25*, 737–45 (1972)

Ho, K.J., Taylor, C.B. & Biss, K. Overall control of sterol synthesis in animals and man. In: *Atherosclerosis. Proceedings of Second International Symposium*, ed. R.J. Jones (Springer-Verlag, New York, 1970)

Hoes, M., Binkhorst, R.A., Smeekes-Kuyl, A. & Vissurs, A.C. Measurement of forces exerted on a pedal crank during work on the bicycle ergometer at different loads. *Int. Z. Angew. Physiol., 26*, 33–42 (1968)

Hokanson, J.E. Psychophysiological evaluation of the catharsis hypothesis. In: *The Dynamics of Aggression*, ed. E.I. Megargee & J.E. Hokanson (Harper & Row, New York, 1970)

Holloszy, J.O. The epidemiology of coronary heart disease: national differences and the role of physical activity. *J. Amer. Geriatr. Soc., 11*, 718–25 (1963)

Holloszy, J.O. Biochemical adaptations to exercise: aerobic metabolism. *Ex. Sports Sci. Rev., 1*, 45–71 (1973)

Holloszy, J.O., Oscai, L.B., Molé, P.A., *et al.* Biochemical adaptations to endurance exercise in skeletal muscle. In: *Muscle Metabolism during Exercise*, ed. B. Pernow & B. Saltin (Plenum Press, New York, 1971)

Holmberg, S., Serzysko, W. & Varnauskas, E. Coronary circulation during heavy exercise in control subjects and patients with coronary artery disease. *Acta Med. Scand., 190*, 465–80 (1971)

Holmér, I. & Åstrand, P.O. Swimming training and maximal oxygen uptake. *J. Appl. Physiol., 33*, 510–13 (1972)

Holmes, T.H. & Rahe, R.H. The social readjustment scale. *J. Psychomat. Res., 11*, 213–18 (1967)

Holmgren, A. Cardiorespiratory determinants of cardiovascular fitness. In: *Proceedings of International Symposium on Physical Activity and Cardiovascular Health, Canad. Med. Assoc., J., 96*, 697–702 (1967)

Holmgren, A. & Strandell, J. Relationship between heart volume, total hemoglobin and physical working capacity in former athletes. *Acta Med. Scand., 163*, 149–60 (1959)

Honey, G.E. & Truelove, S.C. Prognostic factors in myocardial infarction — long-term prognosis. *Lancet* (i), 1209–12 (1957)

Horwitz, L.D., Atkins, J.M. & Leshin, S.J. Role of the Frank-Starling mechanism in exercise. *Circ. Res., 57*, 64–70 (1972)

Horwitz, L.D., Herman, M.V. & Gorlin, R. Clinical responses to nitroglycerin as a diagnostic test for coronary artery disease. *Amer. J. Cardiol., 29*, 149–53 (1972)

Howard, A.N. Recent advances in nutrition and atherosclerosis. In: *Atherosclerosis. Proceedings of Second International Symposium*, ed. R.J. Jones (Springer Verlag, Berlin, 1970)

Humphries, J.O., Kuller, L., Ross, R.S., *et al*. Natural history of ischemic heart disease in relation to arteriographic findings: a twelve year study of 224 patients. *Circulation 49*, 489–97 (1974)

Hunyor, S.N., Flynn, J.M. & Cochineas, C. Comparison of performance of various sphygmomanometers with intra-arterial blood pressure readings. *Brit. Med. J., 2*, 159–62 (1978)

Hurry, J.B. *Imhotep* (Oxford University Press, London, 1926)

Ilmarinen, J. & Fardy, P.S. Physical activity intevention for males with high risk of coronary heart disease: a three year follow-up. *Prev. Med., 6*, 416–25 (1977)

Ingraham, H.S. Public health and fitness — the outdoor life and other antidotes to enemies of fitness. In: *Guide to Fitness after Fifty*, ed. R.H. Harris & L.J. Frankel (Plenum Press, New York, 1977) pp. 39–44

Inman, W.H.W. & Vessey, M.P. Investigation of deaths from pulmonary coronary and cerebral thrombosis and embolism in women of child-bearing age. *Brit. Med. J.* (ii), 193–9 (1968)

Innes, J.A., Campbell, I.W., Campbell, C.J., Needle, A.L., &

Munroe, J.F. Long-term follow-up of therapeutic starvation. *Brit. Med. J.* (ii), 357–9 (1974)

Isacsson, S.O. Venous occlusion plethysmography in 55 year old men. *Acta Med. Scand., 537*, suppl., 1–62 (1972)

Ishiko, T. Aerobic capacity and external criteria of performance. *Canad. Med. Assoc. J., 96*, 746–9 (1967)

Izeki, T. Statistical observation on sudden deaths in sport. *Brit. J. Sports Med., 7*, 172–6 (1973)

Jackson, L.K., Simmons, R., Leinbach, R.C., Rosner, S.W., Presto, A.J., Weihrer, A.L. & Caceres, C.A. Noise reduction and representative complex selection in the computer analyzed exercise electrocardiogram. In: *Measurement in Exercise Electrocardiography. The Ernst Simonson Conference*, ed. H. Blackburn (C.C. Thomas, Springfield, Ill., 1969) pp. 73–107

Jacobs, W.F., Nutter, D.O., Siegel, W., Schlant, R.C. & Hurst, J.W. Hemodynamic responses to isometric handgrip in patients with heart disease. *Circulation 42*, suppl. III, 169 (abstr.) (1970)

Jaffé, D. & Manning, M. Coronary arteries in early life. In: *Proceedings of Thirteenth Annual Congress of Pediatrics* (Vienna, 1971)

James, T.N. Angina without coronary disease. *Circulation 42*, 189–91 (1970)

James, T.N. Mysterious sudden death. *Chest 62*, 454–68 (1972)

James, T.N., Froggatt, P. & Marshall, T.K. Sudden death in young athletes. In: *Exercise and Cardiac Death*, ed. E. Jokl & J.T. McClellan (Karger, Basel, 1971)

James, W.E. & Patnoi, C.M. Instrumentation review. In: *Coronary Heart Disease. Prevention, Detection, Rehabilitation with Emphasis on Exercise Testing*, ed. S.M. Fox (International Medical Corporation, Denver, Colorado, 1974) pp. (7-1)–(7-46)

Jamison, P.L. & Zegura, S.L. An anthropometric study of the Eskimos of Wainwright, Alaska. *Arctic Anthropol., 7*, 125–43 (1970)

Jansson, L., Johansson, K., Jonson, B., Olsson, L.G., Werner, O. & Westling, H. Computer assistance in the e.c.g. laboratory — a new look. *Scand. J. Clin. Lab. Invest., 36*, suppl. 145, 1–43 (1976)

Jean, C.F., Streeter, D.D. & Reichenbach, D.D. Fiber orientation in the normal and hypertensive cadaver left ventricle. *Circulation 46*, suppl., 44 (abstr.) (1972)

Jenkins, C.D. Psychologic and social precursors of coronary

disease. II. *New Engl. J. Med., 284*, 307–16 (1971)

Jetté, M., Campbell, J. Mongeon, J. & Routhier, R. The Canadian Home Fitness Test as a prediction of aerobic capacity. *Canad. Med. Assoc. J., 114*, 680–2 (1976)

Jetter, W.W. & White, P.D. Rupture of the heart in patients in mental institutions. *Ann. Intern. Med., 21*, 783–802 (1944)

Jezer, A. & Warshaw, L.J. Detection and evaluation of heart disease in industry. In: *The Heart in Industry*, ed. L.J. Warshaw (P. Hoeber, New York, 1960) p. 163

Johnson, S.A., Robb, R.A., Greenleaf, J.F., Ritman, E.L., Lee, S.L., Herman, G.T., Sturm, R.E. & Wood, E.H. The problem of accurate measurement of left ventricular shape and dimensions from multiplane roentgenographic data. *Europ. J. Cardiol., 1*, 241–58 (1974)

Johnson, W.D. Coronary bypass surgery: its value in the rehabilitation of coronary patients. In: *Heart Disease and Rehabilitation*, ed. M.L. Pollock & D.H. Schmidt (Houghton Mifflin, Boston, 1979) pp. 203–11

Johnson, W.D., Flemma, R.J., Manley, J.C. & Leply, D. Physiologic parameters of ventricular function as affected by direct coronary surgery. *J. Thorac. Cardiovasc. Surg., 60*, 483–90 (1970)

Joint Working Party. Prevention of coronary heart disease. *J. R. Coll. Phys. Surg. (Lond.), 10*, 213–75 (1976)

Jokl, E. *The Clinical Physiology of Physical Fitness and Rehabilitation* (C.C. Thomas, Springfield, Ill., 1958)

Jokl, E., Jokl-Ball, M., Jokl, P. & Frankel, L. Notation of exercise. In: *Medicine and Sport*, vol. 4. *Physical Activity and Aging*, ed. D. Brunner & E. Jokl (Karger, Basel, 1970) pp. 2–18

Jokl, E. & McClellan, J.T. *Exercise and Cardiac Death* (University Park Press, Baltimore, Md., 1971)

Jones, N. & Kane, M. Inter-laboratory standardization of methodology. *Med. Sci. Sports 11*, 368–72 (1979)

Jones, N., McHardy, G.J.R., Naimark, A. & Campbell, E.J.M. Physiological dead space and alveolar-arterial gas pressure differences during exercise. *Clin. Sci., 31*, 19–29 (1966)

Jones, N.L., Campbell, E.J.M., Edwards, R.H.T. & Robertson, D.G. *Clinical Exercise Testing* (W.B. Saunders, Philadelphia, 1975)

Jones, N.L., Campbell, E.J.M., McHardy, G.J.R., Higgs, B. & Clode, M. The estimation of carbon dioxide pressure of mixed venous blood during exercise. *Clin. Sci., 32*, 311–27 (1967)

Jorgensen, C.R. Coronary blood flow and myocardial oxygen consumption in man. In: *Physiology of Fitness and Exercise*, ed. J.F. Alexander, R.C. Serfass & C.M. Tipton (Athletic Institute, Chicago, 1972) pp. 39–50

Jorgensen, C.R., Gobel, F.L., Taylor, H.L. & Wang, Y. Myocardial blood flow and oxygen consumption during exercise. *Ann. N.Y. Acad. Sci., 301*, 213–23 (1977)

Jorgensen, C.R., Kitamura, K., Gobel, F.L., Taylor, H.L. & Wang, Y. Long-term precision of the N_2O method for coronary flow during heavy upright exercise. *J. Appl. Physiol., 30*, 338–44 (1971)

Jorgensen, C.R., Wang, K., Gobel, F.L., *et al*. Effect of propranolol on myocardial oxygen consumption and its hemodynamic correlates during upright exercise. *Circulation 48*, 1173–82 (1973)

Juergens, J.L., Edwards, J.E., Achor, R.W.P. & Burchell, H.B. Prognosis of patients surviving first clinically diagnosed myocardial infarction. *AMA Arch. Int. Med., 105*, 444–50 (1960)

Julian, D.G. The natural history of ischemic heart disease. In: *Advances in Cardiology*, Vol. 8, ed. P. Halönen & A. Louhya (Karger, New York, 1973) pp. 38–48

Julian, D.G., Campbell, R.W.F. & Murray, A. Predicting and preventing ventricular fibrillation in acute myocardial infarction. In: *Sudden Coronary Death*, ed. V. Manninen & P.I. Halonen (Karger, Basel, 1978) pp. 183–90

Julius, S., Amery, A., Whitlock, L.S. & Conway, J. Influence of age on the hemodynamic response to exercise. *Circulation 36*, 222–30 (1967)

Kahler, R.L., Gaffney, T.E & Braunwald, E. Effect of autonomic nervous system inhibition on the circulatory response to exercise. *J. Clin. Invest., 41*, 1981–7 (1962)

Kahn, H. The relationship of reported coronary heart disease mortality to physical activity of work. *Amer. J. Publ. Health 53*, 1058–67 (1963)

Kala, R., Romo, M., Siltanen, P. & Halonen, P.I. Physical activity and sudden cardiac death. In: *Sudden Coronary Death*, ed. R. Kala, M. Romo, P. Siltanen & P.I. Halonen (Karger, Basel, 1978) pp. 27–34

Kallio, V. Results of rehabilitation in coronary patients. In: *Advances in Cardiology*, ed. K. König & H. Denolin (Karger,

Basel, 1978) pp. 153–63

Kannel, W.B. Habitual level of physical activity and risk of coronary heart disease. The Framingham study. *Canad. Med. Ass. J., 96*, 811–12 (1967)

Kannel, W.B. Cardiovascular disease: a multifactorial problem (insights from the Framingham Study). In: *Heart Disease and Rehabilitation*, ed. M.L. Pollock & D.H. Schmidt (Houghton Mifflin, Boston, Mass., 1979) pp. 15–51

Kannel, W.B., Castelli, W.P., Verter, J. & McNamara, P.M. Relative importance of risk factors in the pathogenesis of coronary heart disease. The Framingham Study. In: *Coronary Heart Disease*, ed. H.I. Russek & B.L. Zohman (Lippincott, Philadelphia, 1971a)

Kannel, W.B., McNamara, P.M., Feinleib, M., *et al*. Unrecognized myocardial infarction. *Geratrics 25*, 75–87 (1970)

Kannel, W.B., Sorlie, P. & McNamara, P. The relationship of physical activity to risk of coronary heart disease. The Framingham Study. In: *Coronary Heart Disease and Physical Fitness*, ed. O.A. Larsen & R.O. Malmborg (University Park) Press, Baltimore, Md., 1971b) pp. 256–60

Kaplinsky, E., Hood, W.B., McCarthy, B., McCombs, H.L. & Down, B. Effects of physical training in dogs with coronary artery ligation. *Circulation 37*, 556–65 (1968)

Karlsson, N., Nordesjø, L.O., Jorfeldt, L. & Saltin, B. Muscle lactate, ATP and CP levels during exercise after physical training in man. *J. Appl. Physiol., 33*, 199–203 (1972)

Karvonen, M.J., Klemola, H., Virkajärvi, J. & Kekkonen, A. on heart rate. A 'longitudinal' study. *Ann. Med. Exp. Fenn., 35*, 307–15 (1957)

Karnoven, M.J., Klemola, H., Virkajärvi, J. & Kekkonen, A. Longevity of endurance skiers. *Med. Sci. Sports 6*, 49–51 (1974)

Kasch, F.W. & Boyer, J.L. Changes in maximum work capacity resulting from six months training in patients with ischemic heart disease. *Med. Sci. Sports 1*, 156–9 (1969)

Kasser, I.S. & Bruce, R.A. Comparative effects of aging and coronary heart disease on submaximal and maximal exercise. *Circulation 39*, 759–74 (1969)

Katila, M. & Frick, M.H. A two year circulatory follow-up of physical training after myocardial infarction. *Acta Med. Scand., 187*, 95–100 (1970)

Kato, K. & Watanabe, H. Haemodynamic response to exercise in patients with coronary heart disease. *Jap. Circ. J.*, *35*, 29–33 (1971)

Kattus, A. Medical versus surgical therapy for ischemic heart disease. *Chest 58*, suppl. 1, 299–304 (1970)

Kattus, A. & Grollman, J. Patterns of coronary collateral circulation in angina pectoris: relation to exercise training. In: *Changing Concepts in Cardiovascular Disease*, ed. H.I. Russek & B.L. Zohman (Williams & Wilkins, Baltimore, 1972)

Kattus, A.A. & McAlpin, R.N. Diagnosis, medical and surgical management of coronary insufficiency. *Ann. Intern. Med.*, *60*, 115–36 (1968)

Kattus, A.A. & McAlpin, R.N. Role of exercise in discovery, evaluation and management of ischemic heart disease. In: *Cardiovascular Clinics*, vol. 1, No. 2, *Coronary Heart Disease*, ed. A.N. Brest (Davis, Philadelphia, 1969) pp. 225–79

Katz, A.M. Effects of ischemia on the contractile process of heart muscle. *Amer. J. Cardiol.*, *32*, 456–60 (1973)

Katz, A.M. *Physiology of the Heart* (Raven Press, New York, 1977) pp. 1–433

Katz, A.M. & Katz, P.B. Diseases of the heart, in the works of Hippocrates. *Brit. Heart J.*, *24*, 257–64 (1962)

Katz, L.J. & Landt, H. The effect of standardized exercise on the four-lead electrocardiogram: its value in study of coronary disease. *Amer. J. Med. Sci.*, *189*, 346–51 (1935)

Katz, L.N. & Feinberg, H. Relation of cardiac effort to myocardial oxygen consumption and coronary flow. *Circ. Res.*, *6*, 656–69 (1958)

Kaunitz, H. Causes and consequences of salt consumption. *Nature (Lond.)*, *178*, 1141–4 (1956)

Kavanagh, T. A cold-weather 'jogging mask' for angina patients. *Canad. Med. Assoc. J.*, *103*, 1290–1 (1970)

Kavanagh, T. *Heart Attack? Counter Attack!* (Van Nostrand, Toronto, 1976)

Kavanagh, T., Pandit, V. & Shephard, R.J. The application of exercise testing to the elderly amputee. *Canad. Med. Assoc. J.*, *108*, 314–17 (1973a)

Kavanagh, T. & Shephard, R.J. The immediate antecedents of myocardial infarction in active men. *Canad. Med. Assoc. J.*, *109*, 19–22 (1973a)

Kavanagh, T. & Shephard, R.J. Importance of physical activity in post-coronary rehabilitation. *Amer. J. Phys. Med.*, *52*, 304–13

(1973b)

Kavanagh, T. & Shephard, R.J. Conditioning of post-coronary patients. Comparison of continuous and interval training. *Arch. Phys. Med. Rehabil.*, *56*, 72–6 (1975a)

Kavanagh, T. & Shephard, R.J. Maintenance of hydration in 'post-coronary' marathon runners. *Brit. J. Sports Med.*, *9*, 130–5 (1975b)

Kavanagh, T. & Shephard, R.J. Maximum exercise tests on 'post-coronary' patients. *J. Appl. Physiol.*, *40*, 611–18 (1976)

Kavanagh, T. & Shephard, R.J. The effects of continued training on the aging process. *Ann. N.Y. Acad. Sci.*, *301*, 656–70 (1977a)

Kavanagh, T. & Shephard, R.J. Sexual activity after myocardial infarction. *Canad. Med. Assoc. J.*, *116*, 1250–3 (1977b)

Kavanagh, T. & Shephard, R.J. Fluid and mineral needs of post-coronary distance runners. In: *Sports Medicine*, ed. F. Landry & W.R. Orban (Symposia Specialists, Miami, Fla., 1978)

Kavanagh, T. & Shephard, R.J. Exercise for post-coronary patients: an assessment of infrequent supervision. *Arch. Phys. Med. Rehab.*, *61* (3), 114–18 (1980)

Kavanagh, T., Shephard, R.J., Chisholm, A.W., Qureshi, S. & Kennedy, J. Prognostic indexes for patients with ischemic heart disease enrolled in an exercise-centered rehabilitation program. *Amer. J. Cardiol.*, *44*, 1230–40 (1979)

Kavanagh, T., Shephard, R.J. & Doney, H. Hypnosis and exercise — a possible combined therapy following myocardial infarction. *Amer. J. Clin. Hypnosis 16*, 160–5 (1974a)

Kavanagh, T., Shephard, R.J., Doney, H. & Pandit, V. Intensive exercise in coronary rehabilitation. *Med. Sci. Sports 5*, 34–9 (1973b)

Kavanagh, T., Shephard, R.J. & Kennedy, J. Characteristics of post-coronary marathon runners. *Ann. N.Y. Acad. Sci.*, *301*, 656–70 (1977a)

Kavanagh, T., Shephard, R.J. & Kennedy, J. Are the benefits of exercise in post-coronary rehabilitation an artefact of patient selection? *Cardiologia 62*, 84–5 (1977c)

Kavanagh, T., Shephard, R.J. & Pandit, V. Marathon running after myocardial infarction. *JAMA*, *229*, 1602–5 (1974b)

Kavanagh, T., Shephard, R.J. & Pandit, V. Marathon running after myocardial infarction. In: *Twentieth World Congress of Sports Medicine, Melbourne, Australia*, ed. H. Toyne (Australian Sports Medicine Federation, Melbourne, 1975a)

Kavanagh, T., Shephard, R.J. & Tuck, J.A. Depression after

myocardial infarction. *Canad. Med. Assoc. J., 113*, 23–7 (1975b)

Kavanagh, T., Shephard, R.J., Tuck, J.A. & Qureshi, S. Depression following myocardial infarction: the effects of distance running. *Ann. N.Y. Acad. Sci., 301*, 1029–38 (1977b)

Kay, C. & Shephard, R.J. On muscle strength and the threshold of anaerobic work. *Int. Z. Angew. Physiol., 27*, 311–28 (1969)

Keefer, C.S. & Resnick, W.H. Angina pectoris: a syndrome caused by anoxemia of the myocardium. *Arch. Int. Med., 41*, 769–807 (1928)

Keegan, D.L. The coronary patient: a psychosocial glimpse. *Canad. Fam. Phys., 19*, 66–8 (1973)

Keith, R.A. Personality and coronary heart disease — a review. *J. Chronic Dis., 19*, 1231–43 (1966)

Kellermann, J.J., Ben Ari, E., Chayet, M., Lapidot, C. Drory, Y. & Fisman, E. Cardiocirculatory response to different types of training in patients with angina pectoris. *Cardiology 62*, 218–31 (1977)

Kellerman, J.J. & Kariv, I. *Rehabilitation of Coronary Patients* (Segal Press, Tel Aviv, 1968)

Kellermann, J.J., Modan, B., Feldman, S. & Kariv, I. Evaluation of physical work capacity in coronary patients after myocardial infarction who returned to work with and without a medically directed reconditioning program. In: *Physical Activity and Aging*, ed. D. Brunner & E. Jokl (University Park Press, Baltimore, Md., 1970) pp. 148–55

Kemple, C. Rorschach method and psychosomatic diagnosis: personality traits of patients with rheumatic disease, hypertensive cardiovascular disease, coronary occlusion and fracture. *Psychosom. Med., 7*, 85–9 (1945)

Kemsley, W.F.F. Body weight at different ages and heights. *Ann. Eugen. (Lond.), 16–17*, 316–34 (1951–3)

Kendrick, Z.B., Pollock, M.L., Hickman, T.N. & Miller, H.S. Effects of training and detraining on cardiovascular efficiency. *Amer. Corr. Therap. J., 25*, 79–83 (1971)

Kennedy, C.K., Spiekerman, R.E., Lindsay, M.I., Mankin, H.T., Frye, R.L. & McCallister, B.D. One-year graduated exercise program for men with angina pectoris. Evaluation by physiological studies and coronary arteriography. *Mayo Clin. Proc., 51*, 231–6 (1976)

Kennedy, J.W., Baxley, W.A., Figley, M.M., Dodge, H.T. & Blackburn, J.R. Quantitative angiography. I. The normal left ventricle in man. *Circulation 34*, 272–8 (1966)

Kentala, E. Physical fitness and feasibility of physical rehabilitation after myocardial infarction in men of working age. *Ann. Clin. Res., 4*, suppl. 9, 1–84 (1972)

Kentala, E. & Sarna, S. Sudden death and factors related to long term prognosis following acute myocardial infarction. *Scand. J. Rehab. Med., 8*, 27–32 (1976)

Kerr, A., Bommer, W.J. & Pilato, S. Coronary artery enlargement in experimental cardiac hypertrophy. *Amer. Heart J., 75*, 144 (abstr.) (1968)

Keys, A. Coronary heart disease in seven countries. *Circulation 41*, suppl. 1 (1970)

Keys, A. Coronary heart disease — the global picture. *Atherosclerosis 22*, 149–92 (1975)

Keys, A., Aravanis, C., Blackburn, H., Van Buchem, F.S.P., Buzina, R., Djordjevic, B.S., Fidanza, F., Karvonen, M.J., Menotti, A., Puddu, V. & Taylor, H.L. Coronary heart disease: overweight and obesity. *Ann. Int. Med., 77*, 15–27 (1972)

Keys, A. & Parlin, R.W. Serum cholesterol response to changes in dietary lipids. *Amer. J. Clin. Nutr., 19*, 175–81 (1966)

Khosla, T. & Lowe, C.R. Indices of obesity derived from body weight and height. *Brit. J. Prev. Soc. Med., 21*, 122–8 (1967)

Kiessling, K.H., Pilstrom, L., Karlsson, J. & Piehl, K. Mitochondrial volume in skeletal muscle from young and old physically untrained and trained healthy men and from alcoholics. *Clin. Sci., 44*, 547–54 (1973)

Kilböm, Å. Physical training with sub-maximal intensities in women. I. Reaction to exercise and orthostasis. *Scand. J. Clin. Lab. Invest., 28*, 141–61 (1971)

Kilböm, Å., Hartley, L.H., Saltin, B., Bjure, J., Grimby, G. & Åstrand, I. Physical training in sedentary middle-aged and older men. I. Medical evaluation. *Scand. J. Clin. Lab. Invest., 24*, 315–28 (1969)

Kinderman, W., Keul, J. & Reindell, H. Cardiac function in sports. In: *Basic Book of Sports Medicine*, ed. G. La Cava (International Olympic Committee, Rome, 1978) pp. 47–58

Kinsey, A.C. *Sexual Behaviour in the Human Male* (W.B. Saunders, Philadelphia, 1948)

Kirchheiner, B. & Pedersen-Bjergaard, O. The effect of physical training after myocardial infarction. *Scand. J. Rehabil. Med., 5*, 105–10 (1973)

Kitamura, K., Jorgensen, C.R., Gobel, F.L., Taylor, H.L. & Yang, Y. Hemodynamic correlates of myocardial oxygen consumption during upright exercise. *J. Appl. Physiol., 32*, 516–22 (1972)

Kivowitz, C., Marcus, H., Donoso, R., Ganz, W., Swan, H.J.C. & Parmley, W.W. Evaluation of cardiac performance with a handgrip dynamometer in patients with heart disease: 'The grip tests'. *Circulation 42*, suppl. III, 122 (1970); *44*, 994–1002 (1971)

Klarman, H.E. Socio-economic impact of heart disease. In: *The Heart and Circulation. Second National Conference on Cardiovascular Diseases, vol. 2, Community Services and Education*, ed. E.C. Andrus (US Public Health Service, Washington, D.C., 1964)

Klassen, G.A, Woodhouse, S.P., Hathirat, S. & Johnson, A.L. The effect of physical training of post-myocardial infarction patients. A controlled study. *Canad. Med. Assoc. J., 107*, 632 (abstr.) (1972)

Klein, H.P. & Parson, O.A. Self-description of patients with coronary disease. Perceptual and motor skills (Southern Universities Press, Birmingham, Al., 1968)

Klein, R.F., Dean, A., Wilson, M., *et al*. The physician and post-myocardial infarction invalidism. *JAMA, 194*, 143–8 (1965)

Klocke, F.J. & Wittenburg, S.M. Heterogeneity of coronary blood flow in human coronary artery disease and experimental myocardial infarction. *Amer. J. Cardiol., 24*, 782–90 (1969)

Kloster, F., Kremkau, L., Rahimtoola, S., Griswold, H., Ritzmann, L., Neill, W. & Starr, A. Prospective randomized study of coronary by-pass surgery for chronic stable angina. *Circulation 52*, suppl. II, 90, 353 (abstr.) (1975)

Klumbies, G. & Kleinsorge, H. Circulatory dangers and prophylaxis during orgasm. *Int. J. Sexology 10*, 97 (1930)

Kober, G., Kuck, H., Lentz, R.W. & Kaltenbach, M. Angiographic evidence of collateral circulation and its effects on left ventricular function in coronary heart disease. In: *Coronary Heart Disease*, ed. M. Kaltenbach, P. Lichtlen, R. Balcon & W.D. Bussmann (G. Thieme, Stuttgart, 1978) pp. 48–54

Kobernick, S.D., Niawayama, G. & Zuehlewski, A.C. Effect of physical activity on cholesterol atherosclerosis in rabbits. *Proc. Soc. Exp. Biol. Med., N.Y., 96* (3), 623–8 (1957)

Koppes, G., McKiernan, T., Bassan, M., *et al*. Treadmill exercise testing. *Curr. Probl. Cardiol., 7* (8), 1–43; 7 (9), 1–45 (1977)

Korsan-Bengtsen, K., Wilhelmsen, L. & Tibblin, G. Blood coagulation and fibrinolysis in relation to degree of physical activity during work and leisure time. *Acta Med. Scand., 193*, 73–7 (1973)

Kötter, V., Von Leitner, E. & Schröder, R. Comparison of effects on hemodynamics and myocardial metabolism of phentolamine, sodium nitroprusside and glyceryl trinitrate in acute myocardial infarction. In: *Coronary Heart Disease*, ed. M. Kaltenbach, P. Lichtlen, R. Balcon & W.D. Bussmann (G. Thieme, Stuttgart, 1978) pp 273–8

Krantz, J.C., Lu, G.G., Bell, F.K. & Cascorbi, H.F. Nitrites. XIX. Studies on the mechanism of action of glyceryl trinitrate. *Biochem. Pharmacol., 11*, 1095–9 (1962)

Kraus, H. & Kirsten, R. Die Wirkung von körperlichen Training auf die mitochondriale Energieproduktion in Herzmuskel und in der Leber. *Pflügers Archiv., 320*, 334–47 (1970)

Kritchevsky, D. Laboratory models for atherosclerosis. In: *Advances in Drug Research*, vol. 9, ed. D. Kritchevsky (Academic Press, London, 1974) pp. 41–53

Kühn, P. Pharmacology of antiarrhythmic therapy. In: *Coronary Heart Disease, Exercise Testing and Cardiac Rehabilitation*, ed. W.E. James and E.A. Amsterdam (Symposia Specialists, Miami, Fla., 1977) pp. 319–24

Kuller, L. Sudden and unexpected non-traumatic deaths in adults. A review of epidemiological and clinical studies. *J. Chron. Dis., 19*, 1165–92 (1966)

Kuller, L., Lillienfeld, A. & Fisher, R. An epidemiological study of sudden and unexpected deaths in adults. *Medicine 46*, 341–61 (1967)

Kurita, A., Chaitman, B.R., & Bourassa, M.G. Significance of exercise-induced junctional ST depression in evaluation of coronary artery disease. *Amer. J. Cardiol., 40*, 492–7 (1977)

Kushnir, B., Fox, K.M., Tomlinson, I.W. & Aber, C.P. The effect of a pre-discharge consultation on the resumption of work, sexual activity and driving following acute myocardial infarction. *Scand. J. Rehab. Med., 8*, 155–9 (1976)

La Due, J.S., Wróblewski, F. & Karmen, A. Serum glutamic oxaloacetic transaminase activity in human acute transmural myocardial infarction. *Science 120*, 497–9 (1954)

Lalonde, M. A new perspective on the health of Canadians

(Information Canada, Ottawa, 1974)

Lamb, L.E. & Hiss, R.G. Influence of exercise on premature contractions. *Amer. J. Cardiol., 10*, 209–16 (1962)

Lamb, L.E., Kelly, R.J., Smith, W.L., LeBlanc, A.D. & Johnson, P.C. Limiting factors in the capacity to achieve maximum cardiac work. *Aerospace Med., 40*, 1291–6 (1969)

Lapiccirella, V., Lapiccirella, R., Abboni, F. & Liotta, S. Enquête clinique, biologie et cardiographique parmi les tribus nomades de le Somalie qui se nourissent seulement de lait. *Bull. WHO 27*, 681–97 (1962)

Largey, L.I. Longevity of college athletes. *Harper's Monthly Mag., 157*, 229–38 (1928)

Larsen, O.A. & Lassen, N.A. Effect of daily muscular exercise in patients with intermittent claudication. *Lancet* (ii), 1093–6 (1968)

Laurenceau, J.L., Turcot, J. & Dumesnil, J.G. Echocardiographic study of Olympic athletes. In: *Proceedings of International Conference on Sports Cardiology*, ed. T. Lubich & A. Venerando (A. Gaggi, Bologna, 1980) p. 705

Laurent, D., Bolene-Williams, C., Williams, F.L., *et al*. Effects of heart rate on coronary flow and cardiac oxygen consumption. *Amer. J. Physiol., 185*, 355–64 (1956)

Lawrie, G.M., Morris, G.C., Hiwell, J.F., *et al*. Results of coronary bypass more than five years after operation in 434 patients. Clinical, treadmill exercise and angiographic correlations. *Amer. J. Cardiol., 40*, 665–72 (1977)

Layman, E.M. Aggression in relation to play and sports. In: *Contemporary Psychology of Sport*, ed. G.S. Kenyon (Athletic Institute, Chicago, Ill., 1970) pp. 25–34

LeBlanc, J. *Man in the Cold* (C.C. Thomas, Springfield, Ill., 1975) pp. 1–195

Lebovits, B., Lichter, E. & Moses, V.K. Personality correlates of coronary heart disease: a re-examination of the MMPI data. *Soc. Sci. Med., 9*, 207–19 (1975)

Lebovits, B.Z., Shekelle, R.B., Ostfeld, A.M. & Paul, O. Prospective and retrospective psychological studies of coronary heart disease. *Psychosom. Med., 29*, 265–72 (1967)

Lee, G., Amsterdam, E.A., de Maria, A.N., Davis, G., LaFave, T. & Mason, D.T. Effect of exercise on hemostatic mechanisms. In: *Exercise in Cardiovascular Health and Disease*, ed. E.A. Amsterdam, J.H. Wilmore & A.N. de Maria (Yorke Medical

Books, New York, 1977) pp. 126–36

Lehtonen, A. & Viikari, J. The effect of vigorous physical activity at work on serum lipids, with special reference to serum high-density lipoprotein cholesterol. *Acta Physiol. Scand.*, *104*, 117–21 (1978)

Leon, A.S. & Bloor, C.M. Exercise effects on the heart at different ages. *Circulation 41/42*, suppl. III, 50 (1970)

Leon, A., Conrad, J. & Hunninghake, D. Effects of a walking program on body composition, carbohydrate and lipid metabolism of obese young men. *Amer. J. Clin. Nutr.*, *32*, 1776–87 (1979)

Leon, A.S., Conrad, J., Hunninghake, D., Jacobs, D. & Serfass, R. Exercise effects on body composition, work capacity, and carbohydrate and lipid metabolism of young obese men. *Med. Sci. Sports 9*, 60 (1977)

Lepeschkin, E. Physiological factors influencing the electro-cardiographic response to exercise. In: *Measurements in Exercise Electrocardiography*, ed. H. Blackburn (C.C. Thomas, Springfield, Ill., 1969)

Leppo, J., Yipintsoi, T., Blankstein, R., Bontemps, R., Freeman, L.M., Zohman, L. & Scheuer, J. Thallium-201 myocardial scintigraphy in patients with triple-vessel disease and ischemic exercise stress test. *Circulation 59*, 714–21 (1979)

Leren, P., Askevold, E.M., Foss, O.P., *et al.* The Oslo study. *Acta Med. Scand.*, *588*, suppl., 1–38 (1975)

Lester, F.M., Sheffield, L.T. & Reeves, J.T. Electrocardiographic changes in clinically normal older men following near maximal and maximal exercise. *Circulation 36*, 5–14 (1967)

Lester, M., Sheffield, L.T., Trammell, P. & Reeves, T.J. The effect of age and athletic training on the maximal heart rate during muscular exercise. *Amer. Heart J.*, *76*, 370–6 (1968)

Lewes, D. Electrode jelly in electrocardiography. *Brit. Heart J.*, *27*, 105–15 (1965)

Lewis, B.M., Houssay, H.E.J., Haynes, F.W. & Dexter, L. The dynamics of both right and left ventricles at rest and during exercise in patients with heart failure. *Circ. Res.*, *1*, 312–20 (1953)

Lichtlen, P., Moccetti, T., Halter, J. & Gattiker, K. Post-operative evaluation of myocardial blood flow in aorta-to-coronary artery vein bypass grafts using the xenon residue detection technique. In: *Coronary Heart Disease*, ed. M. Kaltenbach, P. Lichtlen &

G.C. Friesinger (G. Thieme, Stuttgart, 1973) pp. 286–95

Lie, K.I., Wellens, H.J.J., Downar, E. & Durrer, D. Observations of patients with primary ventricular fibrillation complicating acute myocardial infarction. *Circulation 52*, 755–9 (1975)

Likoff, W. Angina with normally patent coronary arteries. In: *Changing Concepts in Cardiovascular Disease*, ed. H.I. Russek & B.L. Zohman (Williams & Wilkins, Baltimore, 1972) pp. 77–9

Lind, A.R. & McNicol, G.W. Muscular factors which determine the cardiovascular responses to sustained and rhythmic exercise. In: *Proceedings of an International Symposium on Physical Activity and Cardiovascular Health. Canad. Med. Assoc. J.*, 96, 706–12 (1967)

Little, J.A., Shanoff, H.M., Roe, R.D., Csima, A. & Yano, R. Studies of male survivors of myocardial infarction. IV. Serum lipids and five year survival. *Circulation 31*, 854–62 (1965)

Littler, W.A., Honour, A.J. & Sleight, P. Direct arterial pressure, heart rate and electrocardiogram during human coitus. *J. Reprod. Fertil., 40*, 321–31 (1974)

Logan, S.E. On the fluid mechanics of human coronary stenosis. *IEEE Trans. Biomed. Eng., BME22*, 327–34 (1975)

Lopez, A., Vial, R., Balart, L. & Arroyave, G. Effect of exercise and physical fitness on serum lipids and lipoproteins. *Atherosclerosis 20*, 1–9 (1974)

Love, W.D. & Burch, G.E. Influence of the rate of coronary plasma flow on the extraction of Rb[86] from coronary blood. *Circulation Res., 7*, 24–30 (1959)

Lovell, R.R.H. & Verghese, A. Personality traits associated with different chest pains after myocardial infarction. *Brit. Med. J.* (iii), 327–30 (1967)

Lown, B., Kosowsky, B.D. & Whiting, R. Exposure of electrical instability in coronary artery disease by exercise stress. *Circulation 39*, suppl. 3, 136 (abstr.) (1969)

Lundgren, O. & Jodal, M. Regional blood flow. *Ann. Rev. Physiol., 37*, 395–414 (1975)

Mackenzie, G.J., Taylor, S.H., Flenley, D.C., McDonald, A.H., Staunton, H.P. & Donald, K.W. Circulatory and respiratory studies in myocardial infarction and cardiogenic shock. *Lancet* (ii), 825–32 (1964)

Mackintosh, A.F., Crabb, M.E., Grainger, G., Williams, J.H. & Chamberlain, D.A. The Brighton resuscitation ambulances: review of 40 consecutive survivors of out of hospital cardiac arrest. *Brit. Med. J.* (i), 1115–18 (1978)

Maddocks, I. In: *Proceedings of the Sixth International Congress of Nutrition*, ed. C.F. Miles & R. Passmore (Livingstone, Edinburgh, 1964) p. 137

Malleson, A. *The Medical Run-around* (Hart, New York, 1973)

Malmborg, R.O. A clinical and hemodynamic analysis of factors limiting cardiac performance in patients with coronary heart disease. *Acta Med. Scand., 117*, suppl. 426, 5–94 (1965)

Malmcrona, R. Cramér, G. & Varnauskas, E. Haemodynamic data during rest and exercise for patients who have or have not been able to retain their occupation after myocardial infarction. *Acta Med. Scand., 174*, 557–72 (1963)

Malmcrona, R. & Varnauskas, E. Haemodynamics during rest and during exercise at the end of convalescence from myocardial infarction. *Acta Med. Scand., 175*, 19–30 (1964)

Malmros, H. The relation of nutrition to health — a statistical study of the effect of war-time on arteriosclerosis, cardiosclerosis, tuberculosis and diabetes. *Acta Med. Scand., 246*, suppl., 137–53 (1950)

Manley, J.C. Hemodynamic performance before and following coronary by-pass surgery. In: *Heart Disease and Rehabilitation*, ed. M.L. Pollock & D.H. Schmidt (Houghton Mifflin, Boston, 1979) pp. 168–82

Manley, J.C. & Johnson, W.D. Effects of surgery on angina (pre- and post-infarction) and myocardial function (failure). *Circulation 46*, 1208–21 (1972)

Mann, G.V. A factor in yogurt which lowers cholesterolemia in man. *Atherosclerosis 26*, 335–40 (1977)

Mann, G.V., Garrett, H.L., Farhi, A., *et al.* Exercise to prevent coronary heart disease. *Amer. J. Med., 46*, 12–27 (1969)

Mann, G.V., Schaffer, R.D., Anderson, R.S., *et al.* Cardio-vascular disease in the Masai. *J. Atherosclerosis Res., 4*, 289–312 (1965)

Mann, R.H. & Burchell, H.B. Premature ventricular contractions and exercise. *Proc. Staff Mayo Clin., 27*, 383–9 (1952)

Manninen, V. & Halonen, P.I. *Sudden Coronary Death* (Karger, Basel, 1978)

Margaria, R., Aghemo, P. & Rovelli, E. Indirect determination of maximal O_2 consumption in man. *J. Appl. Physiol., 20*, 1070–3 (1965)

Margolis, J.R. Treadmill stage as a predictor of medical and surgical survival in coronary disease. *Circulation 52*, suppl. II, 109 (abstr.) (1975)

Margolis, J.R., Hirschfield, J.W., McNeer, J.F., *et al*. Sudden death due to coronary artery disease. A clinical, hemodynamic and angiographic profile. *Circulation 52–52*, suppl. III, 180–3 (1975)

Maritz, J.S., Morrison, J.F., Peter, J., Strydom, N.B. & Wyndham, C.H. A practical method of estimating an individual's maximum oxygen intake. *Ergonomics 4*, 97–122 (1961)

Maron, B.J. Cardiac causes of sudden death in athletes and considerations for screening athletic populations. In: *International Congress of Sports Cardiology*, ed. T. Lubich & A. Venerando (A. Gaggi, Bologna, 1980)

Marriott, H.J.L. & Myerburg, R.J. Recognition and treatment of cardiac arrhythmias and conduction disturbances. In: *The Heart*, 3rd edn., ed. J.W. Hurst (McGraw Hill, New York, 1974)

Marshall, R.C., Berger, J.H., Costin, J.C., *et al*. Assessment of cardiac performance with quantitative radionuclide angiography: sequential left ventricular ejection fraction, normalized left ventricular ejection rate and regional wall motion. *Circulation 56*, 820–9 (1977)

Marx, H.J, Rowell, L.B., Conn, R.D., Bruce, R.A. & Kusumi, F. Maintenance of aortic pressure and total peripheral resistance during exercise in heat. *J. Appl. Physiol., 22*, 519–25 (1967)

Marx, J.L. Stress: role in hypertension debated. *Science 198*, 905–7 (1977)

Mason, D.T., Amsterdam, E.A., Miller, R.R., Salel, A.F. & Zelis, R. Physiological basis of antianginal therapy: the nitrites, beta adrenergic receptor blockade, carotid sinus nerve stimulation, and coronary artery-saphenous vein bypass graft. In: *Changing Concepts in Cardiovascular Disease*, ed. H.I. Russek & B.L. Zohman (Williams & Wilkins, Baltimore, 1972) pp. 40–64

Massie, E. Sudden death during coitus: fact or fiction? *Hum. Sex 3*, 22 (1969)

Massie, J., Rode, A., Skrien, T. & Shephard, R.J. A critical review of the 'Aerobics' points system. *Med. Sci. Sports 2*, 1–6 (1970)

Massie, J. & Shephard, R.J. Physiological and psychological effects of training. *Med. Sci. Sports 3*, 110–17 (1971)

Master, A.M. Effect of injury and effort on the normal and the diseased heart. *New York State J. Med., 46*, 2634–41 (1946)

Master, A.M. & Jaffe, H.L. Electrocardiographic changes after exercise in angina pectoris. *J. Mt. Sinai Hosp., N.Y., 7*, 629–32 (1941)

Master, A.M., Van Liere, E.J., Lindsay, H.A. & Hartroft, W.S. Arterial blood pressure. In: *Biology Data Book*, ed. P.L. Altman & D.S. Dittmer (Federation of American Societies for Experimental Biology, Washington D.C., 1964)

Masuda, M., Shibayama, H. & Ebashi, H. Changes in arterial blood pressure during running and walking determined by a kind of indirect method. *Bull. Phys. Fitness Res. Inst. (Japan), 11*, 1–16 (1967)

Matell, G. Time course of changes in ventilation and arterial gas tensions in man induced by moderate exercise. *Acta Physiol. Scand., 58*, suppl. 206, 1–53 (1963)

Mathers, J.A.L., Griffeath, H.I., Levy, R.L. & Nickerson, J.L. Effect of ascending an ordinary flight of stairs on the work of the heart. Observations on normal individuals and on patients with coronary heart disease. *Circulation 3*, 224–9 (1951)

Mathur, V.S. & Guinn, G.A. Prospective randomized study of coronary by-pass surgery in stable angina: the first 100 patients. *Circulation 51/52*, suppl. I, 133–40 (1975)

Mattingly, T.W. The post-exercise electrocardiogram. Its value in the diagnosis and prognosis of coronary arterial disease. *Amer. J. Cardiol., 9*, 395–409 (1962)

Mattingly, T.W., Robb, G.P. & Marks, H.H. Stress tests in the detection of coronary disease. *Postgrad. Med., 24*, 419–30 (1958)

Mausner, J.S. & Bahn, A.K. *Epidemiology. An Introductory Text* (W.B. Saunders, Philadelphia, 1974)

Maynard, J.E. Coronary heart disease risk factors in relation to urbanization in Eskimo men. In: *Circumpolar Health*, ed. R.J. Shephard & S. Itoh (University of Toronto Press, Toronto, 1976) pp. 294–5

McAllister, F.F., Bertsch, R., Jacobson, J. & D'Allesio, G. The accelerating effect of muscular exercise on experimental atherosclerosis. *Arch. Surg., 80*, 54–60 (1959)

McAlpine, V., Milojevic, S. & Monkhouse, F.C. Changes in the electrophoretic patterns of euglobulin fractions following activation of the fibrinolytic system by exercise. *Can. J. Physiol. Pharmacol., 49*, 672–7 (1971)

McCrimmon, D.R., Cunningham, D.A., Rechnitzer, P.A. & Griffiths, J. Effect of training on plasma catecholamines in post-myocardial patients. *Med. Sci. Sports 8*, 152–6 (1976)

McDonald, G.A. & Fullerton, H.W. Effect of physical activty on coagulability of blood after ingestion of high-fat meal. *Lancet* (ii), 600–1 (1958)

McDonough, J.R. & Bruce, R.A. Maximal exercise testing in assessing cardiovascular function. In: *Proceedings of National Conference on Exercise in the Prevention, in the Evaluation, and in the Treatment of Heart Disease. J. S. Carol. Med. Ass., 65*, suppl. I, 26–33 (1969)

McDonough, J.R., Danielson, R.A., Wills, R.E. & Vine, P.L. Maximal cardiac output during exercise in patients with coronary artery disease. *Amer. J. Cardiol., 33*, 23–9 (1974)

McDonough, J.R., Haines, C., Stulb, S. & Garrison, G. Coronary heart disease among Negroes and Whites in Evans County, Georgia. *J. Chron. Dis., 18*, 443–68 (1965)

McGee, D. & Gordon, T. *The Framingham Study. An Epidemiological Investigation of Cardiovascular Disease. Section 31. The Results of the Framingham Study Applied to Four Other US Based Epidemiologic Studies of Cardiovascular Disease*, US Department of Health, Education and Welfare Publication, 76–1083 (Washington, D.C., 1976)

McGill, H.C. Comparison of experimentally induced animal atherosclerosis with spontaneous human atherosclerosis. In: *Comparative Atherosclerosis*, ed. J.C. Roberts, R. Strauss & M.S. Cooper (Harper & Row, New York, 1965) pp. 354–9

McGill, H.C. Introduction to the geographic pathology of atherosclerosis. *Lab. Invest., 18*, 465–7 (1968)

McGill, H.C. Abnormalities potentially mediating the effect of cigarette smoking on atherosclerosis. In: *Atherosclerosis IV*, ed. G. Schettler, Y. Goto, Y. Hata & G. Klose (Springer Verlag, Berlin, 1977) pp. 161–5

McHenry, P.L., Fisch, C., Korden, J.W. & Corya, B.R. Cardiac arrhythmias observed during maximal treadmill exercise testing in clinically normal men. *Amer. J. Cardiol., 29*, 331–6 (1972)

McHenry, P.L. & Morris, S.N. Exercise electrocardiography — current state of the art. In: *Advances in Electrocardiography*, vol. 2, ed. R. Schlant & W. Hurst (Grune & Stratton, New York, 1976)

McHenry, P.L., Stowe, D.E. & Lancaster, M.C. Computer

quantitation of the ST segment response during maximal treadmill exercise: clinical correlation. *Circulation 38*, 691–701 (1968)

McIntosh, H.D. & Garcia, J.A. The first decade of aortocoronary bypass grafting 1967–1977. A review. *Circulation 57*, 405–31 (1978)

McNeer, J.F., Starmer, C.F., Bartel, A.G., *et al.* The nature of treatment selection in coronary artery disease. Experience with medical and surgical treatment of a chronic disease. *Circulation 49*, 606–14 (1974)

McPherson, B.D., Paivio, A, & Yuhasz, M.S. Psychological effects of an exercise program for post-infarct and normal adult men. *J. Sports Med.*, *7*, 95–102 (1967)

Medalie, J.H., Neufeld, H.N., Riss, E., *et al. Physician's Fact Book: Selected Measurements on 10,000 Israeli Males* (Central Printer, Jerusalem, 1968)

Medved, R., Volarić and Pavišić-Medved, V. Sudden death of a top-level football player. *Brit. J. Sports Med.*, *7*, 164 (1973)

Mellerowicz, H. *Ergometrie* (Von Urban & Schwarzenburg, Munich, 1962)

Messer, J.V., Levine, M.J., Wagman, R.J. & Gorlin, R. Effect of exercise on cardiac performance in human subjects with coronary artery disease. *Circulation 28*, 404–14 (1963)

Metropolitan Life Insurance Company, New York City. Outlook for men disabled by coronary occlusion. *Statist. Bull.*, *34*, 1–3 (1953)

Meyer, B.M. Methodologic issues and considerations in epidemiologic studies of etiology and prevention of heart disease. In: *Heart Disease and Rehabilitation*, ed. M.L. Pollock & D.H. Schmidt (Houghton Mifflin, Boston, 1979) pp. 57–72

Miettinen, M., Karvonen, M.J., Turpeinen, O., *et al.* Effect of cholesterol-lowering diet on mortality from coronary heart disease and other causes. *Lancet* (ii), 835–9 (1972)

Mikulaj, L., Komadel, L., Vigas, M., Kvetnansky, R., Starka, L. & Vencel, P. Some hormonal changes after different kinds of motor stress in trained and untrained young men. In: *Metabolic Adaptation to Prolonged Physical Exercise*, ed. H. Howald & J.R. Poortmans (Birkhauser Verlag, Basel, 1975) pp. 333–8

Miller, C.K. Psychological correlates of coronary artery disease. *Psychosom. Med.*, *27*, 257–65 (1965)

Milvy, P. Statistical analysis of deaths from coronary heart disease anticipated in a cohort of marathon runners. *Ann. N.Y. Acad. Sci.*, *301*, 610–6 (1977)

Mirsky, I. Review of various theories for the evaluation of left ventricular wall stresses. In: *Cardiac Mechanics: Physiological, Clinical and Mathematical Considerations*, ed. I. Mirsky, D. Ghista & H. Sandler (Wiley, New York, 1974) pp. 381–409

Mirsky, I. and Parmlet, W.W. Force-velocity studies in isolated and intact heart muscle. In: *Cardiac Mechanics: Physiological, Clinical and Mathematical Considerations*, ed. I. Mirsky, D. Ghista & H. Sandler (Wiley, New York, 1974) pp. 87–112

Mirwald, R., Bailey, D.A. & Weese, C. Probleme bei der Einschätzung der maximalen aeroben Kraft der Untersuchung des Wachstums in einer Längsschnittstudie. In: *Motorische Entwicklung*, ed. R. Bauss & K. Roth (Institut für Sportswissenschaft, Darmstadt, 1977) pp. 65–75

Mitchell, J.H. & Wildenthal, K. Left ventricular function during exercise. In: *Coronary Heart Disease and Physical Fitness*, ed. O.A. Larsen & R.O. Malmborg (University Park Press, Baltimore, Md., 1971) pp. 93–6

Mitrani, I., Karplus, H. & Brunner, D. Arteriosclerosis of the coronary arteries in cases of traumatic death. *Isr. J. Med. Sci.*, *3*, 339 (abstr.) (1967)

Mogensen, L. Exercise testing and continuous long-term e.c.g. recording in the detection of arrhythmias and ST-T changes. In: *Coronary Heart Disease, Exercise Testing & Cardiac Rehabilitation*, ed. W.E. James & E.A. Amsterdam (Symposia Specialists, Miami, 1977) pp. 131–41

Moir, T.W. & DeBra, D.W. Effect of left ventricular hypertension, ischemia and vasoactive drugs on the myocardial distribution of coronary flow. *Circ. Res.*, *21*, 65–74 (1967)

Mojonnier, L., Hall, Y., Berkson, D., *et al.* Experience in changing food habits of hyperlipidaemic men and women. *J. Amer. Diet. Assn.* (1978) Cited by H. Blackburn in: *Heart Disease and Rehabilitation*, ed. M.L. Pollock & D.H. Schmidt (Houghton Mifflin, Boston, Mass., 1979)

Moncur, J. A study of fatalities during sport in Scotland (1969). *Brit. J. Sports Med.*, *7*, 162–3 (1973)

Monroe, R.G. Myocardial oxygen consumption during ventricular contraction and relaxation. *Circ. Res.*, *14*, 294–300 (1964)

Monroe, R.G. & French, G.N. Left ventricular pressure-volume relationship and myocardial oxygen consumption in the isolated heart. *Circulation Res., 9*, 362–74 (1961)

Montoye, H.J. Summary of research on the relationship of exercise to heart disease. *J. Sports Med. Fitness 2*, 34–43 (1960)

Montoye, H.J. *Physical Activity and Health. An Epidemiologic Study of an Entire Community* (Prentice Hall, Englewood Cliffs, N.J., 1975)

Montoye, H.J. Epidemiologic studies of exercise and cardiovascular disease. *Physical Educator 34*, 116–21 (1977)

Montoye, H.J., Metzner, H.L., Keller, J.B., *et al.* Habitual physical activity and blood pressure. *Med. Sci. Sports 4*, 175–81 (1972)

Montoye, H.J., Van Huss, W.D., Olson, H., Hudec, A. & Mahoney, E. Study of the longevity and morbidity of college athletes. *JAMA, 162*, 1132–4 (1956)

Montoye, H.J., Van Huss, W.D., Olson, H.W., Pierson, W.R. & Hudec, A.J. *The Longevity and Morbidity of College Athletes* (Phi Epislon Kappa Fraternity, Ann Arbor, 1957)

Montoye, H.J., Willis, P.W., Howard, G.E. & Keller, J.B. Cardiac pre-ejection period: age and sex comparisons. *J. Gerontol., 26*, 208–16 (1971)

Morgan, P., Gildiner, M. & Wright, G.R. Smoking reduction in adults who take up exercise: a survey of a running club for adults. *CAHPER Journal 42*, 39–43 (1976)

Morgan, W.P. Psychologic aspects of heart disease. In: *Heart Disease and Rehabilitation*, ed. M.L. Pollock & D.H. Schmidt (Houghton Mifflin, Boston, 1979) pp. 105–19

Morgan, W.P., Roberts, J.A., Brand, F.R., *et al.* Psychological effect of chronic physical activity. *Med. Sci. Sports 2*, 213–17 (1970)

Morgan, W.P., Roberts, J.A. & Feinerman, A.D. Psychological effect of acute physical activity. *Arch. Phys. Med. Rehab., 52*, 422–6 (1971)

Morgan Jones, A. Heart disease and fitness for work. In: *Work and the Heart*, ed. F.F. Rosenbaum & E.L. Belknap (P.B. Hoeber, New York, 1959) pp. 400–9

Morganroth, J. & Maron, B.J. The athlete's heart syndrome: a new perspective. *Ann. N.Y. Acad. Sci., 301*, 931–9 (1977)

Moritz, A.R. & Zamchek, N. Sudden and unexpected deaths of young soldiers. *Arch. Pathol., 42*, 459–94 (1946)

Moriyama, I.M., Baum, W.S., Haenszel, W.M. & Mattison, B.

Inquiry into diagnostic evidence supporting medical certifications of death. *Amer. J. Publ. Health 48*, 1376–87 (1958)

Morris, J.N. Recent history of coronary disease. *Lancet* (i), 1–7 (1951)

Morris, J.N. The epidemiology of coronary artery disease. In: *International Symposium on Exercise and Coronary Artery Disease*, ed. T. Kavanagh (Toronto Rehabilitation Centre, Toronto, 1975) pp. 76–89

Morris, J.N., Adams, C., Chave, S.P.N., Sirey, C., Epstein, L. & Sheehan, D.J. Vigorous exercise in leisure time and the incidence of coronary heart disease. *Lancet* (i), 333–9 (1973)

Morris, J.N. & Crawford, M.D. Coronary heart disease and physical activity of work. *Brit. Med. J.* (ii), 1485–96 (1958)

Morris, J.N., Heady, J.A. & Raffle, P.A. Physique of London busmen: epidemiology of uniforms. *Lancet* (ii), 569–70 (1956)

Morris, J.N., Heady, J., Raffle, P., Roberts, C. & Parks, J. Coronary heart disease and physical activity of work. *Lancet* (ii), 1053–7, 1111–20 (1953)

Morris, J.N., Kagan, A., Pattison, D.C., Gardner, M.J. & Raffle, P.A.B. Incidence and prediction of ischaemic heart disease in London busmen. *Lancet* (ii), 553–9 (1966)

Morris, J.N. & Raffle, P.A.B. Coronary heart disease in transport workers: progress report. *Brit. J. Industr. Med., 11*, 260–4 (1954)

Most, A.S., Brachfeld, N., Gorlin, R. & Wahren, J. Free fatty acid metabolism of the human heart at rest. *J. Clin. Invest., 48*, 1177–88 (1969)

MRFIT Report of the MRFIT Research Group: contribution of weight reduction to lowering serum cholesterol. *Circulation 56*, suppl. III, 111–13 (1977)

MRFIT Multiple risk factor intervention trial research group: multiple risk factor intervention trial (MRFIT). Smoking cessation procedures and cessation and recidivism patterns for a large cohort of MRFIT participants. In: *Progress in Smoking Cessation*, ed. J.L. Schwartz (American Cancer Society, New York, 1980)

Mulcahy, R., Hickey, N. & Coghlan, N. Rehabilitation of patients with coronary heart disease. *Geriatrics 27*, 120–9 (1972)

Müller, O. & Rørvik. K. Haemodynamic consequences of coronary artery disease with observations during anginal pain and on the effect of nitroglycerine. *Brit. Heart J., 20*, 302–10 (1958)

Mullins, C.B., Leshin, S.J., Mierzwiak, D.S., Matthews, O.A. &

Blomqvist, C.G. Isometric exercise (handgrip) as a stress test for evaluation of left ventricular function. *Circulation 42*, suppl. III, 122 (abstr.) (1970)

Mullins, C.B. & Blomqvist, G. Isometric exercise and the cardiac patient. *Texas Med., 69*, 53–8 (1973)

Multicentre Trial. Propranolol in acute myocardial infarction. *Lancet* (ii), 1434–38 (1966)

Munschek, H. Primary illness of the heart and sudden death by physical activity. *Proceedings of International Congress of Sports Cardiology, Rome*, ed. T. Lubich & A. Venerando (A. Gaggi, Bologna, 1980)

Murphy, J. *The Canada Health Survey* (Health & Welfare Canada, Ottawa, 1980)

Murphy, M.L., Hultgren, H.N., Detre, K., Thomsen, J., Takaro, J. and Participants of the Veterans Administration Cooperative Study. Treatment of chronic stable angina: a preliminary report of survival data of the randomized Veterans Administration Cooperative Study. In: *Heart Disease and Rehabilitation*, ed. M.L. Pollock & D.H. Schmidt (Houghton Mifflin, Boston, Mass., 1979) pp. 228–42

Murray, J.A., Kasser, I.S., Rowell, L.B. & Bruce, R.A. Aortic pressure and oxygen transport responses to upright exercise in angina pectoris. *Circulation 37*, suppl. VI, 145 (abstr.) (1968)

Myasnikob, A.L. Influence of some factors on development of experimental cholesterol atherosclerosis. *Circulation 17*, 99–113 (1958)

Myerburg, R.J. & Davis, J.H. The medical ecology of public safety. I. Sudden death due to coronary disease. *Amer. Heart J., 68*, 586–95 (1964)

Nager, F., Thomas, M. & Shillingford, J. Changes in cardiac output and stroke volume during first four months after cardiac infarction. *Brit. Heart J., 29*, 859–70 (1967)

Nagle, R., Gangola, R. & Picton-Robinson, I. Factors influencing return to work after myocardial infarction. *Lancet 2*, 454–56 (1971)

Najmi, M. & Segal, B.L. Resting and exercise haemodynamics in patients with coronary heart disease with or without previous myocardial infarction. In: *Atherosclerotic Vascular Disease*, ed. A.N. Brest & J.H. Moyer (Appleton Century Crofts, New York, 1967) pp. 321–35

Nakhjavan, F.K., Natarajan, G., Smith, A.M., Drutch, M. &

Goldberg, H. Myocardial lactate metabolism during isometric hand-grip test — comparison with pacing tachycardia. *Brit. Heart J., 37*, 79–84 (1975)

National Diet-Heart Study Research group. The national diet-heart study. Final report. *Circulation 38*, suppl. 1, 428 (1968)

Naughton, J. *The National Exercise and Heart Disease Project. Manual of Operations* (George Washington University, Washington, D.C., 1978)

Naughton, J., Bruhn, J.G. & Lategola, M.T. Effects of physical training on physiological and behavioral characteristics of cardiac patients. *Arch. Phys. Med. Rehab., 49*, 131–7 (1968)

Naughton, J., Shanbour, K., Armstrong, R., McCoy, J. & Lategola, MT.. Cardiovascular response to exercise following myocardial infarction. *Arch. Intern. Med., 117*, 541–5 (1966)

Neill, W.A. Coronary and systemic circulatory adaptations to exercise training and their effects on angina pectoris. In: *Exercise in Cardiovascular Health and Disease*, ed. E.A. Amsterdam, J.H. Wilmore & A.N. DeMaria (Yorke Books, New York, 1977)

Neill, W.A., Duncan, D.A., Kloster, F. & Mahler, D.J. Response of coronary circulation to cutaneous cold. *Amer. J. Med., 56*, 471–6 (1974)

Nelson, R.R., Gobel, F.L., Jorgensen, C.R., Wang, K., Wang, Y & Taylor, H.L. Hemodynamic predictors of myocardial oxygen consumption during static and dynamic exercise. *Circulation 50*, 1179–89 (1974)

Nemec, E.D, Mansfield, L. & Kennedy, J.W. Heart rate and blood pressure responses during sexual activity in normal males. *Amer. Heart J., 92*, 274–7 (1964)

Newman, G. & Nichols, C.R. Sexual activities and attitudes in older persons. *JAMA, 173*, 33–7 (1960)

Niehnes, B., Tauchert, M., Behrenbeck, D.W. & Hilger, H.H. Myocardial oxygen consumption and coronary vascular resistance under the influence of calcium inhibitors. In: *Coronary Heart Disease*, ed. M. Kaltenbach, P. Lichtlen, R. Balcon, & W.P. Bussmann (G. Thieme, Stuttgart, 1978) pp. 279–83

Nielsen, B. Thermoregulation in rest and exercise. *Acta Physiol. Scand., 323*, suppl., 1–74 (1969)

Niinimaa, V., Cole, P., Mintz, S. & Shephard, R.J. Oral augmentation of ventilation. *Respiration Physiol.* (in press,

1980)

Niinimaa, V. & Shephard, R.J. Training and oxygen conductance in the elderly. I. The respiratory system. II. The cardiovascular system. *J. Gerontol., 33*, 354–61 (1978)

Noakes, T., Opie, L. & Beck, W. Coronary heart disease in marathon runners. *Ann. N.Y. Acad. Sci., 301*, 593–619 (1977)

Nolting, D., Mack, R., Luthy, E., Kirsch, M. & Hogancamp, C. Measurement of coronary blood flow and myocardial rubidium uptake with Rb[86]. *J. Clin. Invest., 37*, 921 (abstr.) (1958)

Norris, R.M., Caughey, D.E. & Scott, P.J. Trial of propranolol in acute myocardial infarction. *Brit. Med. J.* (ii), 398–400 (1968)

Nye, E.R. & Poulsen, W.T. An activity programme for coronary patients: a review of morbidity, mortality and adherence after five years. *New Zealand Med. J., 79*, 1010–13 (1974)

Oberman, A., Jones, W.B., Riley, C.P., *et al.* Natural history of coronary artery disease. *Bull. N.Y. Acad. Med., 48*, 1109–25 (1972)

O'Brien, K.P., Higgs, L.M. & Glancy, D.L. Haemodynamic accompaniments of angina. A comparison during angina induced by exercise and by atrial pacing. *Circulation 39*, 735–43 (1969)

O'Hara, W.J., Allen, C. & Shephard, R.J. Treatment of obesity by exercise in the cold. *Canad. Med. Assoc. J., 117*, 773–9 (1977)

O'Hara, W., Allen, C., Shephard, R.J. & Allen, G. Fat loss in the cold: a controlled study. *J. Appl. Physiol., 46*, 872–7 (1979)

Oldridge, N. What to look for in an exercise class leader. *Phys. Sports Med., 5*, 85–8 (1977)

Oldridge, N.B. Compliance with exercise programs. In: *Heart Disease and Rehabilitation*, ed. M.L. Pollock & D.H. Schmidt (Houghton Mifflin, Boston, 1979a) pp. 619–29

Oldridge, N.B. Compliance of post-myocardial infarction patients to exercise programs. *Med. Sci. Sports 11*, 373–5 (1979b)

Oliver, R.M. Physique and serum lipids of young London busmen in relation to ischaemic heart disease. *Brit. J. Industr. Med., 24*, 181–7 (1967)

Olson, R.E. Vitamin E and its relation to heart disease. *Circulation 48*, 179–84 (1973)

Orban, W.R. *Proceedings of National Conference on Fitness and Health* (Health & Welfare Canada, Ottawa, 1974)

Orlando, J., Aronow, W.S., Cassidy, J., *et al.* Effect of ethanol on angina pectoris. *Ann. Intern. Med., 84*, 652–5 (1976)

Osborn, G.R. *The Incubation Period of Coronary Thrombosis* (Butterworths, London, 1963)

Oscai, L.B., Molé, P.A., Brei, B. & Holloszy, J.O. Cardiac growth and respiratory enzyme levels in male rats subjected to a running program. *Amer. J. Physiol., 220*, 1238–41 (1971)

Oscai, L.B., Molé, P.A. & Holloszy, J.O. Effects of exercise on cardiac weight and mitochondria in male and female rats. *Amer. J. Physiol., 220*, 1944–8 (1971)

Oski, F.A, Miller, L.D., Delicoria-Papadopoulos, M., *et al*. Oxygen affinity in red cells: changes induced *in-vivo* by propranolol. *Science 175*, 1372–3 (1972)

Osler, W. Lectures on angina pectoris and allied states. *N.Y. Med. J., 64*, 177–83 (1896)

Ostfeld, A.M. Lebovits, B.Z., Shekelle, R.B. & Paul, O. A prospective study of the relationship between personality and coronary heart disease. *J. Chron. Dis., 17*, 265–76 (1964)

Ostrander, L.D. & Lamphiear, D.E. Oral contraceptives and physiological variables. *Circulation 58* (4), II-91 (abstr.) (1978)

Otis, A.B. The work of breathing. In: *Handbook of Physiology*, Section 3, *Respiration*, vol. 1, ed. W.O. Fenn & H. Rahn (American Physiological Society, Washington, D.C., 1964)

Paffenbarger, R. Physical activity and fatal heart attack: protection or selection? In: *Exercise in Cardiovascular Health and Disease*, ed. E.A. Amsterdam, J.H. Wilmore & A.N. deMaria (Yorke Medical Books, New York, 1977) pp. 35–49

Paffenbarger, R.S. & Hale, W.E. Work activity and coronary heart mortality. *New Engl. J. Med., 292*, 454–550 (1975)

Paffenbarger, R.S., Hale, W.E., Brand, R.J. & Hyde, R.T. Work-energy level, personal characteristics and fatal heart attack: a birth cohort effect. *Amer. J. Epidemiol., 105*, 200–13 (1977)

Paffenbarger, R.S., Laughlin, M.E., Gima, A.S., *et al*. Work activity of longshoremen as related to death from coronary heart disease and stroke. *New Engl. J. Med., 20*, 1109–14 (1970)

Paffenbarger, R.S., Wing, A.L. & Hyde, R.T. Physical activity as an index of heart attack risk in college alumni. *Amer. J. Epidemiol., 108*, 161–75 (1978)

Palatsi, I. Feasibility of physical training after myocardial infarction and its effect on return to work, morbidity and mortality. *Acta Med. Scand., 599*, suppl., 7–84 (1976)

Pařízková, J. *Body Fat and Physical Fitness* (M. Nijhoff, B.V., The Hague, 1977)

Parker, J.O., DiGiorgi, S. & West, R.O. A hemodynamic study of acute coronary insufficiency precipitated by exercise. With observations on the effects of nitroglycerin. *Amer. J. Cardiol.*, *17*, 470–83 (1966)

Parker, J.O., West, R.O. & diGiorgi, S. The haemodynamic response to exercise in patients with healed myocardial infarction without angina. *Circulation 36*, 734–49 (1967)

Parker, J.O., West, R.O., Ledwich, J.R. & diGiorgi, S. The effect of acute digitalization on the hemodynamic response to exercise in coronary artery disease. *Circulation 40*, 453–62 (1969)

Parkes, C.M., Benjamin, B. & Fitzgerald, R.G. A broken heart. A statistical study of increased mortality among widowers. *Brit. Med. J.* (i), 740–3 (1969)

Parkey, R.W., Bonte, F.J., Meyer, S.L., *et al.* A new method for radionuclide imaging of acute myocardial infarction in humans. *Circulation 50*, 540–6 (1974)

Parr, R.B. & Kerr, J.D. Liability and insurance. In: *Adult Fitness and Cardiac Rehabilitation*, ed. P.K. Wilson (University Park Press, Baltimore, Md., 1975) pp. 219–24

Parran, T.V., Hellerstein, H.K., Cohen, D. & Goldston, E. Results of studies at the work classification clinic of the Cleveland area Heart Society. In: *Work and the Heart*, ed. F.F. Rosenbaum & E.L. Belknap (P.B. Hoeber, New York, 1959) pp. 330–9

Paterson, D.H. *Alterations of Cardiovascular Function with Mild and Intense Physical Training of Post-myocardial Infarction Subjects*. Ph.D. Dissertation (University of Toronto, Toronto, 1977)

Paterson, D.H., Shephard, R.J., Cunningham, D. & Jones, N. Influence of age, angina, and time since infarction upon the cardiovascular response to physical training. *Med. Sci. Sports 12*, 100 (1980)

Paterson, D.H., Shephard, R.H., Cunningham, D., Jones, N.L. & Andrew, G. Effects of physical training upon cardiovascular function following myocardial infarction. *J. Appl. Physiol.*, *47*, 482–9 (1979)

Patton, J.F., Morgan, W.P. & Vogel, J.A. Perceived exertion of absolute work during a military training program. *Europ. J. Appl. Physiol.*, *36*, 107–14 (1977)

Paul, O. Physical activity and coronary heart disease. *Amer. J.*

Cardiol., *23*, 303–6 (1969)

Pedersen, A. & Andersen, S.N. Work test with electrocardiogram, analysis by digital computer. In: *Coronary Heart Disease & Physical Fitness*, ed. O.A. Larsen & R.O. Malmborg (University Park Press, Baltimore, Md., 1971) pp. 202–8

Pedersen-Bjergaard, O. The effect of physical training in myocardial infarction. In: *Coronary Heart Disease and Physical Fitness*, ed. O.A. Larsen & R.O. Malmborg (University Park Press, Baltimore, Md., 1971) pp. 115–16

Pedley, F.G. Coronary disease and occupation. *Canad. Med. Assoc. J.*, *46*, 147–51 (1942)

Pell, S. & D'Alonzo, C.A. Immediate mortality and five year survival of employed men with a first myocardial infarction. *New Engl. J. Med.*, *270*, 915–22 (1964)

Pelliccia, A. Influenza del lavoro muscolare sul numero e sulle funzioni delle piastrine. *Med. Del. Sport 30*, 275–82 (1978)

Penpargkul, S. & Scheuer, J. The effect of physical training upon the mechanical and metabolic performance of the rat heart. *J. Clin. Invest.*, *49*, 1859–68 (1970)

Petren, T., Sylven, B. & Sjöstrand, T. Der Einfluss des Trainings auf die Haufigkeit der Capillaren in Herz und Skelettmuskulatur. *Arbeitsphysiol.*, *9*, 376–86 (1936)

Phibbs, B., Holmes, R.W. & Lowe, C.R. Transient myocardial ischaemia. The significance of dyspnoea. *Amer. J. Med. Sci.*, *256*, 210–21 (1968)

Phipps, C. Contributory causes of coronary thrombosis. *JAMA*, *106*, 761–2 (1936)

Pinto, I.J., Thomas, P., Colaco, F., *et al*. Current developments in India. In: *Atherosclerosis II*, ed. R.J. Jones (Springer Verlag, Berlin, 1970) pp. 328–35

Plas, F. Electrocardiography. In: *Basic Book of Sports Medicine*, ed. G. LaCava (International Olympic Committee, Rome, 1978) pp. 61–5

Polednak, A.P. Longevity and cardiovascular mortality among former college athletes. *Circulation 46*, 649–54 (1972)

Polednak, A.P. & Damon, A. College atheletics, longevity, and cause of death. *Hum. Biol.*, *42*, 28–46 (1970)

Pollock, M.L. The quantification of endurance training. *Exercise Sport Sci. Rev.*, *1*, 155–88 (1973)

Pollock, M.L. Physiological characteristics of older champion track athletes. *Res. Quart.*, *45*, 363–73 (1974)

Pomeroy, W.C. & White, P.D. Coronary heart disease in former football players. *JAMA, 167*, 711–14 (1958)

Poortmans, J.R., Luke, K.H., Zipursky, A. & Bienenstock, J. Fibrinolytic activity and fibrinogen split products in exercise proteinuria. *Clin. Chim. Acta 35*, 449–54 (1971)

Poupa, O., Rakusan, K. & Ostadol, B. The effect of physical activity upon the heart of vertebrates. In: *Physical Activity and Aging*, ed. D. Brunner & E. Jokl (Karger, Basel, 1970) pp. 202–33

Powles, A.C.P., Sutton, J.R., Wicks, J.R., Oldridge, N.B. & Jones, N.L. Reduced heart rate response to exercise in ischemic heart disease: the fallacy of the target heart rate in exercise testing. *Med. Sci. Sports 11*, 227–33 (1979)

President's Council on Fitness. National adult physical fitness survey. *Newsletter*. Special edn, pp. 1–27 (May, 1973)

Price, A.B. Disability due to cardiac impairment under the disability insurance program. In: *Work and the Heart*, ed. F.F. Rosenbaum & E.L. Belknap (P.B. Hoeber, New York, 1959) pp. 499–506

Price, L. Myocardial infarction in garment workers. Characteristics and relationship to time lost from work. In: *Work and the Heart*, ed. F.F. Rosenbaum & E.L. Belknap (P.B. Hoeber, New York, 1959) pp. 387–94

Prior, I.A.M. & Davidson, F. Epidemiology of diabetes in Polynesians and Europeans in New Zealand and the Pacific. *N. Z. Med. J., 65*, 375–83 (1966)

Prior, I.A.M. & Evans, J.G. Current developments in the Pacific. In: *Atherosclerosis II*, ed. R.J. Jones (Springer Verlag, Berlin, 1970) pp. 335–42

Profant, G.R., Early, R.G., Nilson, K.L., Kusumi, F., Hofer, V. & Bruce, R.A. Responses to maximal exercise in healthy middle-aged women. *J. Appl. Physiol., 33*, 595–9 (1972)

Pugh, L.G.C.E. Physiological and medical aspects of the Himalyan Scientific and Mountaineering Expedition 1960–61. *Brit. Med. J.* (ii), 621–7 (1962)

Puska, P. *North Karelia Project. A Programme for Community Control of Cardiovascular Diseases*. University of Kuopio Community Health Series A.1 (1974)

Puska, P., Tuomiletho, J. & Salonen, J. Community control of acute myocardial infarction in Finland. *Pract. Cardiol., 10*, 91–100 (1978)

Pyfer, H. Safety precautions and procedures in cardiac exercise rehabilitation programs. In: *Heart Disease and Rehabilitation*, ed. M.L. Pollock & D.H. Schmidt (Houghton Mifflin, Boston, 1979) pp. 630–9

Pyfer, H.R. & Doane, B.L. Aspects of community exercise programs. A. Economic aspects of cardiac rehabilitation programs. In: *Exercise Testing and Exercise Training in Coronary Heart Disease*, ed. J.P. Naughton, H.K. Hellerstein & I.C. Mohler (Academic Press, New York, 1973) pp. 365–9

Pyfer, H.R., Mead, W.F. & Frederick, R.C. Cardiac arrest during medically supervised exercise training — a report of 13 successful defibrillations, *Med. Sci. Sports 7*, 72 (abstr.) (1975)

Pyörälä, K., Kärävä, R., Punsar, S., *et al*. A controlled study of the effects of 18 months' physical training in sedentary middle-aged men with high indexes of risk relative to coronary heart disease. In: *Coronary Heart Disease and Physical Fitness*, ed. O.A. Larsen & R.O. Malmborg (Munksgaard, Copenhagen, 1971) pp. 261–5

Pyörälä, K., Karvonen, M.J., Taskinen, P., Takkunen, J., Kyrönseppä, H. & Peltokallio, P. Cardiovascular studies on former endurance athletes. *Amer. J. Cardiol., 20*, 191–205 (1967a)

Pyörälä, K., Karvonen, M.J., Taskinen, P., Takkunen, J. & Kyrönseppä, H. Cardiovascular studies on former endurance athletes. In: *Physical Activity and the Heart*, ed. M.J. Karvonen & A.J. Barry (C.C. Thomas, Springfield, Ill., 1967b)

Raab, W. Training, physical activity and the cardiac dynamic cycle. *J. Sports Med. Phys. Fitness 6*, 38–47 (1966)

Rakusan, K., Ost'adal, B. & Wachtlová, M. The influence of muscular work on the capillary density in the heart and skeletal muscle of pigeon. *Canad. J. Physiol. Pharm., 49*, 167–70 (1971)

Rasmussen, R.L., Bell, R.D. & Spencer, G.D. Prepubertal exercise and myocardial collateral circulation. In: *Exercise Physiology*, ed. F. Landry &. W.A.R. Orban (Symposia Specialists, Miami, 1978)

Rautaharju, P.M., Friedrich, H. & Wolf, H. Measurement and interpretation of exercise electrocardiograms. In: *Frontiers of Fitness*, ed. R.J. Shephard (C.C. Thomas, Springfield, Ill., 1971)

Read, R.C., Murphy, M.L., Hultgren, H.N., *et al*. Survival of men treated for chronic stable angina pectoris. A cooperative randomized study. *J. Thoracic. Cardiovasc. Surg., 75*, 1–16 (1978)

Rechnitzer, P.A., Paivio, A., Pickard, H.A. & Yuhasz, M.S. Long-term follow-up study of survival and recurrence rates following myocardial infarction in exercising subjects and matched controls. *Med. Sci. Sport 3*, 502 (C) (abstr.) (1971)

Rechnitzer, P.A., Pickard, H.A., Paivio, A., Yuhasz, M.S. & Cunningham, D.A. Long-term follow-up study of survival and recurrence rates following myocardial infarction in exercising and control subjects. *Circulation 45*, 853–7 (1972)

Rechnitzer, P.A., Sangal, S., Cunningham, D., Andrew, G., Buck, C., Jones, N.L., Kavanagh, T., Parker, J.O., Shephard, R.J. & Yuhasz, M.S. A controlled prospective study of the effect of endurance training on the recurrence rate of myocardial infarction. *Amer. J. Epidemiol., 102*, 358–65 (1975)

Rechnitzer, P.A., Yuhasz, M.S., Paivio, H.A., Pickard, H.A. & Lefcoe, N. Effects of a 24-week exercise programme on normal adults and patients with previous myocardial infarction. *Brit. Med. J.* (i), 734–5 (1967)

Redwood, D.R., Rosing, D.R. & Epstein, S.E. Circulatory and symptomatic effects of physical training in patients with coronary artery disease and angina pectoris. *New Engl. J. Med., 286*, 959–65 (1972)

Rees, G., Bristow, J.D., Kremkau, E.L., Green, G.S., Herr, R.H., Griswold, H.E. & Starr, A. Influence of aortocoronary bypass surgery on left ventricular performance. *New Engl. J. Med., 284*, 1116–20 (1971)

Regestein, Q.R. & Horn, H.R. Coitus in patients with cardiac arrhythmias. *Med. Asp. Hum. Sex., 12*, 108–25 (1978)

Reid, E. *Readiness and Modifying Factors in Exercise Adoption*. Ph.D. Thesis (University of Toronto, 1979)

Reindell, H., Kleipzig, H., Steim, H., Musshoff, K., Roskamm, H. & Schildge, E. *Herz., Kreislaufkrankheiten und Sport* (Johann Ambrosius Barth, Munich, 1960)

Reindell, H., König, K. & Roskamm, H. *Funktionsdiagnostik des Gesunden und Kranken Herzens* (G. Thieme, Stuttgart, 1966)

Remington, R.D. & Schork, M.A. Determination of number of subjects needed for experimental epidemiologic studies of the effect of increased physical activity on incidence of coronary heart disease. Preliminary considerations. In: *Physical Activity and the Heart*, ed. M.J. Karvonen & A.J. Barry (C.C. Thomas, Springfield, Ill., 1967) pp. 311–19

Rennemann, R.S. *Cardiovascular Applications of Ultrasound*

(North Holland Publishing, Amsterdam, 1974)

Renson, R., Beunen, G., Ostyn, M., Simons, J. & Van Gerven, D. Soziale Bedingungen von Körperlicher Fitness. In: *Motorische Entwicklung*, ed. R. Bauss & K. Roth (Institut für Sportwissenschaft, Darmstadt, 1977) pp. 140–50

Rerych, S.K., Scholz, P.M., Newman, G.E., *et al.* Cardiac function at rest and during exercise in normals and in patients with coronary heart disease: evaluation by radionuclide angiography. *Ann. Surg., 187*, 449–64 (1978)

Richards, D.W., Bland, E.F. & White, P.D. Completed 25-year follow-up study of 200 patients with myocardial infarction. *J. Chron. Dis., 4*, 415–22 (1956)

Rigatto, M. Mass spectrometry in the study of the pulmonary circulation. *Bull. Physiol-path. Resp., 3*, 473–86 (1967)

Riley, C.P., Oberman, A., Lampton, T.D. & Hurst, D.C. Submaximal exercise testing in a random sample of an elderly population. *Circulation 42*, 43–51 (1970)

Rinzler, S.H. Primary prevention of coronary heart disease by diet. *Bull. N.Y. Acad. Med., 44*, 936–49 (1968)

Rissanen, V. Occupational physical activity and coronary artery disease. A clinico-pathological appraisal. *Adv. Cardiol., 18*, 113–21 (1976)

Rivard, G., Lavallée, H., Rajic, M., Shephard, R.J., Thibaudeau, P., Davignon, A. & Beaucage, C. Influence of competitive hockey on physical condition and psychological behaviour of children. In: *Frontiers of Activity and Child Health*, ed. H. Lavallée & R.J. Shephard (Editions du Pélican, Quebec City, 1977)

Robb, G.P. & Marks, H.H. Latent coronary artery disease. Determination of its presence and severity by the exercise electrocardiogram. *Amer. J. Cardiol., 13*, 603–18 (1964)

Robb, G.P. & Seltzer, F. Appraisal of the double two-step exercise test. A long-term follow-up study of 3,325 men. *JAMA, 234*, 722–7 (1975)

Robinson, B.F. Relationship of heart rate and systolic blood pressure to the onset of pain in angina pectoris. *Circulation 35*, 1073–83 (1967)

Robinson, B.F. Mode of action of nitroglycerin in angina pectoris. *Brit. Heart J., 30*, 295–301 (1968)

Robinson, J.S., Sloman, G., Mathew, T.H. & Goble, A.J. Survival after resuscitation from cardiac arrest in acute myocardial infarction. *Amer. Heart J., 69*, 740–7 (1965)

Robinson, S. Experimental studies of physical fitness in relation to age. *Arbeitsphysiol., 4*, 251–323 (1938)

Robinson, S., Pearcy, M., Brueckman, F.R., Nicholas, J.R. & Miller, D.I. Effects of atropine on heart rates and oxygen intake in working man. *J. Appl. Physiol., 5*, 508–12 (1953)

Rochelle, R.H., Stumpner, R.L., Robinson, S., Dill, D.B. & Horvath, S.M. Peripheral blood flow response to exercise consequent to physical training. *Med. Sci. Sports 3*, 122–9 (1971)

Rochmis, P. & Blackburn, H. Exercise tests. A survey of procedures, safety and litigation experience in approximately 170,000 tests. *JAMA, 217*, 1061–6 (1971)

Rodbard, S., Williams, F. & Williams, C. The spherical dynamics of the heart (myocardial tension, oxygen consumption, coronary blood flow and efficiency). *Amer. Heart J., 57*, 348–60 (1959)

Rode, A., Ross., R. & Shephard, R.J. Smoking withdrawal program. *AMA Arch. Env. Health 24*, 27–36 (1972)

Rode, A. & Shephard, R.J. Cardio-respiratory fitness of an Arctic community. *J. Appl. Physiol., 31*, 519–26 (1971a)

Rode, A. & Shephard, R.J. The influence of cigarette smoking upon the work of breathing in near maximal exercise. *Med. Sci. Sports 3*, 51–5 (1971b)

Rodstein, M., Wolloch, L. & Gubner, R.S. A mortality study of the significance of extrasystoles in an uninsured population. *Circulation 44*, 617–25 (1971)

Rollett, E.L., Yurchak, P.M., Hood, W.B. & Gorlin, R. Pressure-volume correlates of left ventricular oxygen consumption in the hypervolumic dog. *Circ. Res., 17*, 499–518 (1965)

Romo, M. Factors relating to sudden death in acute ischaemic heart disease. A community study in Helsinki. *Acta Med. Scand., 547*, suppl. (1972)

Rook, A. An investigation into the longevity of Cambridge sportsmen. *Brit. Med. J.* (i), 773–7 (1954)

Rose, C.L. & Cohen, M.L. Relative importance of physical activity for longevity. *Ann. N.Y. Acad. Sci., 301*, 671–97 (1977)

Rose, G. Current developments in Europe. In: *Atherosclerosis II*, ed. R.J. Jones (Springer Verlag, Berlin, 1970) pp. 310–14

Rose, G., Prineas, R.J. & Mitchell, J.R. Myocardial infarction and the intrinsic calibre of coronary arteries. *Brit. Heart J., 29*, 548–52 (1967)

Rosenman, R.H. The influence of different exercise patterns on the incidence of coronary heart disease in the western collaborative group study. In: *Physical Activity and Aging*, ed. D. Brunner & E. Jokl (University Park Press, Baltimore, Md., 1970) pp. 267–73

Rosenman, R.H., Bawol, R.D. & Oscherwitz, M. A 4-year prospective study of the relationship of different habitual vocational physical activity to risk and incidence of ischemic heart disease in volunteer male federal employees. *Ann. N.Y. Acad. Sci., 301*, 627–41 (1977)

Roskamm, H. General circulatory adjustment to exercise in well-trained subjects. In: *Coronary Heart Disease and Physical Fitness*, ed. O.A. Larsen & R.O. Malmborg (University Park Press, Baltimore, Md., 1971) pp. 17–20

Roskamm, H. Limits and age dependency in the adaptation of the heart to physical stress. In: *Sport in the Modern World — Chances and Problems*, ed. O. Grupe, D. Kurz & J.M. Teipel (Springer Verlag, Berlin, 1973a)

Roskamm, H. Myocardial contractility during exercise. In: *Limiting Factors of Physical Performance*, ed. J. Keul (G. Thieme, Stuttgart, 1973b) pp. 225–34

Roskamm, H. & Reindell, H. The heart and circulation of the superior athlete. In: *Training — Scientific Basis and Application*, ed. A.W. Taylor (C.C. Thomas, Springfield, Ill., 1972)

Ross, J. Factors regulating the oxygen consumption of the heart. In: *Changing Concepts in Cardiovascular Disease*, ed. H.I. Russek & B.L. Zohman (Williams & Wilkins, Baltimore, 1972)

Ross, J., Gault, J.H., Mason, D.T., Linhart, J.W. & Braunwald, E. Left ventricular performance during muscular exercise in patients with and without cardiac dysfunction. *Circulation 34*, 597–608 (1966)

Ross, R.S. Ischemic heart disease. An overview. *Amer. J. Cardiol., 36*, 496–505 (1975)

Rothlin, M., Gattiker, K., Huber, R. & Krombach, D. Left ventricular function before and after resection of left ventricular aneurysm. In: *Coronary Heart Disease*, ed. M. Kaltenbach, P. Lichtlen & G.C. Friesinger (G. Thieme, Stuttgart, 1973) pp. 219–22

Rousseau, M., Brasseur, L.A. & Detry, J.M. Haemodynamic determinants of maximal oxygen intake in patients with healed myocardial infarction: influence of physical training. *Circulation 48*, 943–9 (1973)

Rousseau, M., Degré, S., Brasseur, L.A., Denolin, H. & Detry, J.M. Haemodynamic effects of early physical training after acute myocardial infarction, comparison with a control untrained group. *Europ. J. Cardiol., 2*, 29–45 (1974)

Rowe, G.G. The nitrous oxide method for determining coronary blood flow in man. *Amer. Heart J., 58*, 268–81 (1959)

Rowell, L.B. Human cardiovascular adjustments to exercise and thermal stress. *Physiol. Rev., 54*, 75–159 (1974)

Rumball, A. & Acheson, E.D. Latent coronary heart disease detected by electrocardiogram before and after exercise. *Brit. Med. J.* (i), 423–8 (1963)

Ruskin, H.D., Stein, L.L., Shelsky, I.M., *et al*. M.M.P.I. comparison between patients with coronary heart disease and their spouses and other demographic data. *Scand. J. Rehab. Med., 2*, 99–104 (1970)

Russek, H.I. Emotional stress, tobacco smoking and ischemic heart disease. In: *Prevention of Ischemic Heart Disease. Principles and Practice* (C.C. Thomas, Springfield, Ill., 1966) pp. 190–200

Russek, H.I. Propranolol and isosorbide dinitrate synergism in angina pectoris. *Amer. J. Cardiol., 21*, 44–5 (1968)

Russek, H.I. Medical versus surgical therapy in angina pectoris. *Geriatrics 25*, 93–102 (1970)

Russek, H.I. & Russek, L.G. Behavior patterns and emotional stress in the etiology of coronary heart disease: sociological and occupational aspects. In: *Stress and the Heart*, ed. D. Wheatley (Raven Press, New York, 1977)

Russek, H.I. & Zohman, B.L. Relative significance of heredity, diet and occupational stress in coronary heart disease in young adults. *Amer. J. Med. Sci., 235*, 266–75 (1958)

Russek, H.I. & Zohman B.L. The natural history of coronary atherosclerosis. In: *Coronary Heart Disease*, ed. H.I. Russek & B.L. Zohman (Lippincott, Philadelphia, 1971) pp. 167–76

Rutishauser, W., Amende, I., Mehmel, H., Krayenbühl, H.P. & Schönbeck, M. Relaxation of the left ventricle in patients with coronary artery disease. In: *Coronary Heart Disease*, ed. M. Kaltenbach, P. Lichtlen & G.C. Friesinger (G. Thieme, Stuttgart, 1973) pp. 167–72

Ryhming, I. A modified Harvard step test for the evaluation of physical fitness. *Arbeitsphysiol., 15*, 235–50 (1954)

Ryle, J.A. & Russel, W.T. The natural history of coronary disease: clinical and epidemiological study. *Brit. Heart J., 11*, 370–89

(1949)

Sagall, E.L. Legal implications of cardiac rehabilitation programmes. In: *Heart Disease and Rehabilitation*, ed. M.L. Pollock & D.H. Schmidt (Houghton Mifflin, Boston, 1979) pp. 640–9

Saltin, B. Physiological effects of physical conditioning. *Med. Sci. Sports 1*, 50–6 (1969)

Saltin, B. Oxygen transport by the circulatory system during exercise. In: *Limiting Factors of Physical Performance*, ed. J. Keul (G. Thieme, Stuttgart, 1973)

Saltin, B. & Åstrand, P.O. Maximal oxygen uptake in athletes. *J. Appl. Physiol., 23*, 353–8 (1967)

Saltin, B., Blomqvist, G., Mitchell, J.H., Johnson, R.L., Wildenthal, K. & Chapman, C.B. Response to exercise after bed rest and after training. *Amer. Heart Assoc. Monograph 23* (Circulation 37–8, Suppl. 7), 1–68 (1968)

Saltin, B. & Grimby, G. Physiological analysis of middle-aged and old former athletes. Comparison with still active athletes of the same ages. *Circulation 38*, 1104–15 (1968)

Saltin, B. & Karlsson, J. Muscle ATP, CP, and lactate during exercise after physical conditioning. In: *Muscle Metabolism during Exercise*, ed. B. Pernow & B. Saltin (Plenum Press, New York, 1971) pp. 395–9

Saltzman, S.H., Hellerstein, H.K., Radke, J.D., Maistelman, H.W. & Ricklin, R. Quantitative effects of physical conditioning on the exercise electrocardiogram of middle-aged subjects with atherosclerotic heart disease. In: *Measurement in Exercise Electrocardiography*, ed. H. Blackburn (C.C. Thomas, Springfield, Ill., 1969) pp. 388–410

Samson, W.E. & Scher, A.M. Mechanism of S-T segment alteration during acute myocardial injury. *Circ. Res., 8*, 780–7 (1960)

Sanders, T.M., White, F.C. & Bloor, C.M. Myocardial blood flow distribution in the conscious pig during steady state and exhaustive exercise. *Fed. Proc., 34*, 414 (abstr.) (1975)

Sanders, T.M., White, F.C., Peterson, T.M. & Bloor, C.M. Effects of endurance exercise on coronary collateral blood flow in miniature swine. *Amer. J. Physiol., 234*, 614–19 (1978)

Sandler, H. & Dodge, H.T. Angiographic methods for determination of left ventricular geometry and volume. In: *Cardiac Mechanics: Physiological, Clinical and Mathematical*

Considerations, ed. I. Mirsky, D. Ghista & H. Sandler (Wiley, New York, 1974) pp. 141–70

Sanne, H. (in collaboration with D. Elmfeldt, G. Grimby, C. Rydin & L. Wilhelmsen). Exercise tolerance and physical training of non-selected patients after myocardial infarction. *Acta Med. Scand.*, *551*, suppl., 1–124 (1973)

Sanne, H., Elmfeldt, D. & Wilhelmsen, L. Preventive effect of physical training after a myocardial infarction. In: *Preventive Cardiology*, ed. G. Tibblin, A. Keys & L. Werko (John Wiley, New York, 1972) p. 154

Sanne, H. & Sivertsson, R. The effect of exercise on the development of collateral circulation after experimental occlusion of the femoral artery in the cat. *Acta Physiol. Scand.*, *73*, 257–63 (1968)

Sannerstedt, R. Hemodynamic response to exercise in patients with arterial hypertension. *Acta Med. Scand.*, *458*, suppl. (1966)

Sarnoff, S.J., Braunwald, E., Welch, G.H., Case, R.B., Stainsby, W.N. & Macruz, R. Hemodynamic determinants of oxygen consumption of the heart with special reference to the tension time index. *Amer. J. Physiol.*, *192*, 148–56 (1958)

Sarvotham, S.G. & Berry, J.N. Prevalence of coronary heart disease in an urban population in Northern India. *Circulation 37*, 939–53 (1968)

Sayed, J., Schaefer, O. & Hildes, J.A. Biochemical indices of nutrition of the Iglooligmiut. In: *Circumpolar Health*, ed. R.J. Shephard & S. Itoh (University of Toronto Press, Toronto, 1976) pp. 130–4

Schad, N. Nontraumatic assessment of left ventricular wall motion and regional stroke volume after myocardial infarction. *J. Nucl. Med.*, *18*, 333–41 (1977)

Schaefer, O. Vigorous exercise and coronary heart disease. *Lancet* (i), 840 (abstr.) (1973)

Scheidt, S., Aschein, R. & Killip, T. Shock after acute myocardial infarction. A clinical and hemodynamic profile. *Amer. J. Cardiol.*, *26*, 556–64 (1970)

Scheingold, L.D. & Wagner, N.N. *Sound Sex and the Aging Heart* (Human Sciences Press, New York, 1974) pp. 137–41

Schettler, G. Keynote address. In: *Atherosclerosis*, ed. R.J. Jones (Springer Verlag, Berlin, 1970) pp. xxvii–xxxii

Schettler, G. Atherosclerosis, the main problem of the industrialized societies. In: *Atherosclerosis IV*, ed. G. Schettler,

Y. Goto, Y. Hata & G. Klose (Springer Verlag, Berlin, 1977)

Scheuer, J. Physical training and intrinsic cardiac adaptation. *Circulation 47*, 677–80 (1973)

Scheuer, J., Penpargkul, S. & Bhan, A.K. Experimental observations on the effects of physical training upon intrinsic cardiac physiology and biochemistry. *Amer. J. Cardiol., 33*, 744–51 (1974)

Scheuer, J., Penpargkul, S. & Bhan, A.K. Experimental observations on the effects of physical training upon intrinsic cardiac physiology and biochemistry. In: *Exercise in Cardiovascular Health and Disease*, ed. E.A. Amsterdam, J.H. Wilmore & A.N. DeMaria (Yorke Medical Books, New York, 1977) pp. 108–21

Schlant, R.C. Altered cardiovascular physiology of coronary atherosclerotic heart disease. In: *The Heart*, ed. J. Willis Hurst (McGraw Hill, New York, 1974) pp. 1017–37

Schmale, A.H. & Engel, G.L. The giving up-given up complex. *Arch. Gen. Psychiatr., 17*, 135–45 (1967)

Schmid, L. & Hornof, Z. Sudden death in Czechoslovakian sports. *Brit. J. Sports Med., 7*, 156–8 (1973)

Schmidt, D.H., Blau, F.M., Carpenter, J.G. & Hellman, C.K. The clinical and research application of nuclear cardiology. In: *Heart Disease and Rehabilitation*, ed. M.L. Pollock & D.H. Schmidt (Houghton Mifflin, Boston, 1979) pp. 183–202

Schnor, P. Longevity and cause of death in male athletic champions. *Lancet* (ii), 1364–6 (1971)

Schwade, J., Blomqvist, C.G. & Shapiro, W. A comparison of the response to arm and leg work in patients with ischemic heart disease. *Amer. Heart J., 94*, 203–8 (1977)

Scott, R.F., Florentin, R.A., Daoud, A.S., Morrison, E.S., Jones, R.M. & Hutt, M.S.R. Coronary arteries of children and young adults. A comparison of lipids and anatomic features in New Yorkers and East Africans. *Exp. Mol. Pathol., 5*, 12–42 (1966)

Scott, R.F., Likimani, J.C., Morrison, E.S., Thuku, J.J. & Thomas, W.A. Esterified serum fatty acids in subjects eating high and low cholesterol diets. A comparative study of serum lipid metabolism in New Yorkers, indigenous poor East Africans and upper class East Africans. *Amer. J. Clin. Nutr., 13*, 82–91 (1963)

Scrimshaw, N.S. & Guzman, M.A. Diet and atherosclerosis. *Lab. Invest., 18*, 623–8 (1968)

Segers, M.J. & Mertens, C. Psychological and bioclinical CHD risk factors, quantitative differences between obese, normal and thin subjects. *J. Psychosom. Res., 18*, 403–11 (1974)

Selye, H. On the real benefits of eustress. *Psychol. Today 11*, 60–70 (1978)

Semple, T. *Myocardial Infarction. How to Prevent, How to Rehabilitate* (Council on Rehabilitation of International Society of Cardiology, Brussels, 1973)

Semple, T. Acceleration of collaterals by physical activity. In: *Critical Evaluation of Cardiac Rehabilitation*, ed. J.J. Kellermann & H. Denolin (Karger, Basel, 1977) pp. 141–2

Seymour, J. & Conway, N. Value of dual reports on routine electrocardiograms. *Brit. Heart J., 31*, 610–12 (1969)

Shah, V.V., Shah, S.R. & Panse, V.N. Nutritional and physical factors in coronary heart disease. *Geriatrics 23*, 99–103 (1968)

Shaper, A.G. Current developments in atherosclerosis in Africa. In: *Atherosclerosis II*, ed. R.J. Jones (Springer Verlag, Berlin, 1970) pp. 314–20

Shapiro, A.P., Schwartz, G.E., Ferguson, D.C., *et al*. Behavioral methods in the treatment of hypertension. A review of their clinical status. *Ann. Intern. Med., 86*, 626–36 (1977)

Shapiro, S., Weinblatt, E., Frank, C.W. & Sager, R.V. Incidence of coronary heart disease in a population insured for medical care (HIP). *Amer. J. Publ. Health 59*, suppl. 1–101 (1969)

Sharland, D.E. Ability of men to return to work after cardiac infarction. *Brit. Med. J., 2*, 718–20 (1964)

Sharma, B., Goodwin, J.F. & Steiner, R.E. Left ventriculography during angina induced by exercise and atrial pacing. *Amer. J. Cardiol., 37*, 172 (abstr.) (1976)

Sheets, M.F., Eckberg, D.L. & Heisted, D.D. Impairment of autonomic heart rate responses by local sinus node hypoxemia. *Fed. Proc., 34*, 420 (abstr.) (1975)

Sheffield, L.T. The meaning of exercise test findings. In: *Coronary Heart Disease. Prevention, Detection, Rehabilitation, with Emphasis on Exercise Testing*, ed. S.M. Fox (International Medical Corporation, Denver, Col., 1974) pp. (9-1)–(9-35)

Sheffield, L.T. & Roitman, D. Systolic blood pressure, heart rate and treadmill work at anginal threshold. *Chest, 63*, 327–35 (1973)

Sheldon, W.C., Rincon, G., Effler, D.B., *et al*. Surgical treatment of coronary artery disease: pure graft operations, with a study of 741 patients followed 3–7 years. *Progr. Cardiovasc. Dis., 18*,

237–53 (1975)

Sheldon, W.C., Sones, F.M., Shirey, E.K., Fergusson, D.J.G., Favaloro, R.G. & Effler, D.B. Reconstructive coronary artery surgery: post-operative assessment. *Circulation 39*, suppl., 61–6 (1969)

Shephard, R.J. Partitional respirometry in human subjects. *J. Appl. Physiol., 13*, 357–67 (1959)

Shephard, R.J. The development of cardiorespiratory fitness. *Med. Services J., Canada 21*, 533–44 (1965)

Shephard, R.J. The oxygen cost of breathing during vigorous exercise. *Quart. J. Exp. Physiol., 51*, 336–50 (1966)

Shephard, R.J. Normal levels of activity in Canadian city-dwellers. *Canad. Med. Assoc. J., 97*, 313–18 (1967a)

Shephard, R.J. The prediction of 'maximal' oxygen consumption using a new progressive step test. *Ergonomics 10*, 1–15 (1967b)

Shephard, R.J. Intensity, duration and frequency of exercise as determinants of the response to a training regime. *Int. Z. Angew. Physiol., 26*, 272–8 (1968a)

Shephard, R.J. Oscillations of acid-base equilibrium during maximum exercise. *Int. Z. Angew. Physiol., 26*, 258–71 (1968b)

Shephard, R.J. A nomogram to calculate the oxygen cost of running at slow speeds. *J. Sports Med. Phys. Fitness 9*, 10–16 (1968c)

Shephard, R.J. Learning, habituation and training. *Int. Z. Angew. Physiol., 26*, 272–8 (1969)

Shephard, R.J. Standard tests of aerobic power. In: *Frontiers of Fitness*, ed. R.J. Shephard (C.C. Thomas, Springfield, Ill., 1971) pp. 233–64

Shephard, R.J. The influences of race and environment on ischemic heart disease. *Canad. Med. Ass. J., 111*, 1336–40 (1974a)

Shephard, R.J. Sudden death — a significant hazard of exercise? *Brit. J. Sports Med., 8*, 101–10 (1974b)

Shephard, R.J. Exercise test methodology. In: *Coronary Disease. Exercise Testing, Rehabilitation Therapy*, ed. S.M. Fox (International Medical Corporation, Denver, Col., 1974c)

Shephard, R.J. *Men at Work: Applications of Ergonomics to Performance and Design* (C.C. Thomas, Springfield, Ill., 1974d)

Shephard, R.J. Future research on the quantifying of endurance training. *J. Human Ergol., 3*, 163–81 (1975)

Shephard, R.J. Coronary artery disease — the magnitude of the problem. In: *Proceedings of International Symposium on*

Exercise and Coronary Artery Disease, ed. T. Kavanagh (Toronto Rehabilitation Centre, Toronto, 1976)

Shephard, R.J. *Endurance Fitness*, 2nd edn (University of Toronto Press, Toronto, 1977a)

Shephard, R.J. Exercise-induced bronchospasm — a review. *Med. Sci. Sports 9*, 1–10 (1977b)

Shephard, R.J. *Human Physiological Work Capacity* (Cambridge University Press, London, 1978a)

Shephard, R.J. *Physical Activity and Aging* (Croom Helm, London, 1978b)

Shephard, R.J. *The Fit Athlete* (Oxford University Press, London, 1978c)

Shephard, R.J. Recurrence of myocardial infarction in an exercising population. *Brit. Heart J., 42*, 133–8 (1979a)

Shephard, R.J. Cardiac rehabilitation in prospect. In: *Heart Disease and Rehabilitation*, ed. M.L. Pollock and D.H. Schmidt (Houghton Mifflin, Boston, 1979b) pp. 521–47

Shephard, R.J. Current status and prospects for post-coronary exercise multicentre studies. *Med. Sci. Sports 11*, 383–5 (1979c)

Shephard, R.J. Current status of the Canadian Home Fitness Test. *S. Afr. J. Sports Sci., 2*, 19–35 (1980a)

Shephard, R.J. Recurrence of myocardial infarction. Observations on patients participating in the Ontario Multi-Centre Exercise-heart Trial. *Europ. J. Cardiol., 11*, 147–57 (1980b)

Shephard, R.J. *Textbook of Exercise Physiology and Biochemistry* (Prager, Philadelphia, 1980c)

Shephard, R.J. Evaluation of earlier studies — Canadian study. In: *N.I.H. Conference on Exercise and Cardiac Rehabilitation, May 1979*, ed. N. Epstein (Bethesda, Md., 1980d)

Shephard, R.J. A critique: coronary disease and exercise stress tests. *Canad. Fam. Physician 26*, 555–9 (1980e)

Shephard, R.J. The sick sinus syndrome. *Med. Sci. Sports* (in press, 1980f)

Shephard, R.J., Allen, C., Benade, A.J.S., Davies, C.T.M., diPrampero, P.E., Hedman, R., Merriman, J.E., Myhre, K. & Simmons, R. The maximum oxygen intake — an international reference standard of cardio-respiratory fitness. *Bull. WHO, 38*, 757–64 (1968a)

Shephard, R.J., Allen, C., Benade, A.J.S., Davies, C.T.M., diPrampero, P.E., Hedman, R., Merriman, J.E., Myhre, K. & Simmons, R. Standardization of sub-maximal exercise tests.

Bull. WHO, 38, 765–76 (1968b)

Shephard, R.J., Corey, P. & Kavanagh, T. Exercise compliance and the prevention of a recurrence of myocardial infarction. *Can. J. Appl. Sports Sci., 4*, 236 (1979a)

Shephard, R.J. & Cox, M. Some characteristics of participants in an industrial fitness programme. *Canad. J. Appl. Sports Sci., 5*, 69–76 (1980)

Shephard, R.J., Cox, M. and Simper, K. *An Analysis of 'Par-Q' Responses in an Office Population* (Fitness & Amateur Sport Branch, Department of National Health & Welfare, 1979b)

Shephard, R.J., Hatcher, J. & Rode, A. On the body composition of the Eskimo. *Europ. J. Appl. Physiol., 30*, 1–13 (1973)

Shephard, R.J., Jones, C. & Brown, J.R. Some observations on the fitness of a Canadian population. *Canad. Med. Assoc. J., 98*, 977–84 (1968c)

Shephard, R.J. & Kavanagh, T. Biochemical changes with marathon running — observations on 'post-coronary' patients. In: *Metabolic Adaptations to prolonged Exercise*, ed. J.R. Poortmans & H. Howald (Karger, Basel, 1975)

Shephard, R.J. & Kavanagh, T. Predicting the exercise catastrophe in the post-coronary patient. *Canad. Fam. Phys., 24*, 614–18 (1978a)

Shephard, R.J. & Kavanagh, T. Does 'post-coronary' rehabilitation increase longevity? In: *Proceedings of International Conference on Sports Cardiology*, ed. A. Venerando (Fondazione Giovanni Lorenzi, Rome, 1978b)

Shephard, R.J. & Kavanagh, T. On the stage duration for a progressive exercise test protocol. In: *Physical Fitness Assessment*, ed. R.J. Shephard & H. Lavallée (C.C. Thomas, Springfield, Ill., 1978c) pp. 335–44

Shephard, R.J. & Kavanagh, T. Patient reactions to a regular conditioning programme following myocardial infarction. *J. Sports Med. Phys. Fitness 18*, 373–8 (1978d)

Shephard, R.J., Kavanagh, T. & Moore, R. Fluid and mineral balance of post-coronary distance runners. Studies on the 1975 Boston marathon. In: *Nutrition, Dietetics and Sport*, ed. G. Ricci & A. Venerando (Ed. Minerva Medica, Torino, 1978a) pp. 217–28

Shephard, R.J., Killinger, D. & Fried, T. Responses to sustained use of anabolic steroid. *Brit. J. Sports Med., 11*, 170–3 (1977a)

Shephard, R.J. & Lavallée, H. Probleme der Längsschnittuntersuchung motorischer Entwicklung. In: *Motorische Entwicklung. Probleme und Ergebnisse von Längsschnittuntersuchungen*, ed. R. Bauss & K. Roth (Institüt für Sportwissenschaft, Darmstadt, 1977)

Shephard, R.J., Lavallée, H., Jéquier, J.C., LaBarre, R., Rajic, M. & Beaucage, C. Seasonal differences in aerobic power. In: *Physical Fitness Assessment: Principles, Practice and Application*, ed. R.J. Shephard & H. Lavallée (C.C. Thomas, Springfield, Ill., 1978b) pp. 194–210

Shephard, R.J., Lavallée, H., Jéquier, J.C., Rajic, M. & Beaucage, C. Un programme complémentaire d'éducation physique. Etude préliminaire de l'expérience pratiquée dans le district de Trois Rivières. In: *Facteurs Limitant l'Endurance Humaine*, ed. J.R. LaCour (Université de St. Etienne, St Etienne, France, 1977b)

Shephard, R.J., Morgan, P., Finucane, R. & Schimmelfing, L. Factors influencing participation in an employee fitness programme. *J. Occup. Med., 22*, 389–98 (1980a)

Shephard, R.J., Rode, A. & Ross, R. Reinforcement of a smoking withdrawal program: the role of the physiologist and the psychologist. *Canad. J. Publ. Health 64*, S41–S51 (1972)

Shephard, R.J. & Sidney, K.H. Effects of physical exercise on plasma growth hormone and cortisol levels in human subjects. *Ex. Sport Sci. Rev., 3*, 1–30 (1975)

Shephard, R.J., Youldon, P.E., Cox, M. & West, C. Effects of a 6-month industrial fitness programme on serum lipid concentrations. *Atherosclerosis 35*, 277–85 (1980b)

Sherman, M. *Diet, Lipid Metabolism and Atherosclerosis* (US Department of Health, Education and Welfare, Bethesda, Md., 1964)

Sidney, K.H. & Shephard, R.J. Physiological characteristics and performance of the whitewater paddler. *Int. Z. Angew. Physiol., 32*, 55–70 (1973)

Sidney, K.H. & Shephard, R.J. Attitudes towards health and physical activity in the elderly. Effects of a physical training programme. *Med. Sci. Sports 8*, 246–52 (1977a)

Sidney, K.H. & Shephard, R.J. Training and e.c.g. abnormalities in the elderly. *Brit. Heart J., 39*, 1114–20 (1977b)

Sidney, K.H. & Shephard, R.J. Maximum and sub-maximum exercise tests in men and women in the seventh, eighth and ninth decades of life. *J. Appl. Physiol., 43*, 280–7 (1977c)

Sidney, K.H. & Shephard, R.J. Frequency and intensity of exercise as determinants of the response to training in elderly subjects. *Med. Sci. Sports 10*, 125–31 (1978)

Sidney, K.H., Shephard, R.J. & Harrison. J. Endurance training and body composition of the elderly. *Amer. J. Clin. Nutr., 30*, 326–33 (1977)

Siegel, G.H. The law and cardiac rehabilitation. A. Legal aspects of informed consent. In: *Exercise Testing and Exercise Training in Coronary Heart Disease*, ed. J. Naughton, H.K. Hellerstein & I.C. Mohler (Academic Press, New York, 1973) pp. 387–413

Siegel, W. Exercise-induced indicators of coronary atherosclerotic heart disease. In: *Coronary Heart Disease. Prevention, Detection, Rehabilitation, with Emphasis on Exercise Testing*, ed. S.M. Fox (International Medical Corporation, Denver, Colorado, 1974) pp. (3-1)–(3-21)

Siegel, W., Blomqvist, G. & Mitchell, J.H. Effects of a quantitated physical training program on middle-aged sedentary men. *Circulation 41*, 19–29 (1970)

Sigwart, U., Schmidt, H., Bonzel, T., *et al.* Biplane cineangiographic evaluation of left ventricular contraction in ischemic heart disease at rest and during bicycle exercise. *Circulation 51/52*, suppl. II, 37 (141) (abstr.) (1975)

Siltanen, P. Mobile coronary care unit and sudden coronary death. In: *Sudden Coronary Death*, ed. V. Manninen & P.I. Halonen (Karger, Basel, 1978) pp. 193–5

Siltanen, P., Lauroma, M., Mirkko, O., *et al.* Psychological characteristics related to coronary heart disease. *J. Psychosom. Res., 19*, 183–95 (1975)

Sim, D.N. & Neill, W.A. Investigation of the physiological basis for increased exercise threshold for angina pectoris after physical conditioning. *J. Clin. Invest., 54*, 763–70 (1974)

Simmons, R. & Shephard, R.J. Effects of physical conditioning upon the central and peripheral circulatory responses to arm work. *Int. Z. Angew. Physiol., 30*, 73–84 (1971a)

Simmons, R. & Shephard, R.J. Measurement of cardiac output in maximum exercise. Application of an acetylene rebreathing method to arm and leg exercise. *Int. Z. Angew. Physiol., 29*, 159–72 (1971b)

Simonson, E. & Berman, R. Myocardial infarction in young people — experience in USSR. *Amer. Heart J., 84*, 814–22 (1972)

Simoons, M.L. *Computer Assisted Interpretation of Exercise*

Electrocardiograms (Bronder-Offset B.V., Rotterdam, 1976)

Simoons, M.L. Computer processing of exercise electro-cardiograms: In: *Coronary Heart Disease, Exercise Testing and Cardiac Rehabilitation*, ed. W.E. James & E.A. Amsterdam (Symposia Specialists, Miami, Fla., 1977) pp. 154–64

Simpson, F.O. Beta-adrenergic receptor blocking drugs in hypertension. *Drugs 7*, 85–105 (1974)

Singer, A. & Rob, C. The fate of the claudicator. *Brit. Med. J.* (ii), 633–6 (1960)

Skelton, M. & Dominian, J. Psychological stress in wives of patients with myocardial infarction. *Brit. Med. J.* (ii), 101–3 (1973)

Skinner, J.S. Sexual relations and the cardiac patient. In: *Heart Disease and Rehabilitation*, ed. M.L. Pollock & D.H. Schmidt (Houghton Mifflin, Boston, 1979) pp. 587–99

Smith, C., Sauls, H.C. & Ballew, J. Coronary occlusion: a clinical study of 100 patients. *Ann. Int. Med., 17*, 681–92 (1942)

Smith, E.B., Evans, P.H. & Downham, M.D. Lipid in the aortic intima: the correlation of morphological and chemical characteristics. *J. Atheroscler. Res., 7*, 171–86 (1967)

Smith, E.E., Guyton, A.C., Manning, R.D. & White, R.J. Integrated mechanisms of cardiovascular response and control during exercise in the normal human. *Progr. Cardiovasc. Dis., 18*, 421–43 (1976)

Smith, E.P. Lipoproteins — steady state aspects. In: *Atherosclerosis IV*, ed. G. Schettler, Y. Goto, Y. Hata & G. Klose (Springer Verlag, Berlin, 1977)

Smoking and Health. Report of the Advisory Committee to the Surgeon General of the Public Health Service. Public Health Service Publication 1103 (US Government Printing Office, Washington, D.C., 1964) pp. 1–387

Smoking in Canada. Health and Welfare, Canada, Bulletin 5 (1973) pp. 101–6

Snow, J. *On the Mode of Communication of Cholera*, 2nd edn (Churchill, London, 1855)

Society of Actuaries. *Build and Blood Pressure Study* (Society of Actuaries, Chicago, 1959)

Sodhi, H.S., Kudchodkar, B.J., Mason, D.T. & Borhani, N. Relationships between metabolism of cholesterol and the turnover of plasma lipoproteins. In: *Atherosclerosis IV*, ed. G. Schettler, Y. Goto, Y. Hata & G. Klose (Springer Verlag, Berlin, 1977) pp. 298–301

Sohar, E. & Sneh, E. Follow-up of obese patients: 14 years after a successful reducing diet. *Amer. J. Clin. Nutr., 26*, 845–8 (1973)

Sonnenblick, E.H. Oxygen consumption of the heart. In: *Coronary Heart Disease and Physical Fitness*, ed. O.A. Larsen & R.O. Malmborg (University Park Press, Baltimore, Md., 1971) pp. 89–92

Sonnenblick, E.H., Ross, J., Covell, J.W., Kaiser, G.A. & Braunwald, E. Velocity of contraction as a determinant of myocardial oxygen consumption. *Amer. J. Physiol., 209*, 919–27 (1965)

Spain, D.M. & Bradess, V.A. The relationship of coronary thrombosis to coronary atherosclerosis and ischaemic heart disease. *Amer. J. Med. Sci., 240*, 701–10 (1960a)

Spain, D.M. & Bradess, V.A. Occupational physical activity and the degree of coronary atherosclerosis in 'normal' men. A post-mortem study. *Circulation 22*, 239–42 (1960b)

Stamler, J. Acute myocardial infarction — progress in primary prevention. *Brit. Heart J., 33*, suppl., 145–64 (1971)

Stamler, J. (With Coronary Drug Project Research Group). Clofibrate and niacin in coronary heart disease. *JAMA, 231*, 360–81 (1975)

Stamler, J. Improving life styles to control the coronary epidemic. In: *Nutrition, Dietetics and Sport*, ed. G. Ricci & A. Venerando (Ed. Minerva Medica, Torino, 1978) pp. 5–48

Stamler, J., Berkson, D.M., Lindberg, H.A., *et al.* Socio-economic factors in the epidemiology of hypertensive disease. In: *The Epidemiology of Hypertension*, ed. J. Stamler, R. Stamler & T.N. Pullman (Grune & Stratton, New York, 1967) pp. 289–313

Stamler, J., Lindbergh, H.A., Berkson, D.M., Shaffer, A., Miller, W. & Poindexter, A. Prevalence and incidence of coronary heart disease in strata of the labour force of a Chicago industrial corporation. *J. Chron. Dis., 11*, 405–20 (1960)

Stary, H.C., Eggen, D.A. & Strong, J.P. The mechanism of atherosclerosis regression. In: *Atherosclerosis IV*, ed. G. Schettler, Y. Goto, Y. Hata & G. Klose (Springer Verlag, Berlin, 1977) pp. 394–404

Steele, P., Battock, D., Pappas, G., *et al.* Effect of patent coronary arterial occlusion on left ventricular function after aortocoronary by-pass surgery. *Amer. J. Cardiol., 39*, 39–42 (1977)

Stein, R.A. The effect of exercise training on heart rate during coitus in the post-myocardial infarction patient. *Circulation 55*,

738–40 (1977)

Steinhaus, A. Chronic effects of exercise. *Physiol. Rev., 13*, 103–47 (1933)

Stensaasen, S. The sport role socialization process in four industrialized countries: comments from a Norwegian perspective. In: *Sociology of Sport*, ed. F. Landry & W.A.R. Orban (Symposia Specialists, Miami, Fla., 1978) pp. 61–5

Sternby, N.H. Atherosclerosis and risk factors. In: *Atherosclerosis IV*, ed. G. Schettler, Y. Goto, Y. Hata & G. Klose (Springer Verlag, Berlin, 1977) pp. 102–4

Stevenson, J.A.F. Exercise, food intake, and health in experimental animals. *Canad. Med. Assoc. J., 96*, 862–6 (1967)

Stiles, M.H. Motivation for sports participation in the community. In: *Proceedings of International Symposium on Physical Activity and Cardiovascular Health*, ed. R.J. Shephard. *Canad. Med. Assoc. J., 96*, 889–92 (1967)

Stokes, W.R. Sexual functioning in the aging male. *Geriatrics 6*, 304–8 (1951)

Strauer, B.E. Studies concerning the effect of nitroglycerin on the contractile and relaxing properties of the isolated human ventricular myocardium. In: *Coronary Heart Disease*, ed. M. Kaltenbach, P. Lichtlen & G.C. Friesinger (G. Thieme, Stuttgart, 1973) pp. 20–4

Streeter, D.D., Spotnitz, H.M., Patel, D.P. & Sonnenblick, E.H. Fiber orientation in the canine left ventricle during systole and diastole. *Circ. Res., 24*, 339–47 (1969)

Strong, J.P. An introduction to the epidemiology of atherosclerosis. In: *Atherosclerosis IV*, ed. G. Schettler, Y. Goto, Y. Hata & G. Klose (Springer-Verlag, Berlin, 1977)

Stroud, M.W. & Feil, H.S. The terminal electrocardiogram: twenty three case reports of a review of the literature. *Amer. Heart J., 35*, 910–23 (1948)

Surawicz, B. The input of cellular electrophysiology into the practice of clinical electrocardiography. *Mod. Concepts Cardiovasc. Dis., 44*, 41–6 (1975)

Tabakin, B.S., Hanson, J.S. & Levy, A.M. Effects of physical training on the cardiovascular and respiratory response to graded upright exercise in distance runners. *Brit. Heart J., 27*, 205–10 (1965)

Takaro, T., Hultgren, H.N., Lipton, M.J., *et al*. The VA cooperative randomized study of surgery for coronary arterial occlusive disease. II. Subgroup with significant left main lesions. *Circulation 54*, suppl. III, 107–17 (1976)

Tauchart, M., Kochsiek, K., Heiss, H.W., Strauer, B.E., Kettler, D., Reploh, H.D., Rau, G. & Bretschneider, H.J. Measurement of coronary blood flow in man by the argon method. In: *Myocardial Blood Flow in Man. Methods and Significance in Coronary Disease*, ed. A. Maseri (Ed. Minerva Medica, Torino, 1972) pp. 139–44

Taylor, A.W. The effects of exercise and training on the activities of human glycogen cycle enzymes. In: *Metabolic Adaptation to Prolonged Physical Exercise*, ed. H. Howald & J.R. Poortmans (Birkhauser Verlag, Basel, 1975)

Taylor, C.B., Farquhar, J.W., Nelson, E., *et al*. Relaxation therapy and high blood pressure. *Arch. Gen. Psychiatry 34*, 339–42 (1977)

Taylor, H.L., Henschel, A., Brozek, J. & Keys, A. The effect of bed controlled trials of the prevention of coronary heart disease. *Fed. Proc., 32*, 1623–7 (1973)

Taylor, H.L., Henscel, A., Brozek, J. & Keys, A. The effect of bed rest on cardiovascular function and work performance. *J. Appl. Physiol., 2*, 223–39 (1949)

Taylor, H.L., Klepetar, E., Keys, A., *et al*. Death rates among physically active and sedentary employees of the railroad industry. *Amer. J. Publ. Health 52*, 1697–1707 (1962)

Taylor, H.L., Parlin, R.W., Blackburn, H. & Keys, A. Problems in the analysis of the relationship of coronary heart disease to physical activity or its lack, with special reference to sample size and occupational withdrawal. In: *Physical Activity in Health and Disease*, ed. K. Evang & K.L. Andersen (Williams & Wilkins, Baltimore, 1966)

Tepperman, J. & Pearlman, D. Effects of exercise and anemia on coronary arteries of small animals as revealed by the corrosion cast technique. *Circ. Res., 9*, 576–84 (1961)

Teräslinna, P., Partanen, T., Oja, P. & Koskela, A. Some social characteristics and living habits associated with willingness to participate in a physical activity intervention study. *J. Sports Med. Phys. Fitness 10*, 138–44 (1970)

Teräslinna, P., Partanen, T., Pyörälä, K., *et al*. Feasibility study on physical activity intervention. Report on recruiting design, training program, and three months' experience. *Work Environ. Health 6*, 24–31 (1969)

Terjung, R.L. & Tipton, C.M. Plasma thyroxine and thyroid-stimulation hormone levels during submaximal exercise in humans. *Amer. J. Physiol., 220*, 1840–5 (1971)

Terjung, R.L. & Winder, W.W. Exercise and thyroid function. *Med. Sci. Sports 7*, 20–6 (1975)

Texon, M. Causal relationships in heart disease in workmen's compensation cases. In: *Work and the Heart*, ed. F.F. Rosenbaum & E.L. Belknap (P.B. Hoeber, New York, 1959) pp. 426–31

Texon, M. Mechanical factors involved in atherosclerosis. In: *Atherosclerotic Vascular Disease*, ed. A.N. Brest & J.H. Moyer (Appleton Century Crofts, New York, 1967) pp. 23–42

Texon, M. The role of vascular dynamics (mechanical factors) in the development of atherosclerosis. In: *Coronary Heart Disease*, ed. H.I. Russek & B.L. Zohman (Lippincott, Philadelphia, 1971) pp. 121–36

Thompson, P.L. & Lown, B. Exercise and coronary occlusion: experimental studies. In: *Proceedings of Twentieth World Congress of Sports and Medicine*, ed. H. Toyne (Australian Sports Medicine Federation, Melbourne, 1975) p. 278

Tibblin, G., Wilhelmsen, L. & Werkö, L. Risk factors for myocardial infarction and death due to ischemic disease and other causes. *Amer. J. Cardiol., 35*, 514–22 (1975)

Tilkian, A.G., Pfeifer, J.F., Barry, W.H., *et al*. The effect of coronary bypass surgery on exercise-induced ventricular arrhythmias. *Amer. Heart J., 92*, 707–14 (1976)

Tomanek, R.J. Effects of age and exercise on the extent on the myocardial capillary bed. *Anat. Rec., 167*, 55–62 (1970)

Tominaga, S. & Blackburn, H. Prognostic importance of premature beats following myocardial infarction. *JAMA, 223*, 1116–23 (1973)

Trautwein, W., Gottstein, U. & Dudel, J. Der Aktionstrom der Myokardfaser im Sauerstoffmangel. *Pflüg. Archiv., 260*, 40–60 (1954)

Tregear, R.T. Interpretation of skin impedance measurements. *Nature 205*, 600–1 (1965)

Treumann, F. & Schroeder, W. Trainingseinfluss auf Muskeldurchblutung und Herzfrequenz. *Z. f. Kreislauff., 57*, 1024–33 (1968)

Triebwasser, J.H., Johnson, R.L., Burop, R.P., Campbell, J.C., Reardon, W.C. & Blomqvist, C.G. Non-invasive determination of cardiac output by a modified acetylene rebreathing procedure utilizing mass spectrometric measurements. *Aviat. Space Env. Med.*, *48*, 203–5 (1977)

Truett, J., Cornfield, J. & Kannel, W. A multivariate analysis of the risk of coronary heart disease in Framingham. *J. Chronic Dis.*, *20*, 511–24 (1967)

Turell, D.J. & Hellerstein, H.K. Six-year average follow-up of 460 consecutive cardiac patients. *Circulation 18*, 790 (abstr.) (1958)

Turpeinen, O., Miettinen, M., Karvonen, M.J., Roine, P., Pekkarinen, M., Lehtosuo, E.J. & Alivirtam, P. Dietary prevention of coronary heart disease: long-term experiment. I. Observation on male subjects. *Amer. J. Clin. Nutr.*, *21*, 255–76 (1968)

Tuttle, W.B., Cook, W.L. & Fitch, E. Sexual behavior in post-myocardial infarction patients. *Amer. J. Cardiol.*, *13*, 140–53 (1964)

Ueno, M. The so-called coition death. *Jap. J. Leg. Med.*, *17*, 33–40 (1963)

Ungerleider, H.E. & Gubner, R.S. Magnitude of the problem of the cardiac-in-industry. In: *Work and the Heart*, ed. F.F. Rosenbaum & E.L. Belknap (P.B. Hoeber, New York, 1959) pp. 417–25

Valentine, P.A., Fluck, D.C., Mounsey, J.P.D., Reid, D., Shillingford, J.P. & Steiner, R.E. Blood-gas changes after acute myocardial infarction. *Lancet* (ii), 837–41 (1966)

Van der Hoeven, G.M.A., Clerens, P.J.A., Donders, J.J.H., Beneken, J.E.W. & Vonk, J.T.C. A study of systolic time intervals during uninterrupted exercise. *Brit. Heart J.*, *39*, 242–54 (1977)

Van Tassel, R.A. & Edwards, J.E. Rupture of heart complicating myocardial infarction; analysis of 40 cases, including nine examples of left ventricular false aneurysm. *Chest*, *61*, 104–16 (1972)

Varnauskas, E. The circulatory adjustment to training in patients with coronary disease. In: *Physical Activity in Health and Disease*, ed. K. Evang & K.L. Andersen (Williams & Wilkins, Baltimore, Md., 1966) pp. 135–45

Varnauskas, E., Bergman, H., Houk, P. & Björntorp, P. Hemodynamic effects of physical training in coronary patients. *Lancet* (ii), 8–12 (1966)

Varnauskas, E. & Holmberg, S. Myocardial blood flow during

exercise in patients with coronary heart disease. Comments on training effects. In: *Coronary Heart Disease and Physical Fitness*, ed. O.A. Lassen & R.O. Malmborg (University Park Press, Baltimore, Md., 1971) pp. 102–4

Vatner, S.F., Higgins, C.B., Franklin, D. & Braunwald, E. Role of tachycardia in mediating the coronary hemodynamic response to severe exercise. *J. Appl. Physiol., 32*, 380—5 (1972)

Vedin, J.A., Wilhelmsson, C.E., Wilhelmsen, L., Bjure, J. & Ekström, J.B. Relation of resting and exercise-induced ectopic beats to other ischemic manifestations and to coronary risk factors. *Amer. J. Cardiol., 30*, 25–31 (1972)

Vedin, J.A., Wilhelmsson,. C., Elmfeldt, D., Säve-Söderbergh, J., Tibblin, G. & Wilhelmsen, L. Deaths and non-fatal reinfarctions during two years' follow up after myocardial infarction. *Acta Med. Scand., 198*, 353–64 (1975)

Venco, A., Saviotte, M., Barzizza, F., Bianchi, C., Tramarin, R. & Zolezzi, F. Electrocardiographic and echocardiographic findings in well-trained athletes. In: *Proceedings of International Conference on Sports Cardiology*, ed. T. Lubich & A. Venerando (A. Gaggi, Bologna, 1980) pp. 717–22

Venerando, A. Electrocardiography in sports medicine. *J. Sports Med. Phys. Fitness 19*, 107–28 (1979)

Verwoerdt, A. & Dovenmuehle, R.H. Heart disease and depression. *Geriatrics 19*, 856–64 (1964)

Vesselinovitch, D., Wissler, R.W., Fisher-Dzoga, K., Hughes, R. & Dubien, L. Regression of atherosclerosis in rabbits. *Atherosclerosis 19*, 259–75 (1974)

Virchow, R. Aus dem pathologisch-anatomischen Curse. *Wien. med. Wschr., 6*, 809 (1856). Cited by D.E. Bowyer & G.A. Gresham. In: *Atherosclerosis*, ed. R.J. Jones (Springer Verlag, Berlin, 1970)

Von der Groeben, J., Toole, J.G., Weaver, C.S. & Fitzgerald, J.W. Noise reduction in exercise electrocardiograms by digital filter techniques. In: *Measurement in Exercise Electrocardiography. The Ernst Simonson Conference*, ed. H. Blackburn (C.C. Thomas, Springfield, Ill., 1969) pp. 41–60

Von Euler, U.S. Sympatho-adrenal activity in physical exercise. *Med. Sci. Sports 6*, 165–73 (1973)

Vuori, I. Studies in the feasibility of long-distance (20–90 km) ski-hikes as a mass sport. In: *Proceedings of Twentieth World Congress of Sports Medicine*, ed. H. Toyne (Australian Sports

Medicine Federation, Melbourne, Australia, 1975)

Wakefield, M.C. A study of mortality amongst the men who have played in the Indiana high school state final basketball tournament. *Res. Quart., 15*, 3–11 (1944)

Wald, A. *Sequential Analysis* (Wiley, New York, 1947)

Wald, N., Howard, S., Smith, P.G. & Kjeldsen, K. Association between atherosclerotic diseases and carboxyhaemoglobin levels in smokers. *Brit. Med. J.* (i), 761–5 (1973)

Walker, J.A, Friedberg, H.D., Flemma, R.J. & Johnson, W.D. Determinants of angiographic patency of aortocoronary vein by-pass grafts. In: *Cardiovascular Surgery 1971.* American Heart Association Monograph 35 (1971)

Walker, W.J. Changing United States life-style and declining vascular mortality: cause or coincidence? *New Engl. J. Med., 297*, 163–5 (1977)

Wang, Y. Reaction to coronary blood flow during exercise. In: *Fitness and Exercise*, ed. J.F. Alexander, R.C. Serfass & C.M. Tipton (Athletic Institute, Chicago, 1972) pp. 51–4

Warnock, N.H., Clarkson, T.B. & Stevenson, R. Effect of exercise on blood coagulation time and atherosclerosis of cholesterol-fed cockerels. *Circ. Res., 5*, 478–80 (1957)

Wassermill, M. & Toor, M. The effects of graded work exercise in 100 patients with ischemic heart disease. In: *Prevention of Ischaemic Heart Disease*, ed. W. Raab (C.C. Thomas, Springfield, Ill., 1966) pp. 348–50

Watanabe, Y. & Dreifus, L.S. Mechanisms of cardiac arrhythmias. In: *Changing Concepts in Cardiovascular Disease*, ed. H.I. Russek & B.L. Zohman (Williams & Wilkins, Baltimore, Md., 1972) pp. 171–82

Weaver, N.K. The selective placement of cardiacs in industry. In: *Work and the Heart*, ed. F.F. Rosenbaum & E L. Belknap (P.B. Hoeber, New York, 1959) pp. 368–74

Weber, G. Regression of arterial lesions: facts and problems. In: *International Conference on Atherosclerosis*, ed. L.A. Carlson, R.A. Paoletti, C.R. Sirtori & G. Weber (Raven Press, New York, 1978) pp. 1–13

Weber, G., Fabbrini, P., Capaccioli, E. & Resi, L. Repair of early cholesterol-induced aortic lesions in rabbits after withdrawal from short-term atherogenic diet. *Atherosclerosis 22*, 565–72 (1975)

Weinblatt, E., Shapiro, S. & Frank, C.W. Prognosis of women with newly diagnosed coronary heart disease — a comparison with course of disease among men. *Amer. J. Publ. Health 63*, 577–93 (1973)

Weinblatt, E., Shapiro, R., Frank, C.W., *et al*. Return to work and work status following first myocardial infarction. *Amer. J. Publ. Health 56*, 169–85 (1966)

Weinblatt, E., Shapiro, S., Frank, C.W. & Singer, R. Prognosis of men after first myocardial infarction: mortality and first recurrence in relation to selected parameters. *Amer. J. Publ. Health 58*, 1329–47 (1968)

Weisman, A.D. & Hackett, T.P. Predilection to death: death and dying as a psychiatric problem. *Psychosom. Med., 23*, 232–57 (1961)

Weiss, E. & English, O.S. *Psychosomatic Medicine* (W.B. Saunders, Philadelphia, 1957)

Wen, C.P. & Gershoff, S.N. Changes in serum cholesterol and coronary heart disease mortality associated with changes in the postwar Japanese diet. *Amer. J. Clin. Nutr., 26*, 616–19 (1973)

Wenger, N.K. Early ambulation after myocardial infarction: Grady Memorial Hospital — Emory University, School of Medicine. In: *Exercise Testing and Exercise Training in Coronary Heart Disease*, ed. J.P. Naughton, H.K. Hellerstein and I.C. Mohler (Academic Press, New York, 1973) pp. 324–8

Wenger, N.K. Does exercise training enhance collateral circulation? In: *Critical Evaluation of Cardiac Rehabilitation*, ed. J. Kellermann & H. Denolin (Karger, Basel, 1977) pp. 143–5

Wenger, N.K., Hellerstein, H.K., Blackburn, H., *et al*. Uncomplicated myocardial infarction: current physician practice in patient management. *JAMA, 224*, 511–14 (1973)

Westling, H. Comnments on mechanism of angina pectoris and effects of drugs. In: *Coronary Heart Disease and Physical Fitness*, ed. O.A. Larsen & R.O. Malmborg (University Park Press, Baltimore, Md., 1971) pp. 119–21

Wexler, B.C. & Greenberg, B.P. Effect of exercise on myocardial infarction in young vs old male rats: electocardiographic changes. *Amer. Heart J., 88*, 343–50 (1974)

Whipp, B.J., Torres, F., Davis, J.A., Wasserman, K. & Casaburi, R. A test to determine the parameters of aerobic function during exercise. *Fed. Proc., 36*, 449 (abstr.) (1977)

White, J.R. EKG changes using carotid artery for heart rate

monitoring. *Med. Sci. Sports 9*, 88–94 (1977)

White, K.L. & Ibrahim, M.A. The distribution of cardiovascular disease in the community. *Ann. Int. Med., 58*, 627–36 (1963)

Widdicombe, J.G. *MTP International Reviews of Science Physiology*, Series 1, *Respiratory Physiology* (Butterworths, London, 1974)

Widmer, L.K., Hartmann, G., Duchosal, F. & Plechl, S.Ch. Risikofaktoren und Gliedmassenarterienverschluss. *Dtsch. med. Wschr., 94*, 1107–10 (1969)

Wiener, L., Dwyer, E.M. & Cos, J.W. Left ventricular haemodynamics in exercise-induced angina patients. *Circulation 38*, 240–9 (1968)

Wikland, B. Medically unattended fatal cases of ischaemic heart disease in a defined population. *Acta Med. Scand., 524*, suppl. (1971)

Wildenthal, K., Morgan, H.E., Opie, L.H. & Srere, P.A. Regulation of cardiac metabolism (symposium). *Circ. Res., 38* (5), suppl., 1, 1–160 (1976)

Wiley, J.F. Effects of 10 weeks of endurance training on left ventricular intervals. *J. Sports Med. Phys. Fitness 11*, 104–11 (1971)

Wilhelmsen, L., Ljungberg, S., Wedel, H., *et al.* A comparison between participants and non-participants in a primary preventive trial. *J. Chronic Dis., 29*, 331–9 (1976)

Wilhelmsen, L., Sanne, H., Elmfelt, D., Grimby, G., Tibblin, G. & Wedel, H. A controlled trial of physical training after myocardial infarction. *Prev. Medicine 4*, 491–508 (1975)

Wilhelmsen, L. & Tibblin, G. Physical inactivity and risk of myocardial infarction — the men born in 1913 study. In: *Coronary Heart Disease and Physical Fitness*, ed. O.A. Larsen & R.O. Malmborg (Munksgaard, Copenhagen, 1971)

Wilhelmsen, L., Tibblin, G. & Werkö, L. A primary preventive study in Göteburg, Sweden. *Prev. Medicine 1*, 153–60 (1972)

Williams, M.H. & Edwards, R.L. Effects of variant training regimens upon submaximal and maximal cardiovascular performance. *Amer. Corr. Therapy J., 25*, 11–15 (1971)

Williamson, J.S., Bauman, D.J. & Tsargaris, T.J. A comparison of hemodynamic and angiographic indices of left ventricular performance in patients with coronary artery disease. *Cardiology 63*, 220–36 (1978)

Wilmore, J.H. & Norton, A.C. *The Heart and Lungs at Work. A*

Primer of Exercise Physiology. (Beckman Instruments, Schiller Park, Ill., 1974)

Wilmore, J.H., Royce, J., Girandola, R.N., Katch, F.I. & Katch, V.L. Physiological alterations resulting from a ten week program of jogging. *Med. Sci. Sports 2*, 7–14 (1970)

Wilson, F.N. The precordial electrocardiogram. *Amer. Heart J., 27*, 19–85 (1944)

Winter, D.A. Noise measurement and quality control techniques in recording and processing of electrocardiograms. In: *Measurement in Exercise Electrocardiography. The Ernst Simonson Conference*, ed. H. Blackburn (C.C. Thomas, Springfield, Ill., 1971) pp. 159–68

Winter, D.A. & Trenholm, B.G. Reliable triggering for exercise electrocardiograms. *IEEE Trans. on Biomed. Eng., 16*, 75–9 (1969)

Wishnie, H.A., Hackett, T.P. & Cassem, N.H. Psychological hazards of convalescence following a myocardial infarction. *JAMA, 215*, 1292–6 (1971)

Wissler, R.W. & Vesselinovitch, D. Animal models of regression. In: *Atherosclerosis IV*, ed. G. Schettler, Y. Goto, Y. Hata & G. Klose (Springer Verlag, Berlin, 1977) pp. 377–85

Wohl, A.J., Lewis, M.R. & Campbell, M.R. Cardiovascular function during early recovery from myocardial infarction. *Circulation 56*, 931–7 (1977)

Wolferth, C.C. & Wood, F.C. Electrocardiographic diagnosis of coronary occlusion by use of chest leads. *Amer. J. Med. Sci., 183*, 30–5 (1932)

Wong, H.O., Kasser, I.S. & Bruce, R.A. Impaired maximal exercise performance with hypertensive cardiovascular disease. *Circulation 39*, 633–8 (1969)

Wood, J.E. The cardiovascular effects of oral contraceptives. *Mod. Concepts Cardiovasc. Dis., 41*, 37–40 (1972)

Wood, P.D. Effect of exercise on plasma lipids and high density lipoprotein levels. In: *Topics in Ischaemic Heart Disease. An International Symposium* (Toronto Rehabilitation Centre, Toronto, 1979)

Wood, P.D., Haskell, W., Klein, H., Lewis, S., Stern, M.P. & Farquhar, J. The distribution of plasma lipoproteins in middle-aged runners. *Metabolism 25*, 1249–57 (1976)

Wood, P.D., McGregor, M., Magidson, O. & Whittaker, W. The effort test in angina pectoris. *Brit. Heart J., 12*, 363–71 (1950)

Woods, J.D. Relative ischemia in the hypertrophied heart. *Lancet* (i), 696–8 (1961)

World Health Organization. *Classification of Atherosclerotic Lesions*, WHO Tech. Rept. 143 (Geneva, 1958)

World Health Organization. *International Classification of Diseases and Causes of Death* (WHO, Geneva, 1968)

World Health Organization. Myocardial infarction community registers. In: *Public Health in Europe 5* (World Health Organization, Geneva, 1976)

World Health Organization. *The Prevention of Coronary Heart Diseases*, WHO Report ICP/CVD 002 (10) (Copenhagen, 1977)

Wright, G.R. & Shephard, R.J. Carbon monoxide, nicotine, and the 'safer' cigarette. *Respiration 35*, 40–52 (1978)

Wright, G.R. & Shephard, R.J. Physiological effects of carbon monoxide. *International Review of Physiology. Environmental Physiology III, 20*, 311–68 (1979)

Wyatt, H.L. & Mitchell, J.H. Influences of physical training on the heart of dogs. *Circulation Res., 35*, 883–9 (1974)

Wyman, M.G. & Hammersmith, L. Comprehensive treatment plan for the prevention of primary ventricular fibrillation in acute myocardial infarction. *Amer. J. Cardiol., 33*, 661–7 (1974)

Wynder, E.L., Lemon, F.L. & Bross, I.J. Cancer and coronary artery diseases among seventh-day adventists. *Cancer 12*, 1016–28 (1959)

Wyndham, C.H. & Strydom, N.B. Körperliche Arbeit bei hoher Temperatur. In: *Zentrale Themen der Sportmedizin*, ed. W. Hollmann (Springer Verlag, New York, 1972)

Yamaji, K. & Shephard, R.J. Longevity and causes of death of athletes: a review of the literature. *J. Human Ergol., 6*, 13–25 (1977)

Yater, W.M., Welsh, P.P., Stapleton, J.F. & Clark, M.L. Comparison of clinical and pathological aspects of coronary artery disease in men of various age groups: a study of 950 autopsied cases from the Armed Forces Institute of Pathology. *Ann. Int. Med., 34*, 353–92 (1971)

Young, M. & Willmot, P. *The Symmetrical Family* (Routledge & Kegan Paul, London, 1973)

Zakopoulos, K.S. Sudden death in football in Greece. *Brit. J. Sports Med., 7*, 165 (1973)

Zaret, B.L. Strauss, H.W., Martin, N.D., Wells, H.P. & Flamm, M.D. Non-invasive evaluation of myocardial perfusion with potassium 43. Study of patients at rest, exercise, and during angina pectoris. *New Engl. J. Med., 288*, 809–12 (1973)

Zebe, H., Mehmel, H.C., Leinberger, H., Mäurer, W., Tillmanns, H. & Kübler, W. Phentolamine: short and long-term effects in the treatment of congestive heart failure. In: *Coronary Heart Disease*, ed. M. Kaltenbach, P. Lichtlen, R. Balcon & W.D. Bussmann (G. Thieme, Stuttgart, 1978) pp. 262–5

Zetterquist, S. Effect of training in intermittent claudication. Redistribution of blood flow due to training. In: *Coronary Heart Disease and Physical Fitness*, ed. O.A. Larsen & R.O. Malmborg (University Park Press, Baltimore, Md., 1971) pp. 158–62

Zir, L.M., Miller, S.W., Dinsmore, R.E., *et al*. Interobserver variability in coronary angiography. *Circulation 27*, suppl. II, 51–52 (1975)

Zohman, L.R. Early ambulation of post-myocardial infarction patients: Montefiore Hospital. In: *Exercise Testing and Exercise Training in Coronary Heart Disease*, ed. J.P. Naughton, H.K. Hellerstein & I.C. Mohler (Academic Press, New York, 1973)

Zohman, L.R. & Tobis, J.S. The effect of exercise training on patients with angina pectoris. *Phys. Med., 48*, 525–32 (1967)

Zohman, L.R. & Tobis, J.S. *Cardiac Rehabilitation* (Grune & Stratton, New York, 1970)

Zonereich, S., Rhee, J.J., Zoneraich, O., Jordan, D. & Appel, J. Assessment of cardiac function in marathon runners by graphic non-invasive techniques. *Ann. N.Y. Acad. Sci., 301*, 900–17 (1977)

Zukel, W.J., Lewis, R.H., Enterline, P.E., Painter, R.C., Ralston, L.S., Fawcett, R.M., Meredith, A.P. & Peterson, B. A short-term community study of the epidemiology of coronary heart disease. A preliminary report on the North Dakota study. *Amer. J. Publ. Health 49*, 1630–9 (1959)

Zwillinger, L. Die Digitalis Entwirkung auf das Arbeits Elektrokardiogramm. *Med. Klin., 31*, 977–9 (1935)

INDEX

α-Blocking agents 276
Abnormal motion 205-6
  see also dyskinesis 211
Absenteeism 282, 319
Acculturation 67
Acetylene rebreathing 160
Activity 24, 38-9, 45-6, 74, 87, 89,
  94-100, 102-3, 294, 306
  emergencies 49 65, 294
  type of 52, 54-60
  see also prescription, exercise,
    sports, work
Activity questionnaires 120
Actuarial ideal mass 261-2
Acute myocarditis 172
Adipocyte sensitivity 82
Adjuvants to exercise 261-78
Advertising 306-7, 320-1
Aerobic performance 190-5
After-loading 202, 211, 224
Age
  animals 88
  man 117, 125-6, 136-9, 144,
    200-1, 208, 212, 219, 220,
    223, 232, 241, 260, 262, 283,
    289, 294
Age appearance 119
Aggression 79
Akinesis 21
  see also dyskinesis
Alcohol 52, 99, 105, 113, 152, 285
Alprenolol see β-blocking agents
Alveolar CO_2 161
Ambulance training 44-5
American Heart Association ecg
  specification 166
Anaerobic threshold 73, 81-2, 195
Analogue averaging 169
Analogy 128
Aneurysm 21, 149-51, 301
Angina 13, 16-17, 18, 21, 24, 36,
  104, 113, 135, 139, 145, 148-57,
  172, 178, 180, 184, 204 212,
  215, 217, 227, 230, 248, 256,
  273, 276, 283, 284, 295, 296-9,
  301
Angiography 73, 134, 165, 180, 182,

229, 297-9
Animal experiments 86-90
Animal fat
  models 86-7
  see also fat, dietary
Antecedents of infarction,
  immediate 58, 65
Anticoagulants 137
Anxiety 60, 64, 174, 190, 197, 281,
  283
  see also stress
Aquabics 296
Arm ergometry 189, 195
Arterial CO_2 161
Arterial pH 216
Arterial sampling 158
Ateriosclerosis 15
Arterio-venous oxygen difference,
  64, 69-70, 75, 80, 81, 206, 208,
  215-16, 275
Assessment 158-98
Åstrand nomogram see sub-
  maximum tests
Asynchrosy 21
Asynerisis 21
Asystole 17, 19-20, 51, 62, 63, 163
  see also dangers of exercise
Atherogenic diet 87
Atherosclerosis 14-15, 87-8, 112-13,
  266, 302
Athletes 67, 105-8, 122
ATP^{ase}, myocardial 211
Atrial tachycardia 174
Atrio-ventricular block 172
Attitudes to exercise 251-60, 296
Attrition, sample 92-3, 99, 130, 134,
  135, 137-8, 139, 140, 145-7,
  249-51, 255-7
Automation 38, 39
Averaging, ecg 169

Back-pressure, CO_2 162
Bassler hypothesis 108
Bed rest 68, 205, 192, 238-9
Behavioural change 47-8
β-blocking agents 45, 137, 194,
  196, 200, 208, 274, 275-6, 285,

287
  withdrawal 276
Beta error *see* Type II error
Bezold-Jarisch reflex 230
Bias 115, 127, 130
  see also methodological bias,
    sampling, selection
Bicycles 38, 45
Biological gradient 127
  plausibility 127
'Black' workers 113-14
Blood pressure 21,33-4, 43, 50, 51,
  64, 70, 74, 80, 92, 94-100, 108,
  109, 115, 116-17, 118-19, 123,
  124, 125, 136-9, 145, 149-53,
  157, 183, 195, 220-5, 277, 278,
  295, 304
  temperature 216
Blue collar 113-14, 138, 145, 156,
  256
  see also social class
Body build 110, 116, 122-3, 124, 126
Body composition 77-8, 263
Body fat *see* fat
Body mass 41-2, 94-100, 105, 115,
  116, 118-19, 157, 261-6
Bradford Hill criteria 125-9
Bradycardia, exercise *see* sick sinus
  syndrome
Breathing exercises 132
Breathlessness 159, 184, 270
British civil servants 122-4
Bronchial spasm 82, 248
Brunner 132
Buerger's exercises 304
Bundle-branch block 173, 176
Bus drivers 24, 114, 115
Business worries *see* stress
By-pass surgery 45, 134, 182,
  299-302, 310-11

Caffeine 174
  see also coffee consumption
Calcification 15, 16, 84
Calcium inhibitors 274, 277
Calcium ions 275
Calibration 188
Calisthenics *see* gymnastics
Camaraderie 79, 84, 258
Canadian experiments 144-7
Canadian Home Fitness Test 192-4,
  233, 236, 237, 308-11
Capillary/fibre ratio 73, 75, 89, 228
Carbon dioxide rebreathing 161

Carboxyhaemoglobin 36, 231, 269,
  271, 298
Cardiac arrest *see* asystole,
  ventricular fibrillation
Cardiac catheterisation 158-9
Cardiac contractility 50, 68-73, 196,
  202-13, 215, 226, 276, 297
Cardiac failure 17, 19, 20-1, 55,
  153-4, 212-13, 215, 225, 238,
  273, 276, 277
  see also regional myocardial
    function
Cardiac glycosides 277
Cardiac hypertrophy 70-1, 83, 89,
  211, 226
Cardiac output 64, 68-73, 158-62,
  213-15
Cardiac reserve 202-13
Cardiac resuscitation *see* resusci-
  tation, cardiac
Cardiac rupture *see* rupture,
  cardiac
Cardiac work 16, 50, 69-73, 80,
  177-8, 196, 225-8, 229, 230,
  276, 297-9, 304
Carotid pulse 164, 234, 237, 239
Car ownership 38-9
Catecholamines 51, 61, 76, 77, 79,
  82, 175, 275
Catharsis 79
Causal association 126-30, 136
Cigar smoking 271
Cigarette smoking 36-7, 42, 46-7,
  58, 62, 74, 78, 92, 94-100, 102,
  103, 105, 108, 113, 116-17, 118,
  122-3, 126, 143, 145, 149-52,
  154, 157, 183, 231, 255, 268-71,
  298, 303, 304, 306, 318
Cineangiography 162-3
Civilisation 28, 36, 42, 100-5
Class leaders 145, 257-8, 311-13
  organisation 242-5
  supervision 243-5, 311-13
Classification, international 22
Clinical assessment 158-9
Clinical diagnosis *see* symptoms
Clofibrate 267
Coagulability 81, 83, 103
Coffee consumption 58, 174
Coherence of explanation 128
Cold weather 17, 58, 65, 74, 78,
  82, 230, 248-9, 304
Collapse of lungs 216
Collateral circulation 19, 72-3, 81,

84, 89, 299
Community surveys 26
Compensation 59-60, 281-2
Competition, avoidance 62, 64, 79,
    86, 255, 281
Compliance, programme 92, 134,
    135, 139, 143, 151-3, 156, 236,
    249-60
    see also motivation
Compliance, ventricular 200
Conduction defect 173
Congenital lesions 15, 52
Consent form 317
Consistency of association 126-7
Contamination, sample 92, 139, 142,
    143, 146, 219
Contraceptive medication 293
Contractility *see* cardiac contractility
Contraindications to exercise 148-57,
    198, 238
Cooper 'points' 234
Cooper test 191
Coronary blood flow 72-3, 74, 80-1,
    89, 165-6, 228-31, 273
    distribution 275
Coronary spasm 15, 229, 274
Cost/benefit analysis 182-3, 305-23
    see also economic factors
CPK *see* enzyme changes
Criterion 23-4
Cross-country skiing *see* skiing
Cross-cultural comparisons 100-5
Cuff size, sphygmomanometer 195,
    220-1
Cycle ergometer 187-9, 193
Cycle ergometer training 132, 140,
    234, 296

Daily routine 234
Dangers of exercise 49-65, 148-57,
    196-8, 259-60, 284, 309, 311-12
    see also cold, humidity, musculo-
        skeletal injuries, running
        surface, traffic hazards
Dead space 161
Death 13, 17, 18, 24-5, 27-8, 49-65,
    98, 112-13, 118, 134-5, 284,
    311-12, 317
    certificates 25, 30
Decrease of coronary disease 42-8
Defares method 161
Degeneration *see* fibrosis
Denial, disability 120, 290
Depression 280, 284, 286-92
Desire, sexual 283

Developed nations *see* civilisation
Diabetes 41, 83, 139, 278, 281, 295,
    303
Diagnosis 18, 24-5
Diagnostic fashions 25, 30
Diastolic filling 200, 202-13, 273
Diastolic phase 81
Diastolic pressure 212
Diet 113, 115, 137
Dietary counselling 95-100, 137
Dietary restriction 78, 89, 265
Digital averaging 169
Digitalis 149-52, 176, 277, 285
Dipyridamole 229
Dissecting aneurysm 16, 19
Diuretics 149-52, 176, 277
Documentation 316
Domesticated animals 88
Duration of training 139, 233
Dye injection techniques 160
Dyskinesis 21, 205-6, 211
Dyspnoea *see* breathlessness
Dysrhythmia 19, 51, 60, 64, 82,
    148, 172-3, 174-5, 186, 235,
    238, 239, 249, 259, 265, 277,
    281, 300
    see also premature ventricular
        contraction, ventricular
        fibrillation, ventricular
        tachycardia

Echocardiography *see* ultrasound
Economic factors 27-8, 92, 156,
    279-82, 289, 305-23
Ectomorph 110
Education, level of 292
Efficiency, mechanical 187-9, 225-6,
    234
Ego strength 284
Ejection fraction 164, 202-13
    time 164
Elasticity 15, 223, 260
Electrical ergometer 188-9
Electrocardiogram 166-84
Electrocardiographic changes
    exercise 167-9, *see also* ST
        segmental depression
    hypoxia 24, 175
    infarction 19, 104
    interpretation 167, 310
    resting 64, 97, 104, 124, 136-9,
        149, 155, 171-3
    technique 166-71
Electrolyte balance *see* potassium
    ions

Electron transport 82
Emboli 16, 55
Emotional strain 55
Employment 279-82
Endocardial hypoxia 227, 229
Endomorph 110
Endurance training *see* training
Energy expenditure 102, 234-5,
    265, 267, 268
Enzyme changes 18, 74, 75, 82,
    208, 211, 216, 303-4
Epidemic, cardiac 23-48
Epidemiology 91-4
Equipment 315
Ergometers 186-90
Eskimos 100, 101-2
Excess body mass *see* body mass,
    obesity
Excitement 297
    see also stress
Exercise log 245
Exercise programmes 61-3, 134, 140,
    239-45
    see also prescription
Exercise testing 60-1, 158-98, 308-11
Experimentation, direct 91-4, 128
Extrasystoles 121
Extroverts 254, 255, 258

Facilities 234, 253-4, 321-3
False ecg changes 176, 277, 310-11
Familiarisation *see* habituation
Family attitudes 152
Family programmes 84, 234
Fat, body 78, 84, 86, 94-100, 101-2,
    115, 127, 157, 236, 261-6, 271
    see also obesity
Fat, dietary 27, 40-1, 47, 101, 157,
    266-8
Fat mobilisation 76, 82
    subcutaneous 83, 195
Fatty acids 267
Fatty infiltration 14
    see also atherosclerosis, plaques
Fat utilisation 75
Female patients 293-6
Fibrinolysis 81
Fibrosis *see* myocardial fibrosis
Fick principle 158
'First-pass' approach 163
Fitness clubs 321-2
Fitness, initial 68, 98, 203, 217,
    280
Fitness vans 308

Flexibility 236, 260
Fluid
    loss 247, 266
    needs 247
Food consumption 38-9
Foreign gas methods 160
Framingham Study 124
Frequency response, ecg 166
    training 233
Frigidity 286

Gallop rhythm 297
Gated camera 163
Genetic factors 67, 102, 103
Geriatric costs 318, 319-20
Girth, abdominal 115
Glucose tolerance 83, 84, 96, 103,
    116-17
    see also diabetes
Glycogen 75
Gothenburg study 124, 140-3
Gottheiner 130
Grafts *see* by-pass surgery
Grip strength 124
Group programmes 254
Growth hormone 77, 82
Guanethidine 194
Gymnasia
    emergencies 61-3
Gymnastics 122, 132. 140, 235,
    243, 254, 321-2

Habitual activity *see* activity
Habituation 67, 80, 195
Haemoconcentration 216
Haemoglobin 77, 216
Halting test, indications 192, 198
Harvard Alumnae Study 121-2
HDL cholesterol 76, 82, 98, 124, 267
Health attitudes *see* health
    consciousness
Health beliefs 184, 253
Health benefits 117-18, 253-4
    see also Cost/Benefit, Risk
        Factor Modification
Health consciousness 78, 84, 113,
    122, 126, 184, 271, 305
Health hazard appraisal 306-7
Health Insurance Plan, New York
    124, 135-9
Health outcomes 184
Heart block 20
Heart loss 83
    see also Humidity, Skin Blood Flow

Heart rate 50, 68, 71, 80, 114, 124,
    192, 196, 199-202, 208-13, 226,
    234, 237, 275, 283
    maximum 68, 177, 191-2,
    199-202
    24 hours 102
Heart sound 164
Heart volume 109, 149-51, 196, 228
Heberden 16
Heller 132-3
Hellerstein 132
Helsinki Study 143
Herrick 18
High risk screening 183
Hippocrates 13
History 13, 16, 28
Homeopathic treatment 140, 145
Home training 144, 243-5, 246, 258, 312
Hormones 77, 293-4
Hospital phase 238-9
Hot showers 51, 243
Household surveys 25
Humidity 51, 58, 65, 243, 246-7,
    259, 264
Humour, sense of 119
Hunter, John 16
Hypertension *see* blood pressure
Hypertrophy
    muscle 75, 78, 80, 83, 208, 211
    see also cardiac hypertrophy
Hyperventilation 176, 195
Hypnosis 144, 272, 290
Hypochondriasis 287-92
Hypokinetic circulation 213-15, 216
Hypotensive drugs 278, 285
Hypoxic tests 229
Hysteria 287-92

Ice 248
Ideal body mass 261-2
Ileal by-pass 83
Impedance, skin 168-9
Impotence 284
Inactivity *see* activity
Incidence 23, 50, 111
Income 113
    see also social class
Increase of disease *see* epidemic
Indians 102
Indirect association 126
Industrial fitness 255, 318
Infarction *see* myocardial infarction
Initial fitness 68, 98, 203, 217, 280
Inotropic effect 208-13

Insudation 14
Insulin 278
Insurance costs 305-6, 312, 317
Intelligence 119
Intensity, occupational activity
    114, 116, 118, 156
    training 234
Intensive care wards 45
Intermittent claudication 303
International classification *see*
    classification
Interval training 203, 219, 221, 274,
    298
Intramural pressure 72
Intravascular pressure 195, 221
Introverts 254, 258
Irregular exercise 156
Ischaemic electrocardiogram *see*
    electrocardiographic changes
Ischaemic heart disease 15-16
Iso-electric line 171
Isometric effort 52, 55-6, 58, 78, 83,
    223-4, 235, 283
    tests 164-5, 203, 206
Israeli studies 130-2

Jewish studies *see* Israeli
Jewish subjects 138
Job categorisation 112, 114, 115
Job transfer 112, 115
Jogging 79, 234, 296, 321-2
    mask 248, 274
    technique 239-45, 246
Jones method 161-2

Kavanagh 133-9
Keeping fit *see* gymnastics
Kellermann 131-2
Kibbutzim 114, 115
Kinetic energy 221
Korotkov sounds 221

Laboratory surveys 25
Lactate, blood 191-2, 195, 222
    coronary 230
Laennec 16
Lag period
    disease 47, 54, 114
    training benefit 140
Laplace's Law 72, 81, 83, 226
Latent period *see* lag period
LDH *see* enzyme changes
LDL cholesterol 76-7, 82, 98, 124,
    267

Leads, ecg 166-8
Lean mass 64, 78
Learning, test 67
Left ventricular failure
    function 148, 164-5, 230, 300
    see also cardiac failure
Leisure activity 45-6, 119, 120-5
    see also activity
Lifestyle
    counselling 314
    see also health consciousness,
        risk factors
Lifting *see* isometric activity
Lipids *see* fatty acids, LDL
    cholesterol, HDL cholesterol,
    triglycerides
Longitudinal studies 67, 130-57
Longshoremen 116-17, 127
Low-risk sample 136

Mail carriers 114
Malpractice suits 316-17
Manual workers *see* blue-collar,
    social class
Maoris 100
Marathon races 108, 134, 141, 219,
    247-8, 291
Masculinity 292, 293
Masters' athletes 109-10, 260, 271
Master test 61, 177
Maximum oxygen intake 68, 134,
    140, 141, 159, 190-5, 216-20,
    240, 241, 244, 284
Meal frequency 265
Meals and heart attacks 285
Mechanisms, preventive 85, 128
Medical problems 145
    see also dangers of exercise
Medical referrals 254
Medical runaround 23
Medical screening 197, 308-11, 316
Medico-legal aspects 281-2, 316-17
Mesomorph 110
Metabolism 74-7, 82-3
Methodological bias 126
Methyl-dopa 194
Migrant studies 103-5
Mineral
    loss 247
    needs 247
Minnesota Multiphasic Personality
    Inventory 286-92
Mitochondria 74
Mixed Venous CO_2 161

Mobitz block 172
Mood 79, 286-92
Mortality *see* prognosis
Motivation 184, 236, 243, 251-4,
    269, 280, 306-7
Multiple risk factors 93
Multivariate analyses 116-17
Muscle blood flow 70, 188, 195,
    208, 223
Muscle strength 195, 235, 236,
    303
Musculo-skeletal injuries 237, 242,
    259-60, 268
Myocardial
    anoxia 16-17, 50, 175, 205-13,
        225, 227, 273, 294, 296-9
    factors 93
    fibrosis 19, 52
    infarction 17-19, 50, 51, 63,
        130-57, 172, 180, 204,
        209-11, 214, 217, 222, 225,
        227
    see also ST segmental depression
Myocarditis, acute 172

Narrowing, coronary 165, 180,
    229-302
Nasal breathing 74, 81-2, 230
National differences 26-7
Negligence, professional 316-17
Nicotine 174, 231, 269
Nifedipine 274, 277
Nitrites 132, 230-1, 273-5, 285,
    298
    see also trinitrin
Nitrous oxide rebreathing 160, 165
Noise, electrical 169, 170
Non-invasive assessment 158-98
Non-randomised studies 130-9
Nuclear cardiology 163-4, 189, 229
Nutrition *see* diet

Obesity 40-1, 236, 261-6
    see also body fat
Observer error 24, 165, 167
Occupation 35, 56, 59, 111-20
    see also social class
Odds ratio 150
Oestradiol 293
On-transients 163, 185, 187, 201,
    215
Orchidectomy 293
Orgasm 283
Osler 16, 35

Oulu Study 144
Out-patient phase 239-45
Over-training 240, 249, 292
Oxygen
   consumption 186, 188, 190
   debt 206, 215, 229, *see also*
      lactate
   extraction 228, 303
   release, red cell 275

Papillary muscles 206
Paramedical tests 309
PAR-Q test 197, 308
Participaction 320-1
Participation 84, 183-4
Pathology 13-22, 50-4, 55, 112
Pedal speed 188-9
Peripheral resistance 211
Peripheral training 75
   vascular disease 302-4
Personality 234, 254, 286-92
Phase-lag 163, 185, 187, 201, 215
Phentolamine 276
Physical activity *see* activity
Physician's attitude 152
Pipe smoking 271
Plaques, atheromatous 165, 229,
   231, 266
Plateau, CO_2 162
Platelet changes 81
Polyfocal PVCs 175
Polynesians 100
Postal clerks 114
Post-mortem findings 52-4, 112
Posture test 203
Potassium ions 51, 58, 110, 174,
   176, 247-8, 265, 275, 277
   isotopes 165
Practolol *see* β-blocking agents
Predictive values 148
Pre-ejection period 164
Preloading 202, 211
Premature ventricular contractions
   21, 36, 51, 98, 109, 149-53, 155,
   169, 174-5, 240, 275-6
Prescription, exercise 63, 64, 67, 84-
   6, 134, 156, 202, 232-45, 276,
   298, 314-17
Pressure rise (dp/dt) 164
Prevalence 23, 112, 179, 181-3
Prevention
   primary 66-90, 314
   secondary 89, 91-129, 314
   tertiary 130-57, 238-45

P-R interval 173
Procaine amide 176
Productive years 27-8
Productivity 319
Prognosis 17-18, 294-5, 298, 300
Progression, disease 256
Progression, training 240, 242
Progressive tests 186
Promotional costs 320-1
Prophylaxis
   exercise catastrophes 63-5
   see also prevention
Propranolol *see* β-blocking agents
P substance 16
Psychasthenia 287-92
Psycho-social problems 145, 279-92
Psychotherapy 290, 299
Public training, resuscitation 44-5,
   50
Pulmonary arterial pressure 213
Pulmonary embolism 172
Pulmonary oedema 216
Pulse counting 64-5
Pump failure *see* cardiac failure
P-wave terminal force 148

Q-T interval 173
Quadriceps overload 188, 200
Quinidine 176
Q-waves 18, 172

Railway workers 127
Ramp-function test 185, 195
Randomised controlled trials 139-57
Raowolfia alkaloids 278
Rate-pressure product 196, 227, 228
Recanalisation 303
Rechnitzer 133
Recidivism 270
Recovery ecg 180
Recovery heart rate 192-4
   stroke volume 203
Recruitment 145, 249-60
Recurrences 133-57, 212, 225, 269
Red cell count 83
   see also haemoglobin
Re-entrant rhythm 20, 175, 275
Refined carbohydrate 41, 266
Regional myocardial function 162-6
Relatives 281
   see also family, wives
Relaxants 278, 285, 299
Relaxation 84, 132, 272
   myocardial 206

Repolarisation 175
Respiratory gas exchange ratio 191-2, 195
Respiratory minute volume 222
    see also hyperventilation
Respiratory system 73-4
Resuscitation, cardiac 44-5, 156, 197, 259, 309, 316
Rhythmic activity 52
Right ventricular failure *see* cardiac failure
Risk factors 33-4, 94
    modification 94-100, 117, 132, 157
    tertiary 148-57
R on T phenomenon 21
Rubidium 165
Running 59, 130-57, 190, 191, 234, 270
    surface 246
Rupture 21, 52, 238
    see also aneurysm

Safety *see* dangers of exercise
Salt 34
Sample selection 95, 99, 110, 115, 133-4, 136, 143
Sample size 93, 140-7
Sampling 25-6
Saturated fat *see* fat, dietary
School instruction 84
Screening 24, 49, 179-84, 308-11
Seasonal factors 67
Sedatives 278
Self-image 255, 284
Self-selection 115, 116, 124
    see also sample selection
Sensitivity 148, 178-9, 183, 310-11
Sequential analysis 146
Severity of disease 215
    see also angina, cardiac failure, myocardial anoxia
Sex differences 30-3, 36, 39, 57, 180, 293-6
Sexual activity 55, 244, 282-6, 289
SGOT *see* enzyme changes
Shoes, running 246
Showers 243, 259
Sick sinus syndrome 192, 194, 200-2, 215
Silent atheroma 14, 50, 63
Sinu-arterial block 172
Skiing, cross-country 45, 52, 61, 106-8, 233, 321

Skills 234, 280
Skin blood flow 70, 75, 80, 208, 216, 264
Skinfold thicknesses 264
Skin preparation, ecg 169
Sleeping 55, 59
Slowing of training *see* over-training
Smoking
    withdrawal 268-71
    see also cigarette smoking
Snow, John 91
Snow shovelling 57, 58, 59
Social class 33, 105, 113-14, 117, 119, 121, 125-6, 138, 145, 156, 280, 321
    mobility 36, 114
Somali 101
Soreness, muscle 249
Southern Ontario Study 145-7
Specificity, association 127
Specificity, test 148, 178-9, 310-11
    speed 234, 242
Specificity, training 67
Spontaneous recovery 219
Sport, benefits from 122, 130
Sport, dangers of 49-65
Spurious association 125-6
Stage One test 185
Stair-climbing 122, 123, 234-5
Starvation 265
Steady state 163
Steady-state test 186
Step test 186-7, 193
Strength of association 126
Stress 34-6, 57-8, 59, 63, 77, 79, 102, 114, 119, 156, 174, 244, 249, 272, 281, 286-92, 297
    see also anxiety
Stress interview 281
Stress testing *see* exercise testing
Stretching 236
Stroke volume 21, 64, 69-73, 80, 202-13, 226, 275
ST-segmental depression 51, 64, 97, 98, 109-10, 149-53, 155, 157, 169-71, 175-84, 185, 215, 229, 239, 244, 259, 270, 281, 294, 297
Sub-maximum tests 177, 185-6, 192-4, 202, 219, 239
Sudden death 13, 19-20, 30, 46, 50, 51-4, 60, 112-13, 116, 135, 174, 285, 311
Sugar *see* refined carbohydrate

Suicide 23
Supine ergometry 189, 203
Surgery *see* by-pass surgery
Sweat 247-8, 268
Swimming 234, 296, 322
Sympathetic drive 70, 81, 173, 174, 200, 208-9
Symptom-limited maximum 177, 184-5, 190, 200, 202, 219, 240
Symptoms 17, 24-5, 158-9, 255, 259, 295
   recognition 65, 239
Syphilitic aortitis 16
Systolic ejection rate 164

Tachycardia 275
Tarahumara 102
Target heart rate 177-8, 184, 234, 240, 241
Technetium 163
Technician, ecg 24
Tecumseh study 125
Telemetry 239, 243, 297
Television 39
Temperature
   blood 216
   body 247
Temporally correct association 127
Tension, ventricular wall 71, 226, 277
   work 225-6
Tension-time index 71, 196
Test safety *see* dangers of exercise
Test yield 181-4
Thallium 163
Threshold *see* training threshold
Thyroxine 77, 83, 87, 267
Time consciousness
   post-infarction 136, 140, 206, 208, 211, 215, 219, 220, 238-9, 258, 279-82, 312
   see also Type A
Tiredness 236, 240
Toronto studies
   non-randomised longitudinal 133-9
   sudden death & exercise 57-60
Traffic hazards 249
Training responses 66-86, 142, 144, 145-6, 208-13, 216-20, 224, 225, 228, 236, 290
   threshold 114, 127, 232-3
Tranquillisers *see* relaxants, sedatives
Trans fatty acids 266

Transit time 164
Treadmill 189-90
Treatment patterns 44-5, 136-7
Triglycerides 77, 84, 101-2, 115, 267
Trinitrin 17, 230-1
Triple product 71, 196
T waves 173
Type I error 126
   II error 140
Type A personality 35-6, 59, 62, 124, 145, 156, 236, 256

Ultrasound 163, 189
Unemployment 279-82
Unifocal PVCs 175
Union influences 115, 116
Urbanisation 119
   see also civilisation

Vagal blockade 201
Variation of tests 24
Vasodilator drugs 304
Vectorcardiography 166
Velocity, shortening 164
Venous pressure 273
Ventilatory equivalent 73
Ventricular fibrillation 17, 19-20, 21, 46, 50, 55, 60-1, 63, 82, 89, 134, 196-7, 243, 259, 275, 277, 311-12
   flutter 61
   tachycardia 60
   see also dangers of exercise
Verapamil 277
Verification, experimental 128
Violent deaths 110, 117
Viral myocarditis 19, 52, 134, 135, 249, 259
Visceral blood flow 75, 216
Viscosity 83
Vital capacity 73-4, 124
Vitamins 268
Voluntary exhaustion *see* symptom-limited
Vulnerable phase 21

Walking 55-6, 59, 79, 122, 303, 323
   prescription 233, 240-5
Wall stress 88, 226
Wall thickness 226, 228
Warm
   down 62, 235, 243, 248, 259, 278

up 62, 186, 235, 243, 248, 259, 274, 298
War-time diet 40
Water, hardness 103
Weather *see* humidity
Weight for height *see* body build, body mass
Weight loss 264-5
    see also body fat, body mass
Wenckeback block 172
Western Collaborative Study 124
White collar 113-14, 138, 145, 156
    see also social class
'White' workers 113-14, 292
Wild animals 88, 89
Wind-chill 248-9

Wives' attitude 283, 289
Wives' programme 243
Women 57, 180, 293-6
    see also sex differences
Work
    classification units 280-2
    see also employment
'Working through' 16, 297
Work-rate 186, 188, 190
World Health Organization
    classification 22
    study 144
Worries *see* stress

[133]Xenon 166
X-irradiation 162-3, 165

THE HUNGRY GHOSTS

KU-757-702

THE HUNGRY GHOSTS

Anne Berry

WINDSOR
PARAGON

First published 2009
by Blue Door
This Large Print edition published 2010
by BBC Audiobooks Ltd
by arrangement with
HarperCollins*Publishers*

Hardcover ISBN: 978 1 408 46050 4
Softcover   ISBN: 978 1 408 46051 1

Copyright © Anne Berry 2009

Anne Berry asserts the moral right to be identfied
as the author of this work

This novel is entirely a work of fiction. The names,
characters and incidents portrayed in it are the
work of the author's imagination. Any
resemblance to actual persons, living or dead,
events or localities is entirely coincidental

All rights reserved.

British Library Cataloguing in Publication Data available

Printed and bound in Great Britain by
CPI Antony Rowe, Chippenham and Eastbourne

*For my matchless husband Anthony,
and my amazing children, Andrea, Antonia,
Ivan and Ruth.
The value of their unflagging support continues
to be of inestimable worth to me*

ACKNOWLEDGEMENTS

My special thanks to my exceptional agent, Judith Murdoch, and my inimitable publisher and editor, Patrick Janson-Smith, also to my editors Patricia Parkin and Laura Deacon.

Be thou a spirit of health, or goblin damn'd,
Bring with thee airs from heaven or blasts from hell,
Be thy intents wicked or charitable,
Thou com'st in such a questionable shape
That I will speak to thee.

WILLIAM SHAKESPEARE, *Hamlet*, Act 1, scene 4

PROLOGUE
Ghost

I am dead. No, strictly speaking that is not the truth. I am neither fully alive nor fully dead. I am 'undead'. I am unable to relinquish my present and consign it to the past. I am unable to accept I have no future. Thus I am static, earthbound, my feet anchored in mud, while my essence, my Chi, is being pulled, tugged, drawn towards the ghosts of my ancestors, towards the dominion of death. Sometimes I feel like a bone being worried at by a dog. This is an appropriate image because that is exactly what happened to me. This 'half-death' does not make for a peaceful spirit. I am troubled and I am trouble. You see I just have to stir things up, play with the laws of physics to prove . . . to prove what? That I may still be the cause and have an effect. When the ancestors clamour I tell them to be patient. I am not prepared for death I say.

My name was Lin Shui. I was the daughter of a fisherman. I lived on the island of Hong Kong and I was not ready to die. But nor were thousands of others, dying all around me every day. This is not what keeps me here. It is my gnawing hunger that fixes me to the earth.

I was murdered on a perfect summer's morning. It was early June, the year 1942. We had seen a black Christmas come and go. Our tiny island was infested with Japanese soldiers. They had invaded our shores. They held us in their vice-like grip.

1

Father told me that the British could not withstand their venom, that, though they fought with courage, a time had come when they buckled and fell. He explained to me in his customary soft voice that our Governor, Sir Mark Young, had gone in person to the Japanese headquarters in the Peninsula Hotel, and surrendered on Christmas Day. I thought that was odd, to hand over our island home in a place where people had once come to dine and dance, and wear fine clothes and sparkling jewels, and talk of nothing in particular. But father told me that everything in the time that was coming would be odd, and often not just odd but terrible as well. He told me the devils of war were unleashed, that we must bear their madness with fortitude. I listened like a child, and feared like the woman rising up within me. Father told me the worst that could happen had happened, that we were an occupied island now, that they could take no more from us. But in this he deceived me, for one day a Japanese soldier was occupying me, and what he took from me was my life.

*　　　　　*　　　　　*

My death is like a tune that plays over and over in my thoughts. I cannot rid myself of the melody.

*　　　　　*　　　　　*

I am alone. My father and our junk have been taken. My mother, who paved my way into this world with her own life, is no more than a shadow to me. For months now hunger has been my constant companion. With each passing day it

2

consumes more of me. I know that soon there will be nothing left. When you are stripped of everything, I reason, it is good to climb a mountain, for then you will see the way ahead. So I slip through the busy streets of Aberdeen dodging the soldiers, ducking out of the way of jeeps, and diving into the maze of alleys. I find the narrow path that winds its way up to The Peak. I will climb this path, I resolve. When I am high up, I will look down on Aberdeen harbour and I will know what to do. Perhaps my spirit mother tries to warn me, but I am headstrong and do not listen. Perhaps the ancestors barrel into me, a wave of consciousness holding me back. But I am stubborn and plough on. Perhaps he has been watching me for days, my murderer, has seen that I am alone, vulnerable, an easy target? Like the hunter he stalks me as I ascend.

It is already warm when I set out. A June day when the sky is clear as glass, and when the sun, as it swells to its zenith, exudes a smouldering heat that makes your skin prickle, and your head throb. The blood drums in my ears. I can feel the sweat pool in the dip between my shoulderblades, and trickle down my back. I can hear birdsong and the sounds of distant traffic. Sometimes a gunshot rings out, and then the birds, startled, fly up from their perches in the thick, green canopy that surrounds me. From time to time I stand at the edge of the path and gaze down the slope, judging how far I have come, how high I am, how much further I have to go before I gain the summit. I look across a tangle of trees and vines and grasses. I am cocooned in confusion. But I am climbing the mountain that will spin lucid strands from all that

3

is dense and opaque, I whisper.

I hear him then, his boot on the dusty ground behind me, and a stone slipping away, falling into the untidy green expanse. I turn but see nothing. Three times I spin round and the third time he is there. Neither of us speak. We both freeze for a moment, statues on the rutted path. Even then I realise I am on the cusp, on the brink of stepping out of time, of sinking in the bottomless well. He glances over his shoulder, and when he is certain we are alone he walks purposefully towards me.

'Run,' cries my mother, wrapping around me. 'Run and together we will shun him.'

There are only a few yards between us now. I can hear his short breaths, and smell his stale sweat. If I face him he will not harm me, I tell my ancestors. They mock softly, but my mother keens. He pauses feet from me, and there is a space between us where our breaths mingle. I can see wet patches on his khaki uniform, under his arms, across his chest, around his groin. He is wearing a cap and his face is partly shaded. He has a rifle slung over his shoulder. He mutters something in Japanese, his voice harsh and dissonant, specks of cloudy spit fires from his mouth. His eyes narrow to thin wet lines. His mouth splits in a yellow-toothed sneer.

Someone will come by and by, and all will be well, I tell myself.

This is in my head as he swings the rifle off his shoulder and rams me in the chest with the butt of it. I feel a shock of pain, a sickening thud, a splintering crack. I reel backwards, lose my footing, and fall against a hard bed of dirt and stones. He has knocked the air out of me. I am

4

gagging, trying to bite in breath. The soldier does not wait for my lungs to fill. He throws the rifle aside along with his cap, leans over me, seizes the top of my blue cotton tunic, and rips it from my body. A slither of oxygen filters into me. Looking down I see my small breasts, the nipples raised, tight and hard against the cedar brown of my flesh. I am going to crawl away, but the pain in my chest blossoms now like a flower. Again the soldier lurches forwards. This time he grasps my trousers. As he wrenches them away my slippers tumble off. My bare feet scrabble in the dirt. I try to draw my knees up to hide my shame, but he lays hold of my legs and thrusts them apart. He thrusts them so wide I think I might split in two. Here, hunched between my open legs, with one hand he frees his penis, with the other he jams fingers inside me, tearing at my soft virgin centre. My scream dies in my throat, paralysed with terror.

He waits a single interminable beat before he drives into me. In that beat his immutable eyes lock with mine, and he brings his fingers up to his mouth. I see they are coated with flecks of blood and matter. While I watch, he sucks at them ravenously. I have found my voice but he smites it with this same hand. My cry is suffocated and becomes no more than a gurgle. I taste myself in the blow, the sea-musk at the core of me, and my own blood, the metallic sweetness of it on the fingers that are clamped across my mouth. As he slams into me I feel rivers scorch and become runnels of ash. With his free hand roughly he kneads a breast, bruising and crushing it, pinching it so hard I am sure his fingers will meet, claw through my soft flesh.

But when the moment comes and he shudders out his power, I cheat him of victory, for I have left my body and am looking down from a great height. My eyes, which have been stretched wide, aflame with fear, are smothered. They set in a dead fish stare. The stare enrages him. He lets go breast and mouth, and sits back heavily. He is gasping, his penis still ramrod straight between his sweat-slicked loins. He clenches a fist and then slams it into my face. The force of the blow breaks two teeth and cuts into my cheek. A trickle of blood courses down it like a single red tear. From above I snigger at him, and the face of that other girl below breaks into a toothless grin, as she joins me, coughing and hacking with laughter. His manhood shrivels then. It becomes a poor thing at the peal of our contempt, and we can see it is no better than a worm. In the same moment he glimpses it too, and his sallow skin is empurpled with fury as he grapples at his belt.

'What have you got for me now?' I taunt him, my voice as light as the breeze at his back. 'You have occupied me and I am still whole. How will you plant your filthy flag with its rising sun now?'

It is then that I see the glint of the knife, the bayonet he has freed from its leather sheath, and I know how he will plant his flag. The red of his sun will be stained with my blood when it flutters in the wind. He thrusts forwards with all his might, up beneath my broken ribs where he hits his mark. My heart gives a mighty shudder, unreels in a final leap and freezes, the blood curdling within it. I watch him come back to himself, caging his demon deep within, hefting out the knife, and springing back before the rush of red that fountains up to

6

meet him. He drags my body to the edge of the path and rolls it roughly into the deep green cavern. But the ragged tear in my chest snags on a branch and my body hangs there. My blood spills onto the bark, cloaking it thickly, dripping darkly, and even now drying to a crisp beneath the unforgiving sun. The soldier cleans his bayonet blade in the earth, slicing the wetness off it, slipping it back in its sheath. He adjusts his uniform, stoops to retrieve his cap, slips it on, takes up his rifle and slings it back over his shoulder. He gathers up my garments and slippers, wipes his hands on them, balls them in his fists and hurls them after my body. They do not snag on the branch but unfold as they spin, performing mid-air acrobatics as they shake off their creases, before landing, hidden in the undergrowth below. He scuffs the pool of blood over with earth, kicking at it, as if the merest sight of his sin is now abhorrent to him. Then he is gone, the beat of his boots ebbing away on the dusty tide.

I watch from my perch in the tree where I rest now, beside Lin Shui's body. Soon all is still once more, but for the 'drip, drip' of my blood against a waxy leaf, scalding red, striking cool virgin green. How easy is it then, this business of dying, the ancestors trumpet, preparing to welcome me into their starry fold. That is when the fury unfurls inside me. I shrink from them.

'I am not ready to go with you,' I say, clinging to my body, smelling the black hair with just a trace of the mineral sea, and the skin, cotton fresh, and blood that oozes still, salt and copper and cloying with sweetness. And when their rhapsody swells and they pluck at me in their impatience, I hiss and

7

lash the air up into a wind. Then they are frightened and disperse.

The flies come first, bent on blood, crazed with the rancid whiff of decay. And while they swarm over Lin Shui, I consider the shame I might bring on my family if I am found like this. If my father returns and discovers me with the blood bubbling between my thighs, it might prove too great a disgrace for him. I reflect over the buzzing of the flies that it would be better if I was never found. I summon all my strength, pushing the flesh that had once been mine, trying to dislodge it, but it is heavy as lead. When the chorus of cicadas start, I implode, gathering up all the spidery range of me. I slip into the branch, where the limb that bears Lin Shui's body angles from the tree. I seep into the taut, woody fibres there, already stretched with the weight of their load. I saw at them, fuelled with anguish, and at last there is a great crack. The branch breaks, and Lin Shui's bloody corpse, *my* corpse, pitches downwards, the green opening up to her like water, and closing over her when she is gone. Now you can no longer see her from the path. She is hidden, a covert child. I slither down to her. She has landed with a twist. She lies on her belly, her head corkscrewing round, her face still wreathed in its broken-toothed smile, crowning her back.

That night the dogs come. At first there is only one, a sad creature, all ribcage and weeping sores, that skulks nervously around my body, snarling and baring his dripping fangs for several minutes before tucking in. He laps and licks the blood thirstily. He tears at sinew and muscle and flesh. He crushes and crunches bones. His teeth grind

8

and grate. The cacophony of his feeding frenzy appals me. He is joined by another. First they scrap, hackles up, wearing what fur they have on their mangy carcasses like ruffs, gnashing their teeth, growling and snapping over their prize. In the end they realise there is enough for both of them, and they settle down together to feast on Lin Shui. I cannot stay here, I think. If I stay here I shall be reminded that I am dead. So I rise up and shiver on the thermals, and see days come and days go. I soar with the birds. But even here there is buzzing, silver planes somersaulting and diving and chattering, and far below me a seething sea, carved up with sail-less pewter ships, all hard lines against the scrolls of the sea. I want somewhere I can repose and gather my wits, some refuge that I can lose myself in.

I know it is ironic for someone cheating death, but I settle at last on a morgue, the morgue of a British army hospital. Perhaps I have more in common with the dead than I realise. It is a gigantic red-brick building, three storeys high, with tiled floors and wide staircases. The patients' wards, the operating theatres, the laboratories and the offices, which nestle within it, are bordered by long corridors, open to the elements but for the arched colonnades that line them. There are smaller barrack blocks standing on the terraced slopes above it. The edifice is reassuringly solid, rooted comfortingly, as I still am, to the earth. It rises grandly from its site in Bowen Road. My morgue lies in a roomy basement at one far end of the hospital. It is quenched of light.

*　　　　*　　　　*

This then is how I come to stave off death, with nothing but my will for weaponry. And it is how, paradoxically, I find myself housed in a sepulchre of death. Above me a battle rages, but I choose to reside below with the defeated. They lie stiffly in the tenebrous ward that all mankind must come to, with their shattered bones and gory stumps. Some have empty red sockets where the jelly of an eye once swivelled, some ragged flesh where once an ear thrilled to the music of life, some scorched bloody caves, where tongues wagged and lips were bellows, pumping the body's elixir of oxygen. Beneath their shrouds I trace the puncture patterns of bullets, reliving the impact of each one, the flesh yielding with a judder to their sting.

These then are my playmates, my companions, these cold rigid cadavers. Sometimes I concentrate very hard and jerk their waxy limbs. I make their petrified, pale eyelids twitch. As I move over their ruined bodies like a lover, my presence soft as gentle rain on their ugly wounds, they tell me their sad tales of death. They speak of lovers left behind, of mothers longed for, and of filth and gore and carnage. They tell me how they grew fluent in the language of horror, of shrieks torn from bodies wracked with pain, of groans dredged up from a Hades of everlasting torture, of grief that had not the luxury to linger. Theirs was a lottery of limbs yielded up to blade and bomb and bullet, their drama, the inestimable tragedy of war. And in turn I croon them to sleep with memories of breath, and the urgency of it, and the beat of blood, and the flood of sensation, and the tick of life. I tell them stories of our junk, *Heavenly Sea*,

10

bucking and pitching across a bowl of liquid gold. I recount how my father, a simple fisherman, was taken by the Japanese, a suspected informer for the Gangjiu Dadui, one of the Chinese resistance forces. I confide my yearning for the inconstant ocean, the salt smack of her rough embrace. I impart that it was the South China Sea that bore me up, when my child's body grew weary with its chores.

So we share our burden of loss, the dead and I, robbed of our lives and of our loves. Once, one of my soldier playmates is brought to the morgue, like me hovering in the half-light between life and death. Before he slips away, he makes a gift to me of his ethereal British army jacket.

'To shield your modesty,' he says, insisting as he departs that he no longer has a need for it.

Then a dawn breaks, that is marked by a ringing silence. Gone is the clattering, booming, jarring disharmony of war. The staccato guns have stopped firing. The crescendo of marching feet is stilled. The medley of horses' hooves is muffled. The dreadful ululation is spent. My dead companions no longer come to see me, and the building above my head grows thick with quietude. I am thinning with loneliness, for dust motes and dried blood make for poor company. Curious, I creep out of obscurity. It is dusk. I alight on a curve of railing. I am aware that time has rolled by and all is changed. I stare down the skirt of the mountain at the harbour, Victoria Harbour. I see it transformed, the dimpled sea freckled with crafts of every imaginable shape and size. Ribbons of road packed with cars and lorries and buses wind about the slopes. There are more buildings

11

beaded with lights than I could ever have dreamt of—buildings so tall they seem to brush the clouds. I am blinded too by the shimmering pictures facing some of the tall towers, pictures that bounce out across the water, luminous sea snakes, electric colours that crackle and spit into the night. Lin Shui's life is faded now, like an old book left in the sun and rain too long. Some days I allow myself to drift towards death. When I do, I think I see a small boy crouching in the shadows, an urchin with hair of spun gold, and skin that shines like varnished teak. He is barefoot and clad in black rags. I start to sink into the soporific infinite blackness at the centre of his eyes. And he stands and smiles, and opens his arms to me in greeting. Like a moth drawn to a flame, I am drawn to him. But always just before he enfolds me, I rouse myself and kick out.

My voice might be weaker but still it cries, 'I am not ready yet. Not yet.'

Then one day the children come. Among them is Alice.

Ingrid—2003

The one person you can reliably guarantee will be missing from a funeral is the deceased. Then why, at the funeral of Ralph Safford, did I have the distinct impression that two people were missing? I suppose that my charge, Lucy Holiday, the deceased's sister, was largely responsible. I had been employed as a carer for Lucy for several years now. Childless, widowed, in her eightieth year and in fragile health, Lucy defied expectations, clinging tenaciously onto life. On the day of her brother's funeral, Lucy, with her wisp of wild, white hair, and bright, periwinkle-blue eyes, was enjoying a rare moment of lucidity. She sat in her wheelchair alongside the pew-end, humming tunelessly to all the hymns, her eyes darting around the congregation, and alighting first on one face then another.

At length, she gestured for me to lean closer, and closer still, then whispered in my ear in her scratchy-record voice, 'Ingrid, where is Alice?'

To which I naturally replied, 'Who is Alice?'

She fidgeted with the fabric of her black polyester dress, and rubbed her matchstick legs before answering, and so long was she that I couldn't help wondering if I'd lost her again.

'Alice is my niece,' she said at last, on a rising note of triumph.

'The daughter of your brother Ralph?' I sought confirmation.

Lucy nodded her affirmation. I was puzzled. As far as I knew, Ralph Safford only had three children. I had met the family a few times since they settled in England four years ago. I recalled the first occasion being held in a party at the Safford's home, Orchard House, to celebrate their return from abroad. Besides this, Lucy had spoken of them, if not often, certainly enough for me to be well acquainted with their names. Jillian was the eldest, and Nicola the middle child, while Harry was the baby of the family. But of this 'Alice', up to now I had heard nothing. With Lucy's customary fits and starts, I had also gleaned a little of the deceased's life, certainly enough to whet my

13

appetite for more. Here, it seemed, was no ordinary man. Apparently Lucy's brother and his family had lived overseas, in the then British Crown Colony of Hong Kong, where he had been employed by the government. 'A high-ranking official,' Lucy had confided to me with a knowing wink, on more than one occasion, often adding enigmatically, 'In the land of the blind, the one-eyed man is king'. Quite what this meant I did not know. However, it only seemed to enhance the impression that Lucy's brother had been out of the ordinary. Apparently too, the Saffords lived at one of the most enviable addresses at the summit of Victoria Peak. This, Lucy had explained, was the highest mountain on the island, and was known locally simply as 'The Peak'. I had also discovered that Ralph and his wife Myrtle only returned to England a year or so after Hong Kong was handed back to China in 1997, though it seemed the children departed some time earlier. But of Alice, until today, there had been no mention. I was intrigued. However, the middle of a funeral service was neither the time nor the place to probe family history, unearthing who knew what skeletons. So when Lucy asked me yet again where Alice was, I did my best to bring the matter to a close for the present.

'I expect she's up at the front with Myrtle, your sister-in-law,' I whispered. Then, without thinking, I added, 'All three children are sitting alongside their mother.' But to my relief Lucy gave another nod, and seemed satisfied.

The priest was offering up prayers now, and a bald patch on the crown of his head loomed somewhat indecently into sight. I could not help

14

noticing that it was a surprising shade of mustard yellow, and gleamed dully with beads of perspiration.

I straightened up, and tried to concentrate on the proceedings once more. Though this was easier said than done, I thought, as the vicar's nasal voice see-sawed on monotonously. But again Lucy beckoned me down to her, frantically flapping her crêpe-paper hand, freckled with age-spots, and roped with prominent, deep-blue veins.

'Four,' she said, and for a moment I was nonplussed.

'Four?' I repeated at a loss.

This time Lucy raised her cracked voice to its very limit. 'Four,' she huffed. And then, when I still looked blank, 'Four children. Ralph had four children.' This last, she said so loudly that several heads turned to glare in our direction.

'I'll find out where she is later,' I hissed, enunciating each word as clearly as I could, without causing further disturbance. Luckily at that moment the organ struck up, and though I could see Lucy was speaking again, her words were drowned out by a thunderous rendition of Onward Christian Soldiers.

And to be honest as the service went on, and, it seemed, Lucy quietened down, I let her supposed concerns slip to the back of my mind. Naturally, with a job like mine, funerals have a way of cropping up regularly. But for the most part these occasions have the sting taken out of them. The death of an elderly person who has lived their life to the full is both inevitable and, in a way, a cause for gratitude. They have managed to reach the end of the game despite the many hazards life would

15

have thrown in their path. Bearing this in mind, my primary concern as a carer for those of advanced years is that my patients make a good end. And yet . . . and yet, the more times I witness death, no matter how peaceful it is, the less comfortable I am with it. These days, I can't help wondering if behind that pallid face, those fluttering breaths, that seemingly limp body, a tussle with death is playing out, fuelled by regrets, opportunities missed, words left unspoken, and last but not least, the indignity of it all.

But for now I abandoned this unsettling train of thought, and cast my eyes around the beautiful old Sussex church. I took in the small sober congregation, clad in their suitably melancholy outfits. These faces were, I noted, no different from the many others I had seen at past services, obviously more unsettled by this grim reminder of their own mortality than distraught with grief at the passing of another. The prickle on the back of the neck, the leaden sensation in the stomach, the feet squirming in their shoes, the longing to be outside filling your lungs with fresh air, the sudden shadow subduing the chirpiest of characters, these were not signs of sorrow, oh no, but of their own disquiet. Nor could I claim that I was exempt from such reflections. Sooner or later, the service, you knew, would be yours. And at sixty-two the 'sooner' undoubtedly applied to me.

Despite this, I let my eyes linger on Ralph Safford's coffin, set to one side of the altar. There was no denying it made a fine spectacle, fashioned in a rosy mahogany, or at least the veneer of it, with flowers draped luxuriously over the lid. I picked out some of my favourites—fragrant lilies, golden roses with tight corollas of whorled petals, fluffy cream carnations, lacy lilac delphiniums, and strident white and yellow gerberas, all arranged in glorious sprays. The soft colours were echoed in the arrangements that were decked throughout the church. The magnificent stained-glass windows drew me too, weathered by time and changing seasons. The summer light, as it poured through them, was transmuted into magical colours, iridescent beams moving over the patina of old wood, transforming the wan faces of the mourners into something unearthly. For a while I became wholly absorbed in a particularly lovely pair of arched windows, depicting two cloaked women in lucent blues and purples and silvery greys.

Then my attention was drawn back to the service again. Nicola Safford was addressing the congregation, delivering a eulogy to her father. Impeccably dressed, she had shown no sign whatever of nerves, or indeed heartache, as she strode confidently up to the lectern. Then, like a consummate actress, she had paused, her eyes sweeping over the pews to ensure she had the full attention of her audience. Now, unsurprisingly, her delivery was flawless—word-perfect, in fact one might almost have said a little too well rehearsed. She spoke of the years of sublime happiness the family spent together in Hong Kong, of her father's absolute devotion to his wife and his children, and of the invaluable contribution he had made on the island.

'He was at the helm in good times and bad, serving his Queen and country without flinching. He faced the challenges of keeping the colony on an even keel throughout the period of unrest that

17

culminated in the riots of 1967. With immense bravery he stood proud, in the front line. He defended the citizens of Hong Kong from the bloodthirsty insurgents who threatened the stability of the island. Under my father's auspices order was restored. And for his exceptional contribution to his monarch, Queen Elizabeth the Second, and to the British Government of the time, he was awarded the OBE, and made an Officer of the British Empire.'

I listened, rapt, as Nicola Safford's clear, well-modulated voice echoed off the stone walls of the thirteenth-century church, revealing yet more admirable facets to her father's character. Finally softening her tone, lowering her gaze, and blinking back tears that very nearly convinced me, she spoke of the love she had for her father.

'I was so grateful . . . grateful for the opportunity to demonstrate the veneration in which I held my father, grateful to be close to such a fine man, doing what little I could to ease his passage through those final years.' Her last words, delivered at a slower pace, the volume swelling, the pitch deeper, resonated like the closing chord of a great symphony. Nor do think I imagined the slightly awkward moment that followed, in which the impulse to applaud had to be quelled by the mourners.

Nicola Safford's address had certainly pushed Lucy's perturbation to the back of my mind. But if I thought I had heard the end of Alice, I was mistaken. In fact it was just the beginning. Later, when the service had finished, and my charge and I joined the little queue, to pay our condolences to Myrtle Safford and the children, Lucy took up the

18

same refrain. Where, she wanted to know, was Alice? She could see Harry, Jillian and Nicola, but surely Alice should be with them. It would have mattered to Ralph that his youngest daughter was here. Alice would have wanted to attend too. Even, more ominously, what had they done with her? There was no doubt about it, I had a Miss Marple kind of curiosity awakening inside me.

I soothed Lucy as best I could, easing her forwards in her chair and plumping up the cushions behind her, checking that she was comfortable. Then, as we neared Harry Safford, I promised her that I would make inquiries about Alice. I shook her nephew's clammy hand, reminded him of my name, told him how sorry I was for his loss, how beautiful the flowers were, and how moved I had been by the service. This over, I had the distinct impression that Harry had already dismissed me from his mind. But once set in motion I am like an ocean liner: it takes considerable effort to stop me. I leaned in towards Harry, resolved not to move on until I had questioned him on behalf of my charge. I took a deep breath. Suddenly I felt nervous. How ridiculous, I told myself, as I sent out the first scout in search of Alice.

'Your Aunt Lucy is feeling a bit anxious,' I told him, pushing my rimless spectacles more firmly up my nose with a fingertip. 'She wants to know where your sister Alice is?' Did I imagine it or was there a flicker of something in his cold, bluish-grey eyes. Recognition? Anger? Or perhaps even fear?

'Alice?' he queried with a dry little laugh. 'Really? Who is Alice?' He placed crossed hands over his rotund belly, almost defensively.

'Forgive me. I thought that Alice might be your sister,' I explained. 'Your Aunt Lucy seems convinced you have another sister. Alice?'

'Well, my aunt is mistaken,' Harry said curtly, looking at my charge with undisguised displeasure. He bent over the fragile form of Lucy and bellowed, 'What rubbish are you talking now, Aunty, getting Ingrid all upset? Ralph would be ashamed of you making up such silly things.' I detected, though subtle, a slightly lazy 'r' in his speech.

'I'm not upset,' I assured Harry Safford. 'It's just that your aunt seems so certain. She keeps saying that Alice should be here. She seems concerned that something may have happened to her.' Harry arranged his features in an expression of extreme bafflement. But I was not to be so easily thwarted. I pointed my next words. 'To Alice I mean. That something may have prevented Alice from coming.'

'What is all this nonsense, Aunt Lucy?' Harry blustered, his face reddening, more with annoyance, I guessed, than embarrassment.

'Why is Harry shouting at me?' Lucy wanted to know, hunching further down in her chair. 'I'm not deaf. But then he always was a bully.'

Now it was my turn to colour. The old, like the very young, do not screen their words, parcelling them up and sending them out in acceptable packages for this world to receive, as most of us do.

'I'm sorry,' I apologised on behalf of Lucy. 'She's a bit tired, and probably a touch overwrought with the emotion of the day.'

'It's quite understandable,' Harry said shortly,

eyes unblinking, giving me a perfunctory smile. He turned away from us then towards his mother and sisters, ruffling back his short ash-grey hair in an impatient gesture.

'It's just that Lucy appears to be quite fractious about . . . well . . . about Alice you see,' I persisted.

Reluctantly Harry turned back. But this time he recruited his sisters to add weight to his own voice.

'Aunt Lucy has been bothering Ingrid with foolish stories about someone called Alice,' he said, with the air of a parent whose tolerance is being pushed to its absolute limits. Again, I thought I saw a furtive glance pass between Nicola and Jillian.

Jillian, a large lady, whose considerable height was diminished by her width, gave a slight shiver before speaking. She tossed back her startling, shoulder-length red hair, greying at the roots. 'Poor Aunt Lucy,' she said at last. 'She gets very muddled.' She reached out a hand tentatively and touched her aunt's bony shoulder. It was hard for me to read the expression in her flint-grey eyes, with her large, square-framed glasses reflecting back the bright sunshine at me. She did not, I observed, have her sister's dress sense. The variation in shade, however slight, from the black tailored trousers, to the dark navy jacket, was disconcerting. Added to this, the jacket appeared rather snug and the trousers at least one size too large.

'That's right,' Nicola chimed in, her tone liberally soaked in pity, 'poor Aunt Lucy hardly knows what day it is, bless her.' She shot me a swift appraising look, critically taking in my own cheap black suit, practical flat shoes, and hurried attempt

21

to pin up my straight salt and pepper bob.

She was a little shorter than her sister, and slimmer in build. From a distance her outfit had looked smart, but close up it was stunning. The knee-length black dress with matching jacket, delicate gold flowers stitched into the fabric, had the unmistakeable sheen of heavy silk. The outfit was finished off with inky stilettos, a designer's golden tag glinting at their heel backs. Her hairstyle was eye-catching too. The overall shade was altogether more natural than her sister's, a deep mocha-brown, aflame with red and gold highlights. It was cut into irregular bangs that suited the fine bone structure of her face. But bizarrely her hands, I noticed, were those of a nineteenth-century scullery maid, rubbed red and raw. Now she fixed me with her own inscrutable eyes, just the colour of the slab of liver I had purchased for Lucy from the butcher's that week.

'You really shouldn't be concerning yourself with Aunt Lucy's ramblings, Ingrid. Surely you're experienced in caring for the elderly? You should know what to expect.' And I could have sworn there was a warning edge to a voice that had an unsettling, forced brightness in it.

'Of course,' I said, understanding that the conversation had been brought to a close.

I pushed Lucy onwards, briefly shaking Myrtle Safford's hand. The matriarch of this family was a tall woman with a proud but guarded face, gimlet eyes, glittering jewels, and outdated clothes which nevertheless screamed quality. However, I barely had time to express my sympathy, before her children whisked her away to speak to a less troublesome mourner. My thoughts in turmoil now, I steered my charge to a quiet spot in the churchyard, beneath the shade of an oak tree encircled with a wooden seat. I tucked a cheerful tartan rug I had brought with me about Lucy's knees, and told her gently that she must be mistaken about Alice. Was she perhaps thinking of someone else, from her husband's side of the family? Another niece or perhaps the child of a friend? When she said nothing, I crouched before her, my hands resting on the arms of her wheelchair, levelling my gaze with hers. For a moment her sharp blue eyes had a promising intensity about them. She opened her mouth and took a shaky but deliberate breath.

'You see, Ingrid, Alice is . . . is . . .'

'Is what?' I urged her eagerly. But the elusive thought had wriggled away, and Lucy's eyes suddenly shut tremulously. 'You're tired. I'll take you home now,' I told her, unable to keep the disappointment from my voice.

But just before I helped her into my car she grasped my bare arm. I had peeled off my jacket by then and was only wearing a short-sleeved cream blouse. Now Lucy's fingers scrabbled against the flesh of my forearm, splayed and light as birds' feet.

'Where is Alice? Alice should have been here. Ralph would be most upset, Ingrid, you know,' she croaked. Shortly after this I bundled her into the car, and she immediately fell into a deep sleep, snoring lightly.

I was staying overnight with Lucy in her small terraced house in Hailsham. After her tea, cottage pie and raspberry jelly, I decided a warm bath might settle her for the night. I never quite got

23

used to the shrivelled bodies I handled daily, with their spun-glass bones and their tracing paper flesh. As I sponged the curve of Lucy's back, knotted and wrinkled as the bark of some ancient tree, my mind played over the events of the day. No matter which thread of thought I plucked at, they all seemed to lead back to Alice, as if by merely uttering her name Lucy had conjured up her ghost. Later, when my charge was tucked into bed, just before I slipped out her false teeth, I tried once more.

'Are you sure your brother Ralph had a fourth child, a child called Alice?' I asked softly.

The last thing I wanted to do was to distress Lucy just before she fell asleep. But I needn't have worried. She looked at me blankly, and then the coquettish smile of a flirtatious young woman wreathed her wizened face.

'Who . . . is Alice?' she said.

For the remainder of the evening I watched a bit of television, and then settled to a crossword puzzle. I like doing crosswords, everything fitting into its correct space, all the words connected, interdependent. Just before turning in, I drew back the green velour curtains, and stared out into the tiny garden. The pane had misted lightly with the cool of the night. I wrote the name 'Alice' very carefully on it with my index finger.

'Alice who?' I whispered and climbed the stairs to bed.

Myrtle—2003

I am sitting in the back room of Orchard House. I am always sitting in the back room waiting for something to happen. And when you sit, as I do, for hour after hour, you find yourself reminiscing. You cannot help it. You begin to wonder about how it all came to pass. The young look forward. The old look backward.

I remember the child I once was, the child who visited Kew Gardens with Mother and brother Albert. I craned my small neck, looking at the red pagoda that rocked upwards, diminishing into the unremitting drabness of an oyster-grey sky. And I dreamed my dreams. All the way home, as the bus rumbled and coughed, and juddered and spluttered, through London traffic, I watched a fly fling itself against a sooty pane of glass. Turning my head, I could see Albert, beautiful Albert, with his piercing ice-blue eyes, sensuous red mouth, and dark curls. And I could see my mother, her brown hair neatly crimped, her own prim mouth, bright with deep pink lipstick, her round cinnamon eyes, dancing with obvious delight. Their heads were touching, mother and son, their voices low and intimate, washed into one another. Close as conspirators they were, oblivious of me, gazing at them from across the aisle. So I turned away, back to the fly buzzing and battering itself against the glass, its frenzy futile. I imagined smashing that pane of glass with a closed fist, hearing it shatter. I pictured the fly bursting out into the infinite space, and whirring away, hardly daring to believe its luck.

I recall how years later, shortly after the war, my gentle giant of a father died. His disease-ridden heart, the organ that had prevented him fighting for his country and earned him a coward's feather, finally gave out in peacetime. It seized up and froze before a plate of pink blancmange. As the breath trickled out of him he keeled over, right into the cold, gelatinous pinkness of it, a single bubble of breath breaking the surface seconds after. I remember my dismay looking on, knowing I had lost my only ally in the gloomy red-brick house in Ealing.

And I recollect my first sight of you, Ralph— dark, tall and dashing, with alert steely-blue eyes, clasping a camera before you. You were covering an amateur show for the local rag, and had come to photograph its parochial stars. I was numbered among them. Gwendolen in Oscar Wilde's *The Importance of Being Earnest*. At best, my performance could be described as lacklustre; at worst, wooden. But you, it appeared, had seen a different play altogether, as you posed me for your photographs, your face so animated, those beguiling eyes of yours sparkling. Next to your striking looks, it was the enthusiasm that captured and held me. It was as if there was nothing you couldn't do with it. Take a shabby little amateur production in a village hall, with threadbare costumes and tatty scenery, and transform it into a glittering spectacle, showcasing the astonishing talent that lay at the heart of a thriving community. Or, perhaps, take a dull British girl destined for banal suburbia and transform her into a shimmering princess?

26

'What a superb show! I don't know when I've laughed so much. And you, well, you were wonderful Miss Lambert, entrancing. I brought Lucy, my sister, along too. And she loved your performance.'

That's what you said to me, as you pushed a strand of hair back from my face and, with a finger under my chin, adjusted the angle of my profile. You were wonderful. I knew I wasn't. Hadn't the director, Ron Fowler, spent eight weeks informing me of the fact? And all the while his invective boomed out, those expressive fingers of his would spear back his leonine mane, and his fleshy cheeks would colour plum-red.

'Do lighten your delivery, Myrtle. This is Wilde at his finest, witty, effervescent repartee. It's a comedy, darling, not a wake. Must you keep clinging onto the furniture, lovey? Anyone would think you were on the *Titanic*, hanging on for dear life, seconds before the bloody thing went down. Sweetheart, do pick up your cues a bit more promptly, you're slowing down the pace to a deathly crawl. Must you keep folding your arms, darling? You look like the genie from Aladdin, not the alluring Gwendolen Fairfax.'

They just kept coming, and the worst of it was knowing the comments were completely justified. I had no talent: my foray into amateur theatre only served to confirm what I had always suspected. I did not have the fascination of the sea about me, no glittering treasure lying undiscovered many fathoms down. It was disheartening to realise the truth. Oh Ralph, I just wanted to shine for a time, the way Albert did, for Mother to be just a little in awe of me . . . as if . . . as if I really was an

27

interesting person. Is that too much to ask?

You did that. Looking back, I think something in your exuberance answered to my reticence. I was self-contained, you were abandoned. Opposites attract, isn't that what they say? But I knew, almost immediately I knew. As I sat there wishing I was not quite so tall, that my hair would not fall so stubbornly straight, that I could instil some mysterious depths into my eyes, like Rita Hayworth or Bette Davis, and your camera clicked and flashed, I knew. You were my ticket out of there, away from Mother and the ever-present reprobation in those grim button eyes of hers, away from Albert, the brother, the boy, the son and heir, who had been given so many gifts that there were none left over for me. And away from the gloomy corners of the red-brick house, and the grey that I felt my soul was steeped in.

I sensed you were attracted to me that first meeting. It was quite enough to be going on with. Had director Ron only known it, I followed my dismal debut as Gwendolin Fairfax with a breathtaking improvisation of Myrtle Lambert, the woman every man wants by his side, his perfect helpmeet, the accomplished hostess, the contented housewife, the adoring lover. I gave it everything I had, because, you see—and here, believe me I am not exaggerating—my future relied upon it. And when you didn't ask for your money back, but seemed entirely swept away by the illusion, indeed, just kept following curtain-call with curtain-call, I knew I had a triumph on my hands. Maybe not worthy of the Oscar which all Hollywood actresses hanker after, but then who wanted some old statue gathering dust on their shelf when instead they could have handsome, dynamic Ralph Safford for their very own. And more, a life as far away from dreary Britain as it was possible to get, thrown in with the bargain.

So we were married—you for love, and me for . . . ah Ralph, for a force much stronger than that: the longing for freedom. I was entirely satisfied with the arrangement, and be honest, so were you, to start with anyway. When you were posted to Africa, Kenya, as a government photographer, I was by your side. You whisked me away, leaving Mother seething far behind in the red-brick house, claiming she had been abandoned by the pair of us.

I used to love sitting on the veranda of our bungalow in Kenya, sipping scotch. I close my eyes and I am there. It is very hot. The air pulses with the heat. The chill of England seems so distant. I open my eyes sleepily, just a fraction, smile and take another sip of scotch. Having a drink together in the evenings was all part of the ritual. Do you recall, Ralph? The servant bringing the bottle of scotch on a tray, together with the ice tub and two glass tumblers, each already filled with chunks of ice. I loved the way the ice cubes chimed as I rolled them round the glass. I loved the whisper of the cold, golden liquid going down, a thread of flame tightening inside me. I was enthralled by the extremes, the last rays of the dying sun scalding through me, the cold of the frosted glass against my cheek. Sunsets were very different in Africa, weren't they, Ralph? The sun was a red fireball that sunk very slowly into the parched red clay. The skies were almost obscenely brilliant—topaz, coral, mauve, malachite, banks of radiance shifting

29

from second to second. Actually, I found the evening displays a trifle vulgar, wasteful, the squandering of so much colour.

It's raining now, an insistent drumming on the rooftop, runnels of rain coursing down the sash windows, the sound of spattering droplets closing in on me. It always seems to be raining here in England. It wasn't like that in Hong Kong, was it Ralph? Except of course during the typhoon season, or when the mists settled on The Peak, and the mizzle closed in.

God alone knows what possessed Nicola to choose that dreadful wallpaper for this draughty room. White flowers plastered over a red background. It calls to mind the new regional flag they've chosen for Hong Kong. An uninspiring design if you ask me. It looks like one of those handheld windmills you buy at a fair, or at the seaside. Hardly something you can take seriously. It can't be compared to the Union Jack. Now there's a flag you can be proud of, a flag that means something.

The roof of this wretched building leaks. Why Nicola persuaded us to buy it I will never know.

'Orchard House. The two of you will love it.' That's what she said, as if we didn't have any choice in the matter. And, quite honestly, looking back, I'm not sure we did.

There are buckets placed at strategic points to catch the drips. I can hear them plinking now. It is a bit like a form of Japanese water torture, waiting for the next plink, watching the buckets and pails slowly fill, wondering when the silvery skins will rupture, and the collected rain will trickle down the sides and soak into the Persian rugs. I think I

30

can say that the state of the roof is the most weighty problem here, but there are others. Damp in general, peeling wallpaper, rotting window-frames and cracked panes, missing floortiles, banging pipes and a faulty central-heating system, to name but a few. I think we may even have a bit of woodworm on the first floor that needs treating. Oh, we have mice too. Larry, my son-in-law, claims he's dealing with them. But I doubt it. He says a great deal, and as far as I can see does very little. And Jillian's not much better. What I wouldn't give for a couple of amahs to set the place to rights. I thought Nicola said that having Jillian and Larry living with us was going to make life much easier, that it would alleviate all our difficulties. What's more, I could have done without the boy being foisted on us. Amos. What a ridiculous name for a child! It's not even as if we're great ones for religion. Besides, I have never been maternal. I can't think why Jillian and Larry spent all that money trying to have a baby. When the doctor told her they had problems (something odd about Larry's sperm, not that I pressed them for any details you understand), in my opinion she should have just accepted it. I would have. Gladly, as it happens!

I'm sorry, Ralph, but you know I never really wanted children. Not all women hanker after a family you know. We aren't all programmed for reproduction. Some of us don't need miniature replicas of ourselves to make our lives complete. Conversely, in Alice's case, far from completing me, she very nearly destroyed me. I had her for your sake you know, so you can't blame me entirely for what happened, what happened to our daughter, Alice. You were determined to have your son, weren't you? Oh, you never put it into so many words, but the understanding was implicit. I did my best, Ralph. You must give me that. I tried my hardest to produce your boy, your heir. And if it did take me four goes, I managed it in the end. Don't judge me, Ralph, wherever you are now. You have no idea what it was like for me producing girl after girl, producing Alice at that hospital in Ealing. I had to feel Mother's scorn at my inability to get a son for my husband—not once, not twice, but thrice. After all, she had managed the feat first time, hadn't she?

We didn't put Alice's name on your gravestone. The children wanted to make a dedication to you, a personal thank-you to their father. We talked about adding her name after theirs, but in the end we decided it wasn't appropriate. We felt she hadn't earned her place there. And Ralph, this once you weren't around to make a fuss. So there it is, Jillian, Nicola and Harry, but . . . no Alice. If you want my opinion, and you never really did when it came to Alice, this is as it should be.

'Is it a boy?' I asked the midwife repeatedly. She was quite terse with me in the end.

'It's a girl,' she snapped. 'I've told you it's a girl, a lovely girl.'

That was an oxymoron to me by then, Ralph. Can you understand that? I'd had Jillian and Nicola, and each of those pregnancies cost me dearly. But as a man you could never appreciate that. Besides, delivering Alice was meant to be my last messy natal performance. I deserved to have a boy. I deserved a son by then. You know what they say, Ralph, third time lucky. Well, it wasn't for me.

Having Alice was the most unpropitious thing that ever happened to me. Our daughter, our third daughter filled me with dread. But not you, oh no. You adored her, didn't you?

The midwife was a big, hearty woman, with apple-red cheeks, and large pink hands, butcher's hands I recall. She reached towards my chest and started fumbling with the tie of my nightie.

'No! No, no!' My voice was pitched too high. It reeked of panic.

'Put her to your breast,' she urged, still pulling at the lacing. She had a slight burr to her voice, though what the accent was I couldn't tell you.

I thrust her hand away. 'I am not feeding it myself. I need a bottle,' I told her succinctly. I had an image of a stray dog then, a dog I had seen on the streets of Nairobi, its dugs heavy with milk, puppies suckling frantically at them. Its eyes were rolled upwards to heaven, you could see their whites, but it lay in the gutter, and was coated with filth.

I suppressed a shudder. She stopped scrabbling at my painfully engorged breasts and nudged the baby forwards instead. I took it awkwardly, as if I thought it might bite me at any moment. I looked into the face. The wispy hair was lighter than Nicola's. The mouth that rooted hopefully towards me was pretty enough. But the eyes unsettled me. They were the rich brown of tobacco, and preternaturally alert. They were needy too. I have been told a newborn cannot focus immediately, but as this child stared steadily up at me I had my doubts. Returning her gaze, what I felt was not a trickle of love, but a wave of cold dislike. 'She' meant that I would have to do it all once more.

She was unnecessary, surplus to requirements. She did not even have the decency to look abashed, as Nicola had done. And quite suddenly, with the smell of disinfectant and warm sweet blood, and the distant muted sounds coming to me from far corridors of rolling trolleys and muffled voices and footsteps, I felt afraid.

'Shall I show your husband in?' asked the determined midwife, her tone brisk, business-like. And when there was no response, she added with unnecessary emphasis, 'To see his beautiful baby daughter?'

For a second I wondered who she meant. Then Ralph, in you came. You took the bundle carefully in your arms, studied it for a moment, and then your face lit up. You looked so delighted.

'It is a girl,' I explained, thinking you had not grasped this. It was the year 1956 and I had given birth to yet another baby girl.

'I know,' you said. 'She's beautiful.' To my amazement, your shining eyes proved the sincerity of your words. The baby seemed to sense this, following the sound of her father's voice. Father and daughter's eyes locked. Ralph, you looked smitten, mesmerised. I felt a pang just under my ribcage and had to turn away.

'I think the name Alice suits her,' you said. 'Oh ... yes, definitely. Alice. What do you think?'

I shrugged indifferently. 'If you like,' I said. I wasn't really bothered one way or another. Alice would do as well as the next name.

There was black magic involved in the coming of my son though. Oh, scientists would say that I was just being fanciful, but I know. I was in my sixth month. We had since moved to the British

34

Crown Colony of Aden. Having developed extreme eczema, blistering and bleeding over your hands and lower arms—a reaction to the chemicals you used in photography—you had been persuaded by George Walbrook, your friend in the foreign office, to apply for a posting in government information services in Honduras. Failing to secure this, you were offered instead the administrative post in Aden. And it was here, in the merciless heat and chaos of this busy port, with its shark-infested harbour, that we settled with our growing family. This time, I had decided not to return to England for the birth. I did not think I could bear Mother's disapproval if yet again I failed to produce the necessary male. Besides, I had been assured that they had the very best of facilities and doctors here in Aden.

We were having a party when it happened. Do you remember, Ralph? We had many friends there, British and Arab. I was wearing a voluminous midnight-blue affair. Quite suddenly a tall Arab gentleman, with sable skin and very white teeth—dressed, I couldn't help thinking, with his turban and glittering tunic, a bit like a fairground magician—seized hold of the hem of my dress, folded himself in half, and with his other hand flung some white powder up under the bell of my skirt. It coated my mound. The gentleman's name was A . . . A . . . Akil, that's right, and he worked with you.

He fixed me with his black hawk eyes, Akil, and straightened up. As I moved away the remaining powder fell softly about my ankles, like a dusting of snow. I was taken aback. I had not been prepared for someone shoving handfuls of unknown substances up my maternity dress, and did not know quite how to react. He bowed to me graciously.

'The baby you are carrying, it shall be a boy now,' he said in a deep, sonorous voice.

I was so delighted with his prediction that I forgot to be annoyed. At least he understood the turmoil inside me. The thought of another girl growing there, another Alice . . . dear God! Later that night as you and I tried in vain to slumber in the heat, you mentioned the encounter. I didn't think you had seen it. Even in my tangle of sheets, hot and bothered, with the child stirring restlessly inside me, as if it too was finding the intense heat unbearable, I was surprised.

'That Akil has a cheek,' you mumbled through a yawn. 'Throwing talcum powder up your dress, and coming up with that mumbo-jumbo about our baby.' You thrust the sheet back from your body, and I saw that your skin was slick with sweat.

We were sleeping beneath mosquito nets, and I found the effect of that claustrophobic haze disturbing.

'He took me unawares,' I responded primly, pushing down my own portion of our sheet, sitting up, and resting back against the pillows. 'He told me that now we will have a son.'

You laughed. 'What, as if it was down to him!'

Outside the netting, the high-pitched whine of a mosquito could be heard, fading and then coming back, as it attempted re-entry.

'It might be true. It might be a boy,' I commented casually, as if I couldn't have cared less.

'And it might be a girl,' you said equably.

36

After that you fell asleep. But I remained awake for some time, my hands exploring my bump, glossy with moonlight. I could not bear to go through this again. There was no choice in the matter, and the child should know this. It had to be male. Our son was born three months later. Clearly he had been paying attention to our Arab friend. But he had obviously been a touch overwrought at the prospect of his much longed-for arrival, and had wound the umbilical cord around his neck like a noose. He emerged not a healthy shade of pink, flushed with his first breaths of life, but milky-blue, his lips an even deeper hue, kissed with death. The doctors were uncertain if he would make it through the night. They took him away to wrestle with the black prince, promising to do their best to snatch my son from his grip. I lay alone in bed that night, in a white nondescript room, in a hospital in Aden. I felt bleak. I had produced a son. Finally I had produced a son, and now he might die. I thought about our three *healthy* children—my firstborn, Jillian, a girl, but welcome for all that, and my second, Nicola, impossible not to like, with her indomitable charm and her discretion. She understood the boundaries so well and never overstepped the mark. And then our third daughter, Alice. Alice had already made it apparent that she did not understand about boundaries. She was colouring outside the lines. I felt annoyed just thinking about her. If I could . . . if . . . I could . . . swap her life for his, then . . . At first the thought was so terrible that it floored me. It had all the menace of dark fairy tales. I will give her up if you will . . .

But gradually in the dullness of that room my wicked thought glowed like a hot coal. You may take Alice but leave me my son. I will never renege on the contract. Take her. Take Alice. Take Alice. Take Alice, was my incantation. She's yours. I shall never want her back, only leave me my son. It seemed the demons were not listening, or perhaps they didn't want Alice either because as it was they both survived. The next day you brought our daughters to see their new brother. You stood, Ralph, and the girls sat on the low wall that surrounded the hospital. They squinted up through the fierce sunlight as I stepped onto the balcony from my second-floor room, my fragile son in my arms. The doctors felt it would be better to keep my sickly babe away from any possible source of infection for the time being, until he grew stronger. They recommended no direct contact with our other children during those first crucial days.

The girls were wearing matching pinafore dresses, with white blouses, Jillian in French navy, her blonde hair in pigtails, Nicola in bottle-green, her dark silky locks cropped short, and Alice in red, blood-red, her mousy-brown bob with a side parting, held back from her face with a grip. The green and blue blended in with the flashing gold of the sun and the cooler acid green of the young palm trees. The girls waved. You waved, Ralph. I looked down at my son and felt pride wash over me.

'Here in my arms are all my hopes and dreams,' I thought.

But the red of Alice's dress hooked me back again. Even then she was a jealous child.

You were reassigned after that, this time to the British Colony of Hong Kong. When you first mentioned it to me, the new posting, I was intrigued.

'How would you like it if I spirited you away to a beautiful island in the Orient?' you asked, jumping up suddenly from the wicker chair you had been sitting in. We were in the bedroom of our bungalow home in Aden. Above our heads a fan rotated noisily, doing its best to hold the heat at bay.

'I should like that very much,' I said, only half listening, concentrating on our blue-eyed, golden-haired boy, wriggling in my arms.

'Then your wish is my command. I shall transport you to Hong Kong,' you shot back, unable to hide your delight.

'Hong Kong?' I said, trying out the name and finding it both familiar and unknown.

You elaborated. 'It's a small island in the South China Sea, not much more than 400 square miles I believe. But then there is the Kowloon Peninsula and the New Territories too, just across the harbour.'

'Oh,' I said, trying to sound enlightened. 'It seems odd that we should own an island so far away.' You smiled knowingly and continued.

'It was leased to Britain after some skulduggery which involved the shipping of a great deal of opium grown by us in India into China. Very lucrative apparently. When China, unsurprisingly, protested and asked that we desist in the trade, we were so outraged we went to war with them.' Here you paused mid-stride and chuckled.

'Ah,' I said, switching my son from one shoulder

39

to the other, and patting his back gently. In a while I would call for his nanny, but just for now it was nice playing mother. You packed tobacco into the bowl of a wooden pipe, then paced thoughtfully around our bed. You used to smoke a pipe back then, though you gave it up when we got to Hong Kong. I rather liked the smell of it and missed it later. 'And we won?' I asked.

'We did, and among the spoils we acquired Hong Kong Island in 1842, and a bit later on, Kowloon and the New Territories, leasehold for 99 years.'

You perched on the side of the bed, Ralph, leant forwards and gently stroked your son's golden curls. Then you placed the stem of the pipe in your mouth, struck a match, and held the flame to the bowl, sucking hard until the fragrant strands of tobacco caught. For a while you puffed contentedly, your expression dreamy. After a bit you removed your pipe, those engaging eyes of yours searching my face. 'So how do you fancy a spell residing on Queen Victoria's ill gotten gains?' you asked, your eyes alight with mischief.

I thought about it for a moment—only a moment, mind. I recalled a red pagoda towering up into the sky, the roof of each diminishing segment looking like an oriental hat, the brim curving upwards into delicate points. I recalled a fly beating its wings against the grubby window of a bus, longing for liberation, and I remembered too the dull greyness that seemed to encroach on everything back then.

'I think I should like that very much,' I said. So we packed our trunks and set off again. In the late spring of 1962 I had my first sighting of Hong

Kong, as we sailed into busy Victoria Harbour. We would come to know that bridge of water between the island and Kowloon as if it was an extension of our own bodies. The dull, green face of the sea was dotted with sampans and junks and ferries. From here, my gaze strayed past the mass of buildings that crowded the waterfront, and on up the verdant slopes looped with winding roads. We had docked off a bustling, mountainous island, the summits veiled mysteriously in dense powder-grey clouds. And it was a short while later up these mountains we wound in a shiny, black chauffeur-driven car.

'Our flat is set almost on the highest point of The Peak,' you told me, Ralph. 'Fabulous views.' We threaded our way higher and higher, into what seemed to me an impenetrable fog. 'That is of course, unless we are temporarily lost in the mist. I understand it can be a real problem here,' came your wry observation.

But any qualms I may have had about our mountain home were soon quelled. Here was a grand, airy, top-floor flat, situated right at the top of The Peak, with the views you had boasted of to be enjoyed from every window. The white, flat-roofed building was only six floors high, double-sided, the central column housing the stairwell and the lift. Our front door opened onto a hall that would have graced any stately home back in England, while doors to either side of it led on the left to a lounge, this in turn giving onto a long, open veranda, and on the right to a dining room, and thence into a spacious kitchen. Beyond the kitchen was a communal sheltered area for drying washing. It led through to the servants' accommodation, six tiny bedrooms in all, with a shared rudimentary bathroom and toilet, and for their use a separate stairwell leading down to the ground floor. Returning to our hall I explored further, the children running ahead excitedly. My high heels clicked smartly on the wooden floors of the long corridor that ran the length of the flat. Light flooded through tall wide windows to my right, while on my left doors led off it into large bedrooms, the first of which had a luxurious en suite bathroom. A second bathroom lay at the end of the corridor from which, on fine days, you assured me, you could look out over Pokfulam and the sea.

There was room aplenty for the Safford family and we had soon settled in. I told you that, for the time being, I could make do with just two servants. So Ah Dang, with her glossy jet-black hair drawn back into a tight bun, her wide girth attesting to her own passion for food, and her glittering gold front teeth, became our housekeeper and cook. And Ah Lee, with her bouncy, dark curls and her constant nervous giggling, juggled the tasks of washing, ironing, cleaning and shopping and, it seemed, found plenty to amuse herself in each. We provided them both with the standard uniform— drawstring black trousers, and plain three-quarter length white tunics. The children were dispatched to English-speaking Little Peak School and Big Peak School respectively, both within walking distance, Alice attending the former, and Jillian and Nicola the latter. Four-year-old Harry, our son, soon followed, so to a large extent, I had my freedom. Quite what we would do when Jillian finished at Big Peak School I did not know, for exclusively English-speaking secondary schools were in very short supply.

Life on The Peak in Hong Kong was punctuated by regular letters from Mother. I had come to dread these epistles. I had forsaken her. I was on the other side of the world, living a life of opulence and indulgence. I never spared a thought for her. In these aspersions, Mother was wrong. I thought about her a great deal. After careful consideration, I decided to make a sacrifice to appease her. I would give her Jillian and Nicola. They would be dutiful in my place. It would soon be time for Jillian to go to secondary school. It made perfect sense to send first Jillian and then Nicola to a boarding school in England—and not just any boarding school, but the convent at which my mother was now employed part time teaching English and Drama. Of course, she had no qualifications for the job, but apparently rearing Albert, now a professional musical actor, was pedigree enough.

'I'll miss Jillian,' you admitted, as we sat sipping scotch on the veranda one evening, watching dusk deepen and the lights of Aberdeen start slowly to glimmer, appearing one by one, as if by magic. You looked shattered. These days your only escape from work was on our boat, *White Jade,* and even then we had been tracked down by the marine police a couple of times with urgent messages.

I freshened up my own drink, and ran the frosted tumbler between my hands before taking a hefty swallow. Cars purred by on the road below. I waited a moment then took another gulp. The whisky seemed very watery tonight; the bite was slow in coming, and the accompanying numbness

43

even slower.

'I'm sure Saint Mary's Convent is a wonderful school, and that the children will relish a bit of time with their grandmother,' I persuaded you.

You sat forward in your chair and sighed. 'I'm just not certain—' you began, but smoothly I interrupted you.

'These insects can be a real problem in the evenings,' I said, swatting away a flying ant. Even paradise has its drawbacks. 'Let's go inside. I'd better check that everything's all right with the amahs in the kitchen. Take your eyes off them for a second and they start doing all kinds of silly things.' I picked up the bottle of scotch and stood up. When you did not move, Ralph, but just sat brooding and staring into your glass, I told you dinner was almost ready and took the lead.

I had thought that sending Jillian and Nicola to boarding school would free me up to devote more time to you and my social duties as wife of an important government servant. I had even looked forward to seeing more of my friend and next-door neighbour, Beth Fielding, and enjoying a leisurely lunchtime drink with her once or twice a week. But this presumption was flawed. Alice, a demanding, insecure child from the outset, was becoming steadily more and more difficult. My mind teemed with a growing tally of unnerving incidents, where her behaviour was both unpredictable and extreme, incidents which no matter how much scotch I drank often refused to melt away.

The part of a king in the school nativity play became a nightmare when I tried to apply shoe polish to her face, in an attempt simply to make her look authentic.

'What are you doing, Mummy? You are making me all brown! It's horrid of you,' she wailed, plucking the crown from her head, and letting it fall to the ground.

My entreaties that it was just for the role she was acting were ignored. 'I don't want always to have a brown face!' she had screamed, so loudly that several other mothers in the school changing rooms looked round and grinned. 'Why have you done this to me, Mummy?'

Painstakingly I explained that with the help of soap and water, the shoe-polish would quickly wash away, but Alice only shot me a disbelieving look and abandoned herself to racking sobs. Finally she tottered onto the stage, her blotchy complexion attesting to hurried attempts at scouring her face of its autumnal hue. But even this did not assuage her histrionics, and she broke down before a baffled Mary, and had to be coaxed from the stage. This scene marked the first of several involving the parents of other children, teachers, and even on one occasion the headmistress. No matter how much I implored, cajoled and pleaded, there was no reasoning with Alice once her mind was made up.

In addition to this, you and I, Ralph, were called upon to attend many performances celebrating Chinese festivals. I had come to loathe these very public outings. Inevitably you would insist that the children attend, though goodness knew why. I felt they would do very well with the amahs at home watching a bit of Chinese opera. Certainly Alice would. But you were immovable on this, as you were on many issues involving our youngest daughter. So there we would be, in VIP seats at

45

the front row for all to gawp at. Harry, of course, would always sit placidly, entranced by the colourful spectacle, Nicola on her best behaviour at his side. But Alice would fidget incessantly. Never content simply to be near me, she would have to keep tugging on my sleeve, stroking me, resting her head on me, reaching for my hand, tickling it, patting the necklace I was wearing, or the bracelet that adorned my wrist, or twisting the rings on my fingers. On one such occasion, a dragon dance by the harbour side, my patience snapped. Oblivious to the massive, bobbing, brilliant, red head of the dragon, with its swivelling, bulbous eyes, only feet from us, I suddenly sprang up, thrusting Alice from my lap where she had been settling herself.

'Oh do stop touching me, Alice, for goodness sake!' my voice rang out over the clanging Chinese music, as Alice tumbled to the floor. 'Leave me alone. For the love of God, get away from me!'

I must have shouted. Faces turned to look at me. Alice righted herself, and gingerly sat once more in her assigned seat between you, Ralph, and me. Locking eyes with you for a second, the look you gave me would have frozen blood. The dragon head bounced and shook, its gaudy finery a blur before me. Its striped body writhed and twisted. Then it froze for an instant, the great head seemingly suspended in the air right before my eye-line. Slowly it blinked its white, fur-trimmed eyelids. And in that moment, I would have liked to dash forwards and gouge its impertinent eyes from their teacup sockets. Like Alice's, their gaze was far too astute. Then the wretched little man who jigged by the serpent's side put his hands on his hips and shook with pantomime laughter. Not satisfied with this, he went on to clasp both hands over the mouth that was slashed into his enormous, lobster-pink, papier-mâché globe of a head. He wagged this monstrous mask from side to side, the focus of his slit eyes on me, the butt of the joke. Briefly I glanced down at Alice. Always she was thinking, the wide, solemn eyes seeing everything. Thinking, thinking, thinking! Then the beast shivered and burst once more into life. My daughter had shown me up yet again, in front of all the important guests in the audience. Even the Governor was there, enjoying the jest I presume. It was a high price to pay for losing my control, for letting my guard slip. Alice had humiliated me publicly, before the most important British official on the island.

Our daughter was making life intolerable, Ralph, whether you were prepared to acknowledge it or not. She went for sleepovers with friends, vowing that she wanted to go more than anything she could think of, only to be returned home, sobbing and distraught in the middle of the night. The cause of these upsets remained a mystery both to you and to me. She was beset with night terrors, where she roamed the flat in strange trances, sometimes dragging her mattress great distances to find rest. And being Alice, she was not content to suffer her insomnia alone. Stricken with fear, and knowing very well that she would get no sympathy from me, she would turn instead to you, her beleaguered father, and make you sit up the night with her. She would beg you to tell her that she was not alone, for she felt, she said, as if she was the only person living in the blackness, and that all

47

the world was dead. As a result, struggling with the demands of your high-profile job and little sleep, you were jaded and consequently short-tempered with me. Her selfishness was astounding. But if you tackled her about these episodes, the resulting dialogue simply revealed Alice to be an irrational child, deaf to reason and common sense. Often in the evenings she would scream for me, and when I came running I would find her peering out of a bathroom window at the corridor's end, mesmerised. She would insist that I look at the sunset, exclaiming that she had never before seen anything so beautiful. She would gasp, and tell me that she could barely breathe at the wonder of it, that it made her want to cry and laugh all at once. After a time, like the villagers charging up the mountain in response to the shrieks of the boy who cried wolf, I would dismiss her summons, or just give her a cursory nod in passing.

I even spoke to you and arranged for Alice to have a dog. Of course at the time I said it would be a family pet and lovely for all of us. It was really for Alice though, to occupy Alice, to absorb her, and perhaps give the rest of us a little peace. We fetched the wretched creature from the Hong Kong SPCA. Alice chose him. If I'm honest I thought him a disagreeable mongrel, quite absurd in appearance—a motley assortment of colours, brown, black, white, grey and even a bit of yellow. He had a feathered tail far too long for the compact body, huge paws, a ragged ear, a long thin snout, and a black tongue which, when it hung out, very nearly trailed to the ground

'Really Alice! Why him?' I asked her, running my eyes over the scrappy mutt. 'There are others that are so much prettier.'

But true to form, never taking her eyes from the dog she had selected, Alice seemed not to hear me.

'I shall call him Bear,' she had announced, as I filled out the paperwork. I resisted the temptation to state the obvious. It was a dog not a bear! I thought it an absurd name. Why not call the thing Rover or Sparky or Rusty? But Alice was adamant. And to be fair, 'Bear' did fulfil his allotted task of providing a preoccupation for Alice. It was not unknown for the two of them to disappear for several hours at a time. Though Alice, when present, remained just as challenging.

Why, I asked myself countless times, couldn't she just take things at face value? Why was she was forever digging under the skin, probing things best left alone. Yet despite this you seemed to relish her company, Ralph. And for her part, Alice would happily have followed her beloved father anywhere. As Alice began her final year at Big Peak School, my relief was palpable. Soon, very soon, she would join her sisters at the convent in England, and then it would just be you, Ralph, and me, and our son of course. I broached this subject one weekend after a particularly good meal, when I knew you were relaxed and mellow and would be most receptive. We were sitting at the dining-room table and enjoying a small cognac with our coffees.

'It's probably time for us to make arrangements for Alice to join her sisters,' I ventured. I waited. There was no response. I took a mouthful of brandy for courage and soldiered on. 'I can hardly believe it, but Alice is in her last year at Big Peak School, and with the problem of finding suitable

49

secondary education here I—'

'I've been thinking about that,' you said, uncharacteristically cutting me off mid-flow.

Had you indeed, I ruminated. You continued.

'I've heard they're opening up a new school on Bowen Road. They're setting it up in the old British Army Hospital while they make a start building new premises on the terraced slopes above. In time they plan to demolish the hospital entirely, making way for further expansion. I want Alice to go there.'

I drew in a breath sharply. You gave me a quick glance. 'Is there a problem?' you asked, a dangerous note sounding in your voice.

I felt stunned, as if I had been slugged over the head and temporarily my eyesight was blurred. I tried to hold onto the salient facts. You had been thinking, you had been thinking about Alice, thinking about keeping Alice here with us, despite the chaos she was causing, Ralph, you wanted to send her to a new school they were building, a school I had heard nothing about.

'But darling,' I said, reaching for the cognac bottle, 'we don't know anything about this school.'

'I do,' you fired back. 'I've been to see the site. Nigel has been telling me all about it. They're considering sending Christopher and Anita there. Actually, I'm surprised Beth hasn't mentioned it to you.'

And so was I. Although this could not quite be classed as deception, my friend and neighbour Beth Fielding's omission to acquaint me with this startling news came a pretty close second in my book. I tipped up the bottle and refilled my glass. 'I see. Well. Well, well, well.'

'Myrtle, be honest with yourself,' you went on as I stiffened in my seat 'it would be a disaster sending Alice to boarding school.' Under your breath you added, 'I'm not at all sure it's been a success for Jillian or Nicola either.'

I sipped my cognac, then cradled my glass, slowly swilling round the amber liquid.

'I feel we should at least discuss it,' was my face-saving remark.

'We have,' you said brusquely, rising from the table.

*   *   *

Tonight Alice is worse than ever. Sometimes you can almost believe she alters with the rising of the moon, a kind of moon-madness. She is like a lone wolf howling and prowling all through the night. Ralph is dealing with her. With Alice his patience is inexhaustible. Harry seeks refuge in my bed. We close our eyes and block our ears. Finally I drift off to sleep. I dream we are on our junk, *White Jade*, which we have moored in a pretty bay. We are floating on a cobalt-blue sea. I feel the gentle rise and fall of the boat like breath coming in and going out, the rhythmic lift and fall of the thing. The sun is shining. We are fanned by a light breeze. And we are fishing, Ralph and Alice and I. We have cast out nylon lines with hooks knotted at the end of them. We have speared wiggling maggots for bait. Time passes. Ralph catches nothing. I catch nothing. Then Alice reels in a fish. It is several inches long, and it flaps dripping over the wooden deck, the silver scales brilliant as coruscating diamonds kissed by the sun. We all point at the fish as it gulps in air, and slaps and slips about. Our faces are masks of delight. Then quite suddenly the fish starts to inflate, like a silver balloon spiked with prickles. It swells up obscenely until it no longer flaps over the deck. It is a motionless bubble. Its prickles become barbs, hooking into the soft flesh of the damp wood.

'It is a puffer fish!' cries Alice in dismay. 'It's poisonous!' She is standing now over the gasping, hideous thing, hypnotised. Then she looks up at me. 'If you eat my fish you will die, Mother,' she says, and I wake.

My hands itch all day. When Alice returns from school we have a row. I do not like rowing. Some people can shrug off rows like a dog shaking water from its coat. I cannot. Brutal words stay with me . . . well . . . sometimes for a lifetime. I keep count of them. I notch them into the bark of my life, so deeply that they will never grow out. I tell Alice she cannot carry on with her deranged nights. My voice is quite calm, quite steady. I tell her they are taking a dreadful toll on her father. I tell her how hard he works, and that she is making him very ill. And when none of this seems to have any effect, I tell her that she is coming between us, that she is forcing us apart, her mother and her father. Alice's voice rises up like a snake with its egoistic jingle-jangle, as if she really is the only person alive in the world, and not just through the long, dark nights but through the long bright days as well. My voice shifts key. I feel the 'demon rasp' tolling in me then, purifying, abrasive, because Alice smiles a foolish smile. The demon is full of wrath, and he spits words out at the smiling, loon-faced child.

We are in the bathroom, the same bathroom

where Alice has summoned me so many times with her games. The window is open and the sky is red. I feel it bleed into me. I am dimly aware that my mouth is still working, and that my voice has grown deep and masculine, a war cry, and that my limbs are flaying. Alice is bold and stands her ground. And still she is smiling, smiling! I want to wipe that smile off her face. I draw back my hand and deal her such a blow across her grinning visage, that she is sent reeling backwards, covering the distance of several feet to the window, sliding down the wall, crumpling on the floor, while incongruously, above her head, Alice's wondrous sunset is framed. I am transfixed by the white face looming through the long brown hair. The eye is already puffing up. The cheek is split with a deep gash. Her blood is such a vivid shade of red. It dribbles from the wound and down her chin. It drips onto her summer school uniform, flowering on the white cotton.

I think: I am wearing my wedding and engagement rings and they must have cut into her cheek, a marital knuckleduster. I think, I have committed a mortal sin, somehow or other the Mother Superior at the convent back in England will know of it. I am envious of Alice. I am envious of my daughter. Alice, who has roared through so many nights, is silent now. I cannot even hear her breathing. I watch the blood spill and grow more copious. It pools in a crease at her neck. This creates the impression, reminiscent of a horror movie, that her head has been severed from her body, and that, if you push it, it will tumble off and roll over the green, marble-effect rubber tiles of the bathroom floor. I wonder what time Ralph will be home. I have an idea he is out tonight and will not be back until late. By tomorrow it will not look so bad. Besides, a story can be told. I feel sure a story will come that fits my purpose. Alice, I know, will never tell. She will hold it all in, keep it contained. Like Iwazaru, one of the three wise monkeys, she will speak no evil. She will gag herself. I gaze unmoved at the sunset, then my eyes slide downwards and hold Alice's.

'At last,' I say, 'when I come, there is something to see.' My voice scrapes the silence. My hands have stopped itching. They are trembling now. I need something to steady my nerves.

NICOLA—1965

I never really grasped why Jillian made such a fuss about boarding school. True, it was a bit of a blow the parents choosing Gran's school, it being Roman Catholic and we being . . . well, heathens. But it didn't really worry me. I knew we would have a laugh. I told Jillian so, as she sat on her bed, in the flat on The Peak. The Easter holidays were drawing to a close, and she was red-cheeked and wretched. She was flying back to England the next day and I was helping her to pack.

'In September I'll be joining you,' I told her with a grin. 'We'll shake things up Jilly.' She managed a weak smile.

'I hate it there,' she said brokenly. 'I'm miserable.' She took off her glasses and I saw her eyes were swimming with tears. 'The nuns are bitches!'

I tossed in a T-shirt with a picture of kittens on it, shunted the case along the bed, and sat down next to my sister. I put an arm over her shoulder. This was an awkward gesture for me. I am not a touchy-feely person. It is nothing personal but I experience a kind of revulsion when things get sloppy. That day there had been a scene at lunch, a spectacular scene. It was a roast dinner. We generally have a roast on the weekends. Jillian, already feeling as if she was fading away, as if she was only half visible, with her return to England imminent, was upset even before we sat down. Alice kept asking her silly questions. What was it like at boarding school? Did she have a boyfriend? Was she excited about the flight tomorrow? That sort of thing. Jillian loathed Alice. She had told me late one night that she would like to slap her, that she could not bear her enthusiasm, her eagerness, her desire to please.

'She can afford to behave like that,' Jillian had said bitterly, screwing up her eyes behind their lenses, as she watched Alice chatting to one of the amahs.

I sympathised with Jillian. From time to time Alice got on my nerves too. But it was plain to me that my elder sister hadn't thought this through. Anyone could see that Jillian's vendetta against Alice did not work in her favour. For a start it maddened Father, who seemed to feel he had to keep riding to Alice's rescue, like some paternal knight in shining armour.

'Why not make a friend of Alice, then make that friendship work for you,' I suggested reasonably to Jillian.

But to no avail I'm afraid. Jillian's revulsion for

55

our little sister knew no bounds. She gave long-suffering sighs when Alice walked into a room. On car journeys she insisted on winding up the window, claiming the draft was blowing her hair out of shape, knowing full well that Alice was prone to travel sickness. And she would stoically ignore our little sister when she bounded up to her full of adoring compliments. How lovely Jillian was looking, Alice would say. How she wished her brown hair was fair like Jillian's, and would Jillian help her pick out some new clothes because she had no idea what was fashionable in London at present. It astonished me that Alice did not seem to realise she was antagonising Jilly. But then she can be a little obtuse sometimes.

So when we all trooped into lunch that day, I had an idea that something was going to happen. Father carved the meat. It was roast beef. Jillian wanted an outside cut and so did Alice. Neither of them liked bloody meat, whereas I liked mine nearly raw. I was happiest with a middle slice, all pink and oozing blood. Father served Alice before her older sister, and Jillian clearly felt the snub. She made up her mind that all the best bits had gone to Alice, and that the cut she was dished up was undercooked. She took father to task over this, complaining that Alice always got the choicest pieces of meat. Mother piled in. As a matter of course, Harry, son and heir, had been taken care of first. Now he looked perturbed by the delay. Catching his mother's eye, he was given the go-ahead to start his meal. So while hostilities were breaking out, Harry was slowly masticating a mouthful, like a cud-chewing cow. All the while, his eyes focused hypnotically on two black and silver angelfish, gliding about in a tank, set up on the dresser behind the dining-room table. Then Alice made matters much worse by offering Jillian her meat. Typical. Why couldn't she just shut up?

'Here Jillian, we can swap plates if you like,' Alice suggested, lifting her plate and offering it to her sister.

'I don't want it now you've touched it,' Jillian cried, shoving the plate back towards Alice, so hard that the piece of crispy outside meat was launched off it, orbited briefly in the air, before landing with a 'plop', quite fortuitously as it happened, on Harry's plate. Harry's eyes rolled from living fish to dead meat, and stayed glued to the unexpected arrival, his jaws temporarily locked.

'That was uncalled for,' Father said angrily, hurriedly flipping over the joint, carving a slice from the other end, and delivering it to Alice's plate.

'No,' pleaded Alice. 'I don't mind really. Jillian can have it.'

'Didn't you hear me the first time?' Jillian shrieked, shooting a slaughterous look in Alice's direction. 'I don't want anything of yours.'

Alice began protesting that she hadn't touched it, so it couldn't be called *hers* yet. Then Mother, who kept running a thumb up and down along the blade of her own knife, where it lay at the side of her plate, told Alice to be quiet and to get on with her dinner. The colour was draining from Alice's face now, and she began clearing her throat as if she had something stuck there. Father wanted to know if she was okay and would she like some water.

'Oh for goodness sake, if you're feeling sick, Alice, leave the table,' Mother snapped. 'You're ruining everyone's dinner. You are making us all lose our appetites.'

As Mother spoke, I saw she had taken up her own knife and fork. She was grasping them about their middles as if they were weapons, and then suddenly she threw them tetchily a little way from her, across the table. Her fork struck a serving dish full of vegetables, and her knife clanged against the metal gravy boat. Alice rose slowly from her chair. She looked bewildered, unsure if she should go or stay. Father smiled kindly at her and told her to stay put. Mother looked livid. Jillian slid malevolent eyes towards her sister, but her head remained motionless. Staying calm amidst the storm, Harry was moving his fork imperceptibly to snag Alice's slice of meat, all his concentration focused then on edging it towards the centre of his plate. At last Alice moved away from her chair and backed out of the room, bumping into the dining-room door once, before turning, opening it and disappearing through it.

'Come back as soon as you feel better,' Father called after her.

Alice closed the door with infinite care, as if terrified she would disturb a sleeping baby. After Alice's departure, I had thought things would improve, and was just tucking into a succulent morsel of red meat when father placed two fat roast onions on Jillian's plate. Now, if it was a fact known to one and all in our family that Jillian and Alice preferred outside cuts of meat, it was also virtually printed on Jillian's birth certificate that she hated onions, that no earthly force could induce her to swallow what she described as a single slimy mouthful of them, that even God would have his work cut out if he wished Jillian to polish one off, let alone two. Jillian eyes were riveted on the onions. Mother made a squeaking noise. Harry jumped, and then started mashing up a roast potato with admirable intensity. Father sat back in his chair, and with immense care loaded tiny portions of meat, potato, vegetables and onion onto his fork, patting the whole into a small, sausage shape with his knife, inspecting it for a second, popping it into his mouth, and chewing energetically before washing it down with a glug of red wine. Mother had more than a glug, polishing off nearly her entire glassful. The appearance and following inquiry from one of the amahs as to whether she should clear away, and were we ready for dessert, was met with sour faces, and she quickly scurried off again.

'I will not eat an onion,' announced Jillian in a voice of reinforced steel.

This was ignored by Father who made a great drama of having forgotten to say grace, something he hardly ever remembered anyway. He bowed his head piously.

'Dear God, we thank you for your bounty, for the food on our plates, for the meat, the roast potatoes, the gravy, the vegetables and the onions—' Father broke off.

He opened one eye. It rotated, taking in Jillian's raised head, her own eyes held wide open, flashing with defiance, and her folded arms. I made sure Father observed my willing participation in this rare ritual, making quite a drama of unclasping and re-clasping my hands. The fingers of Harry's hands were plaited together as well. His eyelids fluttered as he snatched sneaky peeks at his food, clearly distressed that the serious business of eating was being held in abeyance for the present. Mother's head drooped, but I had my doubts that she was lost in prayer.

'Why were you not praying, Jillian?' Father demanded, when at last grace was over.

'I am not thankful,' Jillian retorted. 'I don't want to be a hypocrite.'

Mother refilled her glass, and took several gulps in quick succession.

'I am just going to have a quick word with them in the kitchen,' she said gaily, her eyes a little too bright, her cheeks inflamed. She rose unsteadily to her feet. 'These servants need their hands held if they are going to produce a meal that is half decent you know.' She gave a shout of raucous laughter. No one seemed to share her hilarity. 'You will sit there until you eat those onions,' Father decreed to Jillian.

Mother scratched the palm of one hand with the fingers of the other, a nervous habit of hers I'd observed countless times, then made a dive for the kitchen door and was gone. To her credit Jillian slowly ate up everything on her plate . . . except the onions. Mother reappeared carrying another bottle of wine, hugging it to her under one arm. The remainder of the meal played out in silence, but for the 'pop' of the cork. One by one we were excused from the table, all but Jillian. At four o' clock Jillian was still sitting at the dining-room table, together with her two onions. By now I thought they looked a little dried out. Hovering in the hall, I shot her a sympathetic look through the open dining-room door, which she acknowledged with a flicker of her eyes. Father strode up and down the long corridor seething. Why, he demanded, couldn't Jillian just eat her onions? They were good onions. They had cost money, money that he worked very hard to make. Perhaps Jillian would like to go out, work hard and make money, so that other people could waste the onions she had bought, he thundered.

Alice was nowhere to be seen. Harry was out on his bike. Mother had passed out on her bed, snoring intermittently. And I was watching the *Flintstones* in the lounge, and feeling levels of anxiety uncommon to me, occasionally dashing out to check on Jillian. I would have scoffed the onions up myself if I could have reached them, but sadly Father was still patrolling the No Man's Land of the corridor, beady eyes scanning the hall. Finally, when the tension had reached a pitch that was unbearable, Father marched Jillian and her plate of onions to her bedroom, and said she was to stay there until she had eaten them. He slammed the door and stood vigil outside. At this point something must have exploded in Jillian, because she chose to take the two onions and fling them out of her window. Although I didn't actually see her do it, I certainly witnessed the aftermath. The onions must have gathered momentum as they fell. Beneath Jillian's bedroom window was the much-prized garden of the Everard family, attached to their ground-floor flat. Mr Everard was gardening that afternoon when the onions came hurtling down from above, he told Father later, decapitating several of his prize orchids in the process. He stood on our doorstep, the crushed, pink flowers in one hand, the beige mess of onion-pulp in the other. I had heard the front door and was peeping out of the lounge.

'Really Ralph, this is too bad.' Mr Everard looked deeply offended. 'This is not what you expect from your neighbours when you settle down for a pleasant afternoon of gardening.' Mr Everard very nearly wiped his perspiring brow, but then he caught sight of the squashed onions nestled on his open palm. Mr Everard had a bald patch over which he arranged his nut-brown hair, disguising it carefully. Now his hair was all mussed up and a shiny pink patch of scalp exposed. 'Luckily I just happened to look upwards and I saw them. I saw them come flying out of a window from your flat, Ralph. I leapt out of the way just in time. Imagine that! You simply do not expect onions to start raining on your head on a fine afternoon. I could have been hurt, Ralph, seriously hurt, not to mention the damage done to my orchids.'

I nearly burst out laughing when Mr Everard said this. I imagined Mrs Everard wailing to Mother that her husband had been minding his own business, when he had been flattened by two onions and rushed to Queen Mary's Hospital.

'I'm sorry, Peter,' Father said, wisely in my opinion opting for brevity.

Mr Everard looked down dejectedly, first at his flowers, then at the onion mush. Mother appeared, walking blearily up to the front door.

'Hello Peter,' she greeted our neighbour, her words just a touch thick and sticky. 'To what do we owe this unexpected pleasure?' She smiled graciously, dipping her head. Her bun had come undone and her plait was beginning to unravel.

Her hands went automatically to her hair and deftly she pinned it up again.

'I was gardening, Myrtle, when two onions landed in my garden, just inches from my head,' Mr Everard said without preamble, his tone piqued. A drip of sweat made its way slowly down the side of his face. It trembled on his lower jaw before falling.

'Really!' exclaimed Mother, not batting an eyelid. 'How dreadful for you Peter. You must have been very shocked.' Father looked as if he had been winded. He caved in slightly, and I saw that his cheeks were suddenly glowing. 'I do hope you weren't hurt?' Mother asked solicitously.

'Luckily no, Myrtle. But I might well have been,' Mr Everard reported peevishly, while Mother gave her appearance a quick once-over in the hallway mirror.

'Well, thank goodness for that,' Mother declared fervently, her expression one of immense relief. She snatched a little look heavenwards, as if touching base with God, and expressing her personal thanks to him for looking after her people. As her gaze left the celestial sphere, and returned to the tarnished world of mortals, she became aware of Mr Everard's hands, held aloft and brimming with onion paste and petals.

'Peter, won't you join us for a drink?' she invited smoothly. 'It's a wee bit early I know, but after all it is a weekend, and you've had a terrible scare.' She gave her most beguiling smile and winked at Mr Everard. Mr Everard hesitated. 'Ralph, tell Peter I shall be desolate if he doesn't join us.'

My father, lost for a moment in Mother's consummate performance, roused himself and reiterated her invitation. Mr Everard wavered a second longer and then gave in. The day was won.

'Do let me show you to the bathroom, Peter, to wash your hands,' Mother said, leading the way, Mr Everard, now fully tamed, trotting after her. 'Ralph, be a dear, and fix the drinks.' She paused and waited for Mr Everard to come alongside. 'Don't tell me, Peter . . . let me see, if my memory serves me right your poison is G and T, ice no lemon.' Mr Everard was duly flattered. 'When friends are important to me, I make a point of remembering these things, Peter,' she breathed. Then, as I watched, she tucked her arm through Mr Everard's, careful to avoid contact with the squashed onion, and they ambled down the corridor towards the bathroom. Pausing outside the door Mother leant in to him, and whispered in achingly manicured tones, 'This is such an unlooked for pleasure, Peter.' She was magnificent.

Father never spoke of the matter again. And the next time Jillian returned to England, I went with her.

Harry—1966

Mr Beecham carried me in his arms, holding me like a baby. Although I felt woozy and my eyes kept closing, there were little flashes that I recall, like going to see a play and not watching it all the way through. That's it, each time they opened I found myself in different scenes.

In the beginning there were his curls, the grey of

64

the clouds moments before the rain comes, and the tips of his upper teeth, tinged with a yellowy-brown, digging into his lower lip, and the specks of sweat breaking out on his large nose. I could feel him panting as well, with the effort, feel his lungs pushing against the weight of me. And the jolt, jolt, jolt, of my body held in his arms as he went down the steps, the several flights of them that ran from the playing field to the school building. But mostly I remember his eyes flicking down at me and what was in them. You see, it was fear, I'd recognise it anywhere. We were old friends. Then, in the middle, there were the blocks of blue sky that seemed to go on and on, and the glitter of the sun making my head throb and my skin prickle. And lastly there was the medical room, and me being laid down so carefully on the bed, how firm it was, how solid. You knew, just knew, that bed wasn't going to let you down. It was cool in there after the scalding sun, and quiet too. Like walking into the St John's Cathedral on a hot morning.

'Harry? Harry? It's Mr Beecham. You're going to be fine Harry. You've had an accident but you're going to be fine.' Mr Beecham's the deputy head. He takes me for English. He's kind, doesn't make me feel stupid when I can't answer the questions, the way some of the teachers do. He smoothed my brow as he talked. I could feel his fingers tickling back my damp hair, smell the faint trace of tobacco that clung to them.

And the way he said it, I knew it was true. I was going to be fine. Then he said the doctor was coming and that was alright too. He said the doctor would make it all better, make me well again. I wanted to believe him, that someone,

65

anyone, really had the power to do that. To make it all better. Only when he told me my mother was on her way, I laughed. Of course it was in my head. I couldn't let it out. It would have hurt too much the way my head was pounding. Besides, that would have been telling on Mother, on *them*. I'd never do that, not even if I was dying.

You know what I thought then, in that cool, still room, where other faces were appearing now, like masks hung on the white walls. I thought that if I was really lucky it might be true. I might be dying and then it would be over. I wondered if Alice would come and join the other masks, but then I remembered that she'd had an upset tummy that morning and stayed home. Sometimes my sister Alice doesn't eat for ages. Mother says that's why she gets stomachache so much. Mother said she does it to get attention, starving herself. But I'm not so sure. Still, imagine being able to go without food for an entire day. Amazing!

'Fatty! Fatty! Blubber boy! Harry is a blubber boy! Nah, nah, sweaty Harry! Nah, nah, smelly Harry!'

It was Keith, Bobby and Andrew that morning. Following me around the playing field. They're like the wasps you get on picnics that just won't go away. Every few seconds one of them would dash forwards and push me, or try to grab the roll of fat that shows when my shirt rides up, or they'd run ahead of me, spin round and poke me in the tummy. It isn't so bad. It doesn't really hurt. Sometimes I even like it, because . . . well . . . because it makes me feel alive, the pain. Anyway, they usually get bored after a while and go away. I can read the signs, clear as the time on a

66

wristwatch. The jeering is loud as can be to start with, like a football flying in the air and everyone screaming 'cos they think it's gonna be a goal. Then, after a bit, their voices start to drop, as if they knew this next shot is going to miss. I name it 'the game-over slump', wait for it, 'cos I know it will come, eventually. After that, with a few more feeble taunts, they slouch off.

Nah, I didn't mind them really, the boys. It's the girls that make me go burning red, and want to cry so bad that it takes everything I have to hold it in. They never touch me. They don't have to. Their bright eyes slide over me, over my pockets of fat, over my thick arms, my wobbly tummy, my plump legs, my big bottom. Then they snatch little sneaky glances at one another and smirk. It's like a knife going in, that shared smirk.

I used to imagine it you know, a knife sliding into a slab of my flesh. I used to watch Ah Dang in the kitchen slicing the fat off some huge piece of dripping, bloody meat, and I used to dream that someone could do that for me. Lie me down on a chopping board and trim the oily fat off me, slash, saw, slash. And then I'd get up all slim and lean, and I'd have muscles, and one of those bellies that was hard and dipped in like the other boys'. Then, when we changed for PE, and I pulled on those bright green shorts, shrugged on that white cotton T-shirt, no one would giggle. They'd say stuff like, 'Hey Harry, want to be in our team?' or 'What about being our goalie today,' or 'We're sure to win 'cos Harry's batting for our side, so there!' Sometimes they'd row over me. They would. In my head, they'd squabble and say, 'It's not fair, you had him last week. This week it's our turn with

Harry.' Instead of me standing alone in the playground 'cos no one wants to pick me, with them all rushing to get into pairs, into groups, into teams, just in case they get landed with the fat pig, Harry Safford. And then I'm paired up with the teacher, who makes it worse by pretending to be really pleased about it. You know, 'Lucky me, I get to be with Harry.' Oh yeah, sure! Nobody wants me. It's as if I stank or something. Ah, who knows, maybe I do.

Anyway, it was after the boys got bored and left that the accident happened. There was this roller thing in a corner of the field. I think they use it to flatten the grass. There was no one over there, and it looked kind of peaceful. The roller was all gritty-brown and grey, flecked with pearly-white too, like slithers of soap shining in the sunlight. Attached to it was a thick, black handle, balanced up against the playground's surrounding wire-mesh fence. Round about were tufts of tall green and yellow grass, like it hadn't been moved for ages. So I wandered over. It was more impressive close up, bigger somehow, sturdier. I touched the handle. Ran a finger along the uneven surface. It was metal, iron I think. Then, for a while I just circled the roller, not all the way round 'cos of the fence you understand, but nearly, and then back again. It looked so heavy, like you'd need a giant or something to shift it. After a bit I sat down on it and stared out at the kids in the field, all playing their games, skipping and chucking tennis balls about, shrieking and laughing too, like they were having a really good time. And the girls' hair was flying all about, brown and black and blonde, and their white socks were glinting in the sun.

The roller felt very warm under my backside, through my grey flannel shorts. Not so hot you couldn't stand it, just kind of comforting. The flesh of my thighs spread out against it, like a cushion. I squinted up at the sun, right at it, something Mother says you should never do. 'Because if you do, you'll go blind, Harry', she liked to sing at me. But I didn't care. Then there were dark spots rushing at me and I was so dizzy. It was the way you get when you spin round and round with your arms stretched wide, and you have to throw yourself down on the grass, and the world just carries on spinning, tilting under you. That's when I decided to do it, stand right up on that roller, plant my feet squarely on the warm curve of it, and see how things looked then. I know it's daft, but I wondered if it might be different up there. Perhaps I'd pick out something I'd never seen before, and seeing it would change everything.

I hauled myself up on the hot hump of stone. It was quite difficult actually, higher than you might think. I had a few attempts before I managed it. At first my back was to the playing field, and I was balancing with my arms out. It was great. Just like I'd imagined it would be. Only I couldn't see the field, just through the wire fence and across the slope of road. I glanced back over my shoulder. I couldn't help it, 'cos I wanted to see if any of the girls were watching me. Especially June Mullery. She is so pretty, June, with pale, yellow hair and soft eyes. She never teased me, and once I was sure she smiled at me. At least I think it was me. I suppose it might have been her friends behind me, but anyhow it felt as if it was for me. Her face lighting up and her eyes so sweet and kind. It made

it hard for me to swallow, seeing her smile like that
... At me.

So I tried to turn round but something blinded
me, something like a bit of the sun glaring at me
from the field. I lost my footing, and I was falling,
falling back, and without thinking I made a grab
for the iron handle propped up against the fence.
Only it just fell away with me, like seizing a stick of
bamboo in a landslide. I tumbled backwards on the
field, and the metal bar chased me, the way the
jeering boys had earlier. The long horizontal
handle at the top of it, the thing they grip to push
it about with I guess, came crashing down across
the brow of my head. Then it was pitch black, with
the sound of the bar striking me, tolling inside my
skull, a great underwater bell clanging on and on.
When my eyes opened next Mr Beecham was
carrying me down the steps.

I didn't die. The doctor came and went. Mother
took me to Queen Mary's for X-rays and that was
quite fun. And the doctors there said I was going
to be okay as well. That's when the laugh came
back.

'You're not very good doctors then, are you?'
came the cheeky voice I hear sometimes in my
head, the voice that longs to speak out loud, but I
know never will.

We're back at the flat now. Mother's fussing
loads and kissing me, so that I have red marks
from her lipstick on my face, and have to rub hard
to get them off. I can smell her perfume as well
and that's nice, warm and comforting, like the
roller before it flattened me. Then later she smells
of something else, something sour, the whisky I
guess, and that isn't so nice, because then she gets

70

a bit sloppy. She looks good. If anyone was watching they'd say, 'There's an excellent mother, a mother who really loves her son. The way she strokes and pets him! Oh my, and can you hear the lovely things she says to him.' But what they wouldn't know is that it's not real. It's pretend. Like acting. And you know before long the performance will be over, or the show will be cancelled because the actress doesn't feel very well, and has to go and lie down.

As it happens Mother does have to lie down after a bit. Dad is away, or working late or something. 'Course Mum said she rang him straight away. She said he was terribly worried, but very relieved later to hear his only son was going to be fine. She's always calling me that. 'Only son!' As if that makes such a big difference to how much I'm worth to them. Like, if there were more sons, if say Alice had been a boy, they couldn't possibly have loved me as much. Who knows, if she had been, perhaps they wouldn't have had me at all?

'Harry, you have to know your father would have raced home if it had been serious,' Mother says, staring straight into my face and looking all grave.

And I understand what she means. That if I'd been going to die or if I had died even, he'd have come; my father would have come then, no question.

'He was frantic, Harry,' she tells me, her finger stroking the side of her glass. 'You know how much he loves you. He wanted to come darling, of course he did. He's so busy. Important, clever men like your father always are. But I told him you were being a brave little man, *our* brave little man,

71

and that there was no need.'

She puts down her drink, then gives me one of those funny hugs of hers, a bit awkward, as if she doesn't quite know where to put me. It lasts longer than normal of course, on account of the accident. By then she's on her second drink. Afterwards she holds me at arm's length.

'I'm so proud of you,' she tells me smoothing back my hair, careful not to touch the raised purple line, where the bar struck me. 'My precious only boy.'

'If it had been really bad, you're sure Father would have come?' I want to know. I can't meet her eyes. I might cry if I did, like with the girls at school, might make a big baby of myself. Hmm . . . Mother would hate that. She doesn't like you to show feelings, not real ones in any case.

'Of course he would have, darling!' she says now, her eyes, that glow amber like a cat's sometimes, wide open. 'You know he would have, Harry.'

I want to say that it might have been too late, if I was dying or worse, already dead. If he'd come then, after I'd died, after my heart had stopped beating and I was all white and icy, well . . . there really wouldn't have been much point, would there? But Mother has turned away by then and the drink is in her hands again. We've had supper but that doesn't matter. I'm still hungry. I'm always hungry.

They've got this creepy festival here—actually they've got lots of weird festivals on the island, but this one is the spookiest. Yue Lan. The Festival of the Hungry Ghosts. It's the end of May now, so I guess it'll soon come round. Anyway, for a few weeks in July the Chinese believe that hungry

72

ghosts, the ghosts of their dead ancestors, and people who've been murdered, or died at sea, or in a war and haven't had a funeral or been buried properly, will come tearing back to earth. And these ghosts who swarm back down here at Yue Lan, they're are not just hungry, they're starving, ravenous even. All the stuff they didn't get in life, like marriage and children and love, and all the money and food and houses and cars, and junk like that, for these few days you see they've just got to have them. You know, like nothing will stand in their way.

Sometimes at night, lying in bed watching the orange stripes of light slide across the ceiling as a car drives by on the road below, I picture them, the hungry ghosts. It's bit like the stampedes you get in cowboy movies, the image in my mind. Hordes of ghosts charging towards you, the air thick with the dust their trailing misty feet are stirring up, and their mouths gaping wide open, like the mouths of caves. Gigantic, black, frozen, empty caves, with those gleaming icicle things hanging down and reaching up at the opening, rows of razor sharp teeth, waiting to gobble you up, to gulp down your blood. They save your still beating heart for last, a special treat. Then crunch up your bones until all that's left are a few splinters.

I expect they'd be delighted to find me, Piggy Harry, oink, oink; that I'd make a really tasty meal, keep them going, well . . . for a bit anyway. I see their eyes in my nightmares sometimes, like balls of fire, and the whites of them showing, only they're a dirty green colour, rolling about and all wild and scary in their smoky heads. I understand their hunger, like there's a living thing eating away

73

at them, like they have to feed it, have to! 'Cos I feel it too, feel I can never cram in enough, that no matter how much I stuff into my mouth, chew and swallow and chomp and gnaw, it'll never stop the hunger, it'll never fill up the hole.

The Chinese do some neat stuff to frighten them away though: they make these brilliant paper models, like three-dimensional kites of all those things you need in life. Then they pile them on huge bonfires and burn them to ashes. They say you have to be careful for a whole month, but that the days in the middle are the most dangerous. They steer clear of the sea as well, stay indoors, and get the kids home early, in case the ghosts jump out and get them. Beaches are especially dangerous over Yue Lan. The spirits lurk everywhere, in the curl of a breaking wave, and in the currents that pull swimmers out of their depth, and in whirlpools that swallow up boats. They leave them food and pray, and burn joss sticks, but as far as I can tell they do that all the time anyway. Those joss sticks really smell if you ask me. Make my eyes water. As if that would satisfy them, with the kind of hunger they've got growling in their tummies. It wouldn't satisfy me, that's definite.

Mother is miles away now, on the phone to Beth next door, making her voice all dramatic, the way she does, describing what happened to me. She's talking about me but . . . well . . . the crazy thing is I feel left out, like I'm not really part of her story, that it's another 'only son'. I mooch into the kitchen and tell Ah Dang I'm hungry, and can she fix me something. She likes that. Makes her feel all needed. She always grins and wags her head, as if she understand the appetite I've got, what a beast

74

it is, and her gold teeth glitter sort of magically.

While she's getting a plate together, Alice comes in. Up till then Mum's kept her away. She's always trying to do that, keep Alice and me separate. You'd think Alice was some kind of snake full of poison. And it's true, my sister goes into these fits sometimes, yowling and moaning, and you do tend to feel a bit jumpy about her, 'cos you don't know what's gonna come next. But I get it. I know where all that noise comes from, all that rage. I'm jealous of Alice 'cos I want to scream too, scream until they all cover their ears, and screw themselves up. But I can't. I just can't.

'How are you feeling?' Alice asks then, and she smiles in that shy way she has.

'Oh not too bad,' I mumble, glancing back at her. I don't think Ah Dang put very much butter in my sandwich and it's bothering me.

'Ah Dang can I have some more butter please?' I ask. I'd like to talk to Alice, but if I take my eyes off Ah Dang, even for a moment, who knows what she might skimp on?

'*Ai ya, ai ya!*' mutters Ah Dang, peeling back the top of the sandwich and starting again. She isn't really angry. She fakes it. She tosses her head, making her plait whisk all over the place, and her hands fly about, and she gabbles in Cantonese, but you can tell. In her eyes she's still smiling.

'That's some bruise you're going to have, Harry,' Alice says.

I guess she must have seen it when I turned round. Ah Lee appears then through the back door. She sees all the food out, and me looking worried, and Ah Dang slamming things about. And she gives one of her silly hysterical giggles.

'*Ai ya, ai ya!*' she echoes Ah Dang, and pinches my bare arm. '*Fei zhai! Fei zhai!*' she squeals, and she's off again.

I know what she said. Fat boy. I hear it lots. The Chinese can't resist my chubby arms. Can't stop themselves from pinching me. Even strangers. Pinching me and grinning, '*Fei zhai, fei zhai*'. I might as well be back at school. You know what it makes me think of. The story of Hansel and Gretel. When the witch locks Hansel up in a cage and every day she brings him lots of food, because you see she's fattening him up. Fattening him up for the day of slaughter, when she's going to kill him and chop him up, and pop him into her huge cauldron, and cook him over her roaring fire till he's all tender and delicious. I like closing my eyes and imagining the witch's cottage, imagining being with Gretel, deep in the heart of the dark forest, then suddenly the two of us coming upon it. I think about how hungry we'd both be, our bellies rumbling, hungry and tired, with nothing to eat but dandelions and grass. Then we'd step into this clearing and together we'd gasp.

My cottage isn't made of gingerbread though, because I don't really like it. It's built of cake bricks, chocolate, and plain sponge flavoured at least six different ways, toffee and orange, and lemon and mint, and strawberry and coffee. And the bricks are cemented together with butter icing, and jam and cream. The windows are huge glacier-mint squares framed with marzipan. The front door is made entirely of caramel, and the doorknob is a shiny ball of liquorice. As for the roof, it's tiled in thick slabs of chocolate, milk and dark and white. There's even meringue smoke coming out of a butterscotch chimney. The biggest problem we have is where to start. I run up to it and take the most enormous bite off a corner brick of rich, moist chocolate. Gretel, she walks nervously up to the door and starts licking it, as if it's a ginormous lollipop. In my version we've virtually polished off the entire building before the witch appears; there's only a few spadefuls of cake crumb rubble, and some broken chocolate tiles left. While Gretel and I are clutching our stuffed stomachs, the witch throws back a hatch in the floor, made, incidentally, of royal icing, and pounces.

'*Fei zhai, fei zhai,*' squeaks Ah Lee again. Pinch, pinch.

And I want to ask, in that voice inside me that never speaks up, 'Am I ready now, Ah Lee? Am I ready for the pot? Is my flesh plump and juicy enough yet? Are you sharpening your knives ready to slice me up?' But I don't of course. I glance at Alice. In the story Gretel saved her brother, made him hold out a twig to the short-sighted, croaky, old witch instead of his finger, so when she pinched it she thought he was still all thin and stringy. Still, that's a story isn't it? Not real life. Not like it is here in the flat on The Peak, where none of us can do anything to put off what's coming. I think Ah Lee's finished her pinching now. She's wiping down the sink.

'Hmph!' I grunt. Ah Dang's only put one slice of ham in my sandwich and barely any cheese at all. At this rate I'll never be ready for the pot. 'Ah Dang, I'm hungry!' I wail. I try to imagine what a hungry ghost would sound like. 'I'm really, really hungry! HUNGRY! There's not enough filling in my sandwich, Ah Dang.'

Then Ah Dang's cursing me in Chinese and pounding her drum tummy, and picking up the butter dish and hurling it back down, and going at the lump of cheddar as if she'd like to murder it. I look back at Alice and our eyes meet. And Alice gives a 'hup' of laughter, and then she claps a hand over her mouth and tries to stifle it. Well, that only makes it worse than ever, because now I'm laughing too, a great boom of a laugh that make my tummy jiggle about under my shirt, like it's alive and it wants to escape. Alice falls back against the fridge and she's helpless now, arms limp, head tipping about, and that makes me lose it completely. I shuffle over to her, and my sides are really splitting, my shirt busting at the seams, and Ah Dang's screaming and brandishing the knife with the butter on it, like she's going to stab us both. And just for a second I let my throbbing head rest on Alice's shoulder, and the peals of laughter rock from her into me and back again. It's good, so very good laughing like that with my sister Alice that I want to sob.

Ghost—1967

I watch many children come and go before Alice arrives. I observe them through the grid of an air-vent set high into the wall of the morgue. Their heads are dull and ordinary, and I know they cannot sustain me. True, I am curious. But when Alice comes I am spellbound. She appears one afternoon when all the other children have gone, and lies back on a patch of scrubby grass. She is a slip of a thing, pale as a creaming wave, her long hair always moving, her eyes moons of contemplation. It does not seem to worry her that the building above her is growing silent, that soon she will be alone. For a bit she stares up at the sky, follows the occasional fleecy cloud. Then she rolls over and sits up. As she does so, the golden-haired boy in the shadows fades away, as if he had never been.

Suddenly she notices the yawning mouth of the morgue, for the door is partly ajar. I cannot tell how long her eyes are trained on it, but the shadows are lengthening when at last she climbs to her feet. She walks straight to the entrance and shoulders open the rusty-hinged door. It shudders and grumbles and sticks a bit before swinging back. Alice slips through, under the nebulous mantle. She takes a few steps, and then waits for her eyes to adjust to the gloom. She inhales a long, slow breath of stale, dead air. She fixes stains on the floor with her perceptive eyes. She let her fingers linger on walls where the paint is flaking, where the bricks are impregnated with the transience of life. As she listens to echoes of the past, I slide into her and instantly feel my strength returning. I become the scum in her blood. I garland myself with ropes of silver-stranded veins. And in the resonance of each heartbeat I know her every thought, her every memory, her every experience, her every twist and turn of emotion, often before she does, as if they are my own.

When at last she leaves, I go with her. We dawdle along Bowen Road. We wait for The Peak Tram, a funicular green cab with the cream roof to come and haul us up The Peak. We leave the terminus and stroll up a long road, past a shop called the Dairy Farm, then along a path to Alice's home. All this is new to me. The people hurrying by, their clothes, their colour too, for up here most of them are white-skinned, the cars and buses and lorries, the houses and the flats. Hers is a top-floor flat, as large as a palace. Surely, I think, several families live here. But I am wrong. There is only one. The flat is filled with beautiful things too, the kind that an emperor might own. Carvings and paintings, jade and ivory, snuff bottles and fans, books and carpets, and shelves crowded with fine porcelain. But there is no emperor, just Alice's family, the Saffords, and some servants to care for them, Ah Dang and Ah Lee. When I was alive there was only my father to care for me. And even then, as far back as I can recall, it had really been my job to look after him. Like me, Alice has a father, Ralph, but unlike me she has a mother too, Myrtle. And Alice has a younger brother, Harry, and a small dog she calls Bear. Alice has two sisters as well, who are being educated in England. It seems strange to me that, with so many people about, Alice should be lonely. But she is. I feel it. Still, it is lucky, because it means that she will probably welcome my company.

Together we decide that we do not like attending classes in the school that has been set up in my old army hospital. This is not because I believe education has no worth. My father was a wonderful storyteller and valued learning above all things. When we returned from a night's fishing I would lie down, the rising sun warming the deck under me, and he'd sit beside me. He'd puff on his

80

clay pipe and after a bit the stories would come. He taught me to read and write too, and together we delighted in the words of the great poets and philosophers.

But the smell of death emanating from the morgue has started to make me fret. No, it is life that beckons to me now. I find myself wondering if the novelty of being alive again, albeit through the medium of Alice, will ever wear off. Somehow, I doubt it. So we abandon dusty studies in favour of exploration. We have to be careful where we go, for there is trouble on the island. The tense atmosphere reminds me of the weeks leading up to the outbreak of war. I overhear Alice's father saying that some of the Chinese people are unhappy about working conditions, and that they believe the British are taking advantage of them. Some days there are riots, people shouting slogans and fighting, even bombs exploding and causing dreadful injuries. It seems strange though that this time the enemy is not the Japanese, but the British.

Despite these disturbances, Alice and I do not curtail our outings. We visit the Tiger Balm Gardens, or we take a ferry to one of the outer islands, or we walk the length of Shek O Beach, or Silvermine Bay, kicking up the sand, or we catch a bus to Aberdeen and watch the boat people, my people, for a while. This last stirs up memories of Lin Shui for me. Sometimes I am certain I spot my father, scrambling about the rigging of one of the great junks, the rust-brown sails flapping and rippling under him, his long, silver hair swept up into a bun and skewered with a netting needle, as was his habit. Sometimes I see a young girl, just like me, her life shrunk to the wooden decks that enfold her, her days spent riding the waves, mending nets, patching sails, cooking, washing pots and pans, and doing her family's laundry. And I wonder if she realises how fine this life of hers is, if she values it as she ought. Sometimes too, I see the shadows of my ancestors and I know they are lying in wait for me.

Of course there are some advantages to being 'undead', for example I no longer feel hunger. I share with Alice what it is to need neither food nor drink. She joins me, fasting for long periods, till her head is light as a feather, and she trips about as if she is stepping onto clouds. When she grows dizzy and black shapes detonate before her eyes, I have to remind myself that Alice is only human and must eat to live. I prompt her then to feed, reminding myself that I am leasing her body. But while Alice fasts, her brother Harry feasts until none of his clothes fit him.

The flat on The Peak is emptier than I thought it would be, reminding me sometimes of the morgue. Alice's father is rarely at home, working constantly. Alice's mother, though sometimes in the same room, feels far away. I am envious of Alice having not one but two sisters. But I find even this, when they return home for the holidays, is not as I imagined it. Late one night we chance upon Jillian in the kitchen. She is surrounded by tins and packets and jars. She is stuffing food into her mouth, slices of bread slathered in chocolate spread and jam and peanut butter, cramming in biscuits and cakes and crisps and chocolate. In between mouthfuls she is gulping juice and milk, and brightly coloured drinks that bubble and fizz,

82

as if infused with lifeforce. I amuse myself by causing one of the tube lights in the kitchen to flash for a time. Jillian barely glances up. Instead, as it flickers, Alice's oldest sister looks as if she is jerking about like a gluttonous puppet, her blonde hair flying. Alice is po-faced, but I think it is very funny.

All the while, fearless nocturnal cockroaches scuttle about. Emerging from the drains they feast on smears and crumbs. Most are on the floor, though a few, braver than the rest, scrabble around on the work surfaces. Their antennae swivel. They are well fed these cockroaches, the size of Hong Kong dollars. Their beetle-brown bodies gleam in the glow cast by the fluorescent tubes. Fine hairs sprout from their busy, spindly legs. The wings of one that is trying to clamber up the slippery sides of a glass whirr madly. It lumbers into the air and flies about, rebounding off cupboard doors and tiled surfaces, before landing to gobble afresh on a fast-melting square of chocolate. They look as shiny as vinyl. Alice flinches. Jillian pauses in her gorging, just long enough to bring a clenched fist down on it. We hear the 'squish' as its mushy body is crushed. Jillian glances cursorily at the base of her fist. She wipes off the stuff that looks like yellow pus on a kitchen towel, and starts guzzling again.

'What are you doing?' Alice wants to know, the juices running into her own mouth at the sight of all that food.

Startled, Jillian jumps and turns on Alice. She cannot have known we were here, watching her. 'Shut up,' she hisses, a chocolaty dribble running down her chin. 'Shut up and get out.' The face of one of the amahs appears like a ghostly apparition at the window in the back door. It is Ah Dang, her plait unravelled, the top buttons of her tunic undone. She looks first sleepy-eyed, then amazed, as if she thinks she might still be dreaming. Despite this, her face registers concern, probably at the prospect of the morning's clean-up job. Meeting Jillian's incensed glare, wisely she elects to creep away.

'You'll make yourself sick if you eat all that,' says Alice prophetically.

And that is exactly what Jillian does. When she has eaten so much that she seems barely able to walk and keep it all contained, she flicks off the kitchen light, staggers through the dining room, and down the long, dark corridor to the bathroom. We follow her and see her stumble inside, slam the door, and switch the light on. A thin, yellow stripe at the base of the door filters into the dimness. We hear Jillian lock it behind her. Then she begins to retch. For a long while she vomits and chokes. The sounds are harsh. They splinter the night. I am amazed that no one wakens at the din. Alice crouches in the murk listening to her sister disgorging herself, and her mother snoring. A few times Bear approaches her, but then he senses my presence and slinks away again, hackles high. Several of the corridor windows are open, and a welcome breeze is cooling the flat. The cicadas trill. Their song rhythmically swells and then subsides. The taps snort out water. The toilet flushes. Then silence. The cicadas too are momentarily still, as if in anticipation. The bathroom door slams open, hitting the wall with a resounding 'thwack'. A square of light falls into the darkness, with the silhouette of Jillian squinting at its centre. She is not wearing her glasses.

'Bitch,' she fires into the corridor. She stinks of bile. She wipes the back of a hand over her mouth, gives a brittle laugh and flicks off the light. The darkness springs back. I remember what it is to be starving, the acid ache of it. I remember not knowing if I would eat again. I remember that food haunted my dreams, that it had the power to bewitch me. Jillian feels her way like a blind man past Harry's bedroom to her own, goes in, the door thumping shut behind her. Still Alice huddles in the blackness. Bear growls softly. Some time later, after several unsuccessful attempts, a key turns in a lock and scratches the dark. The front door swings open. Nicola appears with a boy in tow, silhouettes in the lobby light. Entwined they fall back against the front door, closing it with their bodies. They tumble onto the Persian rug in the shadowy hall. There is a lot of grunting and struggling. Clothes are tossed aside. White bits swim into sight. Buttocks, an erect penis, a breast, an upright V of splayed legs. They are made luminous in the moonlight, these infrequently seen body parts. The dog watches cocking his head in puzzlement.

'For Christ's sake stop fucking about and put it in,' snarls Nicola. The tone of her voice is bored and irritable. There is a bit of adjustment, then a good deal of rocking and panting, followed by a breathy cry. A few seconds pass. 'Get off me, Mick. I think I'm going to be sick,' groans Nicola. The boy, Mick, leaps up obediently. He begins tugging on his jeans. Nicola is slower to get up. She pulls on her pants and smoothes down her skirt. 'I'm tired, so can you just fuck off now,' she says opening the front door, unceremoniously showing the boy out, and shutting it firmly behind him. Without bothering to put on the lights she weaves her way down the corridor, never noticing Alice hugging the blackness to her. She vanishes straight into the room she shares with Jillian.

Alice's mother, Myrtle, is on next. Her bedroom door opens slowly, and for a few seconds she stands swaying in the doorway. Then she steps gingerly into the stream of moonlight. She is wearing a pale dressing gown. There is a metallic sheen to it. Her hair is loose, falling about her shoulders. Her gait is unsteady. She finds her way to the bamboo-clad bar in the hall. She also seems to want invisibility, and does not bother with the lights. She fumbles with the sliding door of the bar, grabs a bottle, unscrews the top and takes a greedy gulp. With it clutched to her chest, she treads with the care of a tightrope walker back to her bedroom, and quietly closes the door.

'While my father is away,' whispers Alice, whose father is on a business trip in Singapore, 'the mice come out to play.'

Later Alice drags some pillows and blankets into the corridor, and nestles by a bookcase that borders one of the walls. She cannot see the titles in the half-light, but she touches the hard spines of the books, and follows the contours of the lettering printed on their covers with an index finger. Much later, when I levitate out of Alice to glide along the ceiling, until I am floating just above the drinks cabinet, Bear cautiously nears my host. He sniffs her bedding warily, until he is satisfied it holds no trace of me. Then he nudges his way into the makeshift bed. Not satisfied with his proximity to Alice, he nuzzles at the bent arm at her side. Alice, half asleep, starts, her eyes springing open. Then in a wave of recognition she enwraps Bear, her dog, and draws him close to her. At length they sleep, Alice dropping off first, Bear rolling his eyes upwards and baring his teeth at me once, and then again, before finally settling down. I peer at them with bafflement at first, and then with something very like resentment. Alice's face is calm, like still water. Her arm rises and falls gently as the dog's lungs fill and deflate. Soon their rhythmic breaths interlock, fitting together like pieces of a puzzle, and their two hearts fall to beating in unison. I am covetous of their shared warmth, their joint slumber. Seeing their bodies spooned together makes me recall the taste of the Chinese speciality, Bitter Melon.

On the bar is a cut-glass decanter. Dipped in moonshine, the diamond panes glint like silver sequins. Although the decanter looks heavy, I am positive I can shift it. I condense myself and slither between it and the smooth, plastic surface of the bar. I radiate heat, drawing it from Alice, from the dog, from the air, and concentrating it, as you might do with a glass concentrating the energy of the sun to make fire. I distil the moisture of the night, sucking it up from the dew soaked air. Soon the plastic is wet and slippery. I feel the decanter move then, just an inch or so. After that it is easy, one inch more and more and more. Now nearly half of the crystal sphere hangs over the edge of the bar. The liquid inside it sloshes and slops, a storm in a bottle. I draw every drop of it into the unsupported half of the glittering bulge. The bottle vibrates a moment. Then it arcs and plummets, splitting into pieces against the wooden floor with a heavy crash. The liquid bursts, liberated briefly before it pools. The dog snarls. Alice shifts drowsily. I hear a whimper coming from one of the bedrooms. I think it may be Harry. Then the hush slowly unfurls again.

In the morning though it is anything but quiet. A shaft of sunlight falls on the jagged pieces of the fractured decanter. It makes a wondrous dazzlement of them. I am delighted by the eye-catching trinkets I have brought into being. Surprisingly, Alice's mother is not impressed. She shrieks at Alice. The dog scurries away, head down, tail between his legs. The amahs raise their hands to their mouths, and insist they know nothing of how the decanter came to be broken. But when Ah Lee hunkers down and begins to pick up splinters of glass, Alice's mother grabs her shoulder and gives it a little shake.

'Alice will do this,' she cries. 'She will collect up every bit of it in a bag, and when her father comes home she will show it to him.' She lets go the shoulder and swoops on Alice. 'You will tell him what you have done. Do you understand me, Alice?' Myrtle Safford's face looks flushed. It is fast becoming the colour of raw meat. Her fingers work busily at the embroidered sleeve of her blouse. She is bound to pull a thread if she persists in picking at the fine handiwork, I think.

'I did not break the decanter,' Alice says, on her feet, head held high, facing her mother. She repeats this several times.

'Do not lie to me,' Myrtle interrupts her. Her eyes look dry and sore, the lids drawing in sharply, as if the bright sunshine is hurting them.

Jillian materialises wearing one of her father's old shirts. Her apathetic flint-grey eyes scan the tableau, amahs askance, mother enraged, Alice defiant. She wags her head slowly, knowingly from side to side. 'I have a sore throat,' she grunts, her hand stroking her collarbone. She yawns expansively, steps carefully over the broken glass, pushes past the amahs, and on into the dining room. 'I need some breakfast. I'm starving,' she mutters over her shoulder.

I cannot not help wondering if she will throw it all up again later on. Nicola does not make an entrance. I expect she is tired after the previous night's exertions. Harry peeps round his door, surveys the scene, and vanishes like a timorous mouse. It is plain to me that Alice is agitated. She does not seem the least bit thrilled with my achievement. She stoops and picks up a piece of glass. While her mother is shouting, she pushes the ragged point of it into the tip of a thumb. Ah Lee bursts into a fit of nervous giggles.

'*Mo lei tau!*' Ah Dang mutters.

Alice looks down and notes there is blood on her hand. Her brow creases in confusion, as if she cannot imagine how it got there.

Days later Alice's father returns home and is presented with a bag that rattles when he lifts it up. It is full of my pretties. He asks Alice to join him in the lounge. He tells her that he is not angry with her, but he needs to understand why she has broken the decanter.

'I didn't break it,' Alice insists. Her thumb still hurts, though of course it is no longer bleeding. She rubs it unconsciously.

89

Alice's father looks shattered. He has dark smudges under his eyes. He presses the heels of his hands into his eye sockets for a long moment. I make the chips of glass in the brown paper bag resting on his lap, chink and tinkle. Hearing them sing drops his hands, and his weary eyes rake the room. They alight on a book, a statue, a carved lantern, a record player, a television, on the Chinese carpet that covers most of the floor, finally coming to rest once more on the crumpled, open-necked bag on his lap. He looks, I observe, as if he has just discovered that life is not what he expected it to be. He looks as if he is staring down, not at a shattered decanter in his lap, but at his own shattered dreams.

'I didn't do it,' Alice reiterates. Her little fingers are crooked now, her face clouded. I explain that I did, but only Alice hears me. Her eyes dart about the room. At last they settle on her father's drooping head. 'I'm going to be good now,' Alice says.

Ralph—1967

My first night home this week, I've been sleeping in Central, down at the office. It could erupt at any time, with each passing day it seems we come closer to the point of no return. And what will become of us then, us few servants of Her Majesty Queen Elizabeth, holding the fort while the Apaches circle? I don't hear the approach of the cavalry. We're on our own, chaps, with only our shadows for company. Myrtle has poured me a large whisky. Don't ask me how, but I know this is a prelude to one of her talks. I am colourless with exhaustion. My wife is making yet more demands on me. At the end of this God-awful day, she wants the only thing I have left, my attention. I feel the finger of scotch stroke the back of my throat. I wonder if Myrtle realises that I may very well be a target, on some kind of a hit list, that we all might be come to that. She is talking . . . talking about our daughter, about Alice.

'She has a violent temper,' she accuses bluntly. 'She is destructive.'

I haven't the strength to contradict her. There is violence breaking out everywhere downtown. Real violence. The blood, injury and death kind of violence. The once peaceful streets of the colony blossom with exploding homemade bombs, known to locals as *'boh loh'*, Cantonese for pineapple. Huge banners fly high, damning the British for the pathetically low salaries of the indigenous people, for their draconian working hours, for water-shortages and increasing prices. Curfews that transform the colony into a ghost town, tear-gas, even the threat that troublemakers breaking the restrictions will be shot on sight, serve only to contain the mêlée. But for how long, dear God, for how long? My neck aches and the base of my spine too. I need a hot bath, a good, long soak. There aren't any showers at the office, and I am aware of the stale odour of a couple of days' sweat coming from my armpits, my back, under my collar, between my thighs. On and on she goes, damning our ailing daughter. There is the heavy tick of the clock behind us in the lounge. We are on the veranda. It is early autumn, but still warm enough to sit outside for a short while. I used to love the tick of a clock, used to find it comforting. But now it is just a reminder that time is running out. My eyes are stinging and my eyelids are heavy. I am so shattered that I am breathless. I am sitting down, and I am gulping in oxygen as if I am running a race.

'Frankly Ralph, I'm not at all sure the Island School is such a good idea for Alice. In the few weeks since she started there her behaviour has been worse than ever, more erratic, more . . . well . . . Peculiar. Quite honestly I feel I can't cope much longer.' Myrtle pauses to assess the effect her words are having on me. Then, judging it to be safe, with a swift, flirtatious smile, she proceeds. 'I know you may not altogether agree with me, but please Ralph, hear me out. I really do feel that the structure of boarding school might be just what she needs. Alright, I will concede that perhaps the convent wouldn't be suitable for Alice. But that doesn't rule out boarding school entirely, now does it?'

The cicadas warble. There is the distant hum of passing cars. A horn sounds a long way off. A dog barks and is echoed with an answer. From where I am sitting I can see at least three cars winding their way up The Peak, and twice that many going down, yellow cones of light sliding along the curling tape of grey road that binds the slopes. There is a double-decker bus too, chinks of warm yellow light threading through the dusk, on route to The Peak Tram Terminus I expect. I wonder idly if Myrtle wants to get rid of all our children? Will she carry on until we have none left? The answer is swift, light as warm air, and just as

92

stifling.

She will carry on until Alice is gone. I sip my scotch and watch the coloured lights of Aberdeen harbour winking busily below, and the lambent stars and moon, poised and rigid above. I am so very tired these days. And I am lonely too. It eats like a maggot into my heart, this loneliness of mine. I nod and try to look as if I am taking it all in, as my wife's voice winds around me. I frown pensively. See, my expression says, I am cogitating, entertaining your suggestion, weighing up the merits of such a course of action.

In reality I am far off. I am reliving the unrest, the coiled spring of tension that lays in wait for me with every breaking dawn. I am thinking about the riots, the faces, distorted and ugly, the gaping mouths that stamp out words, hateful, vicious words, those bent on bloodletting. I think about Central, where often I have enjoyed a coffee at the Hilton, or lunch at the Foreign Correspondent's Club. I think of the Cosmo Club too and the Christmas parties we have had there, of the raffles and the paper hats, and of the turkey and Christmas pudding, the thick, steaming gravy, and the viscous yellow custard, so absurd in this land of sun and bamboo and sea. I recall those evil drinking games that I have tumbled unwittingly into after a Cantonese meal, games that have left me legless and the world spinning. I think of my Chinese friends, these men I have grown to love, who understand me better than any Englishman ever could, these men with whom I have spent my precious hoard of free time lavishly, and never regretted a cent of it. I think about the joy I have had rummaging in the alleys, fingering treasures in dusty boxes, imagining who could have created such beauty, such perfection in a past world. I think about the Star Ferries, their dark prows knifing through the sea, how the thrill of that journey over to Kowloon has never quite evanesced for me. I think of the banks and the money rolling in, the obscene amounts of money. And then, I think of the poverty of the locals, of the workforce, the poverty that in truth I have done little to ameliorate.

Finally the image of a small, thin, naked girl, hair, face and flesh ablaze, forces everything else out of my mind. It is a photograph on the wall of the Foreign Correspondents' Club, in its multi-storey setting, high above Central. There are other pictures alongside it but they do not register. It is black and white, this image of the flaming child. The lack of colour does not lessen the horror, rather the stark contrast seems to highlight it. I think she is Vietnamese. I think it was taken during the Vietnamese war. But it really doesn't matter. It might have been anywhere. Her face is split with anguish. Her mouth is racked into an 'O' of agony. She is staring straight into the camera lens as she staggers along the muddy path. Flames lick upwards and outwards from her core, they roar through her silk-black hair, they spark her eyelashes and crackle over her eyebrows, they crust and blister the jelly of her still seeing eyeballs. She holds her hands out pityingly towards . . . who? The cameraman? The soldiers? God? I cannot free myself of this vision tonight. She haunts me this little girl as she staggers forwards, her arms full of fire, offering up all that she has, offering it up to whoever will take it, offering up

94

her hell on earth.

My wife is speaking again. She talks of the pressure I am under in my job during these unsettled times. She maintains it is vital that I am fit for the task of subduing these red rebels, that both Queen and country are relying on me to restore order to the colony.

'You cannot afford to be distracted by Alice at times like this,' Myrtle insists. She takes a slow meditative swallow of her drink before she speaks again. 'Neither can I. How can I support you, Ralph, if I am drained dry by our daughter,' she wheedles, her voice as velvety as moss. 'And it's not just that,' she continues. 'She is putting such a strain on our relationship, darling. You must see that. We need time to ourselves, time free of endless worries and arguments about Alice. Besides, I am very concerned that her disruptive behaviour may eventually rub off on our son, on Harry.'

Now she is praising a school she has found in the Highlands of Scotland, of all places, an establishment founded on strict principles of discipline and regulation. She is describing its location as if she were selling me a holiday home. The cadence of her voice is very nearly poetic. She paints a scene of rolling heather-covered mountains crowned with garlands of mist, spotted with strutting stags, of the blue-black lochs, ice-cold liquid bodies stretched out for miles, mirrors to the scudding clouds above, of the swarms of midges, and of the banks of virgin snow. I picture Alice in this setting, and marvel that Myrtle believes a remedy can be found for our turbulent daughter so far away, as if geography is the answer.

I turn my whisky tumbler around and around in my hands. The peaty aroma I inhale seems most apt. As the marauding gangs charge through the streets of Central, their war cries a united tirade against Colonial rule, my bowels loosen and my legs turn to water. Perched on high in my office I watch the Hong Kong Police, their arms linked, like playground children at their games. Red rover, red rover, let the rioters come over! A human wall barricading the road, poised for the impact that will surely come. A couple of days ago, peering though my binoculars at this brave force, this force whose job it is to repel the wrath of mighty China, I focused on the face of a boy . . . he was no more than a boy I tell you, a Chinese boy, pitting himself against the rabble, against his own people. For this I know he will earn the title of 'Yellow Running Dog', for he has sided with the 'White Skinned Pigs', the European interlopers.

Music thunders out from loudspeakers in Central District, the volume at such a high level you can hear it in the flat on The Peak, as if it is coming from the next room. It drowns out the slogans and propaganda, being broadcast from the communist-owned buildings. People are being attacked. They are being murdered. And a Chinese boy wearing the khaki uniform of the Hong Kong Police Force, stands erect, head held high, and blocks their path, while I, Ralph Safford, representative of the British Government, look down from my safe offices in the sky, my bowels liquid, my heart pounding too fast, and my hands slick with sweat.

'Damned communists!' I recall saying conversationally to a colleague on one of the darkest days. I peered down at the advancing, boiling mass, at the bracelet of police standing firm. They were advancing on the Hilton Hotel. If they break through, I thought, terror jerking at my heart, perhaps they will pour up Garden Road, past St John's Cathedral, and the lower Peak Tram terminus. Then higher, why not, half of the bloodthirsty rabble peeling off up the slopes to Government House to lynch the 24th British Governor of Hong Kong, Sir David Trench, the rest continuing their march on Victoria Peak, where they knew we lorded it over them in luxury.

'Damned Red Guards with their "Little Red Books",' I blustered, trying in vain to steady my voice. I gestured at the angry crowds beneath our windows. 'Not exactly what we Brits would call a Cultural Revolution, eh?' I managed a chuckle, but the sound was hollow. 'We simply can't have this sort of thing. After all, these fellows are making trouble on British territory,' I said, sounding like the stereotype of a stoic British officer in a bad war film. I tried to instil outrage into my voice, fury at this insult to my sovereign Queen. And I very nearly pulled it off. But the sudden slump of my colleague's shoulders made it clear I was fooling no one. About now, I thought, the film camera should pan to the skies above, buzzing with British warplanes come to put an end to this rebellious nonsense. I glanced upwards, a clear, blue sky, a disarmingly beautiful day on the island of Hong Kong. I wondered if the Chinese boy in his man's uniform was glancing up too. I wondered if he was thinking that it was a good day to die, to become a *sei chai lo*, a dead policeman, with no clouds to impede his soul's flight.

97

My mind slides forward in time and I am back on the veranda with my wife. I raise my glass and toss back my drink. Myrtle takes it from me. She doesn't even ask me if I would like a refill. She busies herself with the new decanter, with the ice bucket. I hear the cubes of ice clunk and rattle as they are agitated with the metal tongs. Looking down, I see a brochure Myrtle has deposited in my lap for a boarding school in Argyll. I flip through the pages. They are full of snaps of Amazonian girls with flushed cheeks doing wholesome things. I pause at a shot of one leaping in the air, arms outstretched, hands spread wide. The netball she has just shot is arcing earthwards, about to slip through the goal ring. Her thick black hair is crushed back by the wind. The expression on her face is vicious. I will mow down anyone who gets in my way, it bugles through slit eyes, ballooning cheeks, a funnelled mouth and gritted teeth. There is a malignancy about it, I decide, that I find decidedly distasteful. I toss the brochure onto the drinks table. Myrtle notes my gesture and quickly hands me my drink. She has poured me a stiff measure. If I down this too fast I shall fall asleep. My lips curl upwards longingly at the thought of slumber, of drowning in slumber.

I wonder where it will all end? I overheard talk today of the People's Republic of China seizing control of the island, taking back Hong Kong from right under our noses. Once a remote, even a ridiculous, idea, this now feels tangible, a very real probability, a probability I am living with every day, down there in Central District. Up here on The Peak, to a great extent the family is insulated. As I listen to Myrtle prattle on about how difficult life has become for her, I smoulder with resentment. I cannot help it. I am in the firing line, the thick of it, not her. For the time being at least, she is tucked up safe in the flat on The Peak, with amahs to care for her. Still, foolish though it may be, I like to believe she's safe, that Harry and Alice are safe, that the communist agitators will draw the line at charging up The Peak and laying siege to the flat. After all, we are British subjects. I am fighting the urge to laugh at this notion, this notion that because we are British subjects, servants of Her Majesty Queen Elizabeth the Second, they will tread carefully around us. It will not make an iota of difference to the raging mob down there. No. I take that back. Of course it will make a difference. It will spur them on till they have butchered all the 'White-Skinned Pigs'.

I must stop this. What with a couple of swift ones before leaving the office, and the hefty measures I am getting through now, I've had far too much to drink on an empty stomach. I am growing maudlin. I ignore my own caution and take another slug of scotch. I bare my teeth at the night sky. I can't concentrate on my wife and her tribulations, tonight of all nights. Why is Myrtle bothering me with this, when what I need is pause, time to regroup, to prepare for the next onslaught, for most certainly it will come. How can I think about Alice's future—when I'm not sure if any of us even have one.

'I think it's for the best,' Myrtle says again, taking a gulp of whisky herself. Then, when I turn to her, my face blank, she adds a reminder of the subject under debate, 'Sending Alice to boarding school in Scotland.' She takes up the brochure,

99

leafs through it, and seizes on the very page with the grimacing netball-player that I stumbled on. She brandishes it at me, stabbing a manicured fingernail at the action shot. 'Just look at that,' she urges. 'That girl wants to win. That could be Alice in a few years from now. Think of that!'

I do not tell her this is the very thing that I am thinking of, this is what I am afraid of. I am too weary to argue. Besides, Scotland seems a long way away tonight, as does England. Sometimes I think I have forgotten what England is like, forgotten that it is home, my country. I feel as if I have been trying to create a little England, here, on the doorstep of China, and that anybody who really considers this will see that it is an impossible task, the work of a lifetime. For what? In just three short decades, as the century closes, China will reclaim her island, and she will probably do a very thorough job of obliterating all evidence of the British, as speedily as she can. And who would blame her?

'Ralph? Darling, are you listening?' Myrtle's voice sounds in my rambling thoughts. 'About Alice? Scotland? What do you think?'

From somewhere I find the might to withstand my wife's determination to dispense with Alice. I take a shuddering breath and meet her eyes, my gaze steady.

'No. It wouldn't work out for Alice. She would never settle in a boarding school.' My voice is unwavering.

'But how can you know that, Ralph, when—' Myrtle persists.

'It's too late,' I interrupt. 'She has started at the Island School. She has her uniform, her timetable.

She may have already made new friends.' This last seems an absurd objection even to me, considering she doesn't have any old friends to speak of. But I plough on regardless. 'Moving her now would cause havoc.'

Again Myrtle, eyes alight, starts to argue, and again I break in.

'That is my final word on the matter, Myrtle. The subject is closed. Alice stays where she is.' I lower my head and stare broodingly into my glass, daring my wife to speak again. When several seconds pass and she does not protest, I glance up. She is staring moodily ahead, chin up, mouth set. She is furious and I do not care.

The year is drawing to a close when I hear at last that an order has come from Beijing, reining in the insurgents, effectively curtailing the violence and bombings for the present. It seems the riots, that will come to be known as the Colonial Riots, have finally subsided. I feel as if I have been holding my breath all this while, and now I can release it. Again I am looking down on the streets of Central and they are blessedly safe. Of course there is the accustomed bustle of this overcrowded island, but the faces I spot are benign, and the scurrying people are devoid of menace. I indulge myself. I dare to think the troubles are behind us, that the structure is still solid, and that Her Majesty's Crown Colony has been delivered back to her safe and sound.

I try not to dwell on the lives lost, or on those men, women and children whose futures will forever be blighted by this appalling time. I try to do what I can to improve the lives of ordinary Chinese citizens, driven now by guilt at what I know were the intolerable conditions they had to survive under. I admit, if only to myself, that corruption in both the ruling classes and the police force has been rife. I use what influence I have to combat this. My motives are not entirely altruistic though. I am driven on by guilt.

I have felt the immense might of China bearing down on me, on this tiny island of Hong Kong. And although this servant of the British Empire stood his ground waving the Union Jack, in reality I know that, like King Canute, trying to halt the rising tide, we never had a chance of holding the colony if China had really wanted to take it. Who knows what deals were done behind the scenes to persuade China to stand down when she did. But no matter the reasons, China has decided to let the British play 'I'm the King of the Castle' for a short while longer. There is no question in my mind that we are only able to continue with our precarious little lives on her say-so. For years I will toss and turn through sleepless nights, my dreams crowded with the ghosts of people killed and wounded, while I was on duty. I will wonder if I might have done better, if my actions might have been speedier, if more lives could have been saved. When the pats on the back are a distant memory, I will wonder truly if it was all worth it.

Brian—1970

I cast Alice Safford in the role of Abigail in Arthur Miller's Crucible, because I thought it might bring the kid out of herself a bit. As Head of English and

Drama at the Island School, , the annual play is my baby, as agreed when I took up the post. I select it, direct it, produce it, sort out scenery, costumes, lighting, programmes, and just about anything else you care to mention. In short, I live it for a term. With the school only open three years, there was a lot riding on this first spring production. I couldn't afford mistakes. But I just had a feeling that fourteen-year-old Alice was up to the job. She's so much more grown up than the other girls in her year—intelligent, observant. Even at that first reading there was something in her voice that made me think she could pull it off. Which is more than can be said for Trevor Lang playing John Proctor. But then again, what he lacked in talent he made up for in enthusiasm. And frankly I didn't have much to choose from, well nobody actually. He was the only boy who showed up to the audition.

Alice was captivating from the outset, endlessly changing, one moment the seductress, the next spitting like a cat, then all wide-eyed innocence. In the court scene, where Abigail drives the other girls into a frenzy, she actually had the hairs standing up on the back of my neck. We even had a few visits from worried parents complaining their children were having nightmares, questioning my choice of play. But if I'd hoped that acting was going to help her overcome her shyness, or curtail some of the strange behaviour she'd been exhibiting at school, I was to be sorely disappointed. Throughout rehearsals and following the success of the play, Alice continued to prove difficult.

She's not a favourite among other teachers, that

103

girl. And recently, I can't deny her behaviour has been challenging. But what the heck, I like Alice. I don't mind admitting it either. I like her. Now when I say that, I don't mean I want to fuck her. Not like some of the older girls. And can you blame me? Sun-tanned legs peeping out from under those flimsy, striped, summer shifts. The zip down the front, with the metal ring through it, that looks like the ring-pull on a can of lager. God, the times I've dreamt of easing those zips down, of glimpsing those lacy, little-girl bras, of touching those firm, young breasts and . . . The winter uniform's not much better either, with the chocolate-coloured skirts, so short that you can sometimes see the crease in the girls' thighs, and a hint of their curved buttocks beneath the fabric.

They know it too! Ah, believe me, they know what they're doing to you, as they sashay about this wreck we're having to make do with. A decrepit army hospital full of ghosts. Well, that's what the kids say anyway, whispering horror stories to one another about the morgue. Oh yes, we have our own morgue here at the Island School, very handy if any of the kids expire before close of day. Actually most of the students won't venture anywhere near it. Even Melvin Furse, the Head, hates it, says he can't wait to have the wretched thing demolished.

I've wandered around outside it once or twice, but I've never had the desire or the nerve to enter. There is something really menacing about that place. Gives a whole new meaning to the nicknames the Chinese have for us British. *Gweilo*. A dead corpse that has come back to life, a ghost man, or *gweipor*, a ghost woman. Apparently, so I'm told, years of oppression earned us such unflattering sobriquets. Still, it's easy to see how the Chinese populace first coined them, staring amazed as their new white rulers paraded before them like the living dead. The Chinese are a superstitious race. They believe in ghosts. As for me, before I came here I would have said it was all nonsense. Now, I'm not so sure. This entire building has an unsettling atmosphere you simply can't ignore, a mausoleum, smelling of damp and mould, paint peeling off walls, loggias open to wind and weather. Completely impractical. Furse keeps promising it won't be long before the new premises, currently under construction on the terraced slopes above us, are completed. Though quite honestly there have been so many delays, I am beginning to feel it will be little short of miraculous when its finished.

And yet, I maintain there's something rather sensual about seeing a lovely girl stroll around this ancient ruin. Echoes of the dying and the dead, screams of agony, groans and sighs, rattling last breaths, mingling with the quick footsteps, fits of giggles, yelps of excitement, and whispered secrets, of ravishing young beauties hurrying to class. Like a film set: the girls playing the leading roles, the ghosts providing all the atmosphere. After all, I'm only flesh and blood, and surely there's no harm in just looking. Honestly, what man wouldn't let his eyes rove a bit with those slim hips swinging ahead of him, those breasts glimpsed from open-necked shirts, through the grinning teeth of an undone zipper. Seeing those swells of warm flesh lifting and falling, beads of sweat adorning them like

105

crystal necklaces. They do it deliberately you know. Leaving one too many buttons undone, innocently hooking that ring with a curved little finger and easing it down a few inches, leaning forwards on purpose so that you can't help but look. What can I say? I'm a good-looking, testosterone-fuelled, young man. But don't get me wrong. With Alice it's never like that. She doesn't flaunt herself, not like the rest of them.

Alice has always been quiet, even from that first day in September when the school opened. Worryingly quiet if I'm truthful. But lately . . . well, sometimes I think she'll disappear, drift away if someone doesn't anchor her down. It's peculiar. Every teacher has a different story to tell about her lately. But they all agree on one thing—that Alice is skiving classes regularly, and that, when she does deign to show up, inevitably there is trouble. In maths they tell me she's proving obstinate and unpredictable, that she walked out of class for no reason last week and hasn't been back since. In French apparently she's been deliberately obtuse, pretending she can't understand a word. Last week she smashed a bottle of ink. I'm told it was all over her dress and hands, and that she just stood there staring at it, as if she was in some kind of stupor. At least that's what Christine Wood the French teacher said. In chemistry she very nearly set fire to her desk a month ago, and now Frank Devine has her sitting at the front of the class, where he can keep an eye on her. In art, her still-life painting is anything but still, I'm reliably informed—things flying about all over the place.

Only last week in the staffroom, Karen Manners, her art teacher, cornered me. I was gasping for a coffee and in a hell of a rush too. But when Karen wants to talk, getting away from her is no easy task. Anyway the upshot is that she told me Alice is always painting the sea, junks and boat people, even soldiers. Japanese, she thinks, she recognises the uniforms. I countered this with some crack about women loving a man in a uniform, which Karen swatted down without so much as the suggestion of a smile.

'I find that remark inappropriate. This is no joke, Brian. It's dreadfully serious,' she flared.

These women! Christ! The trouble is they have no sense of humour. Mind you, I've always wondered if Karen mightn't be a lesbian. That would explain her dour exterior. As Head of English the teachers naturally come to me when they have a problem. I understand that. Though sometimes the stuff is so trivial, I can't help wondering why they can't work it out for themselves. Hand-holding. They all seem to need their hands held. But I have to concede that this time the problem, Alice, is a substantial one. I like to tackle things head on, so I naturally went straight to her.

'Alice,' I said, 'if you keep skipping classes you do realise that it's going to have a detrimental effect on your grades, perhaps even your O levels when you come to take them.'

I'd caught her at the end of the day, hovering in her classroom, after everyone else had left. I don't even think she was listening to me. She was staring out of the window, eyes dreamy and distant.

'Alice,' I tried again, 'where do you go?'

Perhaps I should have said 'where are you now?' She just looked right through me, as if . . . as if she was stumped by the question, as if she honestly couldn't remember where she went when she played truant.

As a last resort I called in her mother. And that was the weirdest thing of all. Oh, she came straightaway. She didn't try to put me off the way some of the parents do. She was punctual, too. Smartly dressed, stylish, you know. A belted, pale yellow shift, with a faded rose print in blush pink and gold. It was silk, I'd bet on it. Not Chinese, but that rough Thai silk. Over it she wore a white, short-sleeved jacket with embroidered sleeves. Her shoes were white as well, with very high heels. Not all women could carry off heels like those, but she could. And she had make-up on; not so much that she looked cheap, but applied subtly, giving her class. She was well-spoken too. I can't help but appreciate when an effort is made. It sets the scene I always think. Gives a meeting a professional air. A few of the parents I know, rolling up in jeans and flip-flops could learn a thing or two from Mrs Safford. She was the finished article right down to her painted pearly-pink nails.

Niceties first. Must observe protocol. First, I congratulated her on the OBE Ralph was awarded earlier in the year, in recognition of his dedicated service on the island. I told her that I'd seen the wonderful pictures of him, in full regalia at the presentation ceremony, on the front page of the *South China Morning Post*. Her too. And was it their son Harry by her side? She smiled appreciatively and inclined her head. And that lovely shot of Alice with her father, very moving. All traces of pleasure instantly vanished. I forged on. Weather. Always a safe bet. Then a smattering

108

of politics, perhaps not quite so safe considering the current climate among the natives. Just lately I'd say they were definitely a wee bit restless. Still, it looked as though the riots were behind us, thank God. Hardly surprising they're fed up, considering we've been bleeding them dry for decades. But naturally I didn't say that to Mrs Safford. No, no!

Then I informed her as tactfully as I could about Alice cutting classes, about her erratic behaviour, about her obsession—yes, her obsession with the sea—which seemed to be influencing all her work in art, and closed by voicing my anxieties over her tumbling grades. As I spoke, Mrs Safford nodded and made small sympathetic noises. She didn't try to deny any of it, didn't make excuses for her daughter. Didn't make excuses for herself, come to that. Finally, when she did respond, I was so taken aback, for a moment I couldn't speak.

'Mr Esmond,' she said, 'I appreciate you imparting your concerns to me. 'But,' she continued, her diction frighteningly perfect, 'I'm afraid there is little I can do about it. Alice can be . . . intractable. She doesn't listen to anyone. Certainly not to me.' She fixed me with her unreadable brown eyes.

She left me nowhere to go after that. I recall muttering something about hoping that we could work together from now on. And her response? Mrs Safford bent, lifted her white handbag from the foot of the chair, and delved inside it. She fished out her sunglasses, opened them up and dangled them by one arm. Then she let the other arm rest momentarily on her flame-red lips, the gesture deliberately provocative, before putting

109

them on. Her eyes now concealed, she pursed her lips lightly together, then gave me the kind of supercilious smile that makes a man wither away.

'I understand your frustration, Mr Esmond. In fact, I empathize with it,' she said, rising so that I rose too without thinking, and automatically put my hand into her outstretched one. 'But thank you so much for alerting us to the problem and for giving up your valuable time. Naturally, I will do my best to impress the gravity of the situation upon Alice. And if you could keep us informed, I should be most grateful.' And with that she bid me good afternoon.

I even remember the feel of her skin. It was very soft and cool. And her nails, they were long and sharp like a cat's, one of them scratching my hand lightly as she withdrew hers. When she'd gone, I tried to get on with some marking, but my mind just kept skipping back to our meeting.

'I'm afraid there is little I can do about it. Alice can be intractable. She doesn't listen to anyone. Certainly not to me.'

Those words of hers played over and over in my mind. I've met enough parents now to expect the unexpected. But nothing could have prepared me for that. You see, what struck me so forcibly was that Mrs Safford had spoken about Alice as if she was not her child.

Myrtle—1970

I am sorting through my box of newspaper cuttings, cards and the children's scraps. There is a write-up about the play, *The Crucible*, in the *South China Morning Post*. I'm holding it in my hands, letting my eyes run down the print, picking out the salient points. There is a photograph of Alice too. She is wearing a floor-length dark dress, long sleeves, a square white collar and a white cap. The colours stand out well in the black and white print. Her eyes are fixed upwards, stretched wide in terror at something they see. It is a good review. Well, it would be, wouldn't it? It's Martin Bishop's byline. Ralph's been friends with Martin more or less since we arrived on the island. They're drinking buddies too, so it stands to reason that he'd be extravagant with praise when it came to Alice.

' "Alice Safford's performance as Abigail Williams was electric. She lit up the stage. She was every inch the part." ' Hmm . . .

Actually, I thought she rather overdid it. You can do that you know, overact. They used to love it in Victorian melodramas. Hiss the villain. Great fun. All that screaming and hysteria. I might just as well have stayed at home. At least here it's free.

I screw up the review and bin it. I can't hang on to these things forever. I have other children you know. If I kept all these bits of paper I'd have a roomful by now. I glance down at the next snap. It is of Ralph being presented with his OBE at Government House last spring. What a day that was! I beam. He looks splendid, better than Sir David Trench I think. I've always thought Ralph would make rather a good governor. I don't think I'll hang on to the one of him and Alice gazing down at the medal. No point really when there at so many others.

111

Since the play Alice has been worse than ever. Fancy that silly Mr Esmond trying to tell me what Alice has been getting up to. As if I didn't know. I live with her. Alice's bad behaviour is part of our daily routine in our flat on The Peak, I'm afraid. Doesn't he realise that if I could have waved a magic wand and put her right, I would have done it years ago. She's unmanageable. And he's out of his depth, though he probably doesn't realise it. Of course he is. Most people are with Alice. Why Ralph can't accept there's a problem I do not know. He's blind to it, and nothing I do or say or even show him, makes any difference. Of course I told him about Alice's latest debacle, about being summoned to the school, about her skipping classes. His rejoinder—she was going through a rough patch. Well, if she is, it has lasted fourteen years.

In any case it's not just Alice's scenes I'm concerned about now. She's infected my son, she's infected Harry with her spleen. He used to be such a nice boy, so good-natured and malleable. I need a drink. I know it's early, that the children aren't even home from school yet, but I need to speak to Ralph tonight. I can't put it off any longer. One drink won't do any harm. I'll fetch it myself. I won't ask one of the amahs to pour it for me. They're so mean with the measures. I wish this damn bar door wouldn't make such a loud noise each time you slide it open. It doesn't seem to matter how careful I am.

'It's all right, Ah Lee. I'm fine thank you. Mrs Safford fine, okay? I don't need any help. Not just now. You carry on with the ironing.'

Snooping about. She might spend half her life

112

giggling, but I've noted those sharp, calculating eyes of hers. I know how these servants gossip. That's the trouble with having servants. No privacy. Nowhere is sacred. Damn. No ice. I just can't face going into the kitchen to get some. How many times have I told her to keep the bucket topped up each day? I'll have another word. Ah! That's better. Never mind about the ice. I'll take it into the bedroom. Shut the door. Give myself space to plan what I'm going to say to my husband. In here the sun has been beating down on the bed for most of the day. The purple satin quilt cover is baking hot. I've kicked off my shoes and I'm sprawling out, letting my bare feet slide. The glossy fabric is so slippery. Its touch burns. And the whisky—that burns too. The wound has been cauterized, the flow stemmed. Now I can cope.

Alice has rubbed off on Harry. He is following her bad example, mirroring it. And he's grown, well . . . fat. Harry has become fat.

'Harry is fat.'

There, I've said it out loud. I'd like to call it puppy fat, and believe that one day he'll grow out of it. But really I'm not so sure. He has a double chin now and you can hardly see his neck. I'm constantly having to buy him larger sizes. I can't keep up with it. I tell those stupid amahs over and over not to indulge him, but when my back is turned I know they do—biscuits, chocolate, steamed pudding with syrup, pancakes, fritters. Anyone would think we lived in the North Pole and needed some fat to keep us warm, not that we were roasting on a sub-tropical island. Of course he's being teased at the Island School. Only been there a couple of terms and already he's being

113

picked on. You'd think that would motivate him to diet. But not a bit of it. They yell abuse at him, and at their signal Harry heads for the kitchen.

I've tried to tackle him about it. But that temper of his, charging about like an angry troll, throwing things about the place. And as if I haven't got enough on my plate, there's a problem at the convent. The headmistress believes Nicola and Jillian may be involved in some way. Personally I think it unlikely, but mother's fuming of course. Let's hope it comes to nothing. I could close my eyes and drift off to sleep. Normally I don't like too much sun but today it's pure balm.

Harry charged a glass door the other day. I expect Alice drove him to it. She certainly makes me want to slam into a glass door. The two of them wound up in casualty. Both of them needed stitches, Harry's hands were in ribbons, and Alice had deep gashes in her leg and foot, and a cut to her face just above her lip. We're becoming quite the regulars there. They might as well book out a treatment room once weekly for the Safford family. What must they think? Still, that nice, little Chinese doctor never says anything. And of course he must know who we are, who Ralph is. He always sees us straight away, no matter how many patients are waiting. I tackled Alice about Harry's rages.

'Alice, do you fully comprehend the affect your conduct is having on your brother?' I asked her.

She was standing in the hall. She had just whistled up Bear and was about to set off for one of her rambles.

'Harry is not himself,' she hedged, not daring to meet my eyes.

114

'Harry is not himself because of you, Alice,' I qualified.

Then she did look up. Her eyes kindled into life. She was angry I think. Or perhaps, incredibly, amused. Though it's hard to tell with Alice.

'You are driving my son away,' I said, just so that there was no misunderstanding.

She put her head just slightly on one side then and gave me that measuring look of hers, eyelids half closed but their sense well and truly open. I despise that way she has of saying nothing and implying everything.

'You've no answer to that, have you?' I dredged up. The silent and plainly ludicrous suggestion that I might be contributing to Harry's exhibitions, hung in the air between us. The bloody dog kept yipping, and I would like to have kicked him, hard. He's not been disciplined properly, that dog. Alice indulges him. Now of course, like everything else, it's too late.

'Just go,' I spat.

I wanted her out of my sight. I couldn't bear to be with her for another second. Before she left she had the gall to ask me if there was anything she might pick up for me at Dairy Farm while she was out, as if all this was normal.

I want to send Alice away. But I can't. Ralph won't have it. So because of her I am going to have to sacrifice my son, my only son. Otherwise she will poison him with her venom. I hear the sound of the front door and Ah Lee's greeting. Alice is home. And I know as I roll the empty tumbler on the quilt, and see the faint residue of gold still coating the glass, that it is to Harry I must say goodbye.

Nicola—1970

Funny, now that we know we're leaving, I almost feel fond of the old place. There's no denying we had some laughs here. Jilly doesn't see it that way though.

'It is a vile, hateful school. It's been torture. The best thing they can do is close it down,' she told me yesterday, as we collected together our things. 'I want to forget it, forget we ever had to endure life here, forget it even exists.'

And it was true, there were moments when the wretched convent with its flock of gloomy nuns trotting out endless catechisms, had me a little depressed too. But I wasn't one to let misery engulf me. So after the first few downtrodden years, I put on a happy face, and instigated a programme of near miraculous recovery. Jesus, Mary and Joseph! I like that oath. I've borrowed it from Shauna, one of the Irish students who uses it all the time. I can do a pretty good impression of her accent by now as well. It makes Jilly nearly wet herself laughing. Anyway so, Jesus, Mary and Joseph, let me tell you how I transformed the once dull Saint Mary's Convent, into something rather like a film set for St Trinian's.

'The trick is,' I told my sceptical sister at the outset, 'not to get caught, Jilly.' I remember I uttered these words on our first midnight excursion. Jillian was already crippled with guilt. I never feel guilty. Things only seem awful when you put yourself in someone else's shoes. I never wear anyone's shoes but my own.

'What if we get caught?' said Jillian, brow pinched, eyes anxious, considering the consequences of our actions. I never do that either.

'We won't be,' I asserted with convincing surety.

We took two friends with us. I chose Margery Billingham, a plump girl with buck teeth and frizzy brown hair. My selection was to prove questionable, the window we all had to crawl through being quite small and Margery being quite large. Jillian picked her best friend, Jane Redwood. Jane was unnaturally slim, with a surprisingly narrow mouth set into her oval face. She had shoulder-length hair the colour and consistency of straw, and spots on her protruding chin that occasionally were, I couldn't help noticing, full of creamy pus. It made me feel nauseous just to look at them. I thought she was anorexic, as I never saw her eat anything, but Jillian said she just couldn't stand the convent food, and that she ate loads of chocolate in secret. Anyway, her thinness proved to be her redeeming feature that night. I had to admit two of her could have slipped through that window with no trouble, unlike wide-girthed Margery. The doors were all locked at night and the nuns kept the keys, so the window it had to be.

The window I keep alluding to was in the larder, the larder lay beyond the kitchens, and the kitchens behind the dining block. I had made careful notes on lock-down procedures at night, which nuns walked the beat and when. By midnight they were all abed and snorting through their dreams, so all we had to do was sneak out of the dormitories, climb down two flights of stairs, creep along the corridors past the classrooms, until we arrived at the dining hall. Once there we stole inside, wrinkling up our noses at the lingering, stewed-cabbage smell that seemed to permeate the walls, tiptoed into the kitchens, and from here made our way through to the larder. We climbed, one by one, on the broad, cold, marble shelf, and clambered out of the small window to the rear of it. It was always left open we learnt from Sister McMullen, head cook, in order to keep the air circulating and the food fresh, and the grid insert was easy to remove.

What I hadn't bargained for was how quiet 'quiet' really is, how sounds swallowed up throughout the day, with thumping feet, chattering voices and closing doors, were magnified a thousandfold at night. Nevertheless we soon got the hang of it. Shoes off, avoid boards that creaked, learn to sign, freeze and vanish at the first hint of trouble, and work as a team. The adrenalin rush on those nights was something else. It was like having an electric charge pulsing through me, all my senses heightened, razor-sharp. From the start, getting Margery through the window was a struggle. In the end, Jilly and Jane went first. It seemed the escape route I had picked had one great advantage. Beyond the window, only feet from it, was a bank of earth, and that meant there was no drop. With a combination of pushing and pulling, in the end we managed to ease Margery through. And once I had joined the group, a quick sprint across the convent lawns, followed by a brief if ungainly scramble over the iron railings, and we were free.

From here we bolted around a bend of the road

that took us away from the convent, and that's where the boys picked us up. We met the first lot hanging around outside Woolworths in Ealing, while we were staying with Gran one weekend. Darren, tall and mouthy, with sticking-out ears; James, the cute one, with blond hair and sexy, blue eyes; Patrick, James's older brother who owned the car, a beat-up green Ford Anglia, not so good-looking but, on the positive side, much more experienced; and Boyd, a bit of an oddball, chubby, a gingernut with crooked teeth and bad breath, who we decided would do for Margery. James and Boyd were still at school, but Patrick worked at the Walls factory in Acton and was very grown up. He had money, which after all was the only thing that mattered. Darren had dropped out of school and was just bumming around. He was constantly trying to scrounge off us. What a turn off! Even when I was really drunk, I avoided fucking him.

They brought booze and condoms and fags, and we roared off in their car, sitting on their laps and snogging before we'd even pulled away from the curb, listening to Radio Caroline or Radio Luxembourg, the Stones or the Beatles or the Searchers blaring out. Then it was a race to Richmond Green, or the towpath to Twickenham, or by the river in Kew, where we drank and fucked and smoked, in that order, rushing back to sneak in by 4:30am latest. I didn't mind this physical contact. I don't know why really—if it was the darkness that made it seem thrilling, or the booze, or the nerves, or perhaps it was just that it was illicit sex.

In time the operation grew slick, cushions in

beds, moving with all the stealth of panthers, even smuggling back contraband, booze, fags, rude magazines, and a bit of weed now and again. The Ford Anglia was slowly upgraded to a Jaguar, and it was no longer boys who picked us up beyond the school gates, but men. We dashed across those lawns in all weathers. Warm summer nights where the moonlight was impossibly bright, and we raced like fugitives over the cropped grass. Autumn, when we had to pick our way carefully over crunchy leaves, the wind for once a bonus, mercifully muffling our steps. Spring, where our dash was frequently accompanied by raw, spicy scents, the air pungent with newness. And winter, when we had to be extra vigilant if there had been fresh snow, treading only in the paths already mapped out by pupils and nuns during the day.

Apart from drifting off to sleep once or twice in class, and having to struggle through dismal, interminable prayers with thumping hangovers, we certainly seemed to be getting away with it. Now we had something to look forward to on the long tiresome days, a soap opera peppered richly with sexual encounters, good and bad to talk over, feats of ardour to compare, lewd and gross behaviour to smirk about. Meanwhile, during school hours we kept up a discreet campaign of disruption, hiding books, stealing small personal possessions that we knew the nuns shouldn't have, scribbling rude words over the pages of bibles in indelible ink: fuck, cunt, prick, fellatio, cunnilingus, masturbation, pudenda; even necrophilia. The effect was staggering. Nuns whispering in the corridors, timetables disrupted, classes cancelled, and an atmosphere of disorientation and chaos spreading even to morning assemblies. I learnt that it was easy to be duplicitous, easier still to manipulate people, oiling the wheels with flattery.

Goodness knows how long it would all have carried on for, if it hadn't been for lumpy Margery. She was so fat anyway that I didn't guess, guess that she was pregnant. One night, no matter how hard I pushed and the others pulled, she lodged fast in the larder window, and began to wail about how she was going to have this baby. She wailed so loudly that I began to wonder if she was going to give birth right there and then, and as I was standing next to the end where it would all happen, it was a bit of a worry. This is how Sister McMullen found us, me in a fetching purple mini-skirt, low-cut blouse, fishnet stockings and tons of make-up, Margery screaming like a stuck pig, her vast stomach wedged in the window frame, her legs kicking out as if she was swimming the crawl, a crate that had been on the marble shelf upturned, and root vegetables rolling about noisily around the tiled larder floor.

The next day Jillian broke down in the toilets, and wept over the retribution that she claimed would surely be swift. I handed her a loo roll, and gave her a play punch on the cheek.

'Don't panic, Jilly,' I reassured. 'This looks much worse than it actually is. It's all about the spin we put on our stories.' I was already gambling on the guilt card I would play to Mother. 'We can make all of this work in our favour.' After that, I went to considerable efforts to ensure that our stories tallied.

'If in doubt say nothing and leave it to me,' I advised my sister. 'You just cry.'

Jillian nodded. Tears were easy for her. I didn't bank on Mother Superior wanting to see each of us alone, but I heard Jillian bawling through the door so I wasn't too dismayed. I gave her an encouraging look as she emerged, red-eyed and snivelling. Then it was my turn. Mother Superior wanted to know which one of us was the mastermind behind our nocturnal wanderings. I prevaricated, making it clear how very uncomfortable I felt about telling on my friends, but at last, hanging my head in resignation, I confessed that Jane had goaded us all into it. I explained that I didn't want to get her into trouble, but that Jillian and I had just been swept along by her cunning. Mother Superior looked doubtful. Picturing Jane, gaunt-faced and stick-limbed, her big soulful eyes and her timorous voice, even I had to admit casting her as arch villain required a gymnastic stretch of the imagination.

'Nicola,' Mother Superior said, searching my face with those penetrating grey eyes of hers, 'you do know it's wrong to lie?'

'Of course, Reverend Mother,' I muttered earnestly, hastily dropping my gaze from hers. Mother Superior placed a finger under my chin and raised my face, until our eyes met once more.

'I cannot be sure what you got up to on these nightly escapades, Nicola, but I have a good idea,' she said, withdrawing her finger.

I sighed plaintively. 'Really Reverend Mother, it was just innocent fun until—'

Mother Superior interrupted me. 'Do you know just how serious this situation is, Nicola? Margery's pregnancy is a catastrophe for her. It might very well ruin her whole life.'

I shook my head mournfully. 'I know, Reverend Mother, I know.' I told her I sympathised, though I didn't add that I thought Margery was a bloody fool to get herself knocked up. Further, if I'd been her, I'd have popped off to get an abortion double-quick. But I'd been at the convent long enough to know Catholics were funny about these things. Trust that fat cow to land us in it, I reflected gloomily. Placing my hands together prayerfully, I added, in the tone of voice parents use to encourage a disheartened child, 'Still, a baby, the miracle of life. Sister McMullen says babies bring their very own unique joy into this world, each and every one of them!'

Mother Superior sighed with exasperation, and lowered her head, making it very hard for me to read the temperature of her reaction. Her next remark clarified things a bit though.

'I'm going to expel you and Jillian from St Mary's Convent,' she announced in clipped tones.

I thought about this for a moment, and then shrugged. My gesture appeared to shake Mother Superior's composure, though I was unsure why. She seemed almost to fall against the edge of her desk, and waved me away with . . . well I might be wrong, but I thought it was something like disgust. As soon as I could, I tracked down Jillian in her dormitory, and broke the news. She flayed the air with her hands and, gasping, took a few tiny steps backwards. I told her to sit down and catch her breath.

'We couldn't have hoped for a better outcome, Jilly,' I told her firmly.

She hugged herself and rocked forwards and back. She muttered about Mother and Father, what they would say.

'I can handle them.' My words sounded glib but I was sincere. I gave her a pat on the back. 'We're going to be fine.'

Jillian looked disbelieving as she wiped her runny nose. But I was beginning to feel that familiar rush of invincibility. The summer was upon us. I was sixteen, Jilly, eighteen. Not long ago we had sat O level and A level examinations, half asleep, hung-over, and without any revision. But even the disastrous results I was expecting did not deflate my buoyant mood.

So there it is. Education gained at St Mary's Convent, England, zilch, experience gleaned, Jesus, Mary and Joseph, a lifetime's worth! We are heading back to Hong Kong, the disgraced Safford daughters, and who knows what delights await us there. Life, I've decided, is a bit like a game of cards, it's all about how you play your hand. And if you have to cheat a bit to win . . . . Well, does it really matter?

Ghost—1970

Alice buys herself a diary. The diary is bound in leather the colour of dried blood. It has the words 'My Diary' tooled in gold on the cover. It has a metal clasp and a tiny key. Alice pays out her words on its stiff, creamy pages, like a miser parting with hidden treasure coin by coin. She hunches over it when she writes her secrets, as if she thinks someone is watching her, as if she thinks she can hide what she is doing from me, as if she has a story separate from mine.

Today she writes: 'I don't think I am alone. There is something, someone with me. I want to tell but who would believe me.'

She is a strange little creature, my host. I tell her I am here, of course. I am always here. I scarf myself about her neck and mutter, soft as the rustle of bamboo leaves in the wind, 'Don't worry Alice, you are not alone. We are cohabiting, you and I. Our tale is plaited tight, the strands of our lives forever interwoven.'

Alice frowns and slams shut her diary. Again she crooks a little finger, a sign I now know indicates her distress. Sometimes I find my host's behaviour a little bewildering. But there is no time to dwell on this, for we are spending today, a Sunday, on a friend's boat. It is the start of July. Conditions are ideal. The sky is the very palest of blues, marbled with milky translucent swirls. The sun, burning brightly, seems to swell as it rises in the sky. There is the barest puff of a breeze, that I know from experience will strengthen as we emerge from Aberdeen harbour. This, I understand, will be one of the last seaside outings for brother Harry for some time. In little over a month we are all to travel to Scotland, on the other side of the world, to install him in a boarding school there. On route we are collecting Alice's sisters from her grandmother's house. We are bringing them back with us to the island. So although the flat on The Peak is losing one resident, it is gaining two more.

The boat trip is to Lamma Island. I know it well. And as we set out, motoring past the walls of boulders, wind- and wave-breakers that protect

125

Aberdeen harbour from the excesses of the weather, my spirit lifts remembering *Heavenly Sea*. This is not a junk though, it is a grand sailing yacht, owned by a commercial bank, Mr Safford says. Our host, Phillip Stubbs, is one of their most senior employees. The yacht is named Seahorse. There are four couples out to enjoy the day—the Stubbs, the Saffords, the Birleys and the Gibsons. So often have I heard the names of the other guests on our car journey rolling down The Peak, that by the time I meet them in person, I feel we are old friends. Alice and Harry are the only children present, the rest are away at boarding school, the summer holidays having not yet begun. There are two Chinese boat boys and a Filipino maid on board as well, and a banquet of food and drink. At first, Harry is morose, sulking in the cabin, but gradually he too seems to absorb the atmosphere of this perfect day and creeps out on deck.

Alice thinks that her parents look like movie stars, draped over the streamlined white *Seahorse*. In the flat there is a book full of photographs of Hollywood actresses. They strike glamorous poses in brightly-coloured swimsuits. They clutch beachballs, hook arms through rubber rings and lounge on lilos. Alice's mother holds a drink. Sitting in the stern of the boat, a green and blue flowered headscarf tied at her neck, eyes mysteriously shaded with sunglasses, her mother looks like someone famous, Alice thinks, someone who signs autographs. She watches her mother deport herself like a model, whose picture might appear the next day in the *South China Morning Post*. While her father, Alice decides, is the image

126

of Sean Connery in one of the James Bond films. She remembers the ceremony earlier that year, in which her father was awarded the OBE, Officer of the British Empire, at a grand ceremony in Government House. She pictures him now in his brilliant white uniform, how handsome he looked, and how proud she felt to be his daughter.

Ralph moves around the boat drinking a beer with quietly spoken Phillip, whose hair seems both prematurely grey and thinning. He shares a joke with demonstrative Mike Gibson, his neatly trimmed dark beard, moustache and horn-rimmed spectacles giving the impression of intelligence. He discusses politics with wiry Jack Birley, whose shrewd eyes roam ceaselessly, and whose large nose is made still more prominent by its generous coating of white sun cream. He stretches out on the sundeck next to Christine, Mike's wife. The heavy make-up she has applied seems much more suitable for an evening engagement than a boat trip. Petite Pippa Birley, her hands forever patting, stroking and even squeezing her body, as if needing to reassure herself that it is still there, sips a glass of white wine and sidles up to Myrtle. She begins chatting animatedly about her sons, Jeremy and Luke, both attending the same boarding school in Oxford, and both, she explains to Myrtle, achieving outstanding results.

Though, of all the women on board, it is Amanda Stubbs who commands most attention, and yet who does the least to win it. Her shoulder-length gold hair is worn loose, the sun imbuing it with fascinating strands of light, from coppery red to an almost greenish citrus yellow. She is attentive to her guests, moving gracefully about the craft.

Her voice is disarmingly gentle and kind, so kind in fact, it is impossible to imagine a vindictive word falling from her full lips. However delightful, it is a very foreign concept to me, this idea of coming out on a boat and doing nothing. Distantly, I recall the work was never over on my father's junk. Yet here the Saffords and their friends lounge in the sun, while the boat boys run the *Seahorse*.

Amanda Stubbs spends most of the outward trip in the cabin organising the food. Occasionally she does put in an appearance, checking if anyone needs their drinks topped up, handing out nuts and crisps, and speaking with the boat boys. Alice is drawn by the dazzle of her sunlit hair. Unlike the other women she doesn't have on a hat, headscarf or sunglasses, just a wide magenta hair band. She wears very red lipstick, and a floaty, diaphanous, cream dress over a turquoise bikini. The dress keeps blowing up in the sea breeze, and once or twice she holds it down laughingly. Alice thinks she resembles Marilyn Monroe, in a film she once watched called *The Seven Year Itch*. Yet even when she laughs, Amanda Stubbs's watery-blue eyes seem glassy with sadness. Alice has produced her diary again. As we skip over the waves, she steals off to the very front of the boat with it.

'I like Amanda Stubbs but she has sad blue eyes. They look as if they have had all the fun rinsed out of them,' she writes, letting her feet trail in the sea

The cold sea spray and the frothy bubbles of the breaking bow wave bursting over Alice's bare feet, make her feel exhilarated. I am not sure if the curve of her left arm is designed to shield her diary from the sea, or from me.

'Harry seems very moody today. I do not think

he likes the idea of boarding- school. I am not sure that he will be happy there,' Alice continues, though with the roll of the boat her writing is a bit of a scrawl.

We buck over a large wave. As the *Seahorse* slaps back down, salty droplets freckle the page. The spindly letters bleed into one another and the words blur. For a second, Alice, whose face is also spattered with salty wet spots, thinks it looks as if tears have splashed onto her pages. She slams shut the diary and hugs it to her. Perhaps the thought has occurred to her that I could easily send it flying into the deep green depths, never to be seen again.

The sails are up now and flapping in the wind. The motor is stilled. The deck has stopped vibrating. Apart from the creak of the rigging and slap of the sails, it is surprisingly peaceful. The boat has slowed and the sea appears calmer. Alice scans the horizon, taking in the sparkling sea and the grey-green islands in the distance. She imagines them as the shoulder of a giant, or the belly of an enormous sea monster recumbent on the seabed, staring up through the watery depths at the strange airy world above. For a long while we sit like this. Then the wind drops and Alice is vaguely aware of the boat boys taking down the sails. In minutes we are under motor again, and the chug of the engine seems to rattle through Alice's head.

Rising cautiously, diary clutched under one arm, her other hand feeling its way along the deck rail, Alice moves to the stern of the vessel. Here her attention is caught by her father's antics. He scoops a handful of ice cubes out of the bucket that Amanda is carrying, and strokes her mother's bare thighs with them. Myrtle has pulled up her bottle-green cotton skirt to tan her legs in the sun. Now she gives a little scream as the ice slides along her warm inner thigh. She shoves her husband's hand away. The ice cubes fall to the deck and skitter about. Alice sees one of the boat boys hurrying to retrieve them. Her father grins at her and gives her a little wave. Then he sinks down next to Myrtle, and lays an arm casually about her shoulders. Myrtle pretends to ignore her husband, but Alice can see she is pleased. Amanda Stubbs, whose back is to Alice at that moment, turns to go down into the cabin. Alice locks eyes with her. Amanda turns the corners of her ruby lips up in a smile, but the smile does not reach those sad eyes.

We anchor in a bay off Lamma Island. Alice stows her diary away safely in her beach bag in the cabin. Soon lunch is served on deck by the Filipino maid and the boat boys. Today even Alice wants to eat. The sea air has given her an appetite. She manages a chicken drumstick and some salad, as well as a small bowl of ice cream. After lunch all the adults seem sleepy. No one is very keen when Alice's father suggests a swim to the beach and a walk. Eventually, Amanda pinches her hips with mock dismay and says she could do with the exercise. The two of them dive off the roof of the boat, their bodies darting into the green depths, shining and opalescent beneath the translucent lid of the sea. Myrtle does not like swimming. Alice cannot remember the last time her mother went swimming. Myrtle claims it makes her ears hurt, and that the doctor has said she must not get them wet.

As Alice watches, her father and Amanda strike out for the shore. Their arms plough rhythmically into the water, their legs just breaking the surface as they kick, a spool of white lace unravelling behind them. Alice feels a strange current of apprehension tingling along her spine. She shades her eyes and tracks their progress. She sees them shrink, until they look as tiny as the porcelain figures in her father's lacquer cabinet at home. At last they clamber out of the water. They look so far away now, Alice is unaccountably frightened she may lose them. With her forehead crinkled in a frown, she follows them walking up the beach. Amanda turns back and waves, as if she has suddenly remembered they have an audience. Alice returns the wave, though she is not sure Amanda notices. Then the two of them, her father and Mrs Stubbs, take a path that vanishes in the undergrowth.

Replete after lunch and dozy with drink, Myrtle Safford reclines on cushions in the stern, under the shade of the canopy. Phillip Stubbs sits reading the paper, and smoking contentedly a few feet from her. Mike Gibson and Jack Birley, in deckchairs set up on the foredeck, are engrossed in talk of business. Their wives sprawl on mats, laid out on the roof of the cabin. Christine Gibson appears absorbed in a book, little of her tanned face visible between the broad rim of her straw sunhat, and the rectangular screen of her open book. Pippa Birley's chestnut curls are caught up in a ponytail. She busies herself applying suncream with grim determination, and shifting her position with such alarming frequency, that she makes the curious occupation of sunbathing look exhausting. Harry

131

has chosen to stay in the cabin, claiming that the sun is too hot for him, though Alice is certain he is preoccupied with thoughts of his imminent departure from the island.

We join him for a short while, and Alice tries to persuade him to come for a swim. But Harry wants shade and solitude. So Alice alone changes into her bathing costume, and shrugs on a baggy T-shirt. We find our way back to the bow. Alice nods briefly to the men deep in their chat of sure-fire investments, and then we climb gingerly down the rungs of the swimming ladder. Despite the scorching heat of the sun, or perhaps because of it, when Alice dips a toe in the sea it feels icy cold. She cannot face diving in as she saw her father and Mrs Stubbs do. For a time she clings to the ladder descending very gradually into the water. When Alice is submerged up to her waist, we jump, her cream T-shirt ballooning around us. The cold water closes over us. Then, to my relief, we stop sinking and rise back up. Alice's head bursts from the depths, a sheaf of silver water slipping from it. Her limbs flay. She swims a few strokes back to the ladder, and hangs there, half submerged.

For a while Alice listens to the slap of the water against the hull. She watches the anchor rope, the pale length of it seeming to waver as it descends, until it is erased in the green depths. She looks at the shoreline and decides that it is not too far, that she would be able to swim there if she wanted to. She calls up to Christine Gibson and tells her where she is going. Mrs Gibson leans over the edge of the roof. She lowers her sunglasses and peers at Alice bobbing below in the sea, as if she is trying to remember who she is. To Alice, Christine

132

Gibson's face, hidden in the shadow of the large sunhat, is virtually invisible, a black disc against the white glare of the sun.

'Alright darling,' she says vaguely. 'Do take care, won't you?'

Alice nods. She is about to ask Mrs Gibson to tell her mother where she is when the disc, looming over her from above, rolls away and disappears. Alice hesitates for a moment and then we set off. The harder she swims, the further away the shore seems to be. Once she turns back to the boat, but no one is scanning the ocean, monitoring her progress. She imagines jellyfish, creamy yellow, and the living bruise of the Portuguese Man of War, gulping mouths rushing towards her, trailing their deadly stinging manes. Her heart races and hers arms lash at the sluggish sea. At last she can make out the blurred, trembling shapes of rocks beneath her. She can see her pallid legs bicycling furiously. She reaches out with them, trying to plant her feet on the slimy barnacled rock rearing up under her. But now she sees it is an illusion, that the rock is much deeper than she first estimated. She has to swim several yards more before she is able to stand. As she does so, rubbery, golden-brown, seaweed fans brush her toes, and the soles of her feet. She finds herself anticipating sea urchins, black and spiky, concealed beneath the slimy curtains of weed. In the end she draws her knees up, and determines not to put her feet down until she sees the glint of yellow sand.

At last we stride from the sea and rid ourselves of its guile. As Alice sloughs off her wet skin, so her fright evaporates. The sand is gritty beneath her feet, and so hot that she has to hop and run to the path. And like her father and Amanda Stubbs, as we step onto it we are camouflaged by dusky foliage. Walking along the narrow trail as it winds up the small hill, we catch glimpses of the sea, its glittering belly heaving gently in leaf-fringed frames. Twice there is the flash of the boat, so white it makes Alice's eyes water. Higher and higher we climb, heading inland away from the beach, till eventually the small bay is lost to us.

We come to a temple, tiny, built of wood, with a steeply sloping roof, ornamented with strange wooden carvings at its apex and four corners. The small reddish-brown door, its paintwork splitting to reveal slashes of rough wood, is propped open. Ducking and stepping through it, Alice's nostrils are assailed with the scent of incense, heavy and acrid. The dusty air within is wreathed with smoky curlicues. It takes some time for Alice's eyes to adjust to the dimness, after the brilliance outside. She blinks back the wave of dizziness that washes over her. At last her pupils dilate sufficiently for the indistinct shapes to resolve themselves. At the far end is an altar, graced with a tall wooden statue, ferocious, unyielding, robed in forbidding red and gold, purple and black. There are offerings laid on the altar at the foot of the uncompromising god, oranges and lychees, a blue rice-pattern china bowl filled with sweets, each of them wrapped in shiny paper, and a wad of fake paper money. Tucked away to the right of the altar, is a huge wooden barrel. Treading softly as a cat, careful not to disturb the fierce god, Alice approaches it. Glimpsing over the rim she sees the glint of water. Alice dips a finger in, withdraws it

134

and sucks it. Salt. Seawater. At her movement, the silver face shivers into tiny ripples, and the walnut shell boat she spies in it bobs gently.

'Here is the sea, and here is the boat that sails on the sea,' Alice says softly. Her voice echoes in the still of the temple. 'In that boat is a fisherman, facing the angry winds and the boiling seas. And when he is away, through the empty black nights, his family come here and pray for his safe return.'

Then we step out of the temple and Alice readjusts to the unremitting fever of the sun. On a whim she decides to continue upwards. As we ascend, the path becomes more treacherous. Alice finds herself stumbling over rocks. Once she stubs a toe, and the subsequent stab of pain almost makes her cry out. The soles of her feet are scratched and sore by the time we crest the summit. The seawater has dried on her skin, and left a powdery residue of salt. It feels stretched, taut as the skin of a tambourine. Her eyes are smarting too, irritated by the sea, the smoky incense, and the blast of light beating down on her, and reflecting back up off the metallic greys of the rocks. Directly in front of her, Alice sees a large granite outcrop, flattened on the top and partly shaded by a giant fir tree.

'Standing atop this boulder I shall see everything,' Alice conjectures. 'If I rotate I shall see all around the coastline of my little island. I shall see the *Seahorse* tugging against its anchor rope. I shall see the roof of the temple that houses the angry god. I will be able to follow the shifting shoreline.'

We clamber up, Alice on tiptoe, arms outspread for balance on the flinty hot surface, and see none

135

of these things. What we see instead is Amanda
Stubbs straddling Alice's father in a clearing below
us. They are both naked. We can see the white
imprint of Amanda Stubbs's bikini standing out in
sharp relief against her tanned flesh. The deep
coral-pink of her nipples jewels the pale breasts.
There is a golden haze between her legs. She is
riding Ralph Safford as if he is a horse, thrusting
her hips rhythmically forwards and back. And she
is facing us, her spine arched, her head thrown
backwards, her face raised to the blazing sky. Her
hands are lost, entwined in her glistening golden
hair. Her mouth is open, her eyes closed. Of her
father, Alice can see only the top of his head,
crowned with his crisp, black hair, and the expanse
of his broad chest. He is ramming his groin
upwards into Mrs Stubbs, his hands on her hips,
grasping them firmly, the muscles in his arms
standing out as she bucks against him. Alice recalls
how many times those strong arms have encircled
her. My host no longer wobbles on tiptoes. The
soles of her feet lie flat against the hot rock, and
she is oblivious to the searing pain.

Then Mrs Stubbs cries out, her head levelling.
She opens her eyes, her watery blue eyes that have
had all the fun rinsed out of them, and those sad
eyes meet Alice's. They hold each other. Hearts
hammer, threads of glittering sweat course down
the flushed softness of hidden flesh. The instant
shatters. Alice swings away, slipping down the side
of the rock. I streak after her. She stumbles over
the scree, immune now to the slashes and jabs of
pain. She falls and grazes her knee. But she
ignores the trickle of blood, and the grit that clings
to the sticky wound. A branch whips across her

face, and a twig lashes her eyelid. She winces. Her vision blurs. She rushes on, scarcely aware she is passing the temple. Finally, breaking from the sheltered pathway, we sprint towards the sea.

She craves its icy purity with her whole being. She is not conscious of the broken fragment of shell that has embedded itself in the heel of her foot. As she runs the shard is driven further in. The sand smudges with her blood. She flings herself into the water, opening her eyes to its coldness and salt smack with dreadful eagerness. Only now does she grow aware of her throbbing foot. For a moment she sculls the water, preparing herself. Then she holds her breath, bends beneath the surface, and takes hold of it. She feels for the ridge of shell protruding from the pad of her heel, grips it and yanks it out. Opening her eyes underwater, in the ring of her salt-excoriated, furred vision, she can make out the red tail of blood spiralling outwards. She pushes back the weight of water and bursts through the sea's skin. Blinking back hot tears, she screws her eyes up in disbelief. A white shape lunges out at her. It is the *Seahorse*, suspended over the vast dark green sea. We plunge forwards. Alice settles into her stroke, breaststroke, her legs and arms frantically describing circles. She tries not to harbour thoughts of grey shadows beneath her, her curl of sweet blood baiting them, drawing the monsters of the deep ever closer.

We are both thankful to tread on the solid deck of the *Seahorse*. The men in their deckchairs grunt a perfunctory greeting. We hurry past. Myrtle stirs, disturbed by the slap and vibration of Alice's wet feet. She glances up.

137

'Whatever have you done, Alice?' she remarks, spotting the blood oozing from the wound in her daughter's foot, as Alice hops into the stern. Phillip Stubbs leaps up looking concerned. 'You're leaving a trail of blood,' Myrtle Safford says with a sigh worn out by repetition. 'It may stain the deck.'

Phillip Stubbs is quick to assure her that this is of no consequence, and sees to it that the cut is washed and bandaged. As soon as his wife and Ralph Safford arrive back, he gives the order to weigh anchor and set sail. Alice is restive on the homeward journey, the confines of the boat claustrophobic. Her father notices the bandage, and probes the circumstances that have warranted it. Alice says that she swam to the beach and stepped on a broken shell. Her manner is offhand. She keeps her eyes lowered.

'We didn't see you there,' Ralph Safford remarks, his voice pitched with extreme care on a note that is both friendly and disappointed.

'No. I cut my foot the moment I stepped ashore,' Alice explains to her father. Her eyes move fleetingly over Amanda Stubbs, emerging from the cabin, dressed now in slacks and a blouse, rubbing her blonde hair vigorously with a towel. 'So I came straight back,' she finishes flatly.

Ralph Safford's blue eyes lighten a shade. 'What bad luck,' he says. And then, 'What a pity. We might have met up.'

'Mm,' agrees Alice absently. 'But it really hurt to walk on, so I didn't feel much like exploring after that.'

Her father nods his understanding of Alice's impossible predicament, and there is an almost perceptible relaxing of his broad-muscled shoulders. Once, perhaps twice, Amanda Stubbs seeks out my host with her sad eyes, but Alice has retreated to somewhere she cannot be reached. When we arrive home at the flat on The Peak, my host does not even bother to watch the sun set. She forgot to apply suncream, and now her face, forearms and legs are burnt, dark pink and tender to the touch. Even the cotton sheets seem to rub her raw when she lies back on them. Late that night she crawls from her bed and finds her diary. The curtains are tied back and moonlight is flooding in. Alice makes do without switching on the light. She sits at her desk, opens her diary, and takes up her pen.

'Today I saw my father and Amanda Stubbs fucking on Lamma Island,' Alice writes.

And then, before I have the chance to shuffle its cream leaves and make my host's diary dance for her pleasure, she hurls it across the room. It flies through the air, its pages flapping like the wings of one of the white cockatoos that gather in flocks about the island. The clasp catches the moonlight. It flashes like the parrots' sulphur crests. I am half expecting it to squawk when it hits the door of one of the built-in wardrobes, and with a final flourish of feathers tumbles to the floor. It is obvious after that, that any tricks I was thinking of performing for Alice's delight would be an anticlimax.

Harry—1970

The cabin on the Stubbs's boat was an oven that day. It was like being cooked alive, sitting down there, dripping with sweat in that baggy T-shirt, feeling it pool where my thighs pressed together, between my buttocks, huge smelly patches of it below my armpits, and my skin slippery with it under my fat-boy breasts. The Filipino servant, fussing with bits and pieces, gave me a huge slice of sticky cake, and then stood over me while I ate it. I knew she wanted to pinch my arm, to squeeze the chubby flesh between her slim fingers till I cried out. But she didn't have the bottle. I suppose she wouldn't have said '*Fei zhai*'. She'd have said something else, in her language probably. I heard Alice get back, saw the bottom of her legs through the cabin windows and her clambering into the stern, heard Mum scream at her 'cos she was bleeding onto the deck or something. Alice's legs looked burnt. Must have forgotten to put suncream on. The Filipino hurried away then, returning seconds later to fetch a medical box. And still I sat, baking in the cabin, wondering how long it would be before I was done to a turn.

I shut my eyes sometimes and try to recapture the feeling of that intense heat, the sweat, the awful stillness of the sea, flat as a mirror, but with all those things wriggling underneath it. In Scotland there are lochs and some of them are huge, stretch for mile after mile. But it's not the same. Not like the sea. It's okay though, because I pretend it's happening to someone else, all of it. I just watch, sit back and . . . well, sit back. Picking up Jillian and Nicola was the best part though. Mum and Dad and Gran in the back room, and me listening at the door, and Uncle Albert on the stairs waving his arms about, and taking a bow every so often. There were long silences and then raised voices, Gran's croaky one mostly.

'You have no idea . . . the goings on . . . the Reverend Mother was shocked . . . got herself pregnant . . . defiled herself . . . filthy . . . could easily have been . . . don't know what you expect . . . over there living it up.'

Dad made small sympathetic grunts. Mother's tone was haughty, and once or twice she even laughed, like a dry cough. With a wink of his eye, sinking down at the bottom of the stairs, Uncle Albert suddenly burst into song. 'How Are Things in Glocca Morra?' from *Finian's Rainbow*. I recognised it. I had seen the film the previous year. When I came out of the kitchen, with supplies of chocolate digestives and a milk moustache, he was still going strong. I licked my moustache, crammed two biscuits in my mouth, leant back by the bulldog umbrella stand, and waited for the song to finish.

'Why a boarding school in Scotland . . . you could have left . . . I'd have looked after . . . the boy needs . . .' Gran again.

'It's all settled.' That was Mother.

'All settled,' I echoed miserably through a mouthful of crumbs. Uncle Albert rose slowly to his feet and his voice rose with him. He was building to a crescendo, arms outstretched. I swear there were tears in his eyes. As the last note faded away he searched my face, desperately needing an answer to the lyric he'd been singing.

'Well,' I said, as truthfully as I could, quickly swallowing down the last of my biscuit and nearly choking on it, 'I'm not at all sure about Glocca Morra, Uncle Albert, but things are pretty crap here.'

Uncle Albert nodded as though he understood. I clapped a couple of times to show I appreciated his performance. He glowed a delighted pink at that. Then I ducked under his arms and headed upstairs where the girls were holding a conference, well Jillian and Nicola were anyway. Alice was standing outside Gran's bedroom door, so Jillian must have lost it with her already. A bit later we all piled into the car and drove up North. We broke the journey in a B&B near Carlisle, and by then my stomach was churning. I reckoned it was how a condemned man feels the night before the execution.

'Eurrh, you're not going to have seconds?' Nicola was disgusted. She hadn't eaten any of her breakfast and neither had Alice. We could all hear the lady hawking and sneezing in the kitchen. I must say it was pretty revolting. But I still felt hungry. I could have eaten at least six eggs, twelve rashers of bacon and half a loaf, easy. Mother and Father went to settle up, Jillian and Nicola to get the bags, and then it was just Alice and me.

'Are you alright, Harry?' she asked, not in a soppy way, just straightforward.

I sighed and cleaned my plate with a thick slice of white bread. 'I guess.'

'It might work out better than you think,' Alice tried.

I shrugged, sniffed noisily, and drained my cup

of milk, then wiped my mouth with the back of a hand.

'Oh Harry, I'm sorry. I am so sorry and I can't ... can't—'

I broke in there, and it ended up with me trying to make her feel better. The rest of the journey continued in silence, interrupted occasionally with the radio, or Jillian having a go at Alice, or Mother and Father mumbling to each other all secretively. By the time we arrived at the school-outfitters it was pouring down with rain, and the sky was almost black. The woman in there, well, she was really thin and mean, and she kept tutting as she measured me, and saying that they didn't have such large sizes in stock.

'And the blazer too could be a wee problem. It's no good getting one that's a wee bitty tight. He'll only get bigger.'

She was on her knees with the tape measure in hand when she said this. Mother, she kept talking fast, like when you put a 33 record on at 45, and her face had this fixed smile on it, fixed the way doll has. Father just looked uncomfortable. He started cracking jokes of all things. I tried to laugh, just to please him really, but honestly they weren't very funny. Alice kept fingering the tartan blankets, looking like she wanted to burrow down in one until she was invisible, while Jillian and Nicola were outside, heads together, probably trying to devise a plan. Once I'd gone, they knew they'd have to explain why they were being chucked out of the convent.

St David's Academy outside Stirling, that was where they all left me a few days later, journeying back down South. I rang and spoke to Mother just before they flew back to Hong Kong.

'Mother, please, please don't leave me here. Please Mother,' I whispered into the communal pay phone. When I made the call there had just been me standing in the corridor, but now there was a queue. I cupped the mouthpiece trying to muffle my voice, so that the other boys wouldn't hear. I had brought lots of change with me but as it happened I didn't need it.

'Harry, darling, you're being so silly. You're bound to feel a touch homesick at first, but trust me, you'll soon settle in and start to love it.'

My silent voice spoke in my head then. It was screaming, screaming louder than Alice ever had. 'I hate it! I hate it! I hate it!'

'Mother, I'm . . . I'm begging you,' I mumbled, and it was like someone was inside winding me up tight.

The carrot-top behind me dropped to his knees, hands clasped, mimicking me. 'Mother, I'm begging you, begging you!' As he scrambled up they were all smirking and hooting with laughter.

'Now darling, I simply must dash. I promise to write to you lots and lots. And before you know it, you'll be home for the Christmas holidays.'

There was a long pause then. I didn't say anything.

'Och come on fatty. You've been ages,' carrot-top complained, giving me a shove.

'I've got to go now, Mother,' I said. I was drowning in the tears I could never shed.

Back she came, a famous actress delivering the last line in a play. 'Goodbye my darling, my little man. You know how much we love you. Now make us both proud.' Then the click as the receiver was replaced. Carrot-top didn't even wait for me to hang up, just pushed me out of the way. 'Piss off English piggy,' he sneered, giving me another dig with his elbow.

'Yeah, piss off bog breath,' joined in the tall boy behind him. 'Piss off back to your Mammy.'

Just as I shuffled off, the bell rang. Teatime. I started down the corridor. I could feel my buttock cheeks rubbing, because, in spite of everything, the seat of my trousers was rather tight, pushing them together. One of the masters stopped me and told me off, so I must have been running. I slowed down after that. I could feel the saliva rushing into my mouth and that hollowness in my tummy, and already I was imagining the texture of the food in my mouth, imagining it filling me up until I was rock hard. The boys' sniggers followed me down the stairs but I didn't care. I could smell the food now.

Ghost—1970

It is the day of the party, the party Alice's parents hold each year on Boxing Day. Everyone seems preoccupied. Alice barely gives me a moment's thought. She is thinking about her father, that she will be able to spend time with him now he has a few days off. Over the past year he seems to have been absent even more than usual and Alice misses him. Because of this, she neglects me and I am hurt. That's why I upset the milk at breakfast. As Alice reaches for it, I tip over the large green and white striped china jug. It is very nearly satisfyingly full. The milk sloshes out soaking the tablecloth. Alice gives a gasp and snatches her hand away.

'Ah, so now I have your attention, Alice,' I tell her sweetly.

She pushes back her hair and rises, one of her hands covering an ear. She rubs it forcefully, as if she might like to pull it off. Alice's mother, too busy for breakfast she says, is a witness to my sleight of hand. All in purple, a shade so dark that when she moves into the shadows it appears almost black, Myrtle, on route to the kitchen, halts in her tracks.

'Alice, what have you done, you clumsy girl?' she cries, her voice so strident that I feel Alice's heart give a small jump, and her pulse quicken. She whirls about. Simultaneously, Jillian sitting on the opposite side of the table springs up with a horrified wail, as her lap gets a good drenching.

'I didn't do it,' Alice is quick to protest.

'Of course you didn't,' I tell her gaily. 'I did it. I've been so bored, Alice.'

'God, look at my skirt!' screams Jillian, her outstretched hands gripping the bunched, black-brocade hem of her skirt. 'This is new. Especially for the party. Now it's ruined!'

'Can't it be . . . be wa . . . ashed and . . . w . . . well dried in time,' Alice stutters anxiously. Her little fingers are tightly curled, that nervous habit of hers.

'No,' Jillian bites back, glowering at her sister. 'This very expensive skirt has to be dry-cleaned!' Her voice snags on the last word and is muffled as she clenches her teeth.

146

Nicola pokes her head round the dining-room door.

'I'm off. Taxi's here.' Her voice is upbeat. She scans the scene swiftly.

'Alice has soaked my dress in milk,' Jillian snarls.

Alice drops to her knees. She starts dabbing with a napkin ineffectually at the milk puddle appearing on the floor. She stares in dismay as the puddle widens, fed by a steady drip-drip from the sodden cloth above.

'Oh dear,' says Nicola glancing at her watch. 'I wish I could stay and help but I'm seeing Tom.' She turns to go, calling back to Jillian over her shoulder, 'You can borrow something of mine if you want, Jilly.'

A steady, if light dribble of milk, is also trickling into Alice's loose hair as she scuttles about, crab-like, on the floor. Alice's mother, surveying the scene, very nearly snorts with exasperation. The kitchen door opens a fraction and Ah Lee's head appears. It looks disembodied. Her white teeth show as she giggles nervously, taking in the upturned milk jug, and Alice diving at the milk puddles as they materialise.

'Missy Alice want me to—' But Ah Lee never finishes her sentence.

There is a loud bang, a very loud bang. It is so loud that this time everyone seems to jump. It emanates from the kitchen. Inside Alice, I flinch, remembering the sound of gunshots and what they importuned during the occupation. Ah Lee's head vanishes and we all follow it into the kitchen. Once inside Myrtle Safford makes straight for the small chest freezer. The lid is open, propped against the wall, trails of frosty vapour billowing out of it. She pauses for a heartbeat before she peers over the brim, her hands scooping at the thick, white mist that is bubbling out of it. I think she looks ghostly, standing there, bending over the chest, a few icy crystals clinging to the strands of her hair that have worked their way loose from her bun. She narrows her eyes until they are nearly sealed shut, and peers through the lashes. The contents of the freezer, at first lost in the smoky waterfall, slowly reveal themselves. Myrtle gives an anguished yelp, both hands closing over her mouth, and staggers back. Surely at the very least she has seen a mutilated body, the blood congealed, the flesh grey as dirty clay and hard as ice.

'What . . . is it?' asks Jillian cautiously, clutching her sodden skirt and inching forwards to take a peek.

Mrs Safford lets her hands fall away from her face.

'My magnum of champagne has exploded,' she says at last, her voice chiming out in plangent tones. 'It's . . . all . . . gone. All of it. Every drop.'

She rotates slowly, rooted to the spot, misty trails pooling now at her feet, like a stream of dried ice pouring onto a stage. Majestic. Livid. A frost queen.

'Alice.' She speaks the name slowly, to herself it seems. Repeats it as if she is impelled to let the dreadful resonance of it sound again in her mouth. 'Alice.'

Alice pushes her way past Jillian, leans forwards and looks into the open freezer, catching sight of a few clumps of frozen, golden champagne. She scrutinises the thousand slithers of green glass

148

lodged in the icy crust that coats the freezer sides. 'They are like uncut emeralds,' she thinks, 'just lying in the snow.' She opens her mouth to deny all knowledge of placing the champagne in the freezer. Ah Lee giggles. Bear, lying across the back door that leads to the servants' quarters, yawns, stretches, stiffens and then relaxes. Ralph Safford bursts into the kitchen.

'What on earth is going on?' he demands.

Then all is bedlam, with Alice whining piteously that it isn't her fault, and Jillian screaming about her dress and the spilt milk and how it is ruined, and Myrtle, her face now disturbingly pale for one so angry, thundering that Alice has put the champagne in the freezer deliberately. Ah Lee accompanies this racket with bouts of unbridled mirth, her arms gesticulating wildly as she attempts to explain that she did it, she placed the champagne in the freezer, to keep it cool Mrs Safford she says. No one pays her any heed. Shortly after this Alice flees to her room and throws herself on her bed, her face buried in her pillow.

I listen to the sound of her frenetic breathing for a bit, waiting for her racing heart to steady itself. It is a couple of hours before we emerge. Alice climbs to her feet in slow stages, crosses to her dressing table, and fruitlessly attempts to draw a brush through her hair, but the milk has made it stick together. It is while she is thus occupied that Alice becomes aware of the front doorbell sounding several times. Eventually we slip out of her room to find the party happening without us. Alice nods to a few people she sees scattered throughout the corridor, glasses and platters of

149

food balanced in their hands, chatting spiritedly.

'Alice, dearest.' says one elegant Chinese lady in a silver-grey Cheongsam, with a carved, white-jade pendant on a heavy golden chain at her neck and a thick gold bangle encircling her delicate wrist. 'I was looking for you. I brought you a gift. I put it under the tree.'

Alice mutters her thanks and shoulders her way on down the corridor, through the steadily thickening pockets of guests. A few people embrace her, and one man, tall, with spiky dark hair, stops puffing on his cigar to peck her on the cheek.

'Alice, darling, I'm trying to persuade your father to bring you all to spend a couple of days with us in Macau. He keeps saying that he's too busy. We're all too busy, damn it. We have to make time for ourselves. Perhaps he'll listen to you.'

Alice nods, gives a quick smile and slides on by. We slip into the dining room. The room is transformed. Gone are the breakfast things, all traces of the split milk vanished. The table is laid with a fresh cloth, and piled high with joints of partially sliced ham, turkey and beef, wedges of cheese and bowls filled with golden curls of butter sitting on beds of ice-cubes to keep cool. There are plates of biscuits and bread rolls, towers of fruit and several cakes. Ah Dang and Ah Lee dart to and fro to the kitchen replenishing supplies, scurrying around topping up drinks. We spot Harry filling a paper plate with crisps and wander up to him.

'Did you see what happened to Mother's magnum of champagne?' Alice asks, tugging at a knot of hair that the sticky milk has cemented together.

Harry grunts that he did. 'I think one of the amahs put it there, so you're off the hook,' he offers, uninterested. He shoves a handful of crisps into his mouth and drifts off.

Looking at the heaving table Alice feels a wave of nausea come over her, so we find our way onto the veranda for a breath of air. The jumble of conversation outside rolls over us in waves, reaching a deafening pitch. Then it seems to subside briefly, before once more gathering volume and fresh momentum. Spread hands slice the air, and fingers bend and uncurl, or swoop on some tasty titbit proffered by the giggling Ah Lee, or the solemn-faced Ah Dang, or they are jabbed emphatically, punctuating the speaker's intense dialogue. Spirals of cigarette smoke are ambushed by the breeze and stretched to translucence. Here too glass lenses catch the light as faces are raised, while mouths open and shut, and chew and pout and shake with laughter. The day is bright, and the sun, though thin, combined with the heat of so many bodies, generates a tolerable degree of warmth. Alice leans back against the veranda railing, taking in Jillian sitting on a rattan chair, smoking a cigarette and sipping a glass of wine. Her flint eyes have a brittle starriness about them, her eyelashes glued with blue mascara. She is wearing a dress of Nicola's, the scalloped neckline showing off her cleavage. And she is surrounded by friends all talking excitedly over each other. Myrtle Safford is clearly in her element, sweeping onto the veranda, clasping a glass of red wine. She moves through her guests, falling in and out of conversation with consummate ease. One moment

151

she is gratifyingly amused at a joke she is told, the next, she is listening avidly to the retelling of some drama, her expression changing in perfect time with the altering mood of the speaker. Through the open glass doors that give onto the lounge, Alice sees her father mingling among his guests, always someone at his elbow vying for his attention. As the day wears on, the guests arriving dwindle in numbers, and one or two even prepare to leave.

Alice pushes her body off the veranda railing and strolls inside. Crossing the hall, she veers off her path answering the front door reflexively when she hears it. Phillip and Amanda Stubbs and their two children stand outside. Inside Alice the shock of recognition is palpable. Adrenalin surges around her body, her heart hammering, her mouth bone-dry, blood pounding in her ears. She reprimands herself silently for not expecting this meeting. The Stubbs, she knows, were invited to last year's party. She stands stiff as a scrubbing board and says nothing, while nestled within her, just like the freezing champagne, I am ready to burst.

'Hello Alice,' says Amanda Stubbs in her low, kind voice. 'Merry Christmas.' Her husband grins amiably. Mrs Stubbs gives her children a little push forwards. 'We've brought Oliver and Jemima. Home for the holidays,' she says. Glancing at them, Alice can see that they take after their mother. Both are blue-eyed and golden-haired. The boy looks decidedly uncomfortable, hands thrust deep in his anorak pockets, shifting his slight weight from foot to foot. The girl has a dreamy set to her features, hiding behind her long fair hair. Still Alice's mouth remains clamped shut.

'We're not gate-crashing, Alice. We were invited. Promise,' Phillip Stubbs ventures, his eyes twinkling mischievously. He gives Alice a wink.

At this prompting she seems to remember herself and steps aside.

'Oh yes, sorry. Merry Christmas. Come in,' she says quietly.

As the family file in, Alice and Mrs Stubbs exchange a fleeting look.

'I . . . I . . . Mrs Stubbs I—' Alice stalls.

'Yes, Alice?' Mrs Stubbs asks, turning back.

'Your coats. I'll take your coats,' Alice mumbles. 'They'll be in my . . . my parents' bedroom.'

The Stubbs family shrug off their coats and hand them to Alice.

'What service, Amanda. Isn't she splendid?' Mr Stubbs says ingenuously. 'Oliver, Jemima, I hope you're watching this. Thank you very much, Alice.' He waves at a few friendly faces he has spotted across the hall.

'Yes, thank you, Alice,' Mrs Stubbs says softly. Jemima is hanging back, fingers resting lightly on the back of her mother's arm. Amanda Stubbs turns to plant a swift kiss on the top of her daughter's head. Oliver moves to his sister's side protectively.

Alice clears her throat. 'There's food in there and . . . and drink.' She nods in the direction of the dining room. 'Mother's on the veranda and . . . and Father's through there, in the lounge.' Phillip nods. Just before he steers Amanda through the open lounge door, he hesitates.

'If we have a really fine day, how would you like to come out on the *Seahorse* again, Alice? We had

153

such a marvellous day last time. Do you remember?' When Alice does not reply immediately he adds a little uncertainly, 'You enjoyed it, didn't you, Alice?'

Alice pauses. 'Mm . . . well, yes.'

'Excellent. What say we make it just the Saffords and the Stubbs this time, and you can choose where we go, eh. How about that? What do you say, Amanda? The children would love it.'

'Sounds great, darling.' Mrs Stubbs's sad eyes are hooded. 'But you know Christmas is such a busy time. Alice is probably booked up.'

'Nonsense,' retorts Mr Stubbs cheerfully, already steering his wife through the lounge door with his hand pressed into the small of her back. 'I'll speak to your father, Alice.'

'Oh . . . thanks.' For a moment Alice stands still, then she starts to shoulder her way down the corridor with her armful of coats. She heaps them on her parent's bed with the many others already piled there.

Afterwards she goes to fetch herself a glass of water, and we walk in unwittingly upon her father and Amanda Stubbs in the kitchen. This time neither of them notice her. At first my host thinks they are looking for something in the kitchen cupboards, and then she realises they have found it. Alice's father and Amanda Stubbs are huddled between two open cupboard doors, and the only thing they are searching are each other's faces. Swiftly Alice turns on her heels and retreats to her bedroom. She sits on her bed in a patch of late afternoon sunlight. She stares at the pattern of wood grain on the parquet floor, sees the eye of a lion and the hooked beak of a huge predatory

154

hawk hidden in the swirls. After a while there is a knock on the door. Alice looks up. Before she can invite the visitor in, the door opens and closes, and Amanda Stubbs is standing in Alice's bedroom.

'I was searching for the bathroom,' Amanda Stubbs says.

Alice snatches a hurried look at the immaculately dressed Mrs Stubbs, before casting her eyes down at the floor again. The image of Mrs Stubbs in a buttercup yellow suit, a pencil skirt and matching jacket, her pale gold shoulder-length hair held back with a fawn velvet band, her lipstick freshly applied and very pink, burns on her retina.

'It's at the end of the corridor. Outside my bedroom door and just to the left,' Alice says briefly. She averts her gaze, fearing she might lose herself forever in those melancholy eyes.

But Amanda Stubbs makes no move to find the bathroom. Instead she comes and perches on the side of Alice's bed. They sit in silence for a bit. When Alice looks up she meets Amanda's eyes with hostility. Bear, who has sought refuge in Alice's bedroom from the hordes of people that the flat is currently teeming with, chooses this moment to crawl out from under the bed. He collapses at Amanda's feet with a sigh of fatigue so complete that it speaks for all of us.

'I'm not ever going to tell my mother, you know.' Alice is intransigent. In the distance the faint sounds of the party can be heard. Bing Crosby is crooning about a white Christmas, an unlikely event on the small island of Hong Kong, I muse, no matter how hard you dream about it. The chink of glasses and cutlery, peppered with sudden shouts of laughter or loud exclamations, drift down the corridor. This muted jangle makes the small quiet that now stretches out between Amanda Stubbs and Alice more marked. Alice casts about her bedroom for some distraction. She looks at the poster of the Beatles pop group, and at the small low table to the right of her bed crowded with dream pets, small stuffed animals all the colours of the rainbow.

'Mrs Stubbs, I know you want me to . . . you want me to tell my mother,' Alice says haltingly. Her diction is very precise, the consonants sounding with frightening crispness. 'But I shan't tell, not ever. If you need her to know, if . . . if you need my mother to know that you and my father are . . . you and my father . . . are . . . are fucking, then you must tell her yourself.'

Mrs Stubbs makes a sound, a smothered cry that dies in her throat. Her hands clasp over the nape of her neck seeming to drag her head down, her golden hair sweeping forwards, obscuring her face.

'You can't have him, Mrs Stubbs. You can't have my father,' Alice says. 'Well, I'm not going to give him to you anyhow. If you want him you have to take him.'

Mrs Stubbs's hair glistens in the white winter sunshine. The scent of her is carried on the air. It is a clean, fresh smell. Bear whines in his sleep and paddles his paws against the floor, a bad dream.

'Oh Alice—' Mrs Stubbs starts, breaking off suddenly, her hands falling away, her head coming up fractionally, her wistful, blue eyes seeking out Alice's. There is a pause. The metal arm of one of Alice's bedroom windows, propped open a few inches, rattles softly. The draft lifts a few strands

156

of Mrs Stubbs's golden hair. Then she speaks again. 'Help me. Please. Help me.' It is a monotone, lifeless.

Alice stares into her eyes. She sees they are no longer sad. Now they hold a chilling vacancy. Mrs Stubbs reaches a hand out to Alice, but when she touches her lover's daughter lightly on her arm, Alice recoils. Amanda rises to go.

'Why didn't you tell my father that I saw you, that I saw you together that day on Lamma Island, Mrs Stubbs?' Alice asks as politely, as if she is inquiring if Mrs Stubbs likes sugar in her tea. She detects the faint whiff of sour milk coming from her hair. Her gaze strays outside her bedroom window, losing itself in the pale wash of sky. She sees a bird hanging, seemingly suspended there, frozen midair, wings outstretched, feathers ruffling, dark eye narrowing in on its prey. A kite, Alice guesses, buffeted by the wind, riding the current.

Amanda Stubbs walks towards the bedroom door. She places her feet carefully as if she is very high up, and knows that if she makes one false move she could fall. She rests her hand on the door handle, leaning heavily on it.

'I didn't tell him because . . . because,' she whispers hoarsely, 'because Alice, it would make no difference. There was . . . no . . . no point!' The door clicks shut behind her. The bird drops like a stone.

Jillian—1971

The Boxing Day shindig's over, thank Christ, and I'm just about as far away as I can get from everyone, waking up in a Macau hotel room, with a sailor snoring at my side. Of course Mother thinks I'm staying with a friend, not that she's bothered anyway. Since the party she's been a bit preoccupied. I should say a bit more preoccupied. You always feel she's not quite there, as if she's going through the motions, her voice rising and falling when it should, her expression changing in perfect unison. 'Oh dear, that is a pity,' she says, and, 'Oh darling, you poor thing,' and, 'Of course you look lovely, Jillian,' and, 'Yes, I see exactly what you mean.' Only she doesn't. She's never seen what I mean. No one has. Except Nicola, and even she gets it wrong most of the time.

The sunlight's filtering through the curtains now, fiercely-bright pages slanting through the gaps. You can see sparkling dust motes spinning in it. I'm looking down at my body, quite naked in the bed. I hate my body. It's a bit like a copy of Mother's, only with her all the proportions are just right—tall, voluptuous, fine facial bone structure, a grace about the way she moves. With me everything's just off a bit: too much fat on the hips, the legs not quite as long as hers, cellulite like orange peel clinging the upper thighs, the breasts big, but droopy. I've seen Mum's breasts. Oh, she didn't show them to me, nothing like that. Christ no! It was through the keyhole. Peering through the keyhole, like a peeping Tom, at her magnificent body all steamy and pink in the bathroom. I just suddenly had to know how we compared, mother and daughter. God, can you imagine if I'd asked her?

'Oh Mother, would you mind showing me your tits, your thighs, and actually while you're at it, I wouldn't mind having a look at your pudenda.'

I know all the rude words. We used to look them all up in the dictionary at the convent, before copying them in the nuns' bibles and prayer books. Anyway, that's what I'd say. 'Could I have a quick peek at your pudenda, Mother.' Then, when she looked a bit put out, I'd elaborate. 'You see, Mother, the last boyfriend I had said my labia majora are a bit thin, sort of flappy. I think that's how he described them. He said he liked them "plump as pigeon breasts, squashy, wet lips you have to prise apart to find the treasure hidden within." Very poetical don't you think? The bastard was pissed.'

I'd spew all this out while Mother was resting with a tiny cup of strong coffee after lunch, still a bit tipsy from the drinks she'd had. And I'd be perched on the end of her bed rifling through a magazine, *Woman's Realm* or something.

'Of course darling,' she'd say with that set intonation of hers. 'Nothing easier.'

And she'd leap up and rip off her clothes, and stand there quite naked, while I strolled round her, thoughtfully nodding my head and rubbing my chin. Now of all fantasies you can have, that's got be the most implausible. So . . . so I peeped. And like the eavesdropper who listens in on something he would rather not have heard, I see that unlike me my mother has a near perfect body, that her breasts, though full, moving as she lifts and dips her arms, creaming herself, have great support. At that filthy convent, Jane, my friend Jane Redwood, she said she'd read if you could get a pencil under your tit, and when you let go it stayed there, that you had shit support. Well I could get a whole pencil case under each boob. It didn't matter how many times I raised my elbows and swung them back and forth like a chicken, doing my support exercises, they still hung there like droopy socks. And now I've been told the flaps of my cunt are too thin! Well Jesus Christ, they're the only things that are, then! One more bit of me to worry about, because some drunken git of a boyfriend decides to tell me they're a disappointment!

It was Jane who got me started on the bulimia business. Skinny Jane who ate so much chocolate she was just one great big pimple.

'I've got no willpower,' I told her once. 'I want to lose weight but I just can't.' We'd sneaked behind the woodshed for a quick fag.

'Jesus Lord, you don't want to go worrying about willpower,' she told me grandly. 'Eat what you want and then just chuck it all up again.'

I couldn't quite believe what she was saying. 'You mean . . . mean . . . vomit?'

Jane took a long draw on her ciggie. Her eyes crinkled and she pursed her lips.

'You laughing at me, Jane?' I demanded, stubbing out my own smoke in a fit of pique.

'Don't get your knickers in a twist,' Jane told me like a puffing dragon. 'I'm just surprised you hadn't thought of it yourself. Eat as much as you like, and then stick your fingers down your throat and bring it all up again. And never gain a pound.'

My disgusted face must have said it all. 'Oh, it isn't as bad as you think. After a while you get to be quite tidy and quick. It's just like the way birds regurgitate their food. Peasy.'

Not that peasy I thought, when two weeks later I still hadn't got the hang of it. But practice makes perfect, isn't that what they say. And now, it's second nature. Not so much in the day, but in the evenings, if you've made a bit of a pig of yourself. Brilliant. Well, not exactly brilliant. My throat hurts sometimes. I get headaches too, and I hate that feeling, the compulsion, making you do it. I hate that you can't just digest your food like everyone else is doing. You've got to find a loo quick, and then make sure no one's about to hear you throwing up. Drinking helps. Not alcohol, just liquid, makes it come sliding out more easily. Just when I think I can't bear to do it again, I see Alice, slim, fragile Alice, my little waif of a sister, who never overeats, who never seems to eat at all in fact. A sparrow couldn't survive on the lettuce leaves she nibbles on. And there am I, a big, ugly cow, stuffing my fat face, then spending half my life down a toilet spewing it all up again.

He's snoring, the sailor by my side, prone and snoring like a foghorn. His name's Jack. He's a bit hairy. You know, hair on his shoulders, all down his back, not much of a turn on. And now he farts. Terrific! But he isn't bothered. He isn't lying there worrying about the size of his dick. Oh, you can be sure of that. He woke up in the early hours and wanted to fuck. And so, because it was easier just to give in, we did. But it was one of those times when someone's on top of you, thrusting away with all their might, and you just can't stop your mind

161

from wandering. I lay there thinking about how it's going to be for me here in Hong Kong, thinking about Alice and how I hate myself for despising her, but how I can't help it. I started counting how many times I've seen my father looking at Alice, those steely-blue eyes of his overflowing with love. He's never looked at me like that. Not once. Not one single time. Doesn't matter what she does, Daddy loves Alice.

I rouse myself then and shake Jack. He gropes for me.

'No!' I tell him flatly. 'We're getting up now and we're going out. Take a shower.'

He doesn't argue, just gets up blearily and stumbles into the bathroom. A moment later I hear him pissing a waterfall, then the toilet flushing. We're too late for breakfast but it sort of balances things out. I didn't manage to throw up supper you see. No opportunity. I just want to get outside, get some air. Can't breathe in this stuffy little room.

'What's the matter with you?' says Jack, tamping down his springy, brown hair. He doesn't say it nastily. He's got an Irish accent, soft, southern. His mother comes from Cork he says. He's an okay bloke. Off one of the British ships in the harbour, and wanting nothing more than to spend a bit of money and have a good time. I shrug and he rubs my shoulders. It's quite nice actually. Of course he's married. They're all married. Most of them don't even bother to take off their rings. 'You're beautiful, you,' he says, and pecks me on the cheek.

'Let's just go,' I counter, trying to keep the weariness from my voice. Think of Mother. She

162

would never let the side down by giving the ugly troll skulking under the bridge a hand up.

We go for a coffee, and I'm really starting to enjoy myself. Then Jack says how great it is to have company over the festive season, and so nearly blurts out 'when you're away from home'. I visualise home then, his home, with his wife stirring something yummy on the stove, raising the steaming spoon to her mouth, tasting and smacking her lips. Then calling out to Jack, face aglow, that his dinner's ready, popping the baby in its playpen, and cooing at it, on and off, through the meal.

'I bet you count yourself lucky,' I find myself saying, pushing my coffee cup away. Suddenly it tastes very bitter.

'Sure I do, Baby,' says Jack on cue, reaching for my hand. 'This is,' he breaks off and nods emphatically, a little too emphatically actually, 'this is fantastic. Being here with you.'

But oh dear me, that troll is definitely coming out to play today, like it or not. Look away now, Mother, it's not going to be a pretty sight.

'I should think you're enjoying this a lot more than finding a whore to fuck in *Wan Chai*.'

Poor Jack looks poleaxed. He gobbles at the air like a turkey, before finally managing to come up with a line. And oh Christ, yes, he hesitates for a moment, just to make sure he's got the name right.

'Jillian, what's the matter with you?' he says, giving my hand, still clasped in his, a little shake. 'What are you suggest—'

But by now the troll is out, a knobbly-kneed leg already over the bridge railings.

'Though I expect I'm a little dearer than a

163

prostitute. Though I don't know. I suppose it depends what kind you go to. A five-dollar fuck up against a wall, or a high-class, overnight, hundred-dollar, no holes barred orgy. I've heard that it can be quite expensive to have the works.'

Jack lets go of my hand. He won't meet my eyes now. He clears his throat noisily. He's a smoker. So am I, so I can't really complain. And already his hand is fumbling in his jacket. He taps the packet on the table, offers me one and I decline. Today, for some reason, I am certain that first drag would make me retch. With his lips he pulls a ciggie out of the packet. Again he fumbles for matches, strikes one, holds it to the tip with a steady hand, and lights it. Then he is inhaling deeply, gratefully, oh so gratefully, poor bugger.

'I guess I'm what you call a high-class escort,' I limp on. But the fight has gone out of me, and the troll is already moving back into the shadows under the bridge again. Though I don't apologise. It's not much, but it's something.

Jack surveys me curiously, as if I'm an island native, as if he has never encountered anything quite like me before, even though he has travelled the seven seas. Then he grins, a dog's grin, the kind Bear pins on sometimes, the kind that says, 'I don't understand what the fuck is going on, but hey, let's just go for a walk, have a pee and forget all about it.'

Again that fractional pause. 'Jillian, I'm going to take you sightseeing. Anywhere you want. You just say. After that we're going out for a meal. And we're having champagne, the best French champagne, none of that rice-wine shit. Then before we have to catch the ferry back, I'm going

164

to take you to a market and buy you anything you want. How's that?'

He doesn't wait for a reply, slips the packet of fags in his pocket, produces a wallet, throws a bill on the table and off we go. And we do have a good time, for a couple of hours at least. We visit the Kun Lam Temple and the Ruins of St Pauls, though the Catholic façade freaks me out a bit. For a while I'm back in that gloomy convent, more like a morgue than a house of God. But I have to say we did have a laugh.

'Have you noticed how much weight Sister McMullen is gaining?' Nicola would hiss in an Irish accent. 'Oh mother of God, could she be eating for two?' And on down the line it went, Chinese whispers, Nicola hamster-cheeked by then, hand clamped over her mouth trying to contain her giggles. Or she'd be pencilling in moustaches, sunglasses, ciggies and anything else she fancied on all the pictures of saints in her bible, or surreptitiously passing a foil condom packet down the row. Before long we were all falling about laughing, and the nuns not knowing what it was all about, looking like rows of battleaxes. Nicola's great like that, taking the black stuff and spinning it, until it's as light and sweet as candyfloss. Trouble is, once you've woofed it down, once it's gone, the black comes crawling back. And somehow it's even darker, because of the brief spell of light.

Anyway, apart from that, my sailor and I do have fun. A great meal, and true to his word we *do* have champagne, and the bubbles go up my nose, the way they describe, only it rarely happens. Then sailor Jack, doing everything he can to make me happy, until I find myself thinking, never mind about the hairy back, hails a taxi.

'Market! Shopping! *Fai d La! Fai d La*!' yells Jack at the driver, and off we speed.

And just about then, for a short interval, I really believe that I am that girl on the big screen, on holiday with the boyfriend she's falling in love with, the one who can't take his eyes off her, that before long we'll sail off into the rose-pink sunset. As we get out I'm laughing, shouting with laughter. Jack's laughing too, and I notice he has really gorgeous green eyes, deep green flecked with dark gold. We link arms.

'You can have anything you want my darlin',' says Jack, and I think he's a little drunk because his Irish brogue is getting more pronounced. 'You just point, my sweetheart, an' it yours.'

And I do point. I point at a pale-pink, padded-brocade jacket, and a string of beads that the stallholder says is best green jade, but that I think is plastic. Still, who cares? Jack's paying, so who bloody cares? I'm about to point at a royal blue Cheongsam, when I see that my fingertip has found something else, something several stalls down from us, something very striking indeed. In fact, one of a kind. My divining finger has found my father. But oh no, not just him. It's found a woman accompanying him. I recognise the woman. She has blonde hair, and gentle blue eyes, and a way of smiling that makes you feel as if crying would be more in order. She came to the Boxing Day Party. It's Amanda Stubbs.

Neither of them see me. I duck behind the row of dresses. My heart is running away and I can't

166

stop it, can't contain it. Jack is distracted, fingering a tray of tacky keyrings on the stall across the way, with a pretty young Chinese girl trying to sell him all of her wares. I slip my hands between two silky Cheongsam, red and gold. My fingers and palms meet. To a passer-by I must look as if I'm praying. And perhaps, considering, that wouldn't be a bad idea. When I open my hands, and my eyes, for I realise with surprise they are closed too, my father and Amanda Stubbs are having some sort of altercation. Mrs Stubbs's slim white hands are flying all over the place, and she is not wearing her smile. She is talking urgently, and I am sure I see a tear spill from one eye. I'm sure because it catches the light and I see it move down her face, winking and sending out its SOS.

I can only see half of my father's profile such is the angle, though more of Amanda. People keep jostling past, blocking my vision. But then, in one of the gaps, another tear spills from Mrs Stubbs's eye, and my father turns so I can see his whole face. He leans down and kisses it, kisses her pain away. And it's like a needle being thrust straight into the centre of my eye, a slither of anguish which, I know no matter how many years I live, will never quite go. They turn. They are at a crossroads in the alleys, then they move off down another lane. It was only an instant, a splinter of time, glimpsing into my father's face, into those ice-blue eyes of his. They were rent with love those eyes. Now they are gone, and Jack is hovering behind me.

'Well my darlin' what would you like? You can have anything darlin', anything at all,' he says flamboyantly, his lips tickling my ear. I can smell

167

the booze on his breath. It's not unpleasant, just there.

What would I like? Oh my God, my God, I would like someone, just once, for one brief moment in my sawdust life, to look at me the way my father looked at Amanda Stubbs. That's what I would like.

Myrtle—1971

Amanda Stubbs is dead. She committed suicide last weekend. I am not as surprised as most. She was, as they say, of a fragile temperament. I'm sure some men found that attractive in her, but I found it irritating. Only weeks ago she was at our Boxing Day party with her children. I doubt she ever gave them a second thought. Phillip is desolate of course. Now I suppose everyone will want to know why she did it. They'll be ferreting about to see if they can find a reason, a reason why she would want to leap from a balcony of the Mandarin Hotel, plummeting to her death. I was talking it over with Beth Fielding yesterday, Wednesday. She popped round for a drink. I was all out of vermouth, Beth's favourite tipple, but as it happens it didn't really matter because what we both felt like was a stiff brandy.

'She was so beautiful,' Beth said mawkishly, helping herself to peanuts from a small, lacquer bowl on the drinks table, flicking them in her open her mouth and chomping them up with distasteful enthusiasm. The whole process, from selection to consumption seemed somehow irreverent. 'Yes, very beautiful. No one could argue with that.'

I agreed, but added that some beauty was only skin-deep. And Beth, who was on her second brandy by then, (we both were), seemed to know exactly what I meant.

'Perhaps she was having an affair?' Beth suggested. I shrugged, hands open, as if I thought it unlikely. 'Perhaps,' said Beth ruminatively, 'whoever it was wanted to end it?'

'Perhaps,' I echoed, draining my glass. I took Beth's brandy balloon, topped it up, and poured myself a third drink. Although it was lunchtime we had had a shock so I felt it was warranted. And Beth didn't protest, therefore I must have judged the mood correctly.

'Maybe he told her it was all over,' Beth hazarded, taking the brandy I held out to her. She then tried to eat and drink concurrently. The result was that she very nearly choked, her face scarlet.

'Would you like some water, Beth?' I offered.

'I'll be fine,' Beth croaked. She took a hefty gulp of her brandy. 'This'll do the trick,' she said. There was a hiatus in the conversation while her complexion faded from a fiery red to a florid pink. Then, with a sharp intake of breath, Beth suddenly grasped my wrist. 'Myrtle, do you think he might have been at your party, the man she was seeing I mean?'

I took a swallow of my own brandy. It was Courvoisier and it was good. But Beth did rather guzzle at everything. She couldn't help it, poor dear. 'Unlikely,' I speculated. 'Not with her husband there and the children. Too risky.'

'Quite right,' said Beth nodding thoughtfully,

169

drawing a hand back and patting her brassy curls. 'But I wonder . . . I wonder who it is then,' she went on reflectively. 'You saw it happen, the tragedy?' she probed, her eyes bright with curiosity. Whatever people say, they have a keen appetite for ghoulish details in a situation like this. There seems little point to me in pretending otherwise. Beth certainly did and I was happy to volunteer the information.

I shook my head and explained that Ralph and I had arrived at the reception just afterwards. 'We were late, Beth. Dreadful traffic,' I elucidated as an afterthought. 'It was all over by the time we arrived. Poor Amanda was lying prostrate on the roof of the lobby. Probably just as well she jumped there. Over the lobby I mean. Otherwise she might have fallen on someone. Imagine that.'

Beth made a small grating noise at the back of her throat, and her doughy face crumpled. I patted her on the back consolingly.

'Whatever is that perfume you're wearing, Beth dear? It's simply divine,' I asked pacifically.

Beth looked pleased. '*Diorissimo,*' she told me, her cheeks once more reddening, but with delight. 'Nigel bought it for me.' She had finished the peanuts, and her tongue probed busily for any morsels that might remain lodged in her teeth. The effect was that of a living organism seeking escape from the closed cavern of her mouth.

'He's a sweetheart, your husband,' I told her. Beth preened. 'Can you bear for me to go on?' Beth nodded decisively. Those curls of hers could certainly do with a bit of taming. When she shook them about and they landed all awry like that, she looked perfectly ridiculous. She took a swift gulp

170

of her drink. I made a mental note to talk to her about her hair dye too. In the afternoon light the colour was an unfortunate chrome yellow, the effect of it cheap and tawdry. Misreading my expression of disapprobation, she lowered her glass and gave me her full attention.

I continued. 'Well, her blonde hair was steeped in blood. It was pooling about her head. She'd landed on her back, and although I'm sure her skull under all that hair must have been completely crushed, her face was untouched. It looked quite calm. Not a spec of blood on it. Her eyes were wide open, staring upwards. That was the worst part of it I think. Those blue eyes. Ooh, it makes me shiver just to picture them. She was wearing a long gown. Red it was, very fetching actually, with sequins sewn into it. It must have blown upwards as she fell. There would have been quite a draught you understand. It was all rucked up around her waist. It looked like a red serpent writhing about her. You could see her panties. Cream lace. Her legs were splayed and twisted at odd angles. Broken certainly. Well, they would be wouldn't they? One arm was hidden under her back and the other seemed to be reaching for something. She looked . . . indecent, her legs apart like that and the panties showing. I told one of the policemen to cover her up. He argued at first. Gabbling about it being a crime scene or something. Then Ralph stepped in. He said something in Cantonese, very curt. He can speak a bit of Cantonese you know. I didn't understand what he said, but they covered her immediately and after—'

'Well, Ralph wouldn't stand for any nonsense,

would he Myrtle?' Beth interjected.

I half smiled. My drink was finished and four really would be pushing it. I thought I might ask the amahs to bring in some more snacks to soak up the booze. Otherwise, I decided, not much would be accomplished that afternoon.

'How did Phillip take it?' Beth prompted, breaking into my reverie.

'He was distraught, naturally. Beside himself,' I said. 'He kept saying, all Amanda told him was that she needed a breath of air. She was popping onto the balcony for some fresh air. That she would only be minute. And that . . . poor man . . . was the last time he saw his wife.'

Beth was lachrymose. She shook her head and pressed the well-padded heels of her hands into her fleshy eye sockets. As she smoothed away her tears she smeared her foundation. It was a rather alarming orangey shade that looked even worse in streaks. She rippled the plump fingers of her hands on her equally plump thighs. Her rings, the white-gold wedding band, the sapphire and diamond engagement ring, and that rather fetching platinum eternity ring encrusted with yet more diamonds, looked tight and uncomfortable, as if she would only be able to remove them with the assistance of large quantities of soap and lubricants. And it was my feeling that some people should never wear slacks. Beth was doing herself no favours with her current wardrobe. They were salmon-pink too. Such a bold, attention-grabbing colour. Still, I've always believed that dress sense is something you're born with, not something you acquire. Some might say my observations on Beth were a trifle waspish, but I feel it is your duty when you have a friend making a fool of herself to bring it to their attention.

'How dreadful for Phillip,' breathed Beth, shifting from buttock to buttock and pulling down the legs of her slacks at the knee, presumably to make herself more comfortable.

'Yes, it was,' I acknowledged, leaning forward to rub at an old lipstick smudge I had noticed on my glass 'After the police had spoken to him, we took Phillip back to his flat. Thank God the children had gone back to boarding school.'

Beth nodded her agreement, clearly thinking of hers and Nigel's children, Christopher and Anita, neither of whom had been sent to boarding school. Briefly I recalled Beth's foreknowledge of the Island school, which she elected not to share with me, and reminded myself to proceed with caution. 'That was my first thought. Imagine trying to explain it to them? I poured us all a drink. I couldn't think what else to do. Phillip cried. Like a baby. It was very disconcerting. Racking sobs. His entire body shaking. Ralph held him. The sounds he made were awful, ugly, unnerving. He kept asking why. Over and over again, why would she do it. Wild red eyes. Ashen-faced. Skin sodden with tears, mucus and saliva. He looked awful. The doctor came and left Phillip some pills to help him sleep. Then between us we put him to bed. Ralph gave the flat a quick once-over, in case there was a note, he said. But there was nothing. Ralph decided to stay, said he didn't want to leave Phillip by himself. I called a taxi.'

'He's such a good friend to Phillip.' Beth picked up her brandy and for once sipped it contemplatively. 'Friends like him are few and far between. I heard she'd been having treatment for depression.'

'It wouldn't surprise me,' came my retort. The mantelpiece clock ticked heavily into the sudden silence.

'She never said anything to you about being depressed did she?' Beth's free hand strayed to an ivory pendant at her neck. She worried at it.

'Never. Amanda and I were not close friends. She hardly spoke to me at all.'

'But then she was a bit like that wasn't she? Kept herself to herself. Except of course at your party.' Beth's tone was breezy. I matched it.

'At my party?' I questioned, still rubbing at the lipstick mark on the glass.

'Yes,' said Beth, her hands sandwiched over the folds at her waist. 'I had to nip back across the way to get the address of my tailor for Christine Gibson. She loved the frock I was wearing. The green velvet. You know the one. She told me she wasn't that happy with her own chap. Anyway, Jillian was at the front door seeing off her crowd of friends, such characters I thought, and it seemed rude to elbow through them, so I went the other way. Out of your back door, past the servants' quarters and through to my back door. That's when I saw you, by the laundry rack, with Amanda.' I must have shot Beth a disbelieving look and she took up the challenge. 'Yes. Oh yes I did Myrtle. You had your back to me Myrtle, but I knew it was you, in that divine purple gown of yours. You and Amanda had your heads close together. Hatching a plot were you? Quite a conspiracy going on, I judged. If not that, then a disagreement perhaps? An altercation?' She

174

stroked her belly and flicked me a smile. 'Some topic that you both felt passionately about, certainly. Though this is all guesswork you understand. I didn't listen in to your conversation. Well of course I didn't. I'm no eavesdropper. Besides, your voices were lowered and it was impossible to hear a thing, with the wind blowing through those funny little octagonal openings in the walls. But I do remember Amanda's face. It was white as a lily, with the oddest spots of red on her upper cheeks. And her eyes . . . that was so peculiar, because she normally has, I suppose I should say had, that serene look about them. No, that's not right. I mean pensive. Yes, that's it. They were pensive eyes. But not that day. Oh no, not when I saw her out the back with you Myrtle dear. They were . . . ablaze. Mm . . . that's it. That's what I remember. Her blazing blue eyes.'

The ticking of the clock suddenly seemed inordinately loud. I had abandoned my attempt at wiping off the lipstick. I would mention it to the amahs. They were getting slack. Once or twice recently I had taken fresh glasses from the cupboard, and found them still bearing the faint traces of lipstick about the rim, or smeary fingerprints on the stem or the glass itself. It just wasn't good enough. 'Oh that,' I said at length, my tone insouciant. 'We were discussing boarding schools. Amanda said that they were having a problem with bullying at the one they send Oliver to. She must have been angry about it. In fact now I recall she was rather upset.'

I stood. I waited. Beth picked a speck of dust from the sleeve of her jacket and crushed it between her fingers. 'Oh I see,' she said, stressing

175

'see' needlessly I felt. 'I didn't think it was important. Not something worth mentioning to the police at any rate.' She gave a breathless laugh. She had a tendency to wheeze. I don't think her weight helped her out much there either. If she wasn't careful she could wind up asthmatic. 'I guessed it was something of that sort. Looks can be so deceptive, can't they, Myrtle?' Beth continued. 'There was I imagining all sorts of silly scenarios, and the two of you were just comparing notes on boarding schools.' Now Beth looked up, her greedy, green eyes meeting mine.

I smiled a slow, lazy smile. I hoped to convey nothing so much as complete relaxation. 'I thought I would ask the amahs to bring in some snacks. I'm feeling a bit peckish. How about you Beth?'

'What a horrible way to die,' Beth said. 'It doesn't bear thinking about does it? Fall through all that space and smashing to pieces on the lobby roof of a luxury hotel. Anyone would think, looking at her life . . .' she paused to draw in a husky, faltering breath, 'that . . . that she had everything. But something must have been missing to make her do a thing like that.' Beth suppressed a belch and thumped her chest with a fat fist. 'Excuse me!'

'There, you see I was right. You *are* hungry, aren't you Beth?'

'I could eat something,' said Beth obliquely.

I crossed to the lounge door. 'How about a nice cheese sandwich, and I'm sure we have some of that delicious Christmas cake left?'

'Sounds wonderful,' Beth replied absently. Her focus had shifted to a copy of the *South China Morning Post* on the shelf under the drinks table.

She drew it out, flapped it open and buried her nose in it. 'There's a wonderful article here about the Mayo Clinic Diet, Myrtle. Not that you need to diet. Rather a lot of eggs if I remember rightly. Have you read it?'

'No.' I opened the lounge door. 'I think we might even have a few mince pies that could be warmed up. And I know we have some cream.'

'Mm . . . I just fancy a mince pie.' As I stepped across the hall I found myself musing that my friend Beth was quite a sleuth. My, my, what sharp little eyes you have Beth dear! All the better to see you with Myrtle. Hmm . . . And I'd never noticed it before. She'd probably read one detective novel too much. Still, perhaps it would be best to be a touch more guarded in her company. I wouldn't want to give any more fodder to that over active imagination of hers. As I entered the dining room, making for the kitchen door, Beth's voice followed me.

'I'm not sure I could cope with all those eggs though Myrtle. They do tend to bind me up rather.'

Beth overstayed her welcome that day. I would have liked her to go much earlier, but then it's awkward showing a friend the door, particularly in the light of recent events. Beth made it clear that she needed to talk, to express her sorrow. So I listened, and listened, and listened. I never thought I'd say I was extremely glad to hear Alice arrive home. Beth made tracks shortly after that, and I was able to steal into my bedroom, lock the door and have a bit of blessed peace. Ralph rang in the evening and told me he'd be late again. He's been spending a great deal of time with Phillip

177

over the past week, helping with arrangements to fly the body back to England for the funeral and burial, dealing with the police and so forth. I told him he'd done enough already, that he needed an early night, but he didn't seem to hear me.

'I owe it to him,' he said tightly and refused to be drawn further.

He's not been himself lately. Actually I think he's having some sort of belated reaction to the strain of the riots. I know it was a long time ago now, but these things happen. All that stress was bound to take its toll eventually. But he's adamant he doesn't want to see a doctor. When he finally arrived home he refused dinner, said he had work to do and shut himself up in the lounge. Jillian stays with friends most of the time now. Nicola was out and Alice was goodness knows where, so at least I didn't have to warn the children off. I went in, took him a coffee and asked him if he wanted to talk about it. But he just waved me away and said he was fine. He was so late coming to bed that I fell asleep in the end. After all, it had been quite a day, what with Beth's extended visit. When I woke up and glanced at the bedside clock it was nearly 2:30am. Ralph's side of the bed was empty. I got up and slipped on my dressing gown. I had fallen asleep without drawing the curtains. I often do. Our bedroom is the first one you come to on the long corridor. From its windows you have an excellent view of the veranda jutting out from side of the building. Naturally it was dark, but there was sufficient light spilling out from the lounge for me to be able to see Ralph clearly. He was leaning over the veranda railing, his eyes looking not outwards but downwards. His head was almost lolling on his shoulders. Honestly, for a moment I wondered if he had dropped off to sleep. Then he lifted his face to the moon, slowly, as if it was a great effort, and sighed. The windows were open. It was a fine night and the sound he made was clear as glass. It reminded me of a cat I found just weeks after father died. It was lying in the road outside the house in Ealing. I think it had been hit by a car. Its eyes were pink with blood, and there was blood on its whiskers too, and a sticky mess of yellow fluid oozing from an ear. As I picked it up it gave a sigh, a throaty moan that seemed to have been drawn from its trembling body by some kind of external force. And with that it let go of life.

The following day I called the Public Works Department, the PWD. I had given the amahs strict instructions to tell Beth I was out if she called. I stood on the veranda where Ralph had prowled the previous night. I took hold of the balcony rail, my fingers curling around the painted, white pole. It was cold and hard. I peered down. It was a long way to the ground. It seemed truly astonishing to me that I had never seen it before. Falling from it would be easy. Perhaps it takes a suicide, someone you know crashing to her death from a hotel balcony, to make you understand how close you are to the edge yourself. The gentleman I spoke to at the PWD was Mr Chen, a helpful man if a little dense. I had had dealings with him before. When the flat was being decorated last year, as it is annually, I selected magnolia, playing safe, and came home to find lemon yellow splashed all over my walls. He was very apologetic and sorted it out as quickly as he could. But nevertheless he owed me a favour.

'Mr Chen, this is Mrs Safford, Ralph Safford's wife.' He acknowledged me with his usual deference. 'I should like bars fitted to the windows of our flat on The Peak,' I said without preamble.

'Bars, Mrs Safford?' he queried.

'Yes Mr Chen. I am worried about the children falling out.'

There was a pause. The black telephone receiver seemed inexplicably heavy in my hand at that point.

'Falling . . . mm . . . falling out of the windows, Mrs Safford?' Mr Chen verified.

His tone of incredulity annoyed me a great deal. 'Yes Mr Chen. And off the veranda too,' I added for good measure. There was another pause presumably while Mr Chen took a mental inventory of the ages of our children, whom he had met on several occasions while supervising work on our flat. 'I know they're teenagers Mr Chen, but . . . well . . . you never know do you?' I said in answer to his unasked question. 'Better to take precautions now, before there's a nasty accident, wouldn't you say, Mr Chen?' I tried to instil a ring of maternal zeal into my voice.

'Indeed Mrs Safford, but I am just surprised that you have not made this request until now.'

That made me fume. As if it was any business of his to second-guess me. I was Ralph Safford's wife and I wanted bars on my windows, and that should have been quite sufficient for him to get cracking having them fitted as far as I was concerned. Down the phone line he must have become aware of his own impertinence, because now he stepped in quickly.

180

'Of course, Mrs Safford. How many windows would you like fitted with bars?' I sighed crossly. This fellow really was slow on the uptake.

'Why, all of them, Mr Chen,' I rounded on him, my patience tried to its limit. 'It wouldn't be much good having some with bars and some without. The children could just as well tumble out of one as all of them.

'Yes, I see that now, Mrs Safford.' Mr Chen sounded penitent and I felt marginally appeased.

'And the veranda too. I want a strong metal grid fitted from the veranda railing to the roof.'

There was a barely perceptible pause.

'But Mrs Safford . . .' he tailed off, his courage I suspect failing him.

'Yes Mr Chen?' I prompted him edgily.

'It will make your veranda look a bit like—' This time he ground to a halt. I heard him take a quick gasp of breath. Then in a rush, 'It will make your flat on The Peak look a bit like a cage . . . a cage in the sky, Mrs Safford.'

'Never mind that,' I dismissed his objection peremptorily.

'And when would you like—' Mr Chen began, but I cut him off.

'Oh just *do* it, Mr Chen! Get your coolies up here as soon as is humanly possible and do it,' I snapped. Mr Chen assured me he would have a team working on it by the end of the week. And with that I had to be satisfied.

Ghost—1971

Lots of Chinese men arrive and fit bars to all the windows. They secure a belt of wire fencing between the veranda railing and the roof. They make the flat on The Peak into a prison. Mr Safford seems to be the only one who barely notices the changes. Jillian corners Alice whenever the opportunity presents itself.

'See what you've done,' she hisses, or, 'This is all your fault, Alice,' or 'Poor mother!' Her eyes rake the length of the corridor repeatedly, taking in the tunnel of bars with a groan.

Nicola insists we all look on the bright side. She tells her siblings that, whatever accidents befall them, they may rest assured that plunging to their deaths from our flat won't be one of them. When Harry comes home for the Easter holidays he stares at the barred windows in puzzlement. He moves slowly down the corridor pausing to grasp a bar and give it a good tug, as if he doesn't quite believe they are fixed in place, as if he thinks he might dislodge them, as if he is contemplating escape. At mealtimes shadow bars fall across the faces of the Safford family ranged about the table. Alice takes to gazing out of the dining-room window, her brow furrowed. She watches the sun set through the barred bathroom window. She looks with undisguised envy at aeroplanes and birds and even insects. The amahs grow mutinous.

'Why putting bars on all the windows?' they demand daily as they bustle about the flat. For once Ah Lee does not think this is a joking matter.

She wrings her hands and squints at the bars suspiciously, her high forehead screwed into deep lines, her mouth tightly crimped. She clicks her tongue, 'Tsk tsk,' and she shakes her head.

Ah Dang pauses frequently in her daily tasks, glaring suspiciously from one window to the next, her hands pulled into fists and resting on her wide hips.

'*Ai ya! Ai ya!*' she says. 'How I clean the windowpanes now. This is very, very bad sign. We trapped with a crazy *Gweilo* family. *Zao gao!*'

Even Bear looks shaken, trying to pounce on the ever-shifting slanted shadows, his paws always bewilderingly empty. He eyes them warily as they slide across the floor, growling and backing away from them when they come too close.

Myrtle Safford is the only one who does not seem to be struggling to acclimatise herself to our prison. She is in good spirits, humming and whistling to herself, satisfaction cloaking her face as she surveys the sturdy bars. Of course I can slip through them with ease but Alice is not so lucky. She keeps counting them. Surprisingly she did not seem pleased by the news of Amanda Stubbs's death. When her mother told her that Mrs Stubbs had killed herself, Alice put her diary into the metal wastebin in her bedroom. She struck a match and set light to it. The pages went up in a whoosh, but the leather cover only charred and smoked for a bit. I can still detect an acrid odour in her room. A good storm might clear the air.

Nigel—1971

It is August the 16th. Typhoon Rose is heading for the colony. At around 5am the radio informs me that Signal No. 3 is being hoisted, that she is about 150 miles away to the south. Despite this, I set off as usual for work, as does my next-door neighbour across the way, Ralph Safford. I am hopeful I can sit out the worst of it down town, overnight at the office if necessary. By 10am, Signal No. 3 has risen to the North-east Gale, Storm Signal No. 7. Rose, we are told, is compact and deadly. Just after midday the South-east Gale, or Storm Signal No. 8, warns that the gale-force winds have altered course. It is clear from forecasts that Typhoon Rose means business. During the afternoon my wife rings me three times, urging me to come home. I find myself wishing that the phone lines would go down.

'I've picked the children up from school,' Beth tells me. 'They say it'll really take hold this evening. At a time like this you should be with your family. Come home, Nigel.' This last is a wail.

I ask her if she has seen to it that the amahs board up the windows, put the antiques away, get the candles ready and so forth.

'Yes I have,' she says. Her voice is sulky, like a recalcitrant child's.

'Then you know the best place to stay is in the hall. Centre of the flat. Most secure. No windows to blow out.' Personally I feel a lot safer in the offices in Central during a typhoon than I do exposed on the top of The Peak.

'Ralph Safford is coming home.' Beth is resentful. 'Myrtle has said we should all go over there and shelter.'

Ah, at last we have it. Beth doesn't wish to be shown up, wants Myrtle Safford to know her husband comes to heel just the same as Ralph does. God, I think, we'll be packed like sardines in that hall! The way things are going we could be there all night rubbing up against each other. Besides, I can think of plenty of other places I'd prefer to while away the hours during a typhoon. But I suppose I will never hear the end of it if I don't go back. By the time I get there, a little after 6pm, Rose is just getting into her stride. The skies are black as night. The rain is sheeting down. The wind really is howling. Getting from the garage to the Saffords' flat lobby is a feat in itself. And it's not just the gale-force winds you have to worry about, but all the debris whirling through the air. You'd be surprised what those winds can pick up and toss around. Anything loose. Anything not bolted down. How must the hillside squatters, the ones still waiting to be resettled feel? Poor blighters. At least I have bricks and mortar between my family and the tempest.

Anyway, battered and sodden I finally manage to get the heavy, swing doors of the lobby open. Greeted by Stygian gloom I stumble in. A power failure naturally. It is a laborious process, feeling my way up several flights of stairs to the top floor in near darkness. Everything is rattling and groaning and creaking and sighing, as if the building is on the verge of collapse As I climb I begin to experience that rather unpleasant disconcerting sensation of the floor swaying gently

185

under my feet, the entire edifice yielding to the relentless drag of the wind. I know it's a safety measure built in by architects—that what bends won't necessarily break—but when you're the one rolling about in a vertiginous top-floor flat on The Peak, logic is cold comfort.

Myrtle Safford, an eerie sight, answers my thumps on the door. Her hair, normally swept up in a bun, is loose and flowing over her shoulders. I've never seen it like that before. In her hand she holds a flickering candle. There are more candles placed about the room, on occasional tables and on the bar. The dancing flames make a play of light and shadow on Myrtle's face, and on the surrounding walls. I recall the Garrison Players' production of *Macbeth* that we caught at the City Hall a couple of months ago. Ralph's wife looks the very image of Lady M. in her sleepwalking scene.

'Out, out damned spot, eh?' I jest as I cross the Safford threshold, and am rewarded with a winning smile. She is quite a woman, Myrtle Safford, just the sort who might think nothing of doing away with a King, if it enabled her husband's ascendancy. Or perhaps I'm just jealous. I have not been awarded an OBE like Ralph Safford. And it is just the kind of window-dressing that the in-laws back in old Blighty would love. I glance over at my wife, Beth. She is on her feet, and gabbling something about how worried she's been. Myrtle Safford, eminently—and in my opinion more admirably pragmatic—hands me a towel and offers me a drink. This episode might be just bearable through a haze of scotch I think.

So here we all are, at the mercy of Rose, a

mistress with an incomparable temper. And of ourselves, no doubt. Which force holds more malignancy? I ponder. Faces by candlelight. Shadow puppets. *Zhi ying xi.* Let the play commence. I take my seat next to Beth, who at last has stopped fussing. She makes herself more comfortable, leaving, I note, scant room for me, and testing the load-bearing capabilities of the elegant wicker settee to the very limit. Myrtle busies herself at the bar, pouring and mixing her potions. Watching her, I am unable to shake the theatrical from my mind. A witch perhaps? In a setting not so very unlike a blasted heath. I brace myself for the prophecies to come. Ralph, who arrived only minutes before me I understand, is slumped on a bar stool lost in his own world.

And what of our children? Christopher, ten and horribly precocious, moves about restlessly on the carpet, as if no position his infant contortionist limbs settle into is comfortable. Anita, seven, an insipid child forever on the brink of tears, squats in a corner with the Saffords' old mongrel, the perfect victim for her ceaseless ministrations. Harry, the Saffords' son, hovers by the bar picking at a bowl of peanuts. Nicola, their second daughter, is leaning back against the cloakroom door, wearing, I cannot not help but notice, a very revealing mini skirt. And her top is cut so low that if she raises her arms her boobs will probably fall out. Besides that, even by candlelight I can see she's plastered in make-up. You might be forgiven for mistaking her as a hooker if you saw her strolling in *Wan Chai*. Little trollop! So is it my fault I find myself imagining what it would be like to do her? A white teenager. Oh,I have plenty of

Chinese girls of course, who look as if they have just trotted out of school. But a bit of white flesh straight from the classroom . . . that is a different matter. It would be a real treat. Myrtle says the older sister is staying with a friend in Kowloon. So that just leaves the amahs, theirs and ours. I glimpse them through the open doorway. They are holed up in the dining room, ready to duck under the table if the windows blow in.

Myrtle comes forward and hands me a scotch. Nice generous measure too. I sip it slowly. Time passes. Conversation is desultory. Myrtle hands round snacks, sandwiches, crisps and chocolate. It does not take much to revive Beth's appetite, and she tucks in as if she hasn't had a decent meal for week. Harry likewise, losing his veneer of diffidence in an instant at the prospect of food. My eyes flick over Ralph's bowed back. It appears the indomitable Ralph Safford had a weakness after all. How touching that the tragic death of Amanda Stubbs should have affected him so deeply. I leave him to his own devices. At about 9pm, the radio, which has been quietly updating the news since I arrived, announces that Increasing Gale or Storm Signal No. 9 has been hoisted, and that Rose, 50 miles southwest of the island, is fast approaching. I mull this over, and am just draining my third drink when a thought suddenly occurs to me.

'Where is Alice?' I ask.

My words seem to give even the mad dog, Rose, pause for thought, and a momentary lull ensues. Ralph straightens up. Looking around the hall he appears to focus for the first time. Simultaneously Nicola smiles and I see the whites of her teeth flash. Then she gives a light whistle, audible in the stillness. Harry grunts, folds his arms and moves across the room, nearer the shadows by the front door. Myrtle, for once in her life, appears tongue-tied.

'She's in . . . well, Alice wanted to stay mmm . . . in her . . . there seemed no harm in letting . . .' Her voice peters out and she takes a swallow of her drink.

'Oh my God,' shrieks Beth, grasping my arm with her podgy hands. 'She's not out there is she, Myrtle? She'll be killed!'

'Of course not,' Myrtle retorts scathingly. 'Don't be so silly, Beth.'

'Then where is she, Myrtle? Where is Alice?' Ralph demands, rising, pushing away the drink his wife holds out to him, his voice a dangerously low growl.

Quite honestly I begin to feel I have stepped into the middle of the story. Why on earth is everyone so absurdly uptight at the mention of Alice? Am I missing something here? As far as I know, Alice is the only one of the Saffords' offspring who keeps a low profile on this island, excepting Harry of course. But then he doesn't count any more, tucked away safely in boarding school for most of the year. Poor little bastard! Chubby as a roly-poly pudding. School will have taken him apart piece by piece by now. Still, he seems to find great solace in food. But as for Alice, she's faultless, isn't she? Maybe not. I wonder . . . I wonder what Miss Alice Safford had been up to? It must have been something delightfully wicked to warrant shutting her away in a typhoon. Well, I think, detaching my wife's hands from my arm and settling back on the settee, this might be a great

189

deal more entertaining than first anticipated.

'She's quite safe,' Myrtle manages defensively, in gear at last after a bit of grinding. She draws herself up imperiously. She is wearing a diaphanous floor-length dress; the reflections of the sputtering candle flames wavering on the pale fabric. Still clasping the drink she offered Ralph, eyes wide, mouth jutting forward stubbornly, she seems ready to brazen it out. 'Alice is in her bedroom. By the time I thought to fetch her, several of the windows had blown in along the corridor. It had become a wind tunnel. Glass was flying everywhere. Impenetrable. It was . . . the most . . . the most sensible course of action. To leave her . . . to leave her where she was until the signals start to drop.'

I stare in the direction of the heavy, wooden, sliding doors that,if closed, divide the hall from the long corridor. The flats are identical, ours and the Saffords'. Of course, with furnishings and decoration we all put our individual stamp on them, but the shell remains the same. In the gloom I can see a fat sausage of rolled towels at the base of the shaking doors, to block the draft and mop up the rainwater that would otherwise be flooding in I presume. Behind those doors the fury of the elements batters and thunders, reminding us all how treacherous it would be to venture beyond what seems like an increasingly feeble barrier.

'I'm going to get her,' Ralph states, his voice still low, though a note of unshakable determination has crept into it.

Myrtle begins to say something and then abandons her sentence. Christopher, who is clearly bored, leaps up and volunteers to go with Ralph. I notice Harry shuffle even further back into the gloom. Beth nearly suffocates our son by springing to her feet and clutching him to her ample bosom. Anita, as I might have predicted, starts to cry. Nicola, whose eyes I now become aware, have never left me, lets a hand move against a thigh, easing her already indecently short skirt up a few inches. Someone should take that girl over their knee and give her a good spanking, I decide. The erotic potential of this image rather negates its original conception. But I have little time to dwell on my prurient thoughts. Ralph pushes past Myrtle, through the open doorway into the dining room, where the amahs huddle round the dining-room table. I rise to follow him. Here too candles sputter, spilling their weak light into the gloom.

'Where are you going?' Beth's sharp cry rises above the maelstrom of the typhoon. I feel her hand pulling on my damp shirt. I had slipped off my sopping wet jacket when I arrived.

'For God's sake, Beth!' I push her off, perhaps a little roughly.

'Don't go, Nigel. It's too dangerous. You'll be injured and then what will we do?' she bleats.

The dog growls. Anita, picking up on her mother's distress, turns the volume up on her sobs. In a torrent of emotion she deserts the nervous beast and flings herself at her mother's feet.

'Christ,' I mutter, moving towards the doorway, my empty glass still clutched in my hand. And still that little tart Nicola is giving me the come-on, moving her thighs together and sliding her tongue slowly along her upper lip. Had we been alone, I would have got some respect out of that little bitch. 'Stop fussing, Beth. I'm going to be fine.'

191

Myrtle takes my glass from me as I pass by. For a brief second our eyes meet. Whatever his failings, Ralph Safford's wife is magnificent. The image of my fat, hysterical, and God-help-me, lifelong partner, waddles into my head. Because that's what she is these days, neurotic and overweight. True, I have gone to seed a bit since taking up this post in Hong Kong as well. I am not able to run around Lugard Road as often as I like, and the once well-muscled belly has lost some of its definition. Though I like to think I am still in pretty good shape compared to the other pencil-pushers. And I'm not bad looking either, really. Distinguished, I concluded the other day, when I passed a critical eye over my reflection in Beth's dressing table mirror. A fair, freckled complexion, for the most part unlined; red-gold hair, albeit thinning a bit on top; cool green, poker-playing eyes, a great asset when working for the British government. And still I only have to wear glasses for reading.

I haven't done too badly, certainly better than Beth. These days it is all I can do to manage to fuck her occasionally. She has put on so much weight. Eats too much and drinks too much. But, I console myself, she has money, or at the very least, stands to inherit it. Only daughter of an English lord with a landed estate. That thought never fails to give me a stiffy before I sink into her. When this party here is over (and let's face it, anyone with an ounce of common sense can see it won't go on forever) I intend to continue the fun. They may mock me now with my lardy wife, but they will soon sober up when they see what's waiting for Nigel Fielding back home. One day, my plump pig of a wife will be bringing home the bacon. I am relying on it. Oh yes, big Beth is my contingency plan, and I would be wisest not to forget it.

But you can't condemn a man for dreaming, can you? More and more these days I think of Cynthia Feng. She is sleek as an alley cat, her smooth skin the colour of milky coffee. The coal-black hair that streams down her back is so long she can sit on it with her shapely buttocks. She doesn't talk much. Too busy sucking the tip of my penis, deep, deep down, with such exquisite delicacy that it jerks of its own accord, as if imbued with its own life. Love-making with Cynthia is a journey into the unknown. Easing apart her labia with their curls of dark hair, soft as goose down, and taking her cunt in my mouth until the lychee sweetness of it trickles down my chin . . . sweet Jesus! And when she slips her big toe with its painted toenail, cherry-red or sky-blue or canary-yellow, always a different shade, always tantalizingly sharp, into my rectum, I am in heaven, heaven on earth. And that's good enough for me. As for love—love doesn't come into it. I pay and pay well, and Cynthia is discreet. Besides, my sessions with her make 'love' seem very ordinary by comparison.

I enter the dining room and see Ralph Safford in the wavering candlelight. He is pulling tablecloths out of the dresser drawers, and swathing himself in them, so that very soon he comes to resemble a cross between an oil sheik and an Egyptian mummy. Atop the dresser the water trembles in the aquarium. The fish are dark shapes, gliding through the tangled golden filaments of reflected flames. I can't help but feel marginally superior, when I consider the disaster

Ralph's affair nearly catapulted him into. Just as well Amanda Stubbs was considerate enough to die when she did, unselfish to the last, silly cow. For that, I suspect, judging by the demeanour of Ralph lately, was the *real* thing, the genuine article, the stuff they write about. How do I know about Romeo and Juliet?

I work closely with Ralph. Observing his surreptitious behaviour, I soon guessed he was having an affair. I just wasn't sure who with, until Amanda did the decent thing and topped herself. Give them credit, they did an excellent job of hiding it, quite a feat on the island, though how long they could have kept up the charade I don't know. So long as the papers don't get a sniff of it ... because that could be messy. As for me, I work for the British Government. I keep it zipped, my mouth that is. We don't want to give these commie chinks any more ammunition than we have to. Sleaze and corruption amongst senior-ranking British government officials. A headline we can all do without, thank you very much. Those red bastards in Beijing would lap it up.

'Here, let me give you a hand, Ralph,' I tell him, very nearly shouting to top the roaring of the gales, noisier now we are in the dining room. Wave after wave of dense rain pelts the windowpanes, the din only fractionally muted by the barrier of wooden boards shuttering the windows. It must have been tricky putting them in place with those bars the Saffords have had fitted. Goodness knows what that's all about.

Ralph stands like a child being costumed for his big entrance in a school play. The amahs hug themselves, their Cantonese conversation

194

stuttering on, their voices rising and falling with the pitch and fall of the storm outside. Suddenly there is a loud, splintering crash.

'*Ai ya! Ai ya! Ai ya!*' screams an amah springing to her feet. It's one of the Saffords' servants I think, her black plait lashing about almost comically, her eyes popping, the whites, ghostly amber in the glow of the candles. They are an unsettling sight, piercing our murky cavern as it pitches and rolls in the dark sky. The others pull her back down and jibber at her until she settles.

'Another of the corridor windows,' Ralph says, his tone so ordinary he might be identifying the ring of a telephone.

I am binding his arms. He can use them to ward off slithers of broken glass, as he battles against the wind, trying to carve a passage down the corridor. He might be a fool but I have to admit he is a brave one.

It looks as if his dalliance with Amanda will be contained after all, no note I understand. What a saint that woman was! Oh, far too righteous for me. I like my women a bit more earthy. But nevertheless, it has to be conceded, one of a kind, determined even in death not to be a canker to her living lover. Cherishing him from the grave. All a bit highbrow for my taste, but I have to admit I'm impressed. Ralph Safford. Lucky, then, as well as a fool.

From the hall I hear my wife's voice chiming in, the bell of doom.

'Nigel! Nigel! I'm scared, darling. Please come back. Stay with me. Stay with me and the children. I can't bear for you to leave me.' Then to Myrtle, 'Don't let the men go. Tell Nigel he has to stay. We

195

need one of the men here with us.' Anita is chanting a nursery rhyme over and over again in that high, jarring voice of hers.

> *'London Bridge is falling down,*
> *Falling down, falling down,*
> *London Bridge is falling down,*
> *My fair lady.'*

'Dad, let me come too,' pleads Christopher, materialising out of the dimness in the dining-room doorway. For the first time I notice that he has an odd-shaped head, the silhouette of it looking slightly lopsided. I hiss at him to return to his mother and he slouches off sourly.

> *'London Bridge is falling down,*
> *Falling down, falling down,*
> *London Bridge is falling down,*
> *My fair lady.'*

The dog howls wolfishly. Beneath my feet the floor tips. I bite back acid bile and fight an urge to puke. I might be standing on the deck of a boat tossed on the ocean. I overhear someone telling Anita to shut up. I think it's Christopher, though it might have been Harry, the voices are so hard to decipher above the wind. In the chaos I am dimly aware that Myrtle is uncharacteristically quiet. She is usually centre stage, taking control, managing events. Perhaps this business with Amanda Stubbs has taken its toll, presuming she knew about it. I rummage in the drawer for fresh cloths. All I come up with is napkins. I make do, folding them hurriedly on the diagonal and winding them about

196

Ralph's forearms, then knotting them clumsily. I would never have made a nurse, I acknowledge to myself. Ralph's brilliant blue eyes peer out at me from his mummified face, as we hear that Hurricane Signal No.10 has been hoisted.

'Thanks,' he says.

'I'll come with you,' I tell him, knowing that he will refuse my offer.

'There are no more tablecloths Nigel,' Ralph relays, giving a backward nod in the direction of the empty drawers. 'You can't.'

I don't argue. I help Ralph through to the hall, and we stand side by side before the sliding door. Looking back I catch sight of the amahs ducking under the dining-room table. The dog scoots past us and joins them, spooked by Ralph's appearance. I leave Ralph poised to make his exit into the mouth of hell, and marshal wives, children and all into the small alcove before the front door. I hem them in with the wicker settee and any cushions I can find. Then, fighting the astonishing pressure of the wind, a lethal vortex of swirling water and glass racing back and forth along the corridor, I manage to draw the door back a couple of feet. Ralph forces his way through, curved arms held against his face like a shield. The wind forges past me. The stinging rain drives into my face remorselessly. I struggle to slide the door closed. My fingers are numb and keep slipping on the wet groove of the metal handle. I feel a stab of pain on my cheek, before I finally succeed in shouldering the bloody thing shut. Later I will find that a blade of glass has slashed my face barely an inch from my eye. I will shiver thinking of what might have been. I will swab the blood up with one of Myrtle's

197

silk scarves, smelling of her scent, rich and overwhelming, the only thing to hand. I will sit, drink more whisky, and watch the candles gutter and die. And I will consider how fortunate we all are to have got off so lightly.

Ralph—1971

I keep my head tucked down, my shoulders hunched, my feet shuffling forwards, inches of rainwater sloshing over my shoes, glass crunching beneath my feet. I summon all my strength and plough ahead into the teeth of the wind. Alice's bedroom is the third I shall come to. I feel my way along the wall, a blind man stepping into the unknown. Already the napkins binding my hands and elbows are soaked through. Small things glance off me. Then something larger. It strikes the back of my head, and for a second I reel and nearly overbalance. I recover myself and move on. Progress is painfully slow. I think how many times I have crossed this distance in seconds. Now I must wage war for a couple of feet.

At last I reach Alice's door. As I push my bulky hand down on the handle, it flies open and inwards, slamming into the bedroom wall. The wind pins it there. It picks me up and jettisons me inside. I am panting. My heart beneath my tablecloth wrappings beats erratically. I stagger ahead, trying to yell above the tumult that it is me, Daddy, that I have come to fetch her, to fetch Alice. But here there are no candles, the windows are boarded up, and in front of me is a blackness so absolute that I am unsure if my eyes are open or closed. The wind claws at my back, trying to reclaim me for its own. Now I am dimly aware of prongs of thin, pewter-grey light, cast from behind me through the jagged jaws of smashed windows. My eyes narrow, straining to adjust to the gloom.

Still I have not found Alice. I lurch forwards towards the bed, scattering some stuffed toys, treading down notebooks and files, snapping pencils, crushing pens. As I near it I leap back, for her bedding rears up like a savage beast challenged in its lair, knotting and twisting and writhing. Then the sheets free themselves and flap, stingrays of the storm. They grow pearly, translucent, insubstantial as mist. Revealed beneath them, I see clearly now the dark shape of Alice. She is lying on her belly, her head to one side, turned towards me. As I lean over my daughter her skin seems to shine. I touch her cheek with my exposed fingertips and it is icy cold. I bend over her, tell her that I have come to get her. She does not stir. Panic, cold and corrosive as gall, worms its way through me. I grasp her narrow shoulders and shake her with my bound hands. Her eyes are shut fast. She is limp and lifeless. Again I shake her, more furiously this time, and to my relief she stirs and props herself up on her elbow.

Slowly she opens her eyes and takes in my surprising appearance. Strands of damp hair cling to her face, like seaweed, slick on a rock after a wave has broken over it. Her lips are trembling. She looks disorientated but not afraid. Again I reassure her, yelling that I am going to bundle her up in her bedding, and take her down the corridor

199

to the hall where she will be safe. She says nothing, but when I start to swathe her in blankets she does not resist. I heft her into my arms and am astonished at how light my daughter has grown, as if there is nothing to her, as if when I come to unwrap her in the hall later, I will find that I have returned empty-handed. But my fears are unfounded. For once back behind the sliding doors in the comparative safety of the hall, I open my parcel to find Alice is very much present, chilled flesh and chattering teeth.

Time has passed since our dramatic entrance. Alice says she is fine. She has had some hot chocolate from a flask and is swaddled in dry towels, hugging the dog under the telephone table. And I have emerged from my trappings like an insect shedding a cocoon, and am hunched in a chair sipping coffee. Nicola is sprawled on the floor, panting as if recovering after some great exertion. She reminds me of a harbour swimmer who has just finished the race. Myrtle and Beth are sitting together on the wicker settee, discussing prices at the Ocean Terminal shopping centre. Harry has made a bed for himself with a few cushions to one side of the bar and, impervious to the storm seems to be sleeping soundly. Nigel is leaning against a wall, smoking a cigarette indolently. I suspect he is bored. Anita has also given in to tiredness, curled up by Nicola's side. She snuffles like a puppy. Christopher lying on his back, legs propped up on the cloakroom door, is thumping it with the heel of one foot, at intervals that I judge to be not nearly long enough. Through the open doorway, I hear two of the amahs muttering in Cantonese, though what they're saying is a mystery. Another has collapsed on her seat, resting her head on the dining room table. I think it is Ah Lee: it is hard to decipher in the dwindling light. Their candles are almost out.

Just after 2am, the eye of the typhoon moves over the flat and an unearthly hush descends. We are all tired and talk is sporadic now. The radio tells us that during the night, Rose will continue on a north-westerly trajectory towards Canton, weakening rapidly as she goes. Some time after 4am, Storm Signal No.10 is replaced by No. 6. At this, judging it to be safe, Nigel rouses Beth, their children and amahs, and together they stumble exhaustedly across the lobby to their flat. At 9:15am, while we are all gratefully enjoying fresh hot coffee and gingerly exploring the flat for damage, Strong Wind Signal No. 3 is hoisted. Finally, by noon on August 17th, this is lowered. Rose has done her worst and it only remains for us to count the cost.

Bear refuses to leave Alice's side. He keeps snarling and I see his hackles are up. I expect he is thoroughly out of sorts with the wretched experience. Judging it safe, Alice and I take him for a walk about The Peak in the afternoon. We pass trees torn up by their roots like so many weeds, mud-slides that engulf cars and sheds, bicycles twisted up like scrap metal. Stranger objects too protrude from the mud, or hang in the trees, or simply lie in the roads. Among the wreckage we spot an ironing board, a bent abacus, a fallen tree with a naked, one-legged doll sitting astride a withered branch, a deflated rubber ring, and a dead cat, its yawning, pink mouth twisted in a rictus of terror, its teeth oddly grey, its eyes frozen open, a streak of blood seeping from one nostril. When we return several hours later, Alice is holding a temple carving of a Chinese god. The wood of the god's brow is split, a slice of glass embedded in it, and an arm is missing, the socket ragged with splintered wood. But the bulging eyes are unscathed I notice. We stand on the doorstep of our flat and ring the bell, now working again, and wait.

'Most of the paint has peeled away,' Alice says, holding the temple carving at arm's length, and studying her find. 'It might be impossible now to recognise exactly which god it is.' I nod. I am not inclined this afternoon to be choosy. These days it feels like any god who cares to listen will do.

Later, I discover the staggering cost of Rose's rampage to the colony—the vessels that went aground or collided, the hundreds of boats that sank, the hydrofoils and ferries that were damaged. I learn that the *Fat Shan*, a Hong Kong–Macau Ferry, capsized, and that only a handful of passengers survived. The hurricane gales swept away countless hillside huts, leaving more than a 1,000 families homeless. Buildings collapsed, and there was widespread flooding and numerous landslides leading to road blockages. The dead and the injured numbered in the hundreds. The huge loss of livestock, and extensive damage to crops and fruit trees, would have a crippling effect on the farming community. It would take months, if not years, to undo the spleen of Typhoon Rose. Next to this, whingeing about what we suffered in the solid secure confines of the flat on The Peak, seems risible.

Nicola—1972

It was high time that my little sister had sex, so I invited her to come along to a party in the New Territories. The summer was drawing to a close but the weather was still great, and the guy who was holding it told me his parents were away. It couldn't have been more ideal.

'Want to celebrate passing your O levels and come to a party?' I asked Alice, when at last I found her in the late afternoon.

She was playing on the swing in the communal gardens of our block of flats. It's a single swing and quite substantial as it happens. But even so, a sixteen-year-old on a swing! For a while I just watched her. Then I raised my voice above the *crick-creak* of metal and wood.

'Fancy coming to a party on Saturday?' I tried again. I was beginning to wonder if Alice could hear me, if she even knew I was there. 'Alice, slow down. I want to talk to you,' I shouted. At last she seemed to notice me, and let her legs dangle. The momentum ceased, the swing slowed and eventually stopped.

'It's like flying,' she said, her words tumbling out all in a rush, cheeks flushed, eyes bright. 'I can see everything. Aberdeen. Junks sailing out to sea. The slopes of The Peak. I'm on top of the world.'

I resisted the urge to sigh my impatience. 'I think it's time you had sex,' I said.

Alice nodded but I had the feeling her attention was elsewhere. She closed one eye and began squinting at the sun.

'Look Alice, Dominic, a friend of mine is having a party next weekend, out at his place in the New Territories, and I want you to come. I'm going to take you to Lane Crawford's to buy something to wear, and we'll finish up at The Alleys to get you a new bag and a bit of jewellery. How does that sound?' If I had expected her to gush with gratitude, I was to be disappointed. Alice looked uneasy. She sucked on a strand of windblown hair that trailed over her mouth, then hooked it out of her face with a bent finger. I saw with annoyance she had chewed her nails since the last time I painted them. They looked dreadful, as if some small animal had been gnawing at them. I glanced down at my own perfect painted talons, and smiled smugly.

'I don't have much money at the moment,' she protested.

'Oh, don't worry about that,' I told her airily. 'I know where to lay my hands on some cash.' And I did. A few dollars here and there, Mother would never even miss it.

She frowned with concentration, then her face darkened. 'I don't know if I'd be very good at sex.' She ran a hand up and down the swing chain nervously.

'Oh, sex is simple. Nothing to it,' I assured her with authority. 'You just open your legs and he'll do the rest. Wriggle about a bit, make noises and pretend you're enjoying it. It's easy.'

Ghost—1972

Even without studying the Fortune Telling Sticks, *Kau Chime*, my advice to Alice is to skip the New Territories party Nicola wants her to attend. I see evil spirits hovering over the house. However, despite frantic efforts to communicate my black premonition to Alice, she allows herself to be alternately browbeaten and cajoled by Nicola into going.

She looks like a painted doll when she finally totters out on foolishly high heels to the maroon Hillman Husky that draws up outside the flat lobby to collect us. Nicola has chosen a lime green-mini skirt for her sister, and a skimpy, sleeveless, white T-shirt. She has lent her a cap she said she purchased in Carnaby Street, with the British Union Jack emblazoned on it. The outfit is finished off with white PVC boots that are a size too large, also on loan, and fishnet tights. She has painted Alice's face, applying a thick layer of shiny, green eye-shadow above each eye, and stroking on so much mascara that her eyelashes clump together like dried mud. They feel heavy when she blinks. She wears a slick of crimson lipstick as well that makes her mouth feel all slippery. Nicola has dabbed scent behind Alice's ears and put three condoms in her sister's bag.

'Make sure he wears one,' she advises.

'Hop in,' cries a voice from the front seat of the car moments later. It is the driver, whose name Nicola says is Rory. Following Nicola into the back seat of the car, Alice recognises Alan, her sister's newest conquest, and another boy who introduces himself as Scott. Nicola sits on Alan's lap and they disappear in a clinch, only stopping to come up for air. Before we reach the end of the drive, Scott lifts a bottle out of a rucksack at his feet and offers Alice a swig. Alice raises it to her mouth and gulps. Then she coughs and splutters, and as the bottle is handed round they all laugh amiably. The sensation of warmth and well-being now radiating outward from Alice's stomach is a new experience for her. The back windows of the car are open and the warm night air pours in. The stars seem very large to Alice as the car races down The Peak. They are spinning in the firmament, their silver cores dividing. Then Alice finds herself on Scott's lap. She is kissing him, and he is kissing her back. He has soft, fair hair, and lips that, when she sees them made gold in the aureole of a street lamp, look as if they have been sculpted. Scott's tongue probes inside her mouth. It is rough and dry, and she likes the sandpaper rub of it.

We cross to Kowloon on the Star Ferry. In between kisses, Alice stares at the myriad colours weaving over Victoria harbour. They are reflections of the neon advertisements that decorate the waterfront buildings. They slither over the black fabric of the sea, a basin teeming with phosphorescent eels. They make Alice feel a little light-headed. Minutes later we dock and thread our way on through the busy Kowloon streets. We pass shops open for business despite the late hour, pavements heaving with people. A night sky criss-crossed with poles of laundry hovers over us. Gradually the blocks of shops, businesses, and flats thin, the hubbub of life is quelled, and the lights are extinguished. We seem to have been driving for a very long time when at last we arrive at the party. Rory pulls up on a triangle of grass at the centre of the double driveway. Alice's bottom and thighs feel numb from sitting on Scott's bony knees for so long. We tumble out. Alice's PVC boots crunch on the gravel. The house is grand, Alice decides, her eyes sweeping giddily from ground to rooftop. Light pours from the upstairs windows. Alice's gaze travels unsteadily downwards to the pillared porch. The front door is wide-open, music streaming into the night.

At first Alice is with Scott, pushing her way into the throng, but she soon loses him. Inside the house the ground floor is dark, darker than outside it seems to Alice. And the music is loud, so loud you cannot talk. It feels to Alice as if she is descending into a sea of interlocking people, who have to undo themselves to let her through. At first she tries to search for Nicola, but it is too crowded to spot her. Someone pushes a bottle of beer into Alice's hands, and she drinks it without tasting the liquid. She stands by herself, her back against the wall and sees shapes moving on the settee close to her, and shapes moving on the floor in front of her. Then Alice's head is wheeling, and her cheeks and ears are on fire, and her eyes are watering with the smoke from so many cigarettes. There is a song playing with someone whispering French words. It feels as if the singer is standing next to Alice, crooning right into her ear. A boy takes her empty bottle away and pulls her into the middle of the room.

'You're lovely,' he says.

He is much taller than Alice and speaks into her

hair. She reaches up and realises her Union Jack cap must have fallen off. She wants to go and look for it, but the boy she is dancing with holds her close. She can feel his hands running up and down her body, touching her shoulders, the small of her back, her bottom, leaning over her. Then he is easing his hand into the groove between her buttock cheeks, and on between her thighs. The room is baking hot, like a lit oven. Alice feels sweat pricking all over her body. Her heart is thundering. She feels as if she is being cooked alive. The boy clamps his mouth over hers. The taste of his tongue is sour. He thrusts it deeper and deeper into Alice's mouth until she feels she might gag.

'Sweet,' says the boy huskily. Then, 'Let's go outside.' He tugs us after him without waiting for Alice's reply. She stumbles in her over-large boots, tripping over sprawled limbs. She hears someone swear at her. Outside, the cool air meets her hot cheeks like a splash of water. She notices two people by the side of the porch kissing, and someone, she is not sure if it is a boy or a girl, hunched in the shadows by the drive smoking a cigarette. When they draw on it, the tip glows orange in the blackness. Alice wants to pause to take it all in. But 'he' is still pulling her, gripping her wrist, dragging her over the gravel, around the side of the house, through the back garden. We pass under a lamp and Alice sees that he has a mane of red hair, this boy who is leading her she knows not where. It glistens in the lamplight. It looks magical, like the hair of a sorcerer, hair that has been dipped in molten copper. Something brushes across her face and she swipes it away. We come to a narrow path that leads downwards. I plead with Alice to turn back.

'The evil spirit, I can feel him here, Alice, with us. Go back before it is too late!' And Alice is suddenly afraid. She freezes in her tracks, and tries to dig her white boots into the dirt path. She wishes to go no further.

'I want to go back inside again,' she says, her voice lifting on the night air.

'Don't be silly.'

He draws us further and further down the path. Alice keeps losing her footing in the treacherous boots, slipping and sliding after him.

'I don't know you,' she calls out, but her words feel gummy and unwieldy.

'Of course you do,' the boy retorts gruffly, halting and rounding on her. Then his voice changes. It becomes soft and malleable, the way I know he wants Alice to be. 'I'm Warren. And I know who you are. You're Nicola's sister.'

Alice nods but she doesn't feel very sure, with the party still reverberating in her head, and the French words ringing in her ears, and the velvet blackness all about her.

'You're beautiful,' says Warren. He runs a thumb pad along her heart-shaped jawline

But Alice still resists, shying away from him, trying to free her wrist from his clasp.

'This path leads to a beach, a small beach so pretty it will take your breath away,' coaxes Warren, looking down on her. His face is in shadow. Alice cannot see his eyes. 'Come with me, Alice.'

Then Alice goes, and she is not sure why she does, except that he called her name. The path winds down quite steeply in places, and sometimes Alice feels she is falling. But Warren catches her and steadies her. And when at last we are there, stepping into a tiny cove, a small sickle of sand studded with a single boulder, and sea frills ruffling and sighing on the shore, Alice's breath does leave her body for an instant. She wants to stop. Nothing more. Just stop and be.

But Warren is impatient, urging her on. And soon Warren is lying on the sickle of sand, and he is wrenching Alice's arm until she topples over in the ill-fitting boots, twisting an ankle. She gives a cry at the sudden pain. But the cry is muffled, for now it is hard to breathe, with the weight of Warren pressing down on her. She wants to push him off but he is too heavy. She is scared she may suffocate. The breath is coming to her in tight little gasps, and she has to fight to expand her lungs and draw it in. Her hands flay in the sand, scattering it like a crab bent on burying itself, seeking the sanctuary of a sandy grave. But she is trapped there. Warren's large hands are all over her now, prising her apart like the two halves of shell, looking for the soft inside of her. He is between her thighs, plucking at her spider web tights, tearing them off, pinching at her flesh. A wave of rage so intense blooms in Alice suddenly, a primitive rage, a rage born of some other place, of some other time: the rage of a small Chinese girl who will not relinquish life.

'No, I don't want to,' Alice screams into the night, expelling every atom of air she possesses.

'Shut up!' snarls Warren, rearing up over her, one hand freeing his sex, the other ripping at her pants. 'Are you a little prick-teaser, Alice Safford?

Is that what you are?' Warren shouts as his sex tears into the dew-soaked essence of her, thrusting again and again.

Alice's lips move but no sound comes. His red hair in the moonlight is incandescent, and when he rocks back, a crown of stars adorns his head. From the boulder a little way off I watch. I want to weep, but I am bound in a place where no tears are shed. When it is done, Warren rises to his feet quite calmly. He fumbles with his trousers and zips his fly, standing over Alice.

'Prick-teaser!' he mutters again. Then he saunters off, up the path and back to the party.

For a long while Alice lies still, while the moonlight slides across surface of the dimpled dark water, and the stars glitter down. She listens to the lap and plash and hiss of it, and breathes in the pungent air, flavoured with salt. She is aware of the blood trickling down her inner thighs and soaking into the sand. It hurts when she sits up. She hugs her knees, her little fingers tightly curled. At last she scrambles onto all fours and retches bile and beer, until her stomach is empty. When she is finished she wipes her hand over her mouth, and sits back on her heels. She looks beyond the tiny beach, at the ink black line of the horizon, where water and air seem to fuse. From here her eyes rove over the sea, across the arch of sky, and along the curve of sand. Warren is right, Alice thinks, this is a lovely place.

When she is able she stands. Her boots have come off in the struggle, and now she peels off her shredded tights and her pants. She lifts her lime-green mini skirt and bunches it at her waist, holding it there. She steps into the sea, and squats in the spume. With one hand she washes herself, cupping the seawater to her. Her secret tender places sting and smart but she is anaesthetized to it. Finally she dashes water on her face, and then she steps out of the sea. She stoops for her tights, scrunches them up and places them between her legs to soak up the blood. She pulls her tattered pants up over them. She collects up her white boots, bends stiffly and climbs into them. And as she turns towards the path, taking slow careful steps over the sand on her wobbling legs, I slip off the boulder where I have been perched. I weave round her shaking shoulders and gather her in.

Ghost—1972

The first time I hear it, the sound is as light as the 'plink' of a raindrop falling into the sea. I dismiss it, for bodies can be noisy places to dwell in, the thunderclap of the heart that reverberates through organs and flesh and muscle, the 'shush-shush' of blood endlessly circumnavigating the body, the bubbling of gastric juices. It is a hive of activity day and night. But even so . . . even so, I hear it distinctly, the isolated drop plinking into the sea, there to be swiftly swallowed, and another falling after it. This sound instead of fading away grows in volume. It swells imperceptibly at first and so I take no real account of it. But then the drop in the sea becomes a drop in a lake, and the drop in a lake becomes a drop in a bath, and the drop in a bath becomes a beat, a second heartbeat! Its relentless rhythm jars on my spirit. On further investigation, I discover the interloper burrowing into the rich, red lining of Alice's womb. It might look innocuous with its dumpling head and its seahorse tail, but I soon discover it has barbs sunk deep into my host. I know this, for when I stir up the pocket of water it dwells in, and wrench at the slippery tail, it holds fast and will not budge.

To my consternation, as time passes the minute creature more than doubles in size. It takes all Alice's reserves of energy for nourishment. There is nothing left for me. My host's body turns in upon itself. It is transformed into a cocoon, and this thing is the pupa encased within it. I tell Alice there is a parasite blockading itself inside her, making her body an impenetrable fortress. While she gives it sanctuary, I warn, it plots her undoing. And, more importantly, I feel certain it seeks to obliterate me.

My host is staring at a fish when first she feels the parasite quicken, the flutter of tiny limbs pounding the elastic walls of her uterus. Perhaps now my host will do something to stop this impending disaster, I think. So while Alice follows a fish, as it glides through the water of a tank on the Sea Palace floating restaurant in Aberdeen, within her another fish stirs. The family is attending a special dinner held by Mr Huang, Ralph Safford's boat-builder. Ralph is the guest of honour. While everyone settled themselves about the table upstairs, we slipped away. We are downstairs watching the fish that customers will select for their meals, their fate, an eminently suitable end for our little fish, I conclude sourly.

'There is a baby swimming in a tank inside me,' Alice whispers, the fingers of her hands pressing lightly on the glass side of the tank.

'Soon,' Alice marvels silently as we journey home that night, 'it will be Christmas, and Harry will be home, and there will be another party with mother glittering like a dragonfly, and darting from one guest to another in a wave of perfume. There will be a feast and gifts, and Jillian will scowl at me, and Nicola will bring home new boyfriends. And all the while the child within me will grow and grow.'

Does my host not recall how this squatter came into being? Can she not see that the coming of it does not bode well for either of us? But like a stubborn child who does not attend to the omniscient parent, Alice refutes my truth. Meanwhile I settle back and brace myself for the quake to come, a seism that I know will shake the shared foundations of our world.

Myrtle—1972

It is a fine day. There is a mosaic of sunshine on the tiled veranda floor, grouted with wire mesh shadows. Very pretty really. I intend to make the most of it, though I did pop on a cardigan before venturing outside. I am sitting back on a wicker chair browsing through a recipe book, trying to come up with a few fresh ideas for the Boxing Day spread. I am really looking forward to it this year. Of course, one or two familiar faces will be missing which is sad. Phillip has already spoken to me and explained that he cannot face it. Entirely understandable I told him. Still, such a shame. He will be greatly missed. But who knows, by next year he may be feeling his old self again. You can't go on grieving forever I told him, with just the right balance of sympathy and pragmatism in my voice. Poor dear Amanda would never want that, I assured him. She would want him to go forward and be happy, if only for the children's sake.

For some unknown reason I am feeling elated today, as heady as a girl having her first taste of champagne. Christmas does that to you, doesn't it? The thought of family and friends all together celebrating the festive season, and nobody to spoil it, no cloud to blot out the sun. I must stop rambling and concentrate, plan menus and list ingredients, then explain exactly what I want to the amahs, make sure there are no misunderstandings. I can't afford any disasters this year. Ralph says Charles Yeung the film director is coming, he even hinted the Governor might look in. Mr Gao has promised that my dress will be ready in time, and as I know he won't want to lose my custom I can afford to be optimistic. Ralph wants me to wear the black pearls he bought me for my birthday. They'll finish the outfit off perfectly.

I do hope recent events don't jeopardise the success of the party. It's been a trying fortnight. I had to let Ah Lee go. Such a shame because she's been with us for a good many years, since we arrived now I come to think of it, seen the children grow up. But I simply cannot have a thief in my home. Despicable as it is, Ah Lee has been stealing from me. Goodness knows how long it's been going on for, but I first became aware of it at the close of the summer. And now two hundred dollars gone from my purse! Two hundred dollars!

At the start of last week I withdrew it from my account at the Hong Kong and Shanghai Bank. I wrote it up on my chequebook stub (I'm meticulous about that kind of thing), and tucked it away for the Christmas shopping trip I was planning on the Wednesday with Pippa Burley. Imagine my shock when I fished in my purse to pay for the cab, and found it was missing. Well, I simply could not let that go.

How could I tell it was Ah Lee and not Ah Dang? Easy. Ah Dang was away. Her mother who lived in Shanghai was very ill, and Ah Dang begged leave to visit her, leave I felt obliged to grant despite the inconvenience. Sadly, I believe she did pass away. I'm not sure Ah Dang made it in time to say her goodbyes. But at least she was able to see the rest of her family and be there for the funeral. So you see there can be no doubt about the identity of the culprit. Actually I have been aware of cash going missing for some time now. Ten dollars here, twenty dollars there. It niggles at you, but at first you tell yourself you've been careless, forgotten an expense or two. After a while though it becomes clear that it's more than that. Of course I didn't rush in accusing her until I was certain. I double-checked my purse, my bag, even my coat pockets and the drawers of my dressing table, before I confronted her.

I called her into the lounge and made sure we were not disturbed. I had my purse open on the coffee table when she came in and I caught the unmistakable flash of guilt in those devious, slanted eyes. Still, she denied it of course. Well, she would wouldn't she? Standing there wringing her hands and looking penitent. Quite pathetic really. I think I would have had more respect for her if she'd owned up immediately. But these servants are continually thinking they can hoodwink their employers. I am beginning to believe that it's an inherent condition. Of course I'm no stranger to servants stealing from us. I recall Aden only too well, Ralph simply avoiding the issue in the hope it would disappear. This time I intended to deal with it head-on.

'Mrs Safford, I not take your money. Please, it not me who did it,' she wailed when I asked her outright.

By now tears were streaming down her face, and really I began to feel sorry for the pathetic woman. But I had to dismiss her all the same. It was an impossible situation. I can't have someone in my home stealing from me and lying to me. Think what effect it might have on my children, being exposed to that kind of immorality. I know the silly woman has probably had no education, that as a result she may struggle to distinguish right from wrong. But I can't help that. Perhaps after this she'll acquire a more discerning nature. I told her I was sorry, but I was giving her notice and I wanted her out within the week. I was extremely generous actually, sending her off with an entire month's salary. But as for the reference she begged me for, it was more than I could do in good conscience. How could I write a letter of recommendation for her, when that would be virtually giving her a helping hand in securing another placement, and an opportunity to carry on with her thieving— possibly in the home of someone I know? Simply out of the question.

'I send money home, Mrs Safford, to my family

in China. Please, please let me stay? I very sorry, Mrs Safford. I will work harder. No holidays. Please please. If I cannot get job, Mrs Safford, how can I live?' she begged. No giggling now, I observed dryly.

Well, she should have thought of that before she started pinching cash from my purse. I was firm, I had to be. I'm not a heartless woman, oh no. But there are limits and I'm afraid Ah Lee pushed beyond them. The consequence of this is that a new amah, Ah Wei, starts on Monday. And all this with the party coming up. Quite honestly it's a nightmare for me. But I shall just have to muddle through.

Suddenly I am aware that Alice is standing on the veranda, her back to me. Her arms are stretched wide, the fingers of her hands poking through the wire mesh. I find myself tuning in to the noises that surround me. The murmur of traffic, the distant sound of machinery as some building project goes forward. A dog barking. The lingering notes of a xylophone struck by a Chinese pedlar in the field below. The banter between two coolies returning home down The Peak after a day's manual work. And the patter of Alice's light voice. She stops speaking abruptly, and I realise it is the absence of her speech and not the presence of it that startles me.

'Stuffed pork. It might be nice cold with pickles for Boxing Day. What do you think, Alice?' I ask, with no expectation of a reply, jotting down a few notes on the pad I am resting on the open pages of a large cookbook.

'Mm. I'm going to have a baby,' says Alice.

What strikes me first about this reply is that is

does not fit the question I have posed. Both question and answer revolve slowly in my head. Side by side they are incongruous, an antithesis to each other. Cooking and procreation. The harder I try to match them up, the less sense they make.

'I'm going to have a baby,' Alice says again.

'You're going to have a baby,' I parrot stupidly, following the intonation of her voice exactly, as if I am repeating a lesson with the assistance of a language tape. Why does Alice always have to talk in riddles, I muse? Why can't she just say what she means? I sigh testily, close my book, sandwiching both pad and pencil inside it, and set it down on the glass-topped table at my side. I slip off my reading glasses and let them dangle on the gold chain to which they are fastened . I have been rather enjoying the winter sunshine, the prospect of the party, and of Harry's homecoming for the holidays. But Alice just has to ruin it. 'What are you talking about, Alice?' I demand, my tone nettled.

Bear, who is basking on the warm tiles, stirs in his sleep. Alice withdraws her fingers from the wire mesh, lets her hands crawl like spiders over it for a moment, before spinning round to face me. She repeats for the third time, quietly, and one might almost say pedantically, that she is expecting a baby. I solve the riddle. I sit forward, my back suddenly rigid, as if a steel rod had been thrust down my spine. My hands, resting in my lap, stiffen, the joints lock. I glance over my shoulder to make sure no one is near, not Jillian or Nicola, or one of the amahs eavesdropping, for despite them playing dumb, I suspect they understand a great deal more than they let on. I even stand and check that Beth is not sitting, sunning herself on her veranda next door, as we all know to our cost what sharp little eyes and ears my neighbour has. Then I retake my seat and address Alice.

'How do you know?' I say in a tone low but distinct.

'Because last night at the restaurant I felt it move,' Alice reveals.

She turns away from me again and appears to be looking down on the Chinese pedlar, while her fingers orchestrate his silly little tune. There is a draught. I shiver and do up the cardigan buttons at my neck. My eyes bore into Alice's back and then veer from head to toe. I reappraise my daughter, for clearly while I was not looking she has changed. I observe her jeans, pale-blue denim stitched in strong, white cotton, and note that her legs look extremely thin, giving the impression that they are out of proportion with the rest of her body. My eyes rove over the sweatshirt she wears.

It is a black and purple tie-dye which I believe I saw Alice making. I recall her peeling back the lids of small, silver drums of dye, and emptying the powder into an old fish kettle, swirling the liquid about with a wooden ladle, a ladle now permanently stained the colour lips turn after eating a surfeit of blackberries. I remember too how she tended the livid brew, simmering it slowly over the gas stove. With my sharp intake of breath, the vinegary dry smell of boiling dye returns to me. I even have a vague recollection of seeing her sitting earlier at the dining room table, knotting glass marbles, clear but for a spiral of primary red, yellow or blue, into the white, jersey cotton.

I take in her plain, brown hair as well, loose,

unkempt and dull. She is, I conclude, just an ordinary girl. There is absolutely nothing remarkable or even memorable about her. And yet, as I look on my daughter grown into a teenager, I feel a band of ice tightening about my heart. The years peel away, and I am in the delivery room of a hospital peering into her creased, newborn face for the first time, the same wintry dread closing over me. My hands flutter to my hair, and fidget with a small, tortoiseshell comb tucked there.

'Are you . . . you . . . quite sure?' I falter.

'Yes,' replies Alice, head tilting, ears straining, as if keen not to miss a single note played by the pedlar far below. 'Can I throw him a dollar? He's playing so nicely?' She seems unwilling to tear her eyes away from him.

I tell Alice to stay where she is. I go inside and pour myself a large scotch. I catch sight of Ah Dang in the dining room. I instruct her that I am not to be disturbed under any circumstances, that she is to keep watch over the lounge door. She nods, folding her arms solemnly and moving to stand sentry in the hall. Then, drink in hand, closing the lounge door resolutely behind me, I cross to the centre of the Chinese carpet, and stare out through the glass doors at Alice. I take a slug of scotch. While I wait for it to take effect, I glimpse a future in which Alice does not cooperate, where she has the child, destroys our standing in the community, makes our family the hot topic of gossip on the island, wrecks her father's career, and consigns the Safford family to obscurity. For this is truly the scandal that will bring us all down, down to Alice's level! I glimpse myself too, spending the remainder of my life looking after a brat Alice has spawned.

And all this because my daughter has cheapened herself with some lout. You cannot even guarantee he is white. It will be in the papers. Everyone will know. The governor will be informed. My role as a mother will come under scrutiny. And because the stigma will never vanish, the shame will always be with us. As for my mother, I can already feel the dark, pebble eyes turning on me with triumphant contempt.

I am determined. I stride forward and open the veranda door.

'I think you'd better come inside,' I tell Alice.

'But the man playing the music,' Alice prevaricates, 'shan't we throw him a dollar as he's playing so—'

'Never mind the pedlar, Alice.' I slice through her words smoothly. I take pains to keep my voice steady, cordial. I take my seat on the settee and gesture for Alice to take hers on the armchair opposite me. 'Sit down and shut the door,' I direct her. Alice does as I bid. And even when she springs up immediately to let Bear in, who, realising he has been deserted has begun whining and pawing at the base of the door, still I keep my sang-froid. I set my tumbler of scotch down on the coffee table. To my surprise my hands are rock-steady. I flick my tongue across my lips and manage a taut smile.

'Alice . . . you have been unfortunate and possibly naive,' I say.

There is a pause. The clock on the mantelpiece ticks. The tiny porcelain, jade and ivory people in the glass-fronted lacquer cabinet by the lounge door, seem to have braced their Lilliputian limbs, waiting for something to happen. Alice, intent on running her fingers like a comb through Bear's coat, picking off any burrs she encounters there, makes no response.

'Who . . . who . . . um,' I begin, and then almost immediately flounder. 'Doesn't matter,' I chirp up, as if the identity of the father is a mere technicality, a minor detail of no real import, which is in fact the truth. For the child, as far as I am concerned, is not destined for this world. Child! It is merely a ball of cells, the result of life getting out of hand, proceeding unchecked. The father's name is entirely immaterial. 'No, no, it really doesn't matter.' My splutter of girlish laughter strikes the wrong chord. I try to attain gravitas in my timbre. 'But you must see, Alice, there is no future in this either for yourself or for the . . . mm . . .' The notes of the xylophone come stretched and distorted, tinkling through the closed glass doors, refusing to be excluded. 'But I'm sure you have already come to accept this, Alice, and so . . . and so quite rightly you have come to me, your mother to assist you in . . . well, in sorting this little problem out. You have been sensible, Alice, and I commend you for it,' I throw in recklessly, remembering the value of flattery when dealing with rebellious progeny.

'So I have been naive *and* sensible?' queries Alice. I should like to have slapped her then, hard, across that ordinary face of hers.

I breathe on a smile, but it fails to ignite. I continue, undeterred by this less than promising start. 'I'm sure you must see what a disaster this would be for your father, Alice, in the important

223

position he holds in government in the colony. And not only that, what a disaster it would be for *you* at such a critical time in your education, were you to continue in your . . . condition.' My eyes keep straying to Alice's waist, trying to detect a thickening there. But I can see nothing and this fuels some scrap of hope that it is all a fabrication, a malicious ploy to inflict distress upon me. Though even as I try to latch onto this comfort, intuitively I know this is no sham. 'Alice, this could ruin your father's life. You can't want that.'

Alice says nothing. 'Children, Alice, require enormous self-sacrifice,' I state feelingly. 'Not to mention the financial cost of rearing a family. I'm sure when you are ready and you have found yourself a nice husband you will have a child, well . . . children, if that is what you really want. But surely you see that this is not that moment,' I finish persuasively.

Finally it appears that I have Alice's attention. No doubt the mention of her father has penetrated, even if she is immune to the misery she will inflict on me if she is obstinate. I see the flicker of uncertainty in her face and seize the advantage. 'Alice you don't have to worry about a thing. I'll arrange it all. The sooner the better if you ask me. The first thing is to fix up an appointment with a doctor and get it all confirmed, and then of course have it dealt with speedily.' In the silence that follows I sense it is incumbent upon me to conclude matters with a show of maternal understanding.

'I'm not unsympathetic, Alice, honestly I'm not. These things happen. You're a young lady growing up fast. It's good that you told me.' Alice rises, her eyes registering nothing. 'You leave it to me to explain to your father.' I take her mute show for acquiescence. 'And Alice,' I caution her just before she goes. 'No one is to know about this. No one! Your father's reputation depends on it. Do you understand?'

'He's stopped playing now, the pedlar,' Alice comments regretfully. 'It's too late.'

'Alice! Do you understand how imperative it is that you tell no one?' In this if nothing else my voice is unequivocal.

At the door Alice turns back. 'Oh yes, I understand,' my daughter says. 'I understand everything, Mother.'

'And you mustn't concern yourself you know. This kind of procedure is very commonplace these days. It's all quite safe, and it'll be over before you know it.' I have been running a finger around the rim of my crystal tumbler. The eerie whine it suddenly emits takes me completely unawares. I jump and pull my hand back as if I have been stung. 'Alice, this is for the best.'

But when I glance up, Alice has left, closing the door silently behind her.

The next day, following a thorough examination of Alice, I am given alarming news. My daughter's pregnancy is a good deal more advanced than first suspected, I am informed by Johnny Sheung. He is the gynaecologist I decide it is prudent to deal with, having shown himself to be most circumspect in the past. We are at his home in Causeway Bay, the nature of the meeting meriting complete privacy and confidentiality. While I speak to Mr Sheung in the seclusion of his study, Alice waits in the hall. Any hope I might harbour that Alice's pregnancy is all in her mind, the result of wild, teenage fantasies, is summarily crushed when he delivers his pronouncement.

'I estimate that your daughter's pregnancy, Mrs Safford, is of at least sixteen weeks gestation, maybe more. To terminate it at this stage will be a complicated procedure,' Mr Sheung tells me gravely in his sibilant voice, his elbows propped on his leather inlaid desktop. He laces his long, graceful, effeminate fingers together under his dimpled chin. I shrug, indicating that it cannot be helped. Mr Sheung nods his understanding of the delicate situation we find ourselves in.

We discuss the transfer of a considerable sum of money from my private account, with the Hong Kong and Shanghai Bank, to the account of Grace Sung, Mr Sheung's married sister, avoiding any direct link between us. In addition to this, I obtain Mr Sheung's personal pledge that he will never divulge to Alice's father how far advanced her pregnancy was at the time of the termination. He also gives me his personal guarantee that all records of the procedure will be destroyed. Then Mr Sheung hands me a slip of paper with an address in Kwun Tong, Kowloon printed on it. He tells me to deliver Alice there, late on Friday night.

To my cursory inquiries as to both the calibre of the equipment to be used, and the standards of hygiene employed in the operation, Mr Sheung gives me first an offended look, and second, effusive assurances. Losing Alice, I tell him pithily, is not an option. Finally, well pleased with Mr Sheung's grasp of our predicament, I close by telling him that I feel quite certain that Government funding for the building of his new birth control clinic will be approved. Further, I give my personal guarantee that the right people will be acquainted with the importance of his project. At this a smile passes between us. We both know that an understanding has been reached.

And to Alice I say after the appointment, as I pull out into busy traffic, 'Mr Sheung informs me that it's all going to be fine. Now, isn't that splendid news?'

Ralph—1972

It is crisp, clear night. The chauffeur-driven car purrs round tight bends as it ascends The Peak. I lean back in my seat and sigh tiredly. I am bone-weary. You have days like this in my job, days when you feel nothing more can be wrung out of you. How many times have I repeated this journey home, my mind wrestling with the dilemmas of government office, discarding one problem by the roadside only to gather another, domestic this time, as the car shifts down a gear, the slope steepens, and I near the flat on The Peak. Tonight I can just make out the dusky shapes of the mountains beneath the night sky. It is hard looking at these curves so redolent of the dips and swells of a human body, not to imagine the island alive, a recumbent colossus, ready at any moment to gather up the folds of his garments and shake us all off, into the oil-black ocean. How whimsical I am tonight, as if I am still resonating with the extraordinary events of the day. I rake a hand through my hair and lightly touch my furrowed brow. Glancing at my faint reflection in the polished glass window, I confess to it, that what has primarily absorbed me over the past ten hours, are not matters of state and government, but the nigh on impossible task of keeping the secretaries in my office happy. Am I a fraud I wonder?

Bands of amber light slide over the car seat as we move beneath streetlamps. It is soporific. I close my eyes and picture my personal secretary, Vivian Yau. She has thick, black hair, always drawn back in a ponytail or a bun. It is surprisingly lacklustre, this hair of hers, as if it has been frazzled after one too many perms. Her face is broad, her eyes set a little too wide apart. She wears thick-rimmed, round-framed glasses that rather exaggerate this feature. Her complexion is wan. Occasionally her face erupts into a rash of spots over the bridge of her nose, or under her chin. She looks in dire need of fresh air and fun. Neither are in plentiful supply in government offices however. I recall her as she stood before my desk some weeks ago, arms folded, tight-lipped, glasses propped on the end of her nose, humourlessly peering over the rims. I asked her to sit down and gestured to the chair in front of her. She declined stiffly. I loosened my tie slightly. The temperature was definitely rising in my office. I gave her a brief, questioning smile and was met with an onslaught.

'Mr Safford, my family has very bad luck since we moved to these new offices. My nephew, he breaks his leg falling down a hole, and the doctor says now there are complications and recovery may take long time, several months even.'

'Oh dear, I'm sorry to hear—' I began, my

stomach already in a knot, a sense of foreboding growing in me.

Vivian rushed on. 'And now my father feeling very bad, and coughing all the time, and having to go to the hospital for X-rays, and my sister Christine, seven months pregnant, says the baby not moving last week. The doctor very worried. My brother as well, he loses lots of money on the races at Happy Valley, and he never loses, always wins.' Vivian paused to draw breath and blinked accusingly at me. 'What you going to do about this, Mr Safford?'

I twiddled my cufflinks and made an effort to assemble my features into a suitably grave expression.

'I am very sorry for your troubles, Vivian, truly I am, but I fail to see—' I sallied forth bravely.

Vivian interrupted with another volley of complaints. 'It is this office, Mr Safford. Very bad luck place.' She revolved slowly, her eyes narrowing as they roved around the newly decorated walls. With a sneer she took in the paintings of Hong Kong island as it was when the British first arrived, bought so recently and hung as a finishing touch, the wide window giving on to fabulous views of Hong Kong's skyline, and the harbour, with its busy sea traffic all jostling for space in the crowded waters. She took in the stylish mock-antique filing cabinets, her sharp gaze finally coming to rest on the expensive, plush carpet, fitted only a month ago. She lifted one shoe and examined it carefully, as if she had inadvertently stepped in dog's mess. 'Not good fortune in this office. Better fortune in last office,' was her unwavering conclusion.

Good God, I railed inwardly, one hand kneading the back of my neck. Does Vivian really think I can be held responsible for her nephew falling down a hole, and all her other family mishaps? And if, incredible as it seemed, she did consider me culpable in this tale of woe, what was I supposed to do about it? Did she expect me to vacate the stunning new premises we had been allocated? Was I supposed to insist on moving back to our former, shabbier, far less attractive offices, smack in the middle of Central, hemmed in on all sides?

'You do something, Mr Safford, or I don't know what happen,' Vivian told me curtly, barely veiling the implied threat. She turned on her heels and exited, making it clear she had delivered her ultimatum. If I did not want to find my office in turmoil, I had better act, and fast.

Before the day was up, I had visits from two more secretaries, Valerie and Cynthia. Valerie complaining that she had been plagued with stomach cramps every day since our arrival at the new offices, and that her landlord had suddenly told her he would not renew her lease. While she spoke, she fingered a mysterious rash on her arm that she said had only just appeared. In her wake Cynthia tramped in, reddened eyes welling up with tears, to declare that her fiancée had postponed their marriage for a year.

For the remainder of the afternoon reports lay unread, letters unwritten, and incoming callers were advised that Mr Safford was in an important meeting. In fact I was fully occupied tracking down a geomancer. He assured me he would divine the cause of our troubles at the government offices, and remedy the situation, bringing us *zhu ni hao yun*, good luck. A mutually suitable time was arranged for his visit, though to be honest as the days passed, so uncomfortable was the atmosphere at the office, I would have been prepared to put off the Governor, Sir Murray MacLehose, to restore equilibrium.

So this morning my office was visited by a geomancer, Mr Lee. He was a wizened old man with rheumy eyes, the pupils consumed in his brown irises, a wispy, white beard trailing from his pointed chin. He was clad theatrically in a silky, black Kung-Fu outfit, and he carried a battered, leather bag which I was to discover was full of instruments. These tools of his trade, I found somewhat disappointingly, resembled nothing so much as the protractor and compass I once possessed for use in Maths' class at my childhood school. Without further ado he walked portentously around the office, observing the position of window, doors, desks and filing cabinets, and measuring the angles between them.

He then announced self-importantly, in a surprisingly deep bass, that the plate-glass window must be partially covered with the large portrait of Queen Elizabeth. He had been eyeing this where it hung on the wall, since he arrived. He also demanded that my desk be moved, so that when seated at it, I no longer had the fantastic view of Hong Kong harbour, but rather at an expanse of grey wall. When I set my jaw at this ridiculous suggestion, the geomancer suddenly became very animated. He circled his arms expansively, inhaled deeply and produced a high-pitched nasal hum,

231

reminding me of a mosquito.

'Not cover window, not move desk, bad fortune stay,' he finally proclaimed, hastily packing instruments back into his extraordinary bag.

As the secretaries led by Vivian bustled in, however, I relented. I summoned two colleagues, who I have no doubt were conjecturing privately that I had lost my wits, to heave my large desk into a dark corner, facing nothing more exciting than several yards of grey emulsion. The portrait of Her Majesty was then set up on the windowsill, blocking much of the view and most of the light. I was then asked to part with a considerable amount of cash for the privilege of having this trickster disrupt my offices. As I wrote out the cheque, I swear that the delight Mr Lee was taking in my wretchedness was palpable. He sucked on his crooked front teeth impishly. Then he snatched the cheque from me with one hand, while with the other he smoothed a long whisker that protruded from a mole, growing to one side of his prominent hooked nose.

'Stay like this, very lucky,' he declared magisterially, giving the whisker a final twang, his eyes raking over the office one last time. Finally, to beams of approval from the secretaries, and a promise of a return visit, just to check the fortuitous angles were being maintained, the wily Mr Lee took his leave.

That is the trouble, I reflect, as we round the last bend and start up the long incline of the driveway. I like to think I perform well at times of crisis in government. Riots down town, bodies washed down the river from China, landslides that cut off The Peak, where supplies have to be

232

airlifted up to the residents, a flue epidemic, a visit from the Beatles or a visit from the Pope, both having much the same effect of public hysteria—these events I can cruise through. But it is the mundaneness of life I cannot handle—the plodding, the pettiness, the fusses over nothing, the superstitious secretaries. As we draw up outside the lobby and the chauffeur, a new chap, likeable enough, leaps out to open my door, Amanda puts in an appearance. She does that from time to time these days. Not content with haunting my dreams, now she materialises at the most inappropriate of times.

'Goodnight Sir,' the chauffeur peals out, cap under his arm, his head lowered to me in respect. I shuffle past with a wave, glancing at my watch and being surprised by the lateness of the hour. Amanda follows me to the lift. In the confined space the air is permeated by her scent, that intrinsic yet inexplicable fragrance that is as indescribable as it is particular. I hurry to drink it in, strangely more jealous of her in death than I think I was in life, increasingly unwilling to relinquish my ghostly lover.

As the lift progresses through the floors, we are joined by Alice, this not the anxious teenager to whom I normally return home, but her younger self, stepping out of the past. I see her clearly, as she was then, a small girl. She stands, potbellied, clad in nothing more than a bikini bottom, a turquoise background with an orange fish print, her mouse-brown hair lifting, flying, rumpled by the breeze. She gambols down Stanley beach, her legs seemingly too long, her motion coltish on the stretch of hot sand as she nears the sea. Then suddenly she stops and looks down at the briny wash, bubbling and ice cold, rushing at her feet, tickling splayed, stubby, pale toes, toes that plough in answer, into the pliant, compact, wetly-golden grit. Her narrow shoulders hunch, her chin juts forwards, her lips part, and seed-pearl teeth chatter in delight.

While others strike out for the raft or hover around the smoking barbecues, drinking and eating, engrossed in conversations too trivial to retain, my tiny daughter plays in the shallows, holding court with herself, her treble tones so soft that no one ever hears what she babbles. A miniature heathen, her hair strewn with seaweed, her hands full of shells, her face radiant, enchanted by sea and sky. Later, I rub her cold, small body vigorously with a towel, the way I have seen vets do with a new born calf to bring it round, to remind it that it is of this world, that it must relinquish that other place from whence it came. And Alice reaches for me, bridging the gap, her anemone fingers flowering inside mine, their chill, wrinkled, tentacle tips suctioning against my flesh.

The lift doors spring open and I step out, crossing to my threshold. I insert my key in the lock and pause. I am overtaken by an immediate desire to cry. I try to name the emotion that floods through me, and am stunned to know it as grief. Unaccountably I am overwhelmed with grief for my youngest daughter, for Alice. Soon I will know that the girl on the beach is a woman, and that the swell of her belly is an indication of the child that grows there. And as I struggle to grasp this, my wife tells me that arrangements are already afoot to abort the foetus, that this is without question the best way to proceed, not only for Alice but for all of us. I learn that Jimmy Sheung has agreed to perform the operation privately, and that I may rest assured that his discretion can be wholly relied upon. My hesitant questions about the identity of the father are discouraged. Myrtle insists that as Alice does not want to keep the child, excavating further is unnecessary. I drink down the scotch that Myrtle keeps pressing on me too fast, the stillness of the flat ringing in my ears. She bowls smoothly on, like a leading barrister delivering closing arguments, while my offerings are piecemeal, stilted and eventually even slurred. As the lounge clock chimes 1am I rise unsteadily and stumble to bed.

'So I take it we are agreed,' Myrtle says just before I drift off.

My lips are sealed. I roll away from my wife; my throbbing eyes latching onto the bars of the bedroom window. They have guillotined the full moon into wedges. I trail the silver segments as they fracture and twirl, as they liquefy and dribble into each other, then sink downwards towards the floor. Perhaps, I reflect foggily, in the morning I shall find them in a tangled heap under my bed. This is my last conscious thought before I pass out.

Ghost—1972

This morning I am carefree. I feel as if might almost rise up from Alice, as she lies inert on the bed, ease the metal-framed window open, slide out and ride on the thermals to soar above the island, as I once did so long ago. I nearly believe that I am alive with joy, for this very day the parasite is to be removed from Alice. Soon it will be just the two of us again. We will nurture the perfect synchronism that drew us like magnets from the first. I tell Alice this, I coo it lovingly into the flesh-pink whorl of her ear, the way when I drew breath I whispered into shells. But Alice is oddly unreceptive, merely turning away from me into her pillow. Undiscouraged I try again.

'No matter how deep the barb has been sunk, Mr Sheung will loosen it and draw the creature from you, Alice,' I tell her knowledgeably.

I have heard the gynaecologist speak of his plan to annihilate the leech, with such supreme authority that even I am convinced, and would, if I could, submit to his skilled hands gladly. I smooth Alice's brow, for it is slick with perspiration. 'Then, oh then Alice your strength will return to you. You will recover yourself. And as you do, you will recover me too.' I very nearly add that I have been increasingly poorly of late myself. As the 'thing' has grown, each day staking out another claim on my Alice, I have been ousted, permitted less and less access to the landscape of my friend. The heart that beat so generously for me has grown hostile, shaking me off to ensure 'it' flourishes. Still more perturbing, the shrunken monkey buried deep in Alice has been thriving, increasing in size at a rate that is plainly designed to intimidate me.

I call it a monkey for that is what it has come to resemble, with its wrinkled flesh coated with fine, carrot-gold hairs, and its skin smeared with some waxy, noxious grease. I have scrutinised its bloated head, disproportionate to the shrivelled, tiny body that dwindles into toothpick limbs. The hairs sprout thickest over the dome of that skull, like tufted grass. Its bead eyes are hooded with veined lids, no thicker than rice paper. Its nose lacks definition too, and squats like a pimple on the pellucid flesh. Its mouth is similar to that of a fish—a slit, swollen lips gaping open and shut as it gulps greedily at the fluidin which it basks. Between its hairy spindle thighs, I spy a scrotum dangling like a pair of cherry stones, and I have seen the cord of its monkey penis stiffen and stir, rippling the wetness. Just lately it has taken to sucking on its nib thumb, so contented is it, so secure in Alice.

The room we are in is very dull, white floors, white walls, white ceiling, white blinds. Unremitting whiteness. A nurse appears and tells Alice they are nearly ready for her. By this stage I can barely contain the excitement I feel. I am tempted to send the ceiling light into a paroxysm of flashing and sputtering. But then, I tell myself severely, such behaviour might inadvertently trigger a chain of events, the final link of which could well be the postponement of the operation. And that would never do. Alice has been given an injection that has made her drowsy and silly. She is attached to a drip that feeds a drug into her blood. I sense the sharpness of it as her cells jostle one another, and her womb tightens and then relaxes. At first this tightening is sporadic, then it increases in frequency and intensity. Soon Alice is starting to draw her legs up beneath her in the bed, squirming at the growing discomfort. Within her the monkey winces and gobbles all the harder at its thumb. Alice is wheeled along a corridor into another room, equally white. But this one I am interested to see is filled with equipment. Buzzing machines and enormous, blazing lamps, making the room unbearably hot and bright. I feel rather like an actress making her first entrance onto the stage at the start of a play, a shiver of adrenalin scissoring through her. And look, there is a tray covered with shiny instruments, like silver treasure trove.

There are four of us in attendance on Alice during the extraction, two nurses and Mr Sheung, all dressed fetchingly for the occasion in pale-blue cotton, and myself naturally. I intend to make sure everything goes by rote for Alice's sake, and for my own of course. Although I am increasingly distracted by how very queer my host is starting to look. Her eyes have grown unsettlingly large, and her lips are so dry that they have cracked. She bites down with such a vicious intensity on them that specks of blood fly up. Poor Alice! I home in on Mr Sheung, try to let him know I am watching him hawk-eyed, that he had better not make a false move. Alice's feet have been lifted into stirrups. With her pale, white legs akimbo it is easy to peek inside her and look for the coming, or perhaps I should say going, of the shrunken monkey.

There is an effervescent atmosphere in the

238

room. I am infected with it and can hardly keep still. So it appears is Mr Sheung, chatting away excitedly. He tells Alice that her cervix is dilating nicely. Alice is not very appreciative of this remark I am sorry to say, and just moans. This could be why from now on Mr Sheung and the nurses speak only in Cantonese. I offer to translate for Alice, but she does not appear the least bit interested. In the end she misses all Mr Sheung's enlivening jokes, a passable story about foot-binding, and some entertaining flirtation betwixt nurse and surgeon, with a great deal of eyelid fluttering. Such a pity!

Alice writhes and groans for what feels like hours, until I begin to feel quite alarmed. Then suddenly the place becomes a hive of activity. The nurses rush about, their shoes tap-tapping officiously on the floor. Alice begins to scream. One of them hurriedly administers another shot of something. Not a moment too soon, I find myself thinking. Alice's pallor has taken on an unpleasant green tint, her eyes are bloodshot, and her cheeks, despite their pallid hue, are boiling hot. As the drug races through her bloodstream, thankfully the smouldering coals of my host are smothered, as if by a damp blanket. Yet still her arms flay, and she fights to lift her chest from the bed. The nurses work in tandem to hold her down.

Mr Sheung clucks like an old mother hen dealing with a wayward chick. My attention is seized by a flash of sliver. I see the medicine man slide his sensual hands over the spread of treasure. Of course he is wearing rubber gloves, but they cling to his sculpted, graceful fingers like a second skin. The brilliant lights bounce off them and bestow a mesmerising sheen upon them. It makes Mr Sheung look as if he has shiny worms writhing where fingers once grew. A second later and the sac that the monkey swims in is ruptured. A lake of crystal water starts to seep out, veined with seams of crimson blood. Silver changes hands. A nurse takes the crochet hook from the doctor, the argent metal glinting wickedly beneath the jellied, crimson gobbets that cling to it. She passes on, in return, something I can only liken to an instrument of torture, that she names as forceps. Then Mr Sheung virtually disappears into Alice, foraging about with them, until he manages to grasp one of the monkey's toothpick legs.

'I am turning it into a breech position,' he announces with grandiosity, and both nurses look suitably impressed.

And even I am a touch awed, when, like a conjurer, he pulls both of the spindle legs out of the birth canal. I follow him as he selects a new instrument, sharp as a miniature rapier, and makes a tidy lunge into the base of the monkey skull. This cut he widens by sliding in miniscule scissors and snipping away like the most dextrous of tailors. Next he calls for a suction catheter. I am at a loss as to what purpose this gadget fulfils. But all is soon revealed as he sucks out the monkey brain, as efficiently as Ah Dang vacuums dust off the floor in the flat on The Peak. The skull caves in, and for a second I am worried that Mr Sheung may have made an error. But the appreciative grunt that accompanies what looks a bit like a balloon deflating must, I feel sure, mean that all is going according to plan.

'This will enable the foetus to continue its

240

journey through the birth canal, slipping out as easily as a greased turd,' quips Mr Sheung, and the nurses titter behind their masks.

Blood burnishes everything now—the floor where the nurses have trodden in it with their rubber heels, and spread it with their efficient steps; it blossoms on their starched cotton robes, and thickly coats their shiny gloves. It is even spattered on the white walls like an abstract painting, and coagulates in heavy, sodden swabs piled high on gleaming trays. It pools about Alice, trickling from her gaping vulva, tattooing her bleached belly and thighs with the print of death. There are even two smears of it on Mr Sheung's convex cheeks, which despite being lopsided, give a jolly and avuncular set to his face. Alice has stopped thrashing now, though at intervals she emits a peculiar, feral, guttural cry.

All the dynamic action is hidden from Alice by a small cloth curtain that divides her upper and lower body. I feel this is rather a shame, and may be why Alice is behaving so irrationally. Perhaps she feels left out, I hazard, abandoned, even isolated? Momentarily Alice is dumb and quiet descends in the room, a quiet punctuated only by the beep-beep of some piece of equipment, and my host's rasping breaths. Into the quiet falls a surprisingly loud sound. It is the 'slap' of the tiny monkey body, as it is deposited in an enamel kidney dish. Even if Alice cannot see, she hears very well I console myself. The mess of it reminds me of the mounds of factory waste I have seen in Aberdeen. I picture the twisted plastic limbs of reject dolls poking out of them, some melded together, some bent into curious contorted shapes, some spattered with dribbles of red paint. Alice draws jagged breaths into her lungs, as if she cannot bear to taste the air, air that is spiked now with an odour both salt and sweet and rancid.

I thought things were proceeding well, but now, as my host's eyes roll upwards until all I can see are their whites, I am not so sure. There is no sense of any kind in her now, I realise fretfully. So concerned am I that I scarcely notice Mr Sheung poring over the remains of the monkey, jabbing and prodding it with some steel instrument. Then he turns his attention back to Alice, taking pains to remove the bloody nest from her body, and making sure it is intact. I relax a bit when I see him lift his mask and smile beatifically. I hear him tell the nurses that it has all gone very well indeed.

Shortly after this Alice is wheeled back to her room. My host sleeps as the nurses scurry about, and Mr Sheung pops in and out, keeping a check on his patient. And even when, some time later, my host does awaken, she seems to be in some kind of torpor. She goes through the motions, cooperating with Mr Sheung and the nurses, pliable as wet clay, but apart from this, shows no sign at all that she is present.

Believing that the monkey has been dealt with, we return to the flat that crowns The Peak. However, on our first night back, my attention is suddenly drawn by a dazzle of golden-red. We are in Alice's bedroom, the lights off, my host fast asleep. Turning from Alice's chalky face, I do the spiritual equivalent of a double take, for jiggling before me is another ghostly visage, spectral emanations streaming from it. I recognise the monkey instantly. Of course I do. That hallmark

242

carroty hair, inherited from the beast that fathered him, cannot be mistaken. On closer inspection, I pick out the familiar toothpick limbs grasping at the air, the golden-red down coating the shrivelled body, and the tuberous genitals. Lastly, I take in the deflated-balloon head. It has grown fluorescent, like a glowing light bulb. The onionskin face is pierced with bottle-green glass-chip eyes. They are curiously open, and keenly scanning Alice's bedroom. It lies at the foot of the bed, and then, clearly aware it has an audience, shows off by levitating a few feet in the air and turning three somersaults in quick succession. I am scandalised.

'I thought we got rid of you,' I spit at it.

Its retort is simply to gurgle and chuckle, and grip its glimmering limbs, flexing them with glee. Obviously reasoning with this little ruffian is useless, so I try a more considered approach.

'Anger binds me to this life,' I inform it haughtily. 'And you? What persuades you to loiter here?' I make every effort to quell the animosity I am feeling at the unexpected arrival of this infant demon, this nursery vagabond.

'Guilt,' comes the burble of the miniature orangutan. 'Hers not mine,' it adds with a mischievous wink.

'I am not sure how long we will be able to accommodate you,' I notify it icily. 'Things are quite tight here already.' The cheeky thing just chuckles at this. I decide to speak plainly. 'It might be better for all involved if you simply left.'

Alice tosses in her sleep, and we are both jolted out of what might have developed into an extremely robust altercation. The monkey indicates Alice with a waggle of its head.

'Can't go until she lets me,' it chants happily, giving an apologetic shrug of its slight shoulders.

'Then we had better make the most of things until she dispenses with you,' I tell it acidly. My words, meant to sober the malignant gnome, serve only to increase its mirth. The creature locks its fibrillar fingers behind its head, crows, and begins blowing frothy, scarlet bubbles at me.

For the time being apparently the monkey is here to stay. Meanwhile, as Alice lurches back to life, I am thankfully far too preoccupied to fuss about it. Instead of celebrating our new freedom, my host is saturnine. She refuses food, seldom speaks and spurns her family. She does drink though, imbibing large quantities of alcohol, as well as taking any drugs she can get her hands on. She no longer washes either, is unwilling to change her clothes, and her skin has grown sallow and mottled. There are deep smudges under her eyes, clusters of sores around her mouth, her teeth are furred, her tongue discoloured and her breath sour.

Now we see next to nothing of the school that was once my home. At the flat on The Peak, Alice's family are wary of her, as if they are living with a tiger. Alice's mother has become still more remote, and though Alice's father seeks her out repeatedly, he is always rebuffed. The only member of the Safford household apart from him who does not repudiate Alice, is Bear. He alone stays by her side when he can throughout the day, and sleeps with her at night. So closely knotted together are the two of them, that sometimes, fixing on them from above, it is hard to see where

244

Alice ends and Bear begins.

Then one memorable summer night it nearly all comes to an abrupt end. Taking advantage of the fine weather, the PWD decide to repaint the exterior wall of the flat. Men come, and scaffolding rises up from the ground. It is like a monstrous stick insect that each day grows fresh joints, bound together with twine. From these joints new limbs shoot, reaching higher and higher into the sky. Before long the bones of scaffolding are rising above the top floor, so that it seems to become a cage within a cage, the metal bars of the windows now enmeshed further with thick bamboo poles. Alice stares at them blankly, at the men scaling them with the ease of trapeze artists, unencumbered it appears by their pots of paint and their brushes.

In the dead of night, Alice rises from her bed, shutting Bear in her bedroom, and creeps down the corridor, through the kitchen, past the amahs' quarters and up to the roof. Hovering before her, leading the way like an overgrown firefly, is the monkey. I shadow the pair of them. The door that opens onto the roof from the back stairs has been left unlocked by the workmen. It is a sultry night. The tumult of the cicadas fills the air. Dusty moths bumble towards the floor lights that trace the circumference of the low roof wall, only to rebound, scalded by hot glass, seconds later. Slate-grey cloud tatters scurry over the face of a half dollar moon. A handful of winking stars plot the night's course. So exposed are we on our rooftop perch that the warm breeze buffets us relentlessly.

The roof resembles an enormous insect. Two huge rectangular wings fan out from a central

245

cabin, the blue rooftop door set into it. I estimate the wingspan to be several hundred yards, one reaching towards the west, the other to the east. These are bordered by a wall no more than a few feet high. Suddenly I am distracted by Alice, scampering along the west wing, the one that effectively runs above the ceiling of her flat. Ahead of her flies the shiny copper sphere of the monkey. When she reaches the wingtip, the wall that is flush with her bathroom window, to my horror she springs onto it. Her arms reach upwards, the panting wind flapping at the baggy shirt she is wearing.

'Alice, get down,' I urge, trying to lasso her slim, bare legs, to hold them fast.

But Alice does not get down. Before her, suspended midair, the monkey jigs, all gummy grins. Below her the scaffolding rattles and creaks, the bamboo arms eager to be free of their bindings. Alice swings her head to the left in the direction of Aberdeen, drawn by the sprinkle of lights. She sways precariously on the narrow lid of the wall, then inches her bare feet forwards and slides her eyes slowly down, through the dizzying heights to the field below. She counts the blocks of light that pour from the illuminated bathroom windows.

'Skip, skip, one, two, skip, three. On the ground floor the Everards have left their light on,' Alice whispers. 'I wonder, if I land in his garden, will he come up to complain with bits of me all squashed and muddled, lying in the palms of his hands, as Nicola said he did with the onions. And will mother glide up to the door making sympathetic noises, and take Mr Everard to the bathroom to

246

wash me off, before fixing him a large drink.'

Alice rocks very lightly on her toes. She roots her eyes to the hibiscus bushes that ring the ground-floor flats, their foliage, iron grey, their huge veined flowers, dark apricot, transformed in the eerie light cast by garden lamps. Alice turns, crouches on the wall, grasps the inner lip of it with both hands, and eases herself over the edge. She swings her legs until her feet contact the first of the horizontal bamboo poles. Once she has found a foothold she frees a hand, and gropes for the strut of a second vertical pole, that rises like a stilt to her right. As she grasps it she lets go the other hand, then circles it in the blustery air, as if testing it for resistance. She leans back as far as she can, out into empty space, the free hand scooping the air, as if she might swim to the ground.

'It would be so easy to just . . . let . . . go,' sings Alice, 'like Mrs Stubbs did.' Her words scatter like autumn leaves on the night's breath. She starts to loosen the fingers of her hand on the hard, smooth surface of the thick, bamboo pole.

Instantly I snap Alice's fingers back down, locking them in place. For a long while we battle, she trying in vain to open her hand, while I fight to keep her muscles taut, her digits bent, her palm curved, a job made harder because by now her hands are slippery with sweat. By the time Alice finally relents, the first lance of dawn is streaking across the horizon. Only then does she permit me to guide her benumbed limbs like a puppeteer. I yank her body back from the brink and fold it over the low wall. I take first one hand then the other, make claws of her fingers, and see that they find purchase on the wall's inner lip. I heft her over it,

247

and finally she lands in an untidy heap on the rough surface of the roof. Not until Alice is safely tucked up in bed do I rest. Only then is there time to consider how close we came to losing our life. How vigilant I must be.

Myrtle—1974

I cannot believe it. Ralph has insisted that Alice accompany us to the Rotary Club dinner tonight. The dinner is being held at the Country Club, located between Aberdeen and Deep Water Bay. Ralph is the guest of honour and will be making a speech. The event will be packed with important people. Alice will be a liability. I tell Ralph as much, but he will not listen to reason.

'I want her there,' is his reply to me. 'I want her to hear my speech. I want her to tell me what she thinks.'

I do not like to shatter Ralph's illusions about Alice entirely. I do not want to describe her moronic attitude, prevalent for over a year now , as well he knows. Nor do I wish to remind my husband that our daughter has dropped out of school, that she spends her days loafing about the house, looking like a tramp. We both have eyes to see and ears to hear. Alice is incapable of uttering a single intelligent word at present. These undeniable facts all evidence the likelihood that our daughter will think very little of her father's speech, if anything at all. But Ralph seems to be blinkered when it comes to Alice. And as I have just seen her emerge from the bathroom, in some ill-fitting garment, so loose she might as well have pulled on a bin bag, it looks as if it's all settled.

'Ralph, I think we should be going,' I say, as my husband paces in the corridor outside Alice's door like a fawning spaniel.

'I'm just waiting for Alice,' he replies, as if she is the guest of honour tonight!

So, because I cannot trust myself a moment longer not to say something I will regret, I dash into the bedroom to give my appearance a final check. The dress, floor-length, royal-blue chiffon with a beaded bodice, my most recent acquisition from the Swan Emporium in Central, looks fabulous. I am wearing my lapis lazuli and gold necklace with matching earrings. My hair, though swept up into its usual bun, is worn in a softer style, with tendrils permitted to escape and frame my face. My make-up is perhaps a touch stronger than I normally like it, with silver-blue eye shadow, plenty of mascara and rouge, and poppy-red lipstick. But in the evenings a little extra goes a long way. As I think this, I have no idea just how far it will be expected to go tonight. I give a dab of perfume to my temples, take a tissue from the box on my dressing table and blot my lipstick lightly with it. I am looking at the imprint of my red mouth on the pale-pink tissue, when I hear Ralph summon me. I hurry out of our bedroom, briefing Ah Dang on our late return as I pass her standing in the dining-room doorway. I note with some displeasure that her white tunic looks a little creased, and make a mental note to speak to her about it later. Incredibly I find my husband and my daughter in the lobby outside our front door, pawing at bolts of fabric. Standing in the background beside the pedlar, her baskets bulging with yet more bolts of cloth, is our chauffeur. Quickly he removes his hat and lowers his head.

'Good evening, Mrs Safford,' he greets me. I ignore him.

'What on earth are you doing?' I ask my husband angrily, glancing at my watch, and stepping gingerly over the yards of material strewn about the cream-tiled floor.

'The lift's not working,' Ralph tells me conversationally, not bothering to look up from a piece of mauve and turquoise brocade he is fingering, as I reach my hand towards the button.

'What do you mean?' I demand, pressing the button several times anyway. I note with exasperation that it does not glow red, and that no hum of the approaching lift can be heard.

'I'm afraid the lift has broken down. Apparently it's been down for some time according to Ah Dang,' Ralph fills me in, seemingly unconcerned despite the late hour.

'What do you think of this fabric?' Alice asks, either oblivious to my growing sense of frustration, or delighting in it. I am not sure which. She holds a length of lavender fabric embroidered with silver flowers against herself. Ralph starts to tell her how well it suits her pale complexion. Unable to contain myself a moment longer I explode.

'We do not have time for this now. Are you mad? Ralph you are the guest of honour. You cannot be late!' I add that I am going back inside the flat to report the fault with the lift to the PWD. In the same moment the Fielding's front door swings open and Nigel appears. He is attending the Rotary Club dinner as well, and Ralph has already told me he has invited him to share our car. Beth will not be joining us as she has a meeting of the craft club she attends, making tat as far as I can tell—oven-gloves, aprons, cloth bags and the like, for the Cathedral's summer fête. Just as well, considering that Alice will now be swelling our numbers.

'Myrtle darling, you look gorgeous,' Nigel says, picking his way nonchalantly across a sea of fabric towards me, and pecking me lightly on the cheek. He is immaculately dressed as always, in a black suit, crisp white shirt and Rotary tie. The crease in his trousers is razor sharp. He has the edge on Ralph whose own trousers, now I observe them, look in need of a good press. It is very remiss of the amahs. I will have a word with both of them tomorrow. You can't let your guard down for a second with these servants. 'You smell gorgeous too, Myrtle,' Nigel compliments me, providing some much needed salve for my smarts. 'Ralph, you don't mind if I steal your wife tonight? Mine seems to have deserted me.'

Ralph opens his hands in a 'be my guest' gesture. Nigel links his arm through mine, at the same time noticing Alice wafting about, like some sort of deranged fairy, stroking the lengths of material spread about us.

'And Alice too,' Nigel cries, feigning delight I have no doubt. 'This is my lucky night. Damn inconvenient about the lift, but I've rung the engineers and they promise they'll be here within the hour. I'm afraid that still rather leaves us in the lurch though, so the sooner we start our descent the better really.' Nigel indicates the stairs with a cheery smile.

251

Trust Nigel to be on top of things regarding the broken lift. I cannot help but be drawn under Nigel's spell. Practised charm it might be, but nevertheless it does the trick smoothing my ruffled feathers. The feeling of gloom that has been hovering over me ever since I learnt that Alice is to join us this evening dispels rapidly. I begin to feel that Ralph could learn a thing or two from his colleague. Yet even Nigel's charm does not succeed in luring Ralph and Alice away from the pedlar's wares, until they have purchased several pieces of cloth. The fabric will, I feel sure, simply sit at the back of a cupboard for months on end attracting moths, until in the end I have to pass it on to the amahs. At least the pedlar has the good grace to stand back and let us leave, before she starts trying to negotiate the stairs with all her bundles.

The journey is mercifully uneventful. Nigel sits in the front and we three huddle together in the back. The proximity of our bodies feels uncomfortable. It is cool for the start of April and a squally shower is falling from a louring sky. But I am not overly concerned about the weather. We are members of the country club, and I know that the car is able to draw up under a sheltered colonnade at the entrance, so none of us need get wet.

Despite my worries the evening seems to get off to a good start. Alice drifts away and as far as I can see, though quite honestly I am far too busy socialising with friends to keep close tabs on my errant daughter, she appears to be adopting a low profile. And that is good enough for me. The upstairs clubroom, where the reception is being held, has been beautifully decorated, with lavish floral displays of orchids, arranged artistically about blocks of wood, gleaming metal and lighted candles, all very Ikebana. I am in the middle of a fascinating discussion with Martin Prowse, Chief Fire Officer, on the difficulties of battling conflagrations in multi-storey buildings, and he is in the middle of eyeing my bosom admiringly, when we are called into dinner. Naturally, as guest of honour, Ralph is seated at the head of the table with me at his side, but the late notice means that Alice has been placed towards the table end. Secretly I am very relieved at this, and, as I see that Nigel is sitting next to her, I rest assured she is being well supervised, and give my sole attention to my husband and the splendid meal.

I am just finishing off an absolutely delicious chocolate soufflé, and settling down to listen to Ralph's speech (he has decided to give it on the resettlement of squatters, an admirable topic and one which I feel sure will draw much interest) when Nigel catches my eye. There are at least sixty guests at the dinner, so he is seated some distance from us. At first I am not sure quite what he is trying to communicate, with his raised eyebrows and his sideways tilt of the head indicating Alice at his side. But Ralph is speaking so I put my concerns on the backburner. Things appear to be going splendidly with Ralph just reaching his peroration when we flounder unexpectedly.

'There is no doubt in my mind that the alternatives we are offering to squatters are a first-class um . . . are a first-class um . . . er . . . are a—'

Ralph breaks off. There is some kind of disruption occurring at the other end of the table.

To my horror I see that Alice has spilt a glass of red wine down the front of that frumpy green dress she is wearing, and that she is rising unsteadily to her feet and applauding loudly. All heads turn from Ralph and swivel in the direction of our daughter. The chair she tries to push back falls over, and a waiter rushes forwards to right it. Nigel is on his feet. Deftly he restrains Alice's windmilling arms, leans into her ear and whispers something. I realise that he is guiding Alice, as best he can, in the direction of the door. I stand. I lean into Ralph, assure him that I can deal with this, urge him to continue his speech, and move speedily to Alice's other side. I know I am blushing.

My daughter may be drunk but she is surprisingly strong, I find.

'Let go . . . go . . . of me, mother,' she slurs. 'I am . . . I am . . . I'm perfectly alright. If only you would leave me . . . be . . . and not keep trying to stop me.'

By the time Alice finishes what she is saying, or trying to say, Nigel and I have steered her successfully from the dining room into the reception room, closing the door firmly behind us. Ralph, I can just hear in the background, has resumed his speech. We lead our struggling charge from here into the corridor and down it to the lift. This one had better be working, I think caustically, as we manoeuvre Alice into it. The lift-attendant fixes his attention on the bank of buttons ahead of him, as if he carries drunken girls up and down all day long, and has grown so accustomed to them that he is effectively blind. I wish this were true, but I feel sure Alice has yet again set tongues wagging and dragged our name into disrepute.

'Where are we going?' Alice blurts out, a touch too loudly, squinting at the panel above the double doors, as it indicates our descent with a sequence of lighted numbers.

She collapses against Nigel. He supports her gallantly, and prevents her from slipping into an undignified tangle of limbs on the floor. I wrap my arms around my waist to prevent them from striking her.

'Nigel, I'm so ashamed—' I begin. But Nigel cuts me off genially.

'Myrtle, don't say another word. All teenagers go through it. Not that mine have reached the dreaded teens yet. But I feel sure Beth and I have all this to look forward to. It would be odd if adolescents didn't test you a bit, eh?'

I want to hug Nigel for his understanding attitude, but Alice is sprawled all over him. As we clamber out of the lift Nigel speaks to the attendant in Cantonese, and I presume he scurries off to fetch our driver. Sure enough, by the time we reach the lobby doors he is there, the car's motor thrumming. He leaps out to open the passenger door, and somehow or other we manage to lift Alice into the back seat. But oh no, she cannot leave it at that, she has to do more damage before we speed away.

'You have lots of red hair growing . . . growing out of your nostrils,' she tells Nigel, her head poking out of the rear window. I am crippled with embarrassment. 'You should . . . should trim it.'

And I'm afraid it is out before I can censor it.

'Just shut up Alice for God's sake!'

I take several deep breaths subsequent to this,

255

while Alice withdraws her head back inside the car, like a tortoise disappearing into a shell, from where she mutters something thankfully incomprehensible. Repeatedly Nigel offers to accompany us home. But I refuse graciously. I cannot bear for him to witness another second of my humiliation. I explain to Nigel that I will send the car back for him and Ralph, before thanking him profusely and settling myself in the front seat. My neighbour waves us off and we execute the most graceful move of the whole evening. Our exit.

Alice dozes on the journey home, her head rolling on her shoulders, while I add the tally of this night's exhibition to Alice's already weighty account. I ponder as calmly as I can, how many people have seen the Saffords' youngest daughter, blind drunk, making a spectacle of herself at the Rotary dinner, at which her father was the honoured guest. I allow myself to consider, in addition, those she may have spoken to prior to the dinner, and what she may have let slip in her inebriated state. I let the names of some of those important guests, names that carry with them influence and power on the island, run through my head. I try to calculate how long it will take to repair the damage done, how many weeks, months, years!

Alice has been through an awkward period, and I imagine the process was a little difficult for her. But she should have done something about it the moment she suspected she might be pregnant, instead of letting time slip by, like some gormless half-wit who thinks it will all go away if she forgets about it. She was lucky, her family stood by her. I personally financed the sordid business. And now that it is over I think she owes it to us not to heap more ignominy upon our undeserving heads. I have had just about all I can stomach from my third daughter. By the time we reach Mount Nicholson, I find myself unable to resist the urge to compare Alice's track record with that of her sisters. Apart from a brief spell at boarding school, where clearly they fell in with bad company, Jillian and Nicola have been a credit to us. Whereas Alice, who if anything has had an easier time of it than her sisters, seems to feel that a terrible injustice is being wrought upon her.

So absorbed am I in my reflections, that it comes as a surprise to me to find we are ascending our drive, and pulling up by the exterior lobby doors of the flat. Alice is asleep. The sight of her spread-eagled on the back seat, eyes shut, lost it seems in a guiltless slumber, enrages me almost more than anything else has done this night. Having ensured the evening is a misery for everyone else, now my daughter is set to enjoy her dreams. Well, not if I can help it. I tell the driver to wait, take the lift upstairs, noting cursorily that it has been repaired, and shake the equally dopey dog from its sleep. I ride back down, a confused, mildly disorientated Bear at my side, and tell Alice that we are going for a walk. With the help of the chauffeur, I manage to eject Alice from her seat and get her on her feet. She sways precariously as the car pulls away, the taillights fading into the night.

'I think I . . . I shall go to bed,' Alice mumbles, her voice thick as glue, groping for the brass pole handles of the lobby doors. Bear, a bit more lively now, prances at her feet.

257

'No, I think a bracing walk round Mount Kellett with the dog is a better idea,' comes my tart rejoinder.

'I'm . . . too, far too tired to walk,' Alice breathes heavily, her hands still grappling ineffectually with the door handles.

'I want you to walk,' I repeat with more emphasis, prising Alice off the door and giving her a shove in the direction of the steps that lead down to Homestead Path. At my prompting Alice at last begins to stagger forwards. 'You'd better grasp the railing,' I tell her as we make our way down the steps. I am damned if I am going to carry her drunken weight for another minute. 'You need to sober up, Alice.' It is a misty night but at least the rain has eased off which is something. 'You have to pull yourself together,' I advise my daughter as she shuffles behind me. She is dragging her feet, stumbling every few steps as we approach the end of Homestead Path, and the start of road that skirts Mount Kellett. Neither of us is wearing suitable shoes for this trek. Our high heels click on the wet tarmac. In the stillness the sounds seem to multiply, as if instead of just the two of us quite a crowd is tripping about The Peak, while the invasive fog hangs over them. 'You can't carry on in this fashion. It was a very important evening for your father tonight, *and* Alice, you mortified him with your drunken behaviour.'

Alice makes no reply. I can hear the 'rasp, rasp' of her breath, see the pale vapour of it coming in little puffs on the cool, dank air. Now we stand at the side of the road, and gaze at a car coasting past us and on round the bend ahead with a hiss, its headlights briefly searching out our faces. We begin our faltering progress around Mount Kellett, following in its wake. At intervals we pass sweeping driveways that branch off the main road. These wind up and down the slopes to flats and houses, from where rectangles, and squares, and circles of light spill into the gloom. Just beyond the street lamps, lines of bamboo stand out in bronze relief. The smooth trunks and droopy leaves gleam as if varnished, wavering on the outskirts of the tangerine tepees of light. I hear a dog yap in the distance. A pair of eyes, luminous, golden beads, burn out at us from the gaping, dark hollow of a hillside drainpipe. From time to time the moon emerges from behind the clouds, and a weak trickle of watery, silver light filters across the sooty pavement. We pass a patch of grass that like the bamboo is bronzed with lamplight. Here wooden slatted benches are set out. From this viewpoint on a clear night we would be able to see Pokfulam, and beyond it the sea. But not tonight. The mist seems to be closing in and it begins to feel as if this road, this mount, is all that exists of Hong Kong, that the remainder of the island has been sponged away by the waterlogged clouds.

'Do you understand what I'm saying to you, Alice? Things have to change. *You* have to change. We cannot go on like this.' My voice seems to come from a long way off, as if it belongs to someone else.

Again, Alice does not respond. She has picked up the pace a bit though, so perhaps her reticence is a sign that she is coming to, that the consequences of her night's antics are beginning to dawn on her. She pauses momentarily beneath a street lamp and our eyes fuse. The whites of hers are made yellow in the glow. Her hair is frosted with mizzle and sparkles as if dusted with gold. Damp strands cling to her skin. Her dress is as soggy as mine, if not more so, for Alice has no shawl clasped about her shoulders as I have. It cleaves to her body like a second skin. The green of the dress has been transformed too. It is the colour of mud. The wine stain over her chest has grown black as blood. It looks like an open wound. The dog darts about, now fully awake to the scents released by the moist earth. He seems blithely unaffected by this bizarre nocturnal outing, though from time to time he freezes and growls, his tail stiffens and the hackles rise on his back. It is almost as if he believes we are being followed. But I can see nothing, so perhaps the fog is spooking him as well.

'Do you have any idea how stressful your father's job is, Alice? Do you comprehend how hard he works and how worried you are making him? He has a position to maintain on the island and you are not helping him to do that, are you, Alice? You are hindering him every opportunity you have. I know you've had a bit of a rough time lately, but you have to put it behind you and start afresh.'

We have left Pokfulam behind us now and passed Matilda Hospital. We have nearly reached the railings that border an exposed curve in the road, from where ordinarily we would be able to see Aberdeen harbour. Here the mountain slope falls away sharply. I begin to wish in earnest that I had grabbed our coats from the flat. The whisky which has provided me with an illusion of warmth for most of the evening is wearing off. I am shivering. I can hear Bear panting, but I can no longer see him. Along with the coats, it dawns on me that I should have brought the dog-lead. But it has to be conceded in my defence that I was distracted. Besides, Bear seldom runs off these days, and so far the night seems unnaturally still. Then the dog's barking suddenly seems to rise an octave. He is yipping in excitement. He must have picked up the scent of some small mammal, or a cat, or another nocturnal prowler. Alice halts abruptly at the sound. I stop too, a few feet ahead of Alice. We are standing adjacent to the stretch of railings. They run for several yards, falling between two lampposts. I lean back against the cold bars. I screw up my eyes and peer into the blackness. The dog is nowhere to be seen.

I sigh in exasperation. 'Whatever must Nigel think of you?' I say. My tone is bitter.

'Oh, I know what he thinks of me,' Alice retorts. My jaw, clenched tightly shut, slackens at this. 'He thinks I am a drunk. He told me so. He leant over . . . me when I was . . . sitting at the dinner table tonight, and he whispered . . . it into my ear. Alice you're a drunk, he said.' Her speech is laboured but clear as a bell now. It is as if the words are being forced out of her.

The breath leaves my body in a narrow visible funnel and dissipates. I feel as if someone has struck me a blow in the abdomen. But I am quick to rally.

'Well?' I challenge my daughter. 'What do you expect. That's what you were tonight, a drunk.'

'He said something else,' Alice continues. And suddenly I want very badly for her to be quiet, to swallow her words, to draw back from the abyss.

261

But Alice has never drawn back and so she drives on. 'He said, you're a drunk and Nicola's a whore.'

My slack jaw drops open, and I try to scream but just like in nightmares no sound comes, only an aspirate whimper. It falls into silence. I take two slow ragged breaths. Only then do I feel able to speak.

'You are a wicked, wicked girl, Alice,' I tell the black silhouette of my daughter, her outline rimmed with gold. 'You have a filthy mouth. It is not enough that you are in the gutter, is it? Oh no, you have to bring the rest of us down with you. I will not listen to your vile lies.' I push off from the railings. Absurd as it may seem, I have an overwhelming impulse to run from my daughter, to stoop down and slip off my strappy evening shoes, and gather up the billows and folds of my chiffon dress and race away. I need to escape from this place, from the girl whose every action, whose every word, eats like a cancer into my life. From Alice. At that precise moment Alice turns from me towards the road and her voice rings out, steeped in terror.

'Bear!'

In the same splinter of time a car roars round the corner. A small solid body is paralysed at a point ahead of it, where the two cones of its headlights merge. An insect frozen in liquid amber. The pools of his dark eyes lock, not on approaching death, but on Alice, arms outstretched towards him. There is a screech of brakes. The dog glances off the car's wing with a barely audible thud. The driver does not even register that he has hit something. The car streaks on past, vanishing as quickly as it materialized. For a long moment we listen to the purr of its engine fading away.

Alice is the first to move. She totters off the pavement and into the murk. I can just decipher the outline of her crouching down, her arms gathering up a dense, black mass. Then she is rocking on her heels. She is making strange keening noises. I take a few steps towards her, bend over the two of them.

'He's been hit. He's injured. We need to get help,' Alice says.

Intuition tells me it is too late for help.

'I think,' I tell her slowly, reaching a tentative hand towards the dog, 'that he may be dead.'

'I've checked and I'm almost certain there are no broken bones,' Alice hurries on, her voice brittle as glass, as if she has not heard me. 'Why did I call him? I don't know why I called him. I didn't hear the car. There was no reason to call Bear then. At that . . . that precise moment. He wouldn't have come if I hadn't called. He's warm, but I'm not sure how long that will last. Shock leads to a drop in temperature, doesn't it? We need to wrap him up. Don't his paws feel like sandpaper, and they're so large too. Out of proportion kind of. I've always thought that. And for a small dog just look at his barrel chest. His muzzle is soft as velvet. Softer. Have you noticed the tear in his ear? Of course you have. It was like that when we got him.' All the time Alice speaks her hands move over the dog, her touch soft as a caress.

Then she opens out her arms as if inviting me to make a closer inspection. I note that the grizzled fur of the barrel chest does not stir.

'He is not breathing Alice,' I tell her. 'Bear is dead.'

Still Alice does not seem to mark my words, or if she does they are meaningless to her. One milk-white hand probes the canine skull. She holds the hand out to me, and I see it is covered with blood, black as tar.

'This is where the car caught him. Look. I will need to clean him up to see how bad it really is. Sometimes, once you've wiped away the blood . . . even if it seems very bad . . . you realise it's no more than a scratch.' She is hiccupping in her breaths and her head is shaking fractionally. 'He makes a terrible fuss about pain, Bear does. He's quite the hypochondriac. He's heavy too. Overfed I think. But if we carry him . . . between us we should be alright. We can phone the vet's emergency service . . . as soon as we get him back.'

'Alice, he's . . . dead,' I say flatly. 'You better give him to me.' Alice staggers to her feet still cradling the dog. His crushed head slips from the circle of her arms and dangles, then swings from side to side as she walks towards the next lamplight. Blood drips slowly from it and splashes onto the bronzed pavement stones.

'What are you doing?' I ask her, catching up, then moving in front of her to block her way. Alice does not answer so I speak again, more loudly, more forcefully. 'What are you doing with the dog, Alice?'

'I'm taking him home of course. I'm taking Bear home.' Alice has begun humming tunelessly. 'We can't leave him here in the cold. He'll be frightened. He hated this stretch of the walk anyway. Did you realise that, Mother? The stretch near the railing. As if he knew, always knew something . . . something bad might happen here. We have to get him away you see. Where he'll be safe. We have to look after him.'

'What are you talking about? Bear's dead, Alice. The dog . . . is . . . dead. Nothing can be done for him now.' I do not add that Alice might just as well have been driving the car that killed him, that all this is all her fault. But I think it.

'Hush hush,' Alice croons, and I am uncertain whether this is directed at the dead dog or me.

'What's the matter with you,' I snap. 'Bear's dead. No one can make him better now.'

'I know it,' says Alice, her tone that of mild reproof. 'But we need to take him home now.' I have had enough. I step forwards and wrestle the body out of Alice's hands. For a split second I consider what a devil bloodstains are to remove. Then I lift the dead dog in my arms over to the railings.

'Don't!' cries Alice, who is beside me now. 'Please don't!'

As Bear's head rolls against my hip, I experience the sensation of warm, viscous fluid soaking into my frothy layers of chiffon. I hoist the dog up over the highest railing, letting the metal pole shoulder the weight of him for a second or two. Then I thrust my arms forward and cast the body out as far as I can, hearing the thud of it as it lands in the brush below.

'Come on.' I am brisk. 'The dog is dead. The thing is done. It cannot be changed. Snap out of it!' I take a few steps, pause and look back. In the dim light Alice lingers by the railings. She is prattling. I pick out the word 'tree' and 'branch' and 'soldier' and 'dogs' and something about her father and shame. That much I understand but the rest is all nonsense of course. I move quickly to her, deliver a swift, hard slap across her face. I take hold of her shoulders and shake her. I grab her arm and drag her forwards. In this manner we finish our walk and arrive back at the flat on The Peak.

We stagger panting into the lobby and stand facing each other. Both our dresses are blotted in blood and so are our hands. Alice has a smear of blood across one cheek, and the flaming imprint of my bloody hand emblazoned on the other. There are crimson drops spattered on her white arms. I resist the urge to look at my own reflection in the gleaming brass panel where the lift buttons are set. Better not to know. I summon the lift and, when it arrives, wordlessly we step inside. Just before the doors close we are joined by Fred Macready from flat six, who heads up immigration services. The doors shudder to a close. Like the lift attendant earlier this evening at the Country Club, Mr Macready stares fixedly up at the lighted numbers indicating which floors we are passing. He clears his throat.

'Evening Mrs Safford, Alice,' he greets us with a brief nod. Automatically I lower my eyelids and dip my head. I gather up a few loose strands of hair that have tumbled free from my bun, and make a failed attempt to secure them.

'Good evening, Mr Macready. Inclement weather,' I say.

'Mm . . . mm . . . so it is. Damned mist,' mumbles Mr Macready. Then silence as the lift ascends to the third floor. The doors spring open and Mr Macready gets out. 'Goodnight to you both.' Again he nods courteously but without meeting my eyes. Then the doors shudder closed behind him and we continue up to the top floor.

Ah Dang greets us. Rapidly she appraises our dishevelled appearance, the blood on our clothes, our hands. She cranes her neck, her eyes raking the foyer over my shoulder.

'Where . . . where is Bear, Mrs Safford?' she inquires tentatively.

'Bear is gone,' I reply brusquely, sweeping past her. 'Bear is dead!'

I leave Alice to her own devices.

Only when I have peeled off my blood-soaked garments and handed them over to Ah Dang, whose broad face remains impassive as she bundles up the soiled chiffon, only when I have poured myself a very large brandy and sit nursing it at my dressing table, only when I am meeting my own eyes in the silver mirror, do I let the darkness that has been with me since the accident crawl towards the light. I relive the car speeding around the bend and the thing freezing in its headlights. Only . . . only . . . the shape I am seeing is that of a teenage girl clad in a dull green dress, wearing a wine stain like a wound over her chest, hair wild, eyes huge, just before the moment of impact, when her body will rocket in the air, bounce on the bonnet, then roll off it, landing crumpled by the roadside, quite, quite dead!

Ghost—1974

We have returned from a surprise late-night stroll around Mount Kellett with Alice's mother. It was, if I am truthful, a disappointing ramble, and this not just because of the damp and the fog, or Mrs Safford's unwarranted hostility. Unfortunately there was an accident. Bear is dead. He was foraging about in the scrub when Alice called him. As he stepped into the road a car rounded the bend and struck him. Alice wanted to bring his body home, but Mrs Safford flung it over some railings. So now my host is sitting on her bed hugging her knees. Although one of the amahs finally persuaded her to take off her dress, she has not washed or changed into clean clothes. She is wearing a bra and pants, both stained with red blotches. Her concave belly is smirched with yet more of Bear's blood. At first it was sticky but now it is dry and looks, when she drops her knees, like an enormous flaking scab. The bedroom light is off, but the room is not dark. The sky has cleared, and the moon is shining with indecent brilliance considering the funereal atmosphere.

Because Alice seems rather glum I play jester and try to lighten her mood. I make a supreme effort, sliding the glass of water on her bedside table around and around in tight circles, slowly speeding up until the liquid splashes out of it. And when this does not even elicit a smile, I push it over the edge, causing it to smash into lots of sharp pieces on the floor. They look so pretty glinting in moonlight but Alice barely glances at them. I undulate the curtains next and start to inch them closed, giving up halfway when Alice's only reaction is a gusty sigh. Not to be outdone the monkey performs so many aerial cartwheels that I begin to feel giddy. Then it sucks on each of its ten effulgent toes in turn. But Alice, head slumped back on her pillow only blinks in apparent boredom. She turns away and stares robotically through the gap in the curtains at the barred windowpane.

So here we all are. The jackanapes has given up and is snoozing under the bedcover. Worn out from my exertions, I am draped over the foot of the bed. This is when we hear it. A rapping noise coming, I think, from one of the windowpanes partially hidden by the curtains. Alice, whose eyes, are closed, now opens them. I straighten up. The monkey gives a hollow little gasp and starts vibrating like a purring kitten. As Alice clambers to her feet and moves in the direction of the sound, the knocking increases. She pushes back the curtain, grips the bars and peers out of the window. I join her, while the monkey, curiosity aroused, drifts over to perch on her shoulder like a jaunty parrot. Staring out at a rapidly brightening sky, at first I conclude the events of the previous evening have frayed all our nerves, and left us with overactive imaginations. There is nothing there. A sinking moon and a few pale stars, the colour draining from them as if they are fluxing.

Then Alice peers downwards, though it is hard, thanks to the bars. Nevertheless, as she screws up her tired eyes forcing them to focus, there can be no mistake. Monkey and I can confirm it. Bear! He is only a few feet away. His back paws are suctioned to the wall. His front paws are sliding up the window. He raises one of them and bangs the glass pane. I realise the noise that alerted us initially was the soft thump of his paw pads, and sound of his claws scratching against the glass. He has almost drawn level now, and his feathery tail is waving enthusiastically. His fur, coarse and wiry with the odd patch of mange in life, has acquired a rutilant sheen in death. His eyes, cloudy on good days, opaque on bad, and frequently crusted in the corners with the dried remains of a glutinous discharge, have become a dazzling shade of ultraviolet. The tear ducts glitter like diamonds. The surrounding lids are copper bright, and as clean as if they have been ferociously scoured. Of course the back of his skull is flattened. This gives a curiously two-dimensional look to his face .

Bear, it appears, is dead but not gone, so it seems I shall have to go on sharing Alice. Inwardly I admit to feeling a little envious of Bear's dramatic apparition. By contrast my own disembodied form verges on a dowdy monochrome. But I feel sure that an intelligent observer would consider the wolfish poltergeist rather vulgar. The test of a superior phantom, I console myself, is knowing when to stop, when to set yourself sensible boundaries. Although I have come across only two other entities thus far in my crepuscular existence, I decide both are of the special-effect ilk. On first encounter my discreet luminance might not grab the eye in quite the same way, but I maintain it embraces subtlety and endurance, qualities of which the dog and the monkey can only dream.

Eyeballing each other through the glass, Alice is

the first to speak.

'Bear! Oh Bear! How shall you come in Bear when the windows are barred?'

Bear shakes from head to tail, the way he used to do in life when he came in from a shower of rain.

'Bars are no problem for me now,' he says in a comfortable sort of growl.

Alice sees that he is right. Bear crouches, and then in one fluid motion jumps straight through the glass, and then the bars. He lands on the bed with far more elegance than his live self was capable of doing. The monkey and I join him, letting our emanations fuse for a thrilling moment. Alice gives a sharp intake of breath. She returns to the bed and sits back down on the side of it, a touch timidly. I like to think this is the moment that she has her first glimpse of me. What am I saying? I know it is. There I am, scorched on the back of her retina, a Chinese girl with short, black hair, naked but for a British soldier's jacket several sizes too large for her. Apart from the broken teeth and the bruises, I think it is quite a comely face. Alice tears her gaze away and lets it rest on the dog.

'I was certain,' she says gently to Bear-as-Was, who is rolling one scintillating violet eye, and making a futile attempt with scrabbling forelegs to dig a hole in the mattress, 'that you died last night?'

'I did,' returns the sparkling, ruby-red visitant. 'I was hit by a car and then your mother threw my body over the railings.' He yawns hugely and it is like looking into a furnace, black teeth jutting out of molten fuchsia gums like chips of glittering coal.

'I'm so sorry, Bear—' begins Alice.

But Bear, scratching some kind of spectral itch, interrupts. He insists there is no need for Alice to apologise.

'Does it hurt?' Alice is curious to know.

'Not now,' says Bear with a throaty chuckle.

Alice's voice sinks respectfully, and she indicates me with a discreet tilt of her head. 'Do you know who she is?'

'I've got a hunch but I can't be certain,' Bear confides, rolling over on his back, and offering up his tummy to be tickled. 'I think she's been floating around for some time now.'

'Mm.' Alice nods as if in recognition. After all, it would be odd if she did not know me, considering we have been living together in fairly cramped conditions for several years now. She ripples her fingers nervously over the gelatinous coruscations of Bear's belly, then watches hypnotically as the surface of it breaks and shivers. The dog writhes in ecstasy. At length she glances up at the banana-flesh glimmer of dawn, rising from the depths of a charred sea.

Now the canine spectre sits up and stretches his neck towards the horizon, his nose gleaming like black onyx. 'I have to go,' he says regretfully, as if reminded of some duty he must perform. 'But don't worry, I'll be back.'

'Wait,' calls Alice, as the resplendent, filmy Bear bounds through the bars. 'When will I be able to cry?' But Bear has gone.

The first I hear of the move is later on in the day, when Alice, still neither washed nor dressed, shuffles into the kitchen to fetch a fresh glass of water. She has shrugged on an old dressing gown, far too long for her, and keeps tripping over the hem.

I am not sure how she has concealed it from me, but she has. Perhaps the idea occurs to her on the spot, even as the words form on her lips.

'I'm going away, Ah Dang,' she announces. She drains her glass and sets it down by the sink.

Ah Dang, who is busy rolling out pastry on a wooden board, looks up. She puts down her rolling pin.

'You going shopping, Missy Alice?' Ah Dang asks.

Alice draws the back of her hand across her mouth. 'No, I don't mean that, Ah Dang. I'm leaving Hong Kong.'

'Where you going?' Ah Dang demands suspiciously, narrowing her eyes and raising a floury hand to cup her chin, so that when she takes it away she looks as if she has grown a white beard.

'I'm going to England to live with my grandmother,' says Alice. 'I'm going to live in the red-brick house in Ealing.'

Something about the set of my host's mouth makes it apparent that this is no idle threat. She wanders down the corridor ignoring her sisters as she passes them. Clearly they have been summoned home so that they can be told of Bear's untimely demise. I shadow Alice, still reeling from her announcement that we are leaving the island.

By nightfall any hopes of mine that Alice will change her mind are dashed. She has at last washed, and dressed in jeans and an old shirt. She skips dinner, finds her parents drinking coffee in the lounge and declares her intention to them.

'I'm going to go and live in England for a while.'

273

She stands before them on the Chinese rug, her voice bold, her stance determined, feet apart, straight-backed, arms folded and head held high.

'Where will you stay?' comes her mother's stunned rejoinder.

I give the proceedings my complete concentration. This affects me personally, something Alice has failed to take into account.

'I thought perhaps I could live with Gran, just for a couple of months, till I find my feet.'

To my relief, Alice's father looks aghast. He begins objecting immediately. It is a very different way of life in England. Alice's grandmother will impose much stricter rules than Alice is used to. Alice will be terribly homesick. And besides, what would she do anyway that she might not do here in Hong Kong? Had I been able to, I would have clasped Ralph Safford to my shredded bosom. However Alice's mother, after a moment's thought, seems to take a sudden liking to the madcap scheme. Yes, she says, deliberating out loud, Alice might do very well in England. It would be a new start, the perfect opportunity for their daughter to develop a bond with her grandmother. What, she wants to know, does Alice plan to do by way of employment?

'I'm not sure exactly, but I think I'll start in the retail industry, just to earn a bit of money. Then, when I'm ready, I'll see about taking up where I left off with my A levels.' Alice's tone rings with verisimilitude.

'Oh,' Myrtle exclaims on an upward inflexion. 'That sounds an excellent idea to me,' she enthuses, setting down her porcelain coffee cup in its saucer with a resounding clack. 'A chance to strike out on your own.' What Myrtle Safford does not seem to appreciate is that Alice will not be on her own. I will be with her, and I have no doubt that so will the mischievous monkey, along with the miasmal *canis familiaris*. It is one thing for Alice to live abroad, but a poor Chinese girl in a threadbare jacket, a foolhardy monkey, and a dog with no road-sense? That is another matter entirely. But Myrtle Safford smiles now, the corners of her mouth twitching. I stare at her in bafflement as Alice's plan ferments. The voices about me grow louder, the gestures more expansive, and the clock on the mantelpiece chimes. I hover predatorily over the ivory carving of an elderly man set on a corner shelf. How intricate the work is, his flowing robes engraved with a pattern of flowers and fruits. I cave in, as if I am being compressed into a box far too small for me. When I spring out it is with the speed of a striking cobra. The ivory carving falls to the parquet floor. It breaks into four pieces. The sagacious, old head bowls away and vanishes under an armchair. There is an immediate hush.

Ralph—1974

It is a perfect June day. The sky is a brilliant blue. I shade my eyes against the glare. Turquoise? Azure? No . . . sapphire perhaps? I narrow it down to forget-me-not, an ironic choice as it happens. Here and there the blue is broken with eddies of white cloud. The effects of a blinding sun, which might otherwise be unpleasant, are eased by the palliative effects of a cool sea breeze. The driver has just dropped me at Kai Tak airport. I am here to see Alice off. She is leaving today, flying to England. She will be living for a while with her grandmother.

A plane roars overhead. I can feel the percussive vibrations of its engines pulsing up from the underfoot asphalt through my body. I meditate on the death of the dog. I think that it was, of all possible ways to end a life, not a bad one really. I told Alice as much. I sat on her bed one night a few days after it happened. I said, 'Alice, he was an old dog. He would not have lasted much longer.' I said, 'What happened, him being hit by a car like that and his life being snuffed out, was a mercy. Some might say a blessing.' Alice sat hugging a pillow, her eyes fixed on mine. She didn't blink. I noticed that. She didn't blink. Not once. Not while I was speaking. I said, 'In time we might have had to put him down. It would have been horrible. At least this way . . . ' Then I tailed off. Alice wasn't buying it. I sighed. I wanted to take her in my arms and hug her to me. I wanted to tell her how much I loved her, would always love her, had always loved her. I didn't. Before I left she said she was sorry. Sorry for what? For being a teenager, for being here, for being alive?

I am inside the airport now and I'm seeing stars. My eyes haven't adjusted yet, coming from the brilliant sunshine into the shade. In a moment I will look for a small girl with a large case. Myrtle will be with her chattering away I have no doubt, filling up the silences. God forbid that we should ever have a spell of silence in the Safford family, for then the questions will surely come. I find myself thinking about a man I saw this morning. He clutched my arm and said he couldn't sleep because of the colour of his cell walls. I was visiting new secure accommodation for the mentally ill out at Stanley. This kind of thing is part of my duties as a Justice of the Peace. He had a bald patch, this man, and was pulling out his remaining hairs one by one. He was selecting them carefully, then giving a trial tug, before he plucked savagely at the follicle. When it came free he held it out victoriously for me to see. The officer showing me around started to intervene and send him away, but I held up my hand.

'It's all right,' I stalled him.

Then: 'I am going mad. The walls are sending me mad.'

This is what the balding man said to me. He spoke in Cantonese of course. I tried in vain to follow what he was saying, but one of the attendants in a white coat stepped forward smiling, and translated.

I scrutinised the hair held delicately between the balding man's thumb and forefinger for my inspection. I observed that the root had a tiny plug of brown flesh attached to it. I nodded sympathetically, and asked him what colour the walls were. I was not sure what to expect. Mustard yellow? Magenta? Khaki?

'White,' he said, his face contorted in revulsion at the mere thought of all those blank walls encircling him. He was suffering from etiolation, I concluded, the walls leaching the life out of him. I empathised. I watched the man shuffle off, busy again, rifling through his thinning hair, and picking the one destined-to-be shed, the one that was

277

dispensable. As I watched tears sprang to my eyes and I had to blink fast, move on, start talking before I drew attention to myself. Filling up the silences. Not so very different from Myrtle then.

Myrtle—1974

We are sitting on a low, rectangular, cushioned bench. It has been thoughtlessly upholstered in black plastic. In the heat it sticks to your legs like glue. You have to virtually peel yourself off it. The sweat trickles between my thighs. My flesh feels as if it is expanding. Even my hands stick to the surface of the seat when I lean on them. I fold them in my lap. I have waited here to see Jillian and Nicola and Harry off. I have waited here for Jillian and Nicola and Harry to arrive home. I have never waited here to see Alice off. Despite the difficulties of extricating myself from this horrid seat, I am up and down like a yo-yo. I am restless. Ralph is late. He is hurrying here from a prison-visit out at Stanley. If he doesn't make it, I am afraid . . . I am afraid Alice will hesitate, and will not go.

'Nicola and Jillian said they would try to make it,' I tell my daughter cheerfully. Alice's face, angled at a plug of chewing gum squashed flat on the floor, comes up at this. Her audible exhalation of breath does for a reply. We both know they are not coming. Things have been awkward between the girls since the death of the dog. I know they didn't see Bear that much, but they were devoted to him all the same. It was a dreadful blow to lose

278

him that way. Jillian wanted to know how Alice could do such a terrible thing, and Nicola just shook her head and said how much she would miss the dog, how she had adored walking him, when she found the time of course. I told them there were extenuating circumstances, that they should not judge their sister too harshly, that she never meant it to happen.

'But it did happen,' said Jillian. And I had to concede she was quite right.

Alice is wearing jeans, and a blue sweatshirt with a swirl of sequins on the front. The sequins reflect the fluorescent tube lighting set into the airport ceiling. They keep drawing my eyes, the sequins, green and orange spangles of light. I would have thought she'd be sweltering in it (the air conditioning in this place is less than useless), but she insists that she feels cold. She is wearing a small rucksack on her back, packed with a few things for the plane. I buy her a magazine and a couple of packets of fruit pastels.

'Make sure you suck them during take-off, won't you? It stops the ears popping,' I say, handing them to her. Her head is down as she takes them, her eyes veiled by hair. I notice her hands in her lap, that she's been biting her nails. They look chewed to the quick. I start to say something, and then I think, why bother. Alice nods in thanks for the sweets but never looks up. I glance at my watch. It is already midday. We have checked in her luggage at the BOAC desk already. I thought it was judicious.

'Let's do it now before a queue builds up,' I suggested. Alice shrugged. I led the way and Alice trundled after me with her case. Asked whether she packed it herself, Alice was non-committal.

'She only means I helped her,' I told the smartly-dressed ground stewardess with a fixed smile. And I reminded myself Alice would soon be lifting off. By tomorrow she would be on the other side of the world. I bit my tongue. 'And are there any seats by the emergency exit?' I requested, defiantly upbeat. 'You'd like a seat by the emergency exit, wouldn't you, Alice?'

'What, in case we crash?' Alice said. I scratched the palm of my left hand with my right, pushed Alice aside and took the initiative. I secured her a seat just in front of the emergency exit. I thanked the stewardess and hurried Alice away as fast as I could, explaining chirpily that these seats had more legroom.

Now we are just waiting. I decide to take advantage of this time alone together to give Alice a little advice.

'You will be careful about Granny,' I say. I reach a hand towards the tresses of Alice's hair, loose down her back. I am going to stroke it. Then Alice wheels round and faces me, and I change my mind.

'What do you mean?' Alice demands bluntly.

I rub the palm of my right hand before I respond. 'I wouldn't mention the . . . well . . . you know?'

'No?'

'She's an old woman. She doesn't understand these things.'

'What things?'

I raise my eyebrows suggestively, tuck in my chin. Alice stares blankly back at me. My legs are saturated. I am sure that when I stand up there will be a wet circle on my rear. I might even get a prickly heat rash where my thighs are rubbing, and that is so uncomfortable. I probably have patches of sweat under my arms too. I would love a cool bath now, a cool bath and a cold drink.

'What things?' Alice is mulish. Around us people struggle with their luggage. There is an endless chorus of murmuring voices. From time to time a few notes bounce off the white walls and the tiled floors, played I think on a xylophone, announcing the arrival or departure of a flight. The atmosphere created is similar to that on an ocean liner, when the passengers are summoned to a meal or an activity. It's odd that airports seem to affect people the way churches do. They all lower their voices and go about looking terribly sheepish. I need a drink. As soon as Alice's plane has taken off I will have a double whisky. The remainder of the day will be spent placating Ralph, I forecast gloomily. I will need fortifying. Perhaps I will have two. 'What things?' Alice prompts me yet again.

I clear my throat and speak in hushed tones, as if I too am being subdued by the reverential atmosphere, rather than discussing my daughter's squalid abortion in a public setting. 'The termination,' I whisper.

'Oh . . . that,' says Alice, her whisper of the 'stage' variety. I do not imagine it. She is being deliberately insolent. I wait for her to continue. She slips her rucksack off her back and fiddles with the buckle, but offers nothing more.

'Granny might be upset if you told her. Surely you can understand?' Why doesn't she say something? Is she enjoying this? Revelling in my embarrassment. 'Telling her . . . well . . . it wouldn't serve any purpose now, would it?'

'Wouldn't it?' Alice returns wide-eyed.

I chew the side of my cheek, then rally. 'And come to that, I'd be inclined not to tell her about the death of the dog either.' My words, delivered with deceptive sweetness, hit their intended target. A flicker of emotion lights Alice's eyes. 'Of course we all know it was an awful mishap that could never have been predicted. But being elderly these things can be disturbing.' Alice looks away and nods simultaneously. Her movements are so lethargic, it is as if she can hardly be bothered to execute them. 'And Uncle Albert, I shouldn't—' I decide to quit while I am ahead. I swallow and remember how dry my mouth is. 'Oh never mind. I know you won't let me down, Alice. I'm so happy for you at the start of this great adventure.' I make to grasp Alice's bony shoulders in an embrace, but she stands up. My hands slip off her, unable to find purchase.

'Dad!' she says.

Turning, I see Ralph striding over to us in a grey business suit, his tie askew, the fingers of one hand combing back his dark hair. They sit, huddle together a short space from me, and talk. I might just as well not be here for all the notice they pay me. But as I hear them call Alice's flight, I chastise myself for being miserly with my husband. Surely I can afford to be generous with these minutes, for soon, very soon, she will be gone, and I will have him all to myself. Even so, by the time we listen to the final call, I am on my feet and pacing about the bench.

'Shall we wander over?' I say, trying my hardest to sound casual. 'Best not to leave it too late. We don't want a horrid rush.' Ralph is fussing about money, passport and goodness knows what else. I want to interrupt him. I want to say we have been over and over this a hundred times. But I contain myself, and let this pointless dialogue run its course. At last we troop over to the departure gate. Prematurely I bend to give Alice a peck on the cheek. I miss my mark and find myself kissing my daughter's ear. I delve in my handbag for a handkerchief. Clasping it, I try to wipe away the smudge of red lipstick I have left on Alice's earlobe. My daughter flinches. I shrug, and pop the hanky back in my bag. I feel very cross and quite ridiculous. I hear an odd snicker of laughter and realise it is coming from me. I stand aside while Ralph enfolds Alice, and, making what I cannot help feeling is an unnecessary spectacle of himself, clasps her tightly for at least a minute.

'If it doesn't work out you know you can always come back,' he says, releasing her reluctantly. I hold my breath and wait for her response.

'I know,' says Alice blithely, but she is looking at me, not Ralph I am pleased to note. Then I release the air from my lungs and greedily gulp a breath. I smile at my daughter. We understand each other.

'Do take care, won't you darling,' I call after her as she vanishes through the departure gates. I tell Ralph that I want to see her plane take off. I do not add that I will not believe she is gone until I see her airborne. We make our way to the outside viewing platform on the second floor. The heat is coming in waves off the runway, making a shivering mirage of it all. We have to wait some time before we catch sight of Alice, stepping off the bus that has ferried her out to the plane. She walks up the mobile steps to the aircraft entrance. She turns then and waves. Ralph is grasping the wire-mesh fencing. He looks as if he would like to scale it, clamber down the other side, run over to the plane and fetch Alice back. Glancing from Ralph to Alice, my eyes are stabbed with a momentary flash as the sun catches on her sequinned top.

It seems ages before the plane takes off. The doors have closed yet nothing happens. In order to see it, we are forced out of the narrow block of shade we have found. My throat is parched. The viewing platform is sheltered, and without a breeze the sun is nigh on intolerable. I have forgotten my sunglasses. What with my thirst, my throbbing eyes, how sticky my skin feels, and how fatigued I am, the kind of fatigue an actress experiences after giving the performance of her lifetime I think, I am almost overcome with impatience. Why doesn't it go? Is something wrong? Is there a fault with the engine? Or is there a passenger who is feeling suddenly unwell? A young woman who has changed her mind, and says she wants to get off?

And then, thank God, the engines start up, a rumble that drowns out the thunder of my own apprehension. And suddenly I do not feel the heat or the clammy sweat. I lace the fingers of my hands and shelter my eyes from the glare. I inch forwards. My skin brushes against the hot metal of the mesh fencing. I breathe in the scent of fuel, mingled with dust and sea. I follow the plane as it taxis out to the start of the runway. I stare at the runway strip. From where we are standing it looks no more than a fragile plank stretching out into the sea. The plank sits on a wall of enormous

284

boulders. The sides of the wall splay as they vanish beneath the glittering water. The plane is hurtling down the plank now, picking up speed and then . . . then it lifts off. I can feel the fencing trembling with the force of it. In its own way it is awesome.

'Well, well,' I say, following the jet's trail in the air. 'It looks like Alice is safely away.' Ralph is as taciturn as his daughter was minutes ago. I smile and gently prise his hands from the fence. I link arms with my husband and lead him in the direction of the airport lounge. 'Let's have a quick drink before we dash off,' I suggest. Ralph shakes his head. I start arguing with him. 'What with the heat and—' I begin, and then break off. When you have won you can afford to be magnanimous.

Ghost—1974

On our arrival we are met with the news that space and privacy in the Ealing house is to be at a premium.

'I've taken on a couple of lodgers, so you'll be sharing with me for bit,' Audrey Lambert, Alice's grandmother says, forcing her voice out through the cracks, as she leads the way up a gloomy flight of stairs.

Alice wrestles with her suitcase. She is red-eyed, her skin dry and papery, her mouth enflamed from licking her lips repeatedly in the dry atmosphere of the plane. Having purchased two bottles of vodka in the duty-free shop before leaving Hong Kong, she has taken periodic nips of the stuff throughout the flight. Now, struggling up the narrow staircase, she glances over her shoulder. Her head wobbles, her eyes stretch wide, and her mouth gapes, for here we all are, the dog, the monkey and me, like a bridal train sweeping behind her. The monkey, having slept for most of flight, is just waking up, green eyes crossed in puzzlement as it surveys the scene. Its illuminations flicker weakly, as it bowls hesitantly up the banister. The dog, never one to make a fuss, trots upstairs after Alice, snuffling the worn carpet at her heels with mild interest. I glide decorously after him. From one of the front rooms, Alice's Uncle Albert can be heard, having what sounds like a conversation with himself. He is a flamboyant character, his robes reminiscent of the elaborate garments I have seen actors wear, when they give performances of Chinese opera.

'Carousel,' identifies Audrey, wheezing and patting her chest, as we gain the upstairs landing. She pauses for a moment outside her bedroom door to catch her breath, and gestures to another door adjacent to it. 'The lodgers' bedroom. They really are very nice girls, Geraldine and Yvonne.' She takes in Alice head to toe and sniffs. 'Very nice and very respectable. The smallest bedroom has been converted into a kitchenette for them, and the largest bedroom, well, that's their sitting room now.' Alice nods dully. Her eyelids are heavy, and although it is only lunchtime she would dearly love to go to bed.

George is waiting for us in Audrey's middle-sized bedroom. George is Audrey's budgie. I loathe him from first sight. In the main he is covered in iridescent lime-green and vivid yellow plumage. Sprouting from these opulent colours are two speckled, dirty-grey wings. This grubby pattern extends upwards, capping his silly domed head. He has a curved honey-coloured beak, a blue cere with dark pin-prick nostrils set into it, and a pair of beady black eyes, rimmed in oyster grey. His cage is suspended from a short chain. This in turn is hooked onto the overhanging metal arm of a stand. The stand is set between quilted twin beds. Eyeing us suspiciously, George squawks and flaps against the shiny, silver bars of his cage. He lights on one of three wooden perches skewered through it, dips his long tail feathers, and defecates messily on the golden, gritted paper that lines his tray.

'Remember George?' Audrey says, crossing to the cage, and blowing kisses through the bars at the bemused bird. 'He's a treasure, isn't he?' Alice looks impassively at George. 'Perhaps I hadn't got him when last you visited. But I don't know what I'd do without him now.'

'Mm . . . does he . . . sleep here?' Alice inquires haltingly setting her case down, and watching as George makes his wagging way along a perch. He moves, she observes, with surprising alacrity, speeding to his feeding bowl, from where he seems to do a far better job of spitting birdseed all over the twin beds than depositing it in his feathered belly.

'Oh yes. I'd be lost if he wasn't by my side at nights,' Audrey says. 'He's such good company. Irreplaceable!' She is temporarily overcome with emotion. Her glasses have misted over. She removes them, polishes them energetically on her pinafore and places them back on.

Over the next few days as Alice tries in vain to catch up on her sleep, we find out just how good

George's company can be. Alice observes through smarting eyes that he never seems to tire, that he keeps up his screeching chatter throughout the night. And this, despite her grandmother putting a cover over his cage, signifying that it is time for all living things to rest. While from the back room that looks out onto the tiny, walled garden, or booming out from the environs of his downstairs bedroom, or declaiming satisfyingly in the splendid acoustics of the upstairs bathroom, Uncle Albert can be heard mid-script, mid-song, mid-performance. During the meals that are eaten around a small, oak dining table, seated on yellow formica chairs, the recitals continue. And they continue through television programmes and radio plays. One morning, washing up in the small kitchen, Alice asks her grandmother why her Uncle Albert no longer performs for a living, while we are lucky enough to be entertained all day long by him.

'He jumped on a nail when dancing in a pantomime, dear,' Audrey says, agitating the few bubbles that float on the surface of the warm water, in the white, enamel sink she hunches over. 'He was barefoot you see. The nail was rusty. Fate my dear, that's what it was. Very nasty. All that talent. Such a waste. Now he works part-time selling tickets for the Royal Opera House.'

From the dining room Uncle Albert can be heard blissfully warbling.

'*Funny Girl*,' Audrey sighs, her chest swelling with pride, her gnarled hands occupied scouring out the grill pan.

Then one Sunday evening after a soggy weekend, in which the bird and Uncle Albert compete with one another to see who is the more voluble, Alice announces she is off job-hunting in the morning. I experience an immediate rush of excitement wondering where this hunt will lead us. However, our search proves to be a wretched affair. Fruitlessly we tramp the streets for several hours, being told repeatedly that there are no vacancies. Just when I think Alice would do well to give up, she accepts a job as a shop assistant at small supermarket in the high street. Harrison's.

'I'm just learning the ropes. Of course, I shan't be a shop assistant for very long,' Alice informs her grandmother over coffee later that night. Audrey shoots her granddaughter a mistrustful look. Alice takes a gulp from her cup and scalds her mouth. After a bit she says lamely. 'They're going to train me up for management.'

Recently we have all grown jittery. And can you blame us, considering. The dog hides in the dark cupboard under the stairs, or paces the tiled hallway, claws clicking, or skulks about at the back of the garden shed, leaping out when you least expect it. The monkey mewls through the nights, compounding Alice's exhaustion. And even I, ill at ease in this cold grey country, finally boil over. The first day of her new job, my host scrambles out of bed to see the stand for the birdcage empty. The chain is swinging gently from side to side. The cage is lying upside down on the floor, under the bay window. There is birdseed showered all over the room, water spattered up the newly decorated bedroom walls, papered in a rose trellis design, and a cuttlefish lodged in the light fitting. The bird cowers in a corner under a torn bit of soggy gritted paper, heart rattling, wings flapping ineffectually.

289

True, he has lost a bit of plumage and his remaining feathers are a little ruffled. But apart from that no real harm has been done, certainly nothing that warrants the kind of reaction Alice and her grandmother have seeing George's little mishap. My host screams as she stands over the empty cage, and then begins to jabber unintelligibly, arms thrashing the air. At the sharp cry Audrey's tired eyes spring open, and veer confusedly from the upturned cage to her granddaughter. She flings back her covers, climbs from the bed and totters over to Alice. The lizard skin on her arms and neck trembles violently. Her flaccid face darkens to a bruised purple. Her brow puckers into ugly, uneven ridges. She sucks in her lips and her eyes flare.

'George my baby! What have you done to George?' she howls.

Audrey—1974

I do not have insomnia. If my rheumatism would only let up, I know I would sleep and sleep. It's the pain that keeps waking me. It settles in the joints. My knees are the worst, then my hips and then my hands. I am wearing my glasses, kept to hand at my bedside. I scrutinise my swollen knuckles. They look like witch's hands now, twisted as the trunk of some old tree. I've put on my sidelight, but I'm afraid it's got George going a bit. Chinks of light must be getting through underneath his cage. He's started chirping, very softly it's true, but I'd best go downstairs if I can't rest. Across from me Alice is asleep. I shall not say fast asleep, for she tosses and turns and mutters.

My hands are bad because I began a letter to Myrtle yesterday. When you are young, you cannot contemplate a world where writing a letter could levy such a high price from you. I did not finish it. Alice returned home, and as the subject of my missive was sensitive enough for me not to want my granddaughter to see it, I put it away carefully in my writing folder. Not satisfied with this I came upstairs, and tucked the folder in the bottom drawer of my dressing table, beneath my undergarments, hidden from sight. No one saw me.

Then in the middle of the night my pain woke me. Even turning on the bedside lamp was a struggle, but I managed in the end. In the subdued lighting, at first I could not believe my eyes. Items of my underwear were strewn across the room. My writing folder was lying wide open on the floor. The two pages of my letter lay screwed up a yard or so from the bin, as if someone had aimed to toss them in, missed and left them scattered, wide of their mark.

I did not cry out. I am getting used to such happenings. I made my slow way over to the bin, bent painfully and retrieved them. I returned with them to my bed, eased myself down on the edge of it, smoothed out the creased paper and read.

Dear Myrtle,
For some months now I have been deeply worried by Alice's behaviour. I have tried to keep my anxieties from you, but we are rapidly descending into mayhem. I feel the

situation can no longer be ignored. Do not
misunderstand me when I say that Alice's
manner is a cause for concern. I do not mean
that she is rude or difficult. In every respect
she appears compliant and polite.

However, although I have never caught
Alice making mischief we live daily with the
consequences of her actions. Lights fuse, the
bath floods, the toilet refuses to flush, the
television has broken down no less than five
times.

I have done all I can to help you in the
past, Myrtle, and this, despite the problems
with Jillian and Nicola, and us having very
different ideas about family life. But
something's not right with Alice.

I have just learnt that my sister-in-law,
your Aunt Deirdre, now living in Haywards
Heath, is gravely ill and has asked for me. I
feel I would never forgive myself if I did not
go to her.'

This was when I left off writing. Now I look at
my scrawl on the crumpled sheet, and see that in
some places it is very nearly illegible. I fold it and
place carefully under my pillow. I can't face
copying it out on a fresh sheet. I will try to
complete it tomorrow or after I get back from
Deirdre's. My eyes rove round the room. I do not
have the energy to tidy away my undergarments
for the moment. It will have to wait until morning.
The shadow of the birdcage looms large on the
wall, and as I watch it begins to shift, just a few
inches at first, and then more, until it is jerking and
swinging. My eyes snap back to the cage.

Motionless. Alice, on her back now, looks as if she is trying to shift some heavy object from her chest. She grunts with the effort. Not for the first time I feel a finger of unease trace my spine. I climb laboriously back into bed and pull the blankets up. In a while I will snap off the light. Though in the dark, some nights I hear strange noises, the thump of a book falling perhaps, the scrape of a chair-leg, the clatter of a saucepan lid. Maybe it's the lodgers I tell myself? Still, why not just this once try to sleep with the light on, eh?

The following day, a Friday, I tell Alice about my sister-in-law, that I must go to her. I inform her that a cab is coming for me on Saturday at noon, and that all being well, I should only be away overnight, returning on the Sunday. I tell her I will leave a number by the phone in the hall, and that she can ring me if there are any problems at all. I add that the lodgers, Geraldine and Yvonne, are visiting their respective parents for the weekend. I have already spoken to Albert. Alice is very sympathetic.

Over and over on the morning of my departure I tell her to make sure the gas is switched off, that all the electrical appliances are unplugged. I tell her to be especially careful if she is cooking. 'Don't worry Gran,' she sings out, as she waves me off and I leave my home behind, 'I'll take care of everything.'

293

Ghost—1974

After Audrey leaves, the house seems very quiet, as if it is waiting for something to happen. Uncle Albert vanishes back into his bedroom. Though Alice pauses outside his door for a time, all continues silent. She goes into the kitchen and pours herself a glass of orange squash. She checks she has turned the tap off several times before she is finally persuaded that it is only dripping, not leaking. Then she sits in the back room, in her grandmother's wooden rocker. For what feels like an age she rocks her slight weight forwards and back, the motion reminding her of sitting on the swing in the gardens of the flat on The Peak. She thinks about England and how it does not feel like her home at all, no matter how much she wants it to. My host feels, she imagines, the way an immigrant does, coming here to settle, leaving their country far behind them, coping with a new life, new ways of doing things. And always searching for that sense of belonging, but not necessarily finding it.

As she rocks, Alice thinks about the Queen, pictures her sitting on her throne with her sparkly crown perched on her head, just like the portraits she has seen so many times in Hong Kong. Alice wonders what she might say to her if she was ushered into her throne room by a beefeater with a crimson jacket and tall busby hat.

'Your Majesty,' Alice imagines saying, after curtseying, 'although I know I'm British, at least that's what's stamped on my passport, I don't feel right here. I feel like a kind of non-immigrant, as if I should fit but I don't.'

She is certain that the Queen would be very gracious about it, but explain in that special voice of hers that it cannot be helped.

'Alice Safford, you are a child of the colonies, and I'm afraid as my empire shrinks, they are vanishing fast. So, wee, wee, wee, my overseas subjects are bound to find their way home. In time, Alice, I feel sure you'll acclimatise and, just like a stick of Brighton Rock, feel British through and through.'

But Alice is not so sure. I remind her that if she is finding the adjustment hard, how difficult does she think it's proving for us! Eventually brooding on this, she falls asleep. The preternatural quiet is harrowing. The dog and the monkey are nowhere to be seen. Even they would have provided welcome companionship at present. But deliverance from this enforced solitude comes from a surprising quarter, for it is Uncle Albert's singing that wakes Alice up. Still dazed, she looks at the clock over the mantelpiece and shakes her head. She stares at the lengthening shadows in the garden. Cool indigo fingers extending over the small expanse of grass, and over the beds, where late summer flowers bob their heads, and on up the brick walls that encase the small plot. Alice rises and we creep into the hall. She is barefoot, and the pretty tiled floor, a geometric design of cobalt blue, nut-brown, saffron yellow and cream, is cold to the flesh. Uncle Albert's bedroom door opens off the hall. Alice stands outside it. We spot the monkey sliding down the banister.

'Wheee!' it squeals.

'Shush!' hisses Alice, a finger to her lips. The daredevil monkey glowers and scampers up the stairs, vaults onto the newel post, and, pipe-cleaner legs astride, starts sliding down again.

Bear-as-Was shuffles out of the under-stairs cupboard, a woebegone expression on his long face, tail between his legs. His shiny steel claws click on the tiles. Alice raises her eyes and shakes her head. Taking the hint, the dog slopes off back into the shadows. Then another sound rings out. It is Uncle Albert again. He is in good voice today. The lyrics of a light opera thunder out, interspersed with what sound like grating sobs.

Alice begins to obey a well-mannered impulse to leave her Uncle to play out his misery in private. She turns away from the door and takes a couple of steps towards the stairs. But we have never been in Uncle Albert's room, and I for one am curious. Without giving Alice time to think I steer her back again. By now, so abandoned is his weeping that it cannot be ignored for any reason. Alice taps softly on his door, and when this draws no response she knocks more loudly. Light comes in coloured shafts, blue and green and brown, falling through the small stained-glass panel set into the front door. It shifts over Alice's white face, giving her the look of a woodland sprite. The leaded panes make up the picture of a boat, making us both feel homesick.

'Uncle Albert, it's me. It's Alice. Can I come in?'

There is a hiatus in the wails, but no summons for her to push open the door. On a whim, for which I must take responsibility, Alice decides she will enter without an invitation. We shut the door

296

in the monkey's naughty face. The scene that meets us could not have been more fantastical. The curtains are tightly drawn against the fading day. A glowing bulb suspended from the ceiling, protrudes from a beaded, pink shade. A bedside lamp set on a table, with a frosted-glass shade shaped like the petals of a flower, also illuminates the fair-sized room. The alchemy of electric light falling on the plain, yellow satin curtains transforms them into bands of shimmering gold. In the room is a bed, one side of which is buttressed against the dividing wall, separating bedroom from hallway. There is a tall, ornately-carved wardrobe, and a chest of drawers with a freestanding mirror set upon it. The mirror comprises three hinged panels, each framed in dark wood, and standing on clawed feet. Here light bounces between the silver planes, the reflections multiplying and splintering, giving you the impression that the room is never-ending.

Uncle Albert lies supine on a decorative, flower-patterned rug, hugging his knees. His face is plastered with thick make-up, a foundation of peach greasepaint, cheeks rouged as red as ripe apples, mouth smeared with scarlet lipstick, eyes ringed with bands of peacock-blue and weighed down with thick, spider-leg lashes. His hair, which normally sits like a pudding basin over his head, dun grey, with a space for his face snipped out, has been tucked up into some sort of net, and clipped firmly down. He is shedding real tears. Seeing them triggers a distant memory of the sensation of weeping in me, the dragging feeling in the chest, the eyes brimming over unbidden, the lungs shuddering in painful breaths, desperate for air but unable to expand, as if squeezed by invisible hands. I follow the progress of Uncle Albert's tears, mesmerised as they roll, not down his cheeks but across them, such is the angle of his head. The tears cloud as they gather specks of peach foundation, blue eyeshadow, black mascara and cherry-red rouge, coursing along the fleshy pads and bony hollows of his cheeks. Mucus is also dribbling from his pronounced Roman nose, and running into the colourful tears. Funny—the sight of his sorrow reminds me that I have never seen my host cry.

He is wearing a willow-green, full-length, mandarin-style robe, with copper fruits embroidered on it. Beside him on the floor lies a blonde wig, sprawled out, as if it has recently faced combat, and is now making the most of a few minutes respite. Albert's bed is unmade. His bedding, together with a tangle of coloured shawls, tumbles over it. They spill onto the wooden floor beneath it. The mirrored door of his wardrobe is flung wide. Several outfits lie in a jumble at the bottom of it, fighting for space with brocade slippers, and pairs of glittery high-heeled shoes. A cigarette in a turquoise enamel cigarette holder, still smoking, balances on the side of a glass ashtray, atop the chest of drawers. Its pearly trail snakes up towards the ceiling. Alongside it are several well-thumbed scripts, and an open wooden box crammed with make-up. A drooping auburn moustache loops over one corner of it. Tubes of greasepaint are just visible, and two false beards, one black and one white. Piled in an oval china dish in front of the make-up box are glittering rings and bangles, shiny beaded necklaces, and pairs of spangled, dangly earrings. Set to one side of the mirror is another wig, a mass of electric-blue curls propped on a wig-stand. Scents of tobacco, incense, perfume and sweat permeate the air. It feels to me like an actor's dressing room, a place of disguise and magic, which I suppose, after all, is what it is.

Then Uncle Albert suddenly spreads his arms wide. Staring straight at the ceiling he gives a prolonged, nasal groan. As Alice approaches cautiously, her nostrils are assailed with the heavy odour of jasmine. When she reaches him she squats down, and leaning over him, speaks in a whisper.

'What's the matter, Uncle Albert?'

Uncle Albert gives another heartfelt sob. He tears his sodden eyes away from the ceiling, and rests them on his niece's features.

'Uncle Albert, do tell me what's wrong? I can keep secrets you know.'

Uncle Albert licks his clown mouth and says falteringly, 'I . . . am . . . I am in love.' Alice nods encouragement. 'I am in love . . . with . . . with a married . . . man.' You can tell he is an actor, I reflect admiringly. His modulation is perfect. He pauses. When Alice does not move, and her steady gaze does not waver, he continues. 'His name is Reginald and he has decided . . . decided that he must go back to his wife and his two children. He has left me, to return to the sham that is his marriage.'

Again the tears rush to his eyes, and his chest heaves up and down. But now he weeps silently, and his anguish seems so much more poignant for the entombment of its sound. Alice draws even

299

closer, lightly touching his shoulder.

'I do not think I can bear the pain. I think I would rather die,' confesses Uncle Albert elongating his words dolorously.

'Perhaps,' says Alice, taking hold of her Uncle's arms, and pulling him up with care until he is sitting, 'we should have a party.'

Uncle Albert slumps, wet-faced on the worn rug, while he absorbs this suggestion. He is still sitting when Alice returns with a brand-new bottle of vodka.

'Let's have a drink, Uncle Albert,' she says, breaking the seal and unscrewing the top.

Uncle Albert has stopped crying, and is looking intrigued. Alice brings in a yellow Formica chair from the dining table in the front room. She goes back and fetches two cream and blue striped mugs. She sets them down on the floor. She pats the chair invitingly. She fills the mugs with generous measures of vodka.

'You sit here, Uncle Albert. I am going to touch up your make-up, and put your wig back on, and soon you will be all beautiful again.'

When Uncle Albert has made himself comfortable on the chair, Alice hands him a mug. She takes her own mug in her hand, and clinks her mug to his with a winsome grin.

'The devil take Reginald,' is her toast. 'Now down it in one, and then I'll pour us another.'

So while Uncle Albert drinks his vodka, Alice redoes his make-up with the utmost care. She decks him with beads and bangles and earrings, till he sparkles. She eases on his shoulder-length blonde wig. She selects a pair of glamorous shoes for him, and with determination tugs them on his large, unwieldy feet. She chooses a mandarin-style jacket from Uncle Albert's wardrobe for herself. It is black, with huge, extravagant, roseate peonies appliquéd on it. She pulls it on over her shirt, and does up the fiddly cord buttons. Then she covers her own face with greasepaint, smoothing it on with her fingertips. She dabs bright spots of rouge onto her cheeks, paints on eye-shadow, strokes mascara through her eyelashes. She sweeps lipstick over her mouth, and, as an afterthought, she seizes the electric-blue wig from the dresser, and pulls it on over her own mousy-brown hair. And when she is finished she tells Uncle Albert that now they are both ready for the party. Uncle Albert takes two, long, thoughtful swallows of vodka, and the corners of his clown mouth turn up in a broad smile.

'Let's dance, Uncle Albert,' Alice proposes.

So Uncle Albert gets up and tries out a few experimental steps. His blonde hair swishes around his face. They push back the chair, lift the vodka bottle and the mugs onto the chest of drawers out of harm's way, link arms and jig about the floor.

'Let's dance the tango?' Uncle Albert proposes.

'I'm not sure I know the tango,' Alice says, frowning.

'It doesn't matter. We'll make it up as we go along,' Uncle Albert reassures her. 'Performers often fake it,' he adds with a professional wink of one heavily-lashed eye. So Alice speeds into the garden and picks a late rose. It sheds a few flesh-pink petals as she rushes back with it, holding it in her clenched teeth. After weighing up the effect Uncle Albert nods his approval. Then, he grasps

301

his niece in a clinch. After the tango they do some ballet. Alice stands on tiptoes and totters around the room circling her arms gracefully. Uncle Albert does proper turns, executed with as much precision as he can manage in his high-heeled shoes. His eyes fix on a spot. Then he spins, his head flicking round and catching up with the rest of him in a flurry of blonde hair a second later. He wiggles and concertinas himself and jumps.

'I do not have the freedom I am accustomed to in a leotard,' he says apologetically. But Alice only applauds the louder.

Then Alice reveals shyly that she has always wanted to fly, and Uncle Albert tells her that it can be arranged.

'I did it once with the aid of a belt and wires in *Peter Pan*, Alice,' he says. 'It was simply stupendous.' He helps Alice onto the bed. When he raises his hand, the agreed signal that he is ready, Alice leaps into the air. Uncle Albert catches her, his open arms closing on her small, air-borne frame.

'I've had to catch all manner of women in my time, and some of them weighed a ton,' volunteers Uncle Albert, wincing at the memory.

'I wasn't too heavy was I?' Alice asks anxiously.

'Not you,' replies Uncle Albert, dismissing Alice's concerns with a flowery wave. 'You are light as a bird, dear lady.' He bows genteelly and Alice giggles.

It is the mention of the bird that gives me the idea. They are having such a fun time, Alice and her Uncle, and I am beginning to feel excluded. I watch them as they collapse onto the rug and share some more vodka together. I ruminate on how I might contribute to the party spirit.

'Reginald can be a pompous twat sometimes, and a bit of a killjoy,' Uncle Albert declares audaciously, finishing off his sentence with a loud raspberry, his tight, red lips flapping as the air is forced out. They both shriek with laughter, making me feel even more keenly that I have been left out in the cold. The private joke just seems to get funnier and funnier. The two of them roll about on the floor and laugh and laugh. They laugh until different tears course down their cheeks. I recognise them as tears of joy. I feel bitterly jealous then. That is when my idea becomes a compulsion, and I force it into Alice's happy head.

'Why don't we set George free?' Alice blurts out excitedly, topping up their mugs with vodka, taking up hers and handing Albert his. They both take several sips as they consider the idea. 'He must hate it cooped up in that little cage. He must want more than anything to spread his wings and fly.'

Uncle Albert listens to what his niece says with his head on one side, and his blonde hair spilling over one shoulder.

'That . . . that . . . is a most ex . . . excellent plan,' he concurs. His voice has become sticky as plum jam.

At last the two of them weave their way upstairs with much hilarity, having drained the bottle, still hugging their now empty mugs. The monkey at the top of the stairs scouts ahead. The dog slouches after them. I slide elegantly along the ceiling. Once we are all in Audrey Lambert's bedroom Alice switches on the light, and with a flourish produces a second bottle of vodka from under her bed. My host and Uncle Albert refill their mugs.

303

'I shall . . . shall endeavour to . . . to sing I am the very modern model mo . . . jor general,' announces Uncle Albert. But he keeps tripping over his words and spluttering with laughter. Alice, overcome with mirth as well, lies on the floor and kicks her legs against the floorboards, until the din of drumming makes the little bottles on Audrey's dressing table tinkle. The monkey sits on the edge of the mantelpiece over the small fireplace clapping its rubiginous star hands, and swinging its spindly legs. Bear-as-Was rolls on his back galloping his diaphanous crimson paws in the air. Then Alice rises unsteadily, and staggers over to the budgie cage. With my guidance she opens its door. George squawks nervously. He hooks his beak on the bars in agitation. He clambers round and round his cage three or four times, as if making sure it is still there, still safe. Uncle Albert says they should forget George, because he is making a drama of escaping.

'We haven't got all day to . . . to wait around for . . . for that daft budgie to take off,' he protests.

Uncle Albert is right because dusk is setting in. Soon the day will be gone and the night will descend. He slips off his high-heeled shoes, and with difficulty mounts Audrey's bed. He climbs unsteadily to his feet and begins to jump. Following his lead, Alice springs on her own bed. They try their hardest to get a rhythm going. The monkey thinks this is a great laugh and joins them, bouncing so high that once or twice it hits the ceiling. The dog makes do with racing round the beds until he is so dizzy he flops down. And because I think it might be amusing I nudge Alice. She clambers dutifully off the bed, and fetches the packet of birdseed from the top of Audrey's dressing table. They fill their hands with hundreds of seeds, and while they bounce clumsily, they throw them up at the ceiling.

'It's raining birdseed!' Alice squeals, alight with merriment as seeds shower down on her head.

Uncle Albert even catches some in his mouth and pretends to crunch on them, as if they are really delicious. But Bear-as-Was and the ghoulish monkey are riveted by something else now. While it is raining birdseed they bound over to the birdcage, their ghostly eyes trained on George. Tempted perhaps by the flying feast, he ventures nervously out of the open cage-door. He flutters around the room, a radiant flash of green and yellow. He trills happily, gobbling seed wherever he finds it. Alice and Uncle Albert are half way through a rendition of 'Three Little Maids from School', which Uncle Albert says is from *The Mikado*, when they notice George has vacated his cage. They point and gaze at the bird for a short period, as he circles the room. By now they are making substantial inroads into the second bottle of vodka, and both are beginning to feel a bit sleepy. Neither of them realise that there is a sizable gap at the bottom of one of the sash windows. I have been inching it up for some while now. I like to keep busy. By the time George discovers it and falls out, Alice and Uncle Albert are so drunk it is hard to think straight.

'George,' Alice slurs, 'has . . . has fall . . . fall . . . en oh . . . oh . . . out of the window.'

'Ah, that is . . . to . . . ooo bad,' is Uncle Albert's only comment, before he blacks out on the floor with a thud.

Alice stumbles over to the window and joins me, the dog and monkey following curiously. The monkey spies a walking stick propped up in a corner of the room, and uses it to pole-vault onto the window ledge. And the dog bounds up and rests his paws either side of the little imp. I mould myself economically to the window-frame. Alice takes up her unsteady position under me and adjacent to the dog and monkey. From here we spot George, illuminated by the bedroom light, sitting in a tree only feet away. It is a large magnolia tree with huge, waxy, dark leaves. Against them, George's dazzling plumage is shown off to great advantage, even in the waning light. Alice slides her hands under the gap in the sash window, and after several attempts manages to push it up at least another foot. She lowers her face to the rectangle of deepening blue, and talks into it in a murmur. She is fighting to keep her eyes open. The image of George keeps splitting in two, and Alice has to concentrate very hard to merge them back into one.

'Fly Georges, fly. Go on, fly away Georges.'

But George only swivels his head, blinks his beady eyes, and nibbles experimentally on one of the large leaves. Then Alice too passes out, close to her uncle, the empty vodka bottle rolling out of her hand, and over the seed-covered floor, before finally coming to a halt by the bird stand, where the empty cage swings gently. We three ghosts curl up beside her.

And this is where Audrey finds us, bathed in the dapple greys of dawn, her son Albert, in his make-up and blonde wig and robe of mandarin splendour, and her granddaughter Alice, crowned with a mass of electric-blue hair, the tips of it sodden from the pool of vomit in which she lies, and me lounging close by. Alice's face is wet with bile. It has soaked into her black jacket, and stained two huge pink peonies a sickly mud-brown. Audrey stands in the doorway and surveys the carnage of her bedroom, her spine rigid, her breath coming in harsh gulps, her heart beating erratically. She has rushed home early, driven by a dark premonition, she mumbles brokenly.

Sensing rather than hearing a presence in the room, Alice opens her eyes. Her throat is parched. Her head hurts and the taste in her mouth is vile. Her skin is crawling. Only inches from her eyes, floating on the brown pool of bile her head lies in, is a fluffy feather, yellow edged with lime green. Now her eyes swim up and beyond it. The first thing she fixes upon is her grandmother's face, puckered and pale as milk skin. Alice sees she is swathed in a coat, standing only feet away. She tracks a line of drool, running from the corner of her grandmother's slack mouth down her chin. Fleetingly Alice meets her pinched, agonised eyes, notes the sweat beading her brow, her eye sockets, her cheeks. Finally her gaze drops to her grandmother's cupped hands. The hands are angled towards her, the rheumatic fingers bent awkwardly about some treasure. The sight makes Alice think suddenly of the three kings presenting their offerings to baby Jesus in the stable. She stares at the gift, stares at the yellow and green plumage streaked red. She sees that George's head has been bitten clean away, a single drop of blood blistering over the ragged stump, swelling and swelling, till at last it is liberated and splashes to the floor.

Dear me, I think resignedly, what a very silly bird not to fly away when it had the chance. Instead it must have hung about, making itself easy prey for the next door's cat. Such a pity! The dog and the monkey at my side nod in agreement.

The very next week we move out, all five of us. Yes, five. It pains me to tell you, but as we climb into the taxi I see a flash of green and yellow in the wing mirror. It seems headless George intends to join us, regardless of how welcome he is. I am not overly impressed with our new domicile either, a bed-sit by Ealing Broadway station. Apart from anything else it is very cramped, consisting of a small combined bedroom and kitchenette, and an even smaller bathroom. It is situated on the second floor of an old Victorian house. It is a hovel compared to the flat on The Peak.

Ghost—1975

The day everything changes dawns like any other. Christmas has been and gone, with Alice refusing an invitation from her father to fly home for the holidays, claiming work could not possibly manage without her.

'I'm afraid Harrison's needs me, Daddy. I couldn't leave them short-staffed during their busiest period,' she told her father on the communal payphone in the hall.

It is January. In Hong Kong soon there will be celebrations for Chinese New Year, the volley of firecrackers in the streets of Kowloon, a riot of coloured fireworks bursting and starring the night sky, homes chiming with laughter, filled with the steaming aroma of appetizing dishes, families and friends visiting with each other. Here, we are on our way to work. Overhead is a canopy of slate-grey cloud, from which drizzle has been falling for some hours. The streets are crowded with people bundled up in coats and hats. Some steer prams and pushchairs, hold umbrellas, or grasp baskets of shopping or briefcases, as they hurry by. Alice has forgotten her coat. She is shivering in her damp clothes, little puffs of her warm breath misting in the cold air. Cars and buses, their headlights raking the gloom, their spinning tyres sending up fans of muddy water, rumble noisily on by. Horns blare, brakes grind, engines grumble, voices blur into one another, and the lights from traffic and shops bounce and scissor over the dark puddles.

Predictably we are late arriving, my host looking unequal to the demands of her job. Hanks of damp tangled hair cling to her cheeks and forehead. There are blue shadows under her glassy eyes and deep grey hollows beneath her pronounced cheekbones. The sores at the corner of her mouth are weeping pus. She looks emaciated. Her clothes are creased and ingrained with dirt. Even her green overall has stains on it. She now slips the quarter bottle of vodka she always carries in her bag into the large pocket stitched at the front of it before making her entrance on the shop floor. The floor-supervisor, Janice, looks askance at her and steams over.

'You don't look well, Alice,' she observes economically. 'P'raps you ought to go home.'

'No . . . no, I'm fine,' Alice insists, swaying

slightly on her feet, and pulling on a lump of matted hair at the back of her head.

'You better stay out of the way this morning then, and do a bit of shelf-stacking. Aisle three,' Janice orders. And then, when Alice hesitates, she tells her to be quick about it. As Alice wanders off, she follows her stilted progress with disapproving eyes, and a shake of her head.

Sure enough, in aisle three we find a trolley loaded with cardboard boxes. Alice prises them open and lifts out the cans she finds, one by one, her muddled brain trying to recall what she needs to do with them. Making painfully slow progress, she begins lifting them onto the shelves. But as she works the monkey does its best to sabotage her efforts, tipping them over. A few fall to the floor, and the dog bats them playfully about the aisle with his scarlet forepaws. Sensing sport, the bird puts its feathered shoulder to a packet of Weetabix, thrilling at the domino effect it manages to achieve. One by one, the entire row of cereal boxes tumble to the floor. I do what I can to curtail this ghostly horseplay, but they are incorrigible.

As we near Alice's lunch-break, my frazzled host can think of little else but the bottle of vodka in her pocket, and how badly she needs a pull on it. At this inopportune moment, a disgruntled customer accosts Alice in an abrasive impatient tone.

'Where are the tins of red salmon? I've been looking all over the place. I do wish they'd stop moving things about. It makes it very difficult when you're in a rush.' She pauses, her sharp mud-brown eyes absorbing Alice's slovenly appearance. She fingers the pearls at her neck irritably. 'I

310

especially need red salmon for a Fanny Cradock recipe I'm making this evening.' Alice scans the tins, trying hard to focus on their labels. She starts ineffectually shuffling them about, then with a trembling hand offers one to the customer

'No, no, that's tuna!' The lady is irate. Her backcombed grey hair sits on her head like a bird's nest, wobbling as her ire rises. Her voice climbs steeply. 'I said salmon, red salmon! Are you deaf? Do I have to keep repeating myself?'

Alice is contrite. She apologises, and after several attempts, thwarted yet again by the monkey, who is once more haunting the shelves, slots the can she is holding back in place.

'There they are,' the customer declares, pointing a manicured finger at the topmost shelf. 'Up there.' The monkey materialises among the cans of salmon she is indicating. 'You'll have to lift one down for me. I can't possibly clamber about in this skirt.'

The monkey grips the shelf edge with its spidery fingers, and peers down at Alice, devilry dancing in its refulgent green eyes. The dog stands on his hind-legs, and places his forepaws on the middle shelf, eager to help. The budgie who has been wheeling overhead, collides with a tower of special offer toilet rolls, and sends several tumbling to the floor. The sudden series of thumps as they impact on the tiles, makes the customer jump. Returning her gaze to Alice, she appraises my host critically.

'Well,' she demands, 'are you going to assist me?'

Alice's head wobbles in assent. She eyes her goal blearily, working out she will need to stand on the bottom shelf in order to reach it. The monkey hides, crouching down behind the tiers of canned fish. I lean back against the shelves, spectral arms entwined, interested to see how this will play out. Alice clears a space for a foothold, and steps onto it. With one hand she grips the second shelf, with the other she reaches towards the third, and makes a grab for the can of salmon. The monkey's riposte is to pitch three tins back at her. One strikes Alice hard on the head, another hits her shoulder, and a third lands on her foot. She yelps, leaps back and ducks. As she bends, arms flaying, the bottle of vodka tumbles out of her pocket and smashes on the floor. Instantly my host dives after it.

'Nooooh!' she wails. Her head swings up. She holds the customer's stunned, brown eyes with her own venomous ones. 'Look what you've done you stupid cow!'

She is kneeling on the broken glass in a paroxysm of rage, more wild, unholy sounds streaming from her mouth. The monkey, emerging from behind a can, peers down in astonishment at Alice crawling on the floor. The dog sticks its beetle-black nose in a puddle of vodka, and crunches experimentally on a shard of glass. The bird, having succeeded in prising the lid off an egg-carton on the opposite shelf, squats hopefully on a large brown egg. The customer clutches at her pearls and starts screaming.

Then they are all running towards Alice, customers and staff alike. They come from the cheese and the meat counter, from the fruit and veg, from the bakery, and from the other aisles. Harrison employees in their green tunics, customers, men and woman, old, middle-aged and young, swell the numbers, wheeling trolleys and clutching shopping baskets and bags. Janice the supervisor is one of the first on the scene, almost as if she has been expecting an accident. She is followed by the manager, who in turn is followed by the new security guard, Bert. As they near Alice, they all freeze and stare. They are agog. My host is on her knees, groping about on the wet floor, among the jagged pieces of glass. The customer, who wanted the salmon for her recipe, slumps against a shelf whimpering. Somebody steps forward to calm her down. Suddenly Alice scoops up a fragment of the bottle that still holds some vodka. She raises it to her mouth and drinks greedily, lapping at it with her tongue.

'Do something, Mr Valler!' cries Janice, her eyes veering from Alice to the manager. 'For God's sake!'

But the manager stands as if paralysed, his mouth gaping open, his eyes glued to my host. As Alice's tongue whips about the fragment of the bottle, it is lacerated on the razor-sharp edges. It begins to bleed copiously. Blood and saliva dribble down Alice's chin, and plop onto her supermarket tunic. They spatter on the tiled floor, making patterns.

'The vodka . . . has gone!' Alice keens, tapping into a deeper register, the plaintive ululation sounding more like a growl. 'There is none left. Look. Can't you see, there's none left.' She sucks desperately on the ragged glass slicing the moist membrane of her inner cheek.

'What shall I do, Mr Valler?' begs Bert, shifting his weight uneasily from one hip to the other, looking anxiously for guidance.

Janice the floor supervisor tries to take

313

command. She steps forwards, arms folded. She stands over Alice. 'Get up!' Alice does not move. 'I think you'd better call the police, Mr Valler!' she barks. A baby starts grizzling. A child bursts into tears. And a guide dog, a golden Labrador, suddenly spots Bear-as-Was floundering beside Alice. The effect is instantaneous. His owner is knocked to the floor as the dog slathers and prances, a handful of customers rushing to his aid.

Alice, head bent, eyes raised, expression demonic, grins at Janice, widening her bloody mouth to reveal wet, red teeth. Then she lowers her face to the floor and begins to lap up the spilt vodka, meticulous as a cat with a dish of cream. The dog, parodying his mistress, joins in. The monkey shimmies down a supporting shelf-column, seizes the cap of the vodka bottle, and scoots off through the crowd with its find. The budgie, flustered by the unfolding hysteria, sticks a clawed foot straight though the egg and gets soaked in yolk.

'Christ!' yells Janice. 'She's mad. That girl's out of her mind. Call the police, Mr Valler.' The look on her face is victorious, her cheeks flushed, her eyes radiant. 'If you don't call them, Mr Valler, I will!'

'What's happening to her? Mr Valler, call an ambulance! Why is the guide dog snarling? She's sick, poor thing. I've never seen the like in Harrison's. Has the girl flipped? I only called in for some jam tarts. Can't somebody get hold of that damn dog! Are you going to leave her in that state? For God's sake, call the police!' come a chorus of shouts from solicitous bystanders as my host continues to grovel on the floor. And then a

314

strident voice booms out above the rest.

'What d'you want to go fetching the police for, getting this child into trouble?'

Her rich sonorous tones roll over us like breaking waves. Bear-as-Was immediately sits to attention, the monkey hurdles back over the sea of bobbing heads, to perch on his rosy brow. Even the budgie, still wrestling with the egg, feels the vibrato rippling through it. Rotating, eggshell hat over stumpy neck, it turns in the direction of the voice. The speaker is a tall, plump woman of middle years, with skin the colour of milk chocolate. Her face is open, her nose broad, her eyes percipient, the irises dark as burnt toast. These features are fringed with hair black as crow's feathers, thick and curly. There is a gilt clip fastened in it, fashioned in the shape of a butterfly, studded with green, yellow and purple plastic gems. She is wrapped up in a mauve coat with a fake fur collar. Her ankle boots, slick with mud, have left prints on the tiled floor of the supermarket. All eyes search her out as she hovers on the fringe of the circle, and in front of her a path clears. Even the guide dog is returned miraculously to its former placid self.

Alice's head comes up fast. She locks eyes with this mystifying woman. In that very second something snaps in my host. The stone heart thaws and the tears finally come. She climbs shakily to her feet. Glass particles adhere to the sticky blood at her knees and a crystal splinter protrudes from the palm of one hand. The woman moves forward.

'Help me. Please.' It is a barely audible whisper, but I see from the light that kindles in the woman's eyes that she has heard it. She moves forward and

315

folds Alice into her coat. She pays no heed to the blood which seeps into the mauve fabric, and which edges the fur collar.

'I'm going to call the police,' Janice declares, pointedly ignoring the remonstrations of this new arrival. 'They need to take Alice away, to sort her out.'

'There's no need for police here,' the woman retorts. 'I know this child. I know Alice. I'll take her home. There's no real harm done.' She starts to guide us all down the aisle.

After that things happen quickly. Janice, the manager and the security guard trundle after us, as do several of the customers. Alice stares blankly ahead. Our new chaperone maintains yet again that she knows Alice, that she is a friend, a good friend, that she will look after her. The manager seeks confirmation of this and, to my amazement my host nods vaguely. The monkey, atop the dog, the dog, walking to heel, shake their heads adamantly. The headless budgie, roosting on Alice's shoulder makes a chopping gesture with its wings, signifying a denial. I bellow in my host's ear that this is a stranger who may lead us into terrible danger.

However, everyone seems so keen to be rid of Alice that they probe no further. In the confusion no one even asks this woman her name. At her request, the manager hurriedly shows the way to the ladies' room. Once inside 'she' lifts off the bloodstained overall, removes the glass splinter and cleans Alice up with paper towels from the machine.

'We do not know this lady,' we importune, all but the budgie. It simply bobs up and down

316

frantically, in mute expostulation.

'It is insane to trust her. If we go with her who knows what might befall us,' I add, my ectoplasm streaked puce with panic. But Alice, still foggy with drink, docilely submits to this stranger's administrations.

'Don't you worry about her. She's gonna be just fine. And as soon as she's feeling better, I'm sure she'll come to see you, to sort this all out,' the interloper tells the manager presumptuously, as we emerge from the ladies' room. 'Oh yes, I'll look after her now.' She wags her head, and the plastic gems in the butterfly clip spark under the supermarket's pearly lights as if they were priceless jewels. Then she grasps Alice's arm firmly and leads us out of the store. My host trots along with her willingly. We share dismayed looks. In this unlikely guise, our expressions say, is a force to be reckoned with.

Audrey—1975

'I said Alice is missing!' I shout into the mouthpiece of the phone. I find it hard to trust this business of long-distance phone calls, speaking to your daughter who is over 8,000 miles away as if she is in the same room. Although I am told it is unnecessary, I cannot break myself of the habit of raising my voice. I speak too with exaggerated clarity. Despite my efforts, Myrtle asks me to repeat myself and I do, even more emphatically.

'What do you mean missing?' Now my daughter's voice matches mine for volume.

'She hasn't been to work for some weeks. Alice's manager rang me, a Mr Valler. He said there had been some trouble, and so he thought . . .'

'You mean there has been more trouble since . . . since the accident with the bird?' Myrtle interjects.

There is a strange delay on these long-distance phone calls that peppers the conversation with momentary silences, or results in two voices sounding at once, speaking over each other. Sometimes I think an entire call is wasted simply trying to achieve sequential communication. I feel every one of my seventy-six years today. My back aches and I am so very tired. I sit down on the chair by the hall table.

'Mother? Mother, are you still there?'

'Yes. I don't really know the details, Myrtle. Her manager was a bit vague about it. I think she may have been intoxicated at work.' I am sure I hear my daughter utter an expletive under her breath. 'Anyway, she cut herself or something. He said it was nothing too serious but he sent her home . . . well, to her bed-sit, and some lady who knew her went with her.' I pause to take a breath. My chest feels tight this afternoon and every inhalation is an effort. My eyes prick too, particularly the left one. Perhaps I have the beginning of a stye. I am a little light-headed as well. I did not manage any lunch today. The talk with that 'Creepy Joe' landlord earlier on has left me feeling strangely disquieted, and yes, if am honest, marginally culpable in this peculiar business. 'Mr Valler said that he didn't call Alice for a couple of weeks, as he felt she might need time to recuperate, though what he meant by that I'm not quite sure. But when

318

eventually he rang she wasn't there. He kept trying, always unsuccessfully. Naturally he became worried, and using her original details that he still had on file, he contacted me. And then . . . and then . . .' Despite sitting down I am feeling dizzy. I lean heavily on the telephone table to steady myself.

'And then? And then *what*, Mother?' comes Myrtle's impatient voice down the line. Always minded of the expense of long-distance calls, I try to gather my thoughts.

'I took a taxi round to her bed-sit this morning and her landlord was there, a Mr Fitch. A most unpleasant gentleman if you ask me. Anyway, he said Alice had been late with her rent, and he'd come over to see what was what. When she didn't open the door he let himself into her room. Well, Myrtle, he said it was empty. Picked clean as a bone. Those were his very words. He said there was no question in his mind that she'd skedaddled, leaving him out of pocket. He seemed to think I was going to reimburse him. The cheek of it. The thing is, Myrtle, she's not been in touch with me either. It's been quite a while since anyone's seen her. She's vanished.' My hand alights on my chest where I feel my heart fluttering wildly, a trapped bird. Remembering George, I shiver. 'I thought you and Ralph would want to know. Do you think I ought to go to the police?'

There is a pause at the end of the line all those thousands of miles away. It lasts several seconds. I wonder if we've been cut off or if there is some kind of interference. I shake the receiver clutched in my hand, hopeful that the line may clear. Then Myrtle's voice sounds again.

319

'No, of course you shouldn't go to the police, Mother. Don't be ridiculous. And we'll settle up with the landlord, so don't fret about that either. I'm sure it's nothing to be concerned about. She probably didn't like her job and, rather than do the responsible thing, she just walked out and found herself somewhere else to live. I don't doubt when she needs money she'll let us know. In the meantime please don't go upsetting yourself. Alice ought to be ashamed of herself. She's put you through quite enough. I am sorry I burdened you with her, really I am.' An audible sigh carries clearly over the line. 'You are not to worry, Mother.' This last comes to me like an order.

'If you . . . you . . . say so,' I falter. I am still uneasy. I should like to dismiss this as Myrtle has, but a deep-rooted instinct tells me there is something more sinister afoot. 'I'll let you know if there's any news.'

'I'd appreciate that. But don't you go getting caught up in this thing. Do you hear me, Mother? In the meantime we'll try to bring forward our leave. We'll be with you as soon as we can, and then hopefully we can sort Alice out once and for all. I'll ring you next week if I don't hear from you before then. Goodbye Mother.'

'Goodbye Myrtle.'

Carefully I place the receiver in its cradle. Throughout the afternoon I listen out for the ring tone of the telephone, feeling at one moment expectant, despondent the next. Albert is late home this evening, and listens with an unreadable face to the news I impart that his niece Alice is missing. My son barely touches his plate of food—rissoles, one of his favourites that I have prepared

320

especially. He pushes it away and walks out of the room without uttering a word.

Ghost—1975

Predictably the headless budgie is the first to take flight. No staying power, that chicken-hearted bird. We're better off without it, I console myself. Our kidnapper races ahead, dodging shoppers and pedestrians, Alice's arm tucked firmly in hers. I streak after them, while the monkey and the dog bring up the rear. I am the only one to spot it. Oh, it is no more than a quick burst of lime-green and butter-yellow, breaking the monotony of a dull grey sky. But I know that that flash signals we've been deserted by the headless budgie, that we ghosts are reduced again to a trio.

'Go on then. Scram,' I holler after it. 'You were never one of us anyhow.'

Then I turn my attention to Alice and plead with her.

'This woman could be a *mo gwei,* a demon in disguise. Who knows where she's taking us?'

But Alice, clutching a tissue to her still bloody mouth with her free hand, indicates her refusal to listen with a stubborn shake of the head. On we go, threading through the crowds, trudging past shops, until we sweep into Ealing Broadway station. Here this busybody purchases tickets for herself and my host, then hurries us onto a train. As we roll away, I realise that it is too late to turn back. The carriage rumbles and rattles along, first above ground, then whistling and screaming through pitch-black tunnels beneath it. It bumps us about until the monkey covers its eyes, the dog buries its muzzle in the grubby upholstery, and I . . . I huddle down into my army jacket and wish us far away. I lose count of the stations we pass through, until at last, when we grind to a halt and the doors judder open, she bundles Alice off. As we slither after them, a voice rings out telling us to 'mind the gap' between the train and the platform. It is a poignant reminder of how vulnerable we all are, how easily we might slip away into ether. We exchange worried looks and plough on through underground passageways. Before long we board another train. When this one screeches to a standstill the meddler hauls Alice out, and on we dash, moving upwards now. We come upon a girl with three shiny silver rings piercing her nose, and scuffed blue boots on her feet, plucking disconsolately on a battered guitar. The woman pauses and rummages through her bag. She drops a handful of coins into the open guitar-case. The girl, still playing, nods her thanks as we pass by.

At last we leave the warm fug of the tunnels, and enter a twilight world dotted with lights. We hurry along pavements hemming wide roads busy with traffic. Brakes scream, engines judder, horns blare. Then these narrow and grow quieter, before we turn into a residential street that looks as if it has one long house snaking the length of it. I soon realise that the snake is divided into segments, and that each of these segments is a home. We stop before a black wrought-iron gate, and 'she' opens it and pushes Alice through. Frantically I try to penetrate Alice's woolly mind, to make her see sense.

322

'This woman,' I whisper persuasively 'could be a madam, a *qian po*. She could be a mistress of whores. She espied you, Alice, with your pliant young body, and plans to cajole you into working for her. If you go into her house you could be raped every day and never escape. Think of that!'

Alice hesitates. She frowns and blinks slowly. But already the woman has opened her front door and is beckoning her inside. I pull hard on each of my host's limbs in turn, trying to dissuade her from entering. The dog and the monkey cower under a low privet hedge which lines the front path, no help at all. Alice glances back over her shoulder. She follows the progress of a large red car as it purrs by and recedes into the distance, and watches an elderly man leaning heavily on a stick as he crosses the road. Her head rolls back. She stares up at a pale gold smudge of moon through a pearly film of cloud.

'Alice, come inside and warm yourself,' says our abductor.

And Alice, with the beginnings of a serene smile touching her lips, straightens up, walks forward and enters the house. Clearly a little abstracted, Alice shuts the front door in our lambent faces, and we have to push through it to join her. Lights have been switched on, two overhead and one standard lamp, illuminating our path. There is no hallway I note. We slide straight into a room much larger than the bed-sit we have grown accustomed to. There are some hooks on the wall by the door where the lady's mauve coat now hangs, her muddy boots standing side by side on a shoe rack under it. A three-piece suite and a television are ranged about a fireplace at one end of the rectangular space, with a dining table and chairs at the other. It is ordered and clean with bright furnishings. A carpet patterned with swirls of gold and blue runs the length of the floor, lemon yellow throws cover both the settee and armchairs, while the curtains, drawn back from the windows at either end of the room, are a shade of deep mustard flecked with white dots. The tiled fireplace is recessed in the honey-coloured walls, knotted newspaper and kindling laid ready in the grate. Above it, set on the dark wood mantelpiece, is a brass carriage clock surrounded by photographs. There are four in all, three of which have carved wooden frames. The largest is of a man in a suit and a woman in a frothy white dress and veil, both smiling widely. A wedding photograph I presume. Scrutinising it closely, I see there is the semblance of our captor about the happy bride. In the next picture she appears again, looking older, standing on a small bridge with a teenage boy on one side, and a girl, a little younger, on the other. Another image has at least a dozen faces crowded together, all of different ages, including a new baby wrapped up in a white cocoon. I have a terrible shock when I look at the last photograph though. Silver-framed, it is the colour portrait of a teenage girl with large brown eyes and long dark hair. Despite her skin tone, the likeness to Alice is uncanny.

'Why don't you sit yourself down, Alice, and I'll fetch us a nice cup of tea.'

Still reeling, I fly about to see the woman watching Alice. She is wearing beaded pink slippers now and an orange, brown and cream striped dress. She bustles through an open doorway at the back of the room, through which I glimpse a kitchen. Still dazed, Alice sits down on one of the four ladder-back chairs arranged round the square dining table. I scud speedily to my host's side, annoyed that I let my attention wander in such a potentially serious situation. I try to communicate my fears to Alice, but her eyelids are heavy and keep closing on me. We hear drawers scraping open and closed, the chink of cutlery on china, and that rich voice I am already learning to dread rising in song, before the whistle of a kettle seems to jolt Alice awake.

'By the way, my name is Reta, Reta Okello,' the women tells Alice, emerging from the kitchen with two steaming mugs of tea. She puts both of these down on the embroidered tablecloth, one before Alice, then turns and fetches a tin from a sideboard. Finally she takes her seat, joining Alice at the table. My host lowers the bloodstained tissue from her mouth and tucks it away in a pocket. Dried blood crusts her swollen lips. Her tongue is thick and her inner cheek is still tingling where she nicked it with the broken glass, though no longer bleeding.

The woman beams, the butterfly clasp in her hair giving its rainbow wink in the glow of the room.

'Much better,' she says approvingly, casting her eyes over Alice's drawn face. 'By tomorrow it'll be all gone. You see.' Cautiously my host fingers her mouth and gives a shy half-smile.

'That's if you live that long, Alice,' I glower. 'If any of us do. Of course it's highly likely that the brew she has made is drugged,' I warn my host, indicating the tea with a hyaline finger. The

325

monkey, occupied inspecting the shiny tin, the dog, nose in the coalscuttle, nod together lugubriously. The dog, not surprisingly feeling insecure in these new surroundings, pads over and lies down at Alice's feet. Tipping Alice's mug over would seem a wise move to me at this juncture. But Alice disagrees, grasping it firmly with both hands the moment I tug it.

'I don't know if you take sugar, Alice, but as you've had a bit of a shock I popped a couple of teaspoons in anyway. It'll do you good,' Reta Okello clucks. Alice nods and blows shakily on the hot liquid. 'I want you to call me Reta, Alice. I'm your friend.'

'Alice does not need any more friends,' I shrill. 'Why on earth would she want you when she has us.' Judging by Reta's smug, self-satisfied expression, she does not hear me. Alice does though. She flinches. I am delighted to see the liquid in her cup slopping over the rim.

'Oh, I'm sorry,' breathes Alice hastily, her eyes immediately anxious.

'Don't worry about it. That's what washing machines are for, Alice,' Reta reassures, her tone easy. She leans forwards and pulls the lid off the tin, sending the unsuspecting monkey flying. It bounces twice and plummets over the edge of the table, landing on the dog's highly sensitive nose. He yelps, and bats the pest off with a paw, bowling it over the carpet. Alice's eyes widen at the spectacle, but Reta notices nothing. She offers Alice a biscuit. At least my host declines this. Then she studies Alice's face carefully for a long moment, reaches over the table and sandwiches Alice's hand in hers.

'You remind me of someone, Alice,' she says, her tone suddenly hushed. Even in her comatose condition I see a flicker of interest in Alice's red-rimmed eyes. After a moment Reta continues, although she does not appear to be focusing on my host, but on a spot a little way above her shoulder. 'Her name was Kesia, my niece Kesia. She was a wild child. Always in trouble. Always so angry with the world. We couldn't tame her, Alice. She found life . . . hard. I think you understand what that means, to find life hard.' Again Alice nods, as if very slowly the words she is hearing are penetrating her reason. 'My sister tried everything to help her daughter. We both did. But Kesia didn't want to be reached. We lost her, Alice. We couldn't hold onto her. She slipped away from us.'

Reta pauses and takes a deep ragged breath. She shuts her eyes, lifts one hand to her mouth and presses two fingers against her trembling lips, holding them there for several seconds before letting them fall away. Still she waits, swallows, takes a slow steadying breath. When she speaks her voice is flat with sorrow. 'I will never forget seeing her lying on that table. She was freezing, poor child. Her fingers were black with the cold. I told them, shouldn't we fetch her a blanket, rub her hands and feet, get the circulation back into them. I wanted to lie down next to her, give her the warmth of my body.'

'Dead?' I suggest to the dog and the monkey.

'Dead,' they chorus back enthusiastically. If there is one thing we three are experts in identifying, it is the signs of death.

'Such a light she had, Alice, such a fierce bold flame. I couldn't believe her fire was gone, that our

Kesia played with ghosts.' She snatches a quick breath and her eyes spring open and come to rest on Alice. She gives my host's hand a little squeeze and grins, a crooked finger wiping moisture away from the corner of her eye. 'I think you would have liked her, Alice. I think you and Kesia would have been great friends. She looked a lot like you. I have a photograph of her on the mantelpiece. When you are feeling better I'll show it to you.'

Reta lets go of Alice's hand. She picks up her mug of tea and sips it thoughtfully. Alice tugs on a strand of hair, pulls it forward in front of her face, teases it apart.

Three times she takes a breath and tries to speak, frowning as she attempts to formulate words in her head, to anchor them down before they drift away.

'You mean . . . you mean,' she begins breathlessly, 'hmm . . . hmm . . . that your niece, Ke . . . Kesia, your niece Kesia is dead?' she asks at last.

Reta, arranging biscuits on a plate, pauses, nods her head and smiles sadly at Alice.

Alice scoops back the strand of hair and for the first time stares straight into Reta's face at the grief etched there. I know she is struggling to master speech, the heat of the vodka still melting her words, making her lips numb, her limbs heavy.

'And now . . . now Kesia . . . plays with ghosts all the time?' It is barely a whisper but it is edged with urgency. Again Reta nods and her shining dark brown eyes glisten anew with tears.

From the houses either side an undercurrent of muffled noise can be heard, the jumping beat of music, distant voices rising and falling, cars, engines firing, turning over, coughing. Underneath the table Bear-as-Was whines. The monkey, who has managed to scale a chair, now gains the summit of the table and takes a running jump into the biscuit tin. Alice's mouth falls open. Then she sees me, sitting at her side desperately trying to attract her notice. I shrink into my army jacket until my head disappears. Normally I would never resort to such silly tactics to get Alice's attention, but Reta, weaving her sad story to inveigle my host, is being unscrupulous. Now I pop my head up through the neck of the army jacket and give my best gap-toothed grin. At the very least I expect a giggle, but to my surprise Alice looks at me with huge frightened eyes, then hurriedly drops her gaze.

'Am I dead, Reta?' she asks quietly.

Reta Okello leaps up giving us all a nasty shock, rushes to Alice, leans over her and embraces her. The dog is on his feet in a flash, teeth bared. The monkey's squashed sorrel head inches into sight above the rim of the biscuit tin. I shudder. We all find this overt display of emotion embarrassing. Besides, this Reta woman has only just met Alice and cannot possibly care for her the way we do. I expect Alice to be appalled and shrug her off. But my host lets herself be pawed, and even starts to respond in kind, swivelling in her chair, her own arms reaching tentatively around the stout lady. The scene repels me so much that I have to look away. The monkey high- jumps over the rim of the biscuit tin and capers about the tabletop wobbling like a jelly. The dog groans, rolls his violet eyes and slumps down on the carpet in disgust.

'No, Alice, you are not dead,' Rita tells my host

firmly, though why Alice has to seek confirmation of this from her, I do not know. She need only have asked us. We would have informed her she was very much alive—after all didn't we all depend on it? Reta starts stroking Alice's hair, a gesture of such intimacy that I want to slap her hand away. 'What makes you say that, eh?' She pulls back from Alice and looks at her with concern.

Alice squirms in her chair. She cannot hold Reta's penetrating gaze. Her eyes veer from her to us. The dog wags its magnificent maroon tail, the monkey waves and makes a vulgar noise, and I nestle closer to my host, lacing my misty legs. 'Because of the . . . the . . . the—' Alice gives a small frustrated cry.

'Because of what, Alice?' echoes Reta Okello.

'The gho-gho—' Alice seems to give up and slumps forward on the table, hiding her face in the crook of her folded arms.

She appears distressed. We exchange baffled looks. But Reta Okello straightens up. Her head wheels round slowly, and with half-hooded eyes she rakes the room. We three freeze instinctively. I cannot be certain, but when she looks in my direction for one weird moment I think she sees me. For a few seconds she is very still, as if she is not only seeing me but hearing me as well, tuning in to my ghostly frequency. I feel violated by this intrusive trickery. She behaves in an identical manner towards the others. Then she hisses through her teeth and with an index finger draws what looks like a five-sided star in the air.

'*Tano*. Five for protection,' she mumbles softly.

Slowly circling the table, she repeats this three more times. As she speaks and draws her stars, we

330

find our ghostly skeins elongating, then tangling into each other and drawing into tight knots. What remains when she has finished her work is a globe of writhing spectral fibres, silver blue, flame red, scintillating foxy-brown, rolling about on the carpet. We are unable to separate ourselves into separate entities for a good quarter of an hour. And while we wrestle to free ourselves, dip and sway like a junk in a typhoon, that dreadful enchantress with her wicked fingertip magic, calmly settles down to drink her tea with Alice.

Despite my ghostly exertions, I force myself not to break contact with my host. A lapse in concentration could prove fatal. So as I arch and dip and gyrate, incessantly trying to gather up my frayed edges and plait them back together, I listen avidly. I discover that Reta is a nurse employed at a local hospital. Despite my uncomfortable condition, I spare a thought for the poor wretches she cares for, and wonder how many, if any, survive. Her husband, she explains pensively, was killed in a car accident many years ago. She lives here alone, though she has children—a son, Kosey, and a daughter, Subira. She tells Alice that she wants her to meet them both. She adds that her son lives in France where he runs a small business exporting fine French foods.

'He is coming to visit in a few weeks. Isn't that lucky, Alice?' Reta says. Our enmeshed emanations let out a unified wail. We share the same horrified reaction. The spawn of this witch might well be more of a threat to us than she is. When we finally succeed in unravelling our ectoplasm, we overhear Reta telling Alice that she looks very tired, that she needs to rest.

Up the sorceress gets and off she goes, my Alice gullibly following her. Disorientated, I barely have time to gather my spirit-wits together. The dog, elated to be liberated from our ghostly quagmire, is currently in fruitless pursuit of his lashing burgundy tail.

'There is no time to waste,' I caution him. 'The witch is leading Alice upstairs. Don't you understand we are in serious danger of being annihilated.' He halts abruptly, buries his nose deep in his pelt and bites frantically on a spectral mite. This is not the reaction I had hoped for, and just serves to illustrate that all apparitions are not of the same calibre. I make a thorough search for the monkey. It is hiding under the table.

'Exactly what are you doing?' I ask, feeling the chances of us being routed increasing fast. The monkey glances up and blathers something unintelligible. I blink back frosty ghost eyes incredulously. The imp is parting chestnut hairs on its wee potbelly and picking off specks of glitter.

'At this rate we are done for,' I muse sombrely, as I shepherd the pair of flat-headed phantoms upstairs. Here, in a small bedroom, we find the hell-cat practising her sophistry on my host, distorting her mind, probing our secrets. I know she intends to destroy my relationship with Alice. But then she does not know how close we are, how insoluble are the ties that bind us. Surely Alice will not abandon me, any more than I will abandon Alice. But if it's a fight the hag wants . . .

She gives my host a nightgown, and I find myself wondering if she has impregnated it with poison. She draws the curtains with their striking pattern of green and red ellipses, and points out the location of the bathroom. While she waits we disappear into it and emerge moments later, my host wearing the nightie, holding her folded clothes. These she lays at the end of the bed before climbing into it. Reta leans over her and tucks the blanket in around her. The dog retreats under the bed, and the monkey wraps itself up in a fold of the curtains. When the witch makes to leave, pausing for a moment at the door, my host begins protesting. For once we ghosts are in harmony. Not before time, we concur telepathically.

'Reta . . . things . . . things come to me in the dark. Bad things.'

I am not quite sure what to make of this. But Reta does not seem phased at all. She gives a brief understanding nod, and as her eyes rake the gloom I am measurably diminished. Once more I experience the uncomfortable sensation that they are alighting on me, tracing my outline. Before I know it, she is revolving on the spot.

'*Tisa*, nine for protection,' she mutters, as her finger strokes the air. '*Nisaidi, tafadhali*. Help me, please.' I see the number nine, red as blood, suspended in the air. Again her finger sketches a figure. '*Saba*, seven for protection.' And there it is, the number seven branded in front of me in a deep dazzling blue. Lastly, her hands move above Alice's prone body making the star with five points. '*Tano*, five for protection,' she whispers. The number five, black and threatening, extends its inky limbs over Alice, encasing her as if in a cage. '*Enda twendle*, go.' I am not sure if my host sees the ominous spidery scrawl looming over her, but her eyes, looking up, are peaceful, drowsy.

Incredibly she is untroubled by this display of evil spell casting. But before I have time to react, I sense invisible flames rearing up from nowhere, starting to scroll across the bedroom floor. As they leap over me it is as if I have taken a sleeping draft. I feel myself sinking and condensing into a puddle. Although I make frantic efforts to whip myself up again, they are futile.

'Don't you worry yourself, Alice,' the crone's voice sounds above me. 'I'll sit with you while you sleep. I won't leave you, I promise.' I make one more attempt to rear up, vowing I will be a maelstrom roaring through Reta Okello's tidy house and leaving devastation in my wake, but to no avail. I manage little more than a ripple.

I feel Alice put her head down on the pillow, a great breath sighing out of her. Within seconds my host is drifting off to sleep. Soon Alice's breathing alters, becoming deep and rhythmic. A sensation of unimaginable relief settles on me as Reta Okello rises and leaves the room. But in minutes she returns clasping a small red velvet purse and a tiny pair of shiny silver scissors. I watch as she bends over the sleeping form of Alice and snips off a lock of her hair, then puts it into the red purse. Next, with immense care she clips a nail from the little finger of one of her hands outstretched on the pillow. This too she places in her purse. Now she rifles through the pile of Alice's clothes and snips a scrap of fabric off the hem of her skirt. She thrusts this into the pouch also, pulling the drawstring neck tightly closed. Then she lays it flat on the palm of her left hand and rubs it with a circular motion of her right, quietly speaking Alice's name jumbled with incomprehensible words.

Lastly she slips a hand between the bed-head and the wall, feeling for something. The glint of the iron nail is reflected on my mirrored surface. She hooks the bag on this before retaking her seat and dozing in the bedside chair. The greys of dawn are edging through the slits in the curtains before I am able to re-form. Having accomplished this I make a few cautious moves, rustling the sheets, flipping the pages of a magazine on the bedside table, levitating the floor rug a few inches, testing my strength. But every time those alert eyes of hers flash open, and almost as quickly she squeezes them into tight slits and pouts, then 'pahs' out a breath. It may not sound like a lot, but believe me it throws my concentration and I am all translucent thumbs. Meanwhile the dog and the monkey are of no assistance whatsoever. Despite my entreaties, they show their cowardice by remaining cloistered throughout the hours of darkness.

Over the next few days it seems to us that Alice does nothing but slumber. I overhear Reta saying to her daughter, Subira, on one of her frequent visits, that Alice sleeps like a baby. Well, if she does, it is news to us. The Alice we know roams through the nights like a caged animal. At first I comfort myself that when Reta goes to work we will have ample opportunity to undo the damage. But I soon find out that Reta never leaves the house without scratching one of her strange signs on the wall and muttering her rhymes. This is one among many unpleasant rituals the witch performs. Tiny gauze pockets of berries are hung from small golden hooks over the windows and doors, red dust appears sprinkled on the threshold of the house, pungent green leaves and soporific herbs are tucked in all the corners of the rooms. In addition to this, when Reta is at home candles burn continuously—candles with peculiar symbols carved into their wax. The results for us are cataclysmic. We loll about in sorry little patches of icy mist, unable to do anything except summon up a drip every so often. It is very worrying not having any idea what the future holds for Alice, for the dog, the monkey and me.

Subira starts to call Alice one of her mother's strays, hugging her as she does so. This enrages me. Alice is no stray. She belongs to me. She is my property, and Reta is as good as stealing her from me. But I am so lethargic, so attenuated that I haven't the energy to put up a fight. I cannot smash a glass, or make a light wink, or even turn on a tap. I am like the opium addicts I used to observe in Hong Kong stumbling out of their shady dens, dizzy and stupid with their poppy juice. I stew frostily as I observe, not once but countless times, Alice confiding in Reta in a way she has never done with me. Oh, I know everything there is to know about Alice. Her mind is transparent to me. But how much does she share willingly with me the way she does with Reta? She talks freely to her, a virtual stranger, about her family and how it was back in Hong Kong in the flat on The Peak. And Reta nods as if she empathises, though she cannot possibly understand the way I do. I was there, seeing Alice through every storm. Most of all, Alice talks of her father, what an incredible man he is and how deeply she loves him. She tells Reta that in time she may contact him, let him know she is safe and well. Reta seems overjoyed by this.

'I was visiting an old friend in Ealing and I popped into Harrison's for some teabags, and found you. How lucky was that, Alice,' Reta says, beaming. Watching them together my essence curdles.

Weeks slide by, and before long we cannot help but observe that Alice is changing. She bathes and brushes her hair daily. Reta pours nasty infusions into the warm bathwater—salt and vinegar, lavender, frankincense and sandalwood, marjoram and sage—until I can no longer detect Alice's distinctive bitter welcoming odour. Her clothes, for the most part lent to her by Subira, may be a poor fit but are clean and pressed. The sores around her mouth have vanished, and her complexion has cleared. Though still pale, there is hint of peach occasionally in her cheeks. She has found an appetite too and is in danger of making a habit of meals. While Alice apparently thrives within Reta's portals we decline.

I am exuberant on the morning that Alice returns to the bed-sit in Ealing, convinced we are saying our goodbyes. Off we four go, and even if Bear-as-Was does look badly neglected, his coat hanging in greasy, lustreless strings, his tail between his legs, and the monkey is forever sulking, I refuse to be downcast. But it turns out to be a fleeting visit with some mad old lady who lives on the ground floor. Before we know it we are back in Reta's house, with no prospect of decamping. Unexpectedly the next day Subira arrives to take us out. As we strive to keep up, we overhear her telling Alice that she mustn't be nervous, that she will be made to feel welcome as soon as we get there. Instantly we become apprehensive.

Like her mother, Subira is tall. She has short wiry black hair, streaked with mahogany-brown, and a wide gap between her two gleaming white front teeth. She laughs a great deal and so does Alice in her company. They make an exhibition of themselves all the way to the church Subira takes us to. It is a dingy, antiquated building, the stone walls cloaked in lichen, vines, and unkempt rambling roses, though they are not yet in bloom. One or two tiles are missing from the moss-ridden roof, and likewise from the steeple that reaches up, weather-worn, into the sky.

I feel a touch constrained as we walk through the graveyard. I don't know what it is about the dead that both attracts and repulses me. We do not enter the church though, but loop around the back of it and pile into a small room. We are greeted warmly on the way in, though I say 'we' advisedly. The jolly woman in the purple pantsuit looks right through the dog, the monkey and me. Inside the room many chairs are set out in rows, all facing towards a wooden desk, while a further two are set behind this. School, I conclude confidently, remembering the Island school my host and I attended in Hong Kong. There is no disputing that it is a very nice school. The pupils are being handed tea and coffee through an open hatch in the wall, and offered biscuits from a plate. They are even permitted to smoke. I take an inventory of the other students. They are all different, in age, colour, shape and size. Some are smartly dressed, some of average appearance, and still others look scruffy and untidy, all mingling and chatting together.

Suddenly the two teachers take their places behind the desk, the remainder of the class filling up the surrounding seats. I float uneasily at the back of the room beside the dog. Disturbingly, he seems to have taken on the appearance of a cobweb, foggy and disjointed, with tiny holes appearing here and there. Seconds later the monkey joins us, its expression glum, its thumb very nearly chewed off. Then one of the tutors launches into a monologue, centering unrelentingly on his own life. Considering that his only major achievement, as far as I can fathom, was downing the equivalent of the South China Sea in wine, I am surprised he is so eager to publicise it. In any case, I am bored stiff, quite an achievement for a vaporous apparition I feel. I start to drift off, but, before I do, I observe my host's expression. There is no misreading it. She is enthralled. After what seems like an age, coupled with an unnecessary amount of kissing, hugging and hand-shaking, Subira leads the way to the door.

This is when I chance to regard the dog more closely. He has grown . . . well, invisible in patches, and this not the healthy lucidity of a hale and vivacious entity. Even as I peer at him he starts to disintegrate.

'Alice! Alice look at your dog! There is something amiss with your dog. He's losing cohesion.' Alice marches past me without a pause. I chase after her, just managing to grab the monkey by the scruff of its neck, and bring it along with me. But by the time we reach the church gate the dog is nowhere to be seen. I glance back and see it hovering in the air over a holly bush. It is fizzing, dissolving, much like the Alka-Seltzer tablets Myrtle Safford sometimes popped into a glass of water, and drank down in the mornings in Hong Kong. There are no better words to describe the unfortunate process poor Bear-as-Was is undergoing.

'Hurry up,' I beckon, conscious that I cannot loiter with the pace Subira is setting. It shakes its ragged two-dimensional head, then turns dolefully away and slopes off, melting into the nacreous sky. I am sorry to see it go. I have grown accustomed to the old brute.

We repeat this unfortunate exercise several days later, and this time the sickly pallor of the infant monkey alerts me instantly. Moment by moment it is becoming more vitreous. Finally it flickers like a tawny sparkler for a couple of seconds, before fading away without so much as a charred wisp to mark its parting. Alice hurries down the church path, oblivious to me and to the unfolding tragedy.

'Alice,' I cry, tracking her with difficulty, 'the monkey has gone. We must search for it. We cannot possibly desert it.'

She pauses as if listening to me. I wait to see her face blench aghast, but to my astonishment she gives a tremulous smile. Then she links her arm through Subira's and with a jaunty step skips away towards the gate, very nearly leaving me behind too. Kosey arrives the following day. He is even taller than his mother and athletic in build. He has keen dark eyes, chiselled features and a fuzz of black hair cropped close to his skull. For two weeks his deep voice and rumbling laugh fill the small house. Subira seems to be over nearly every day. She is tickled when she finds evidence of her mother's sorcery everywhere in the house.

'Oh Mother, more of your nonsense,' she says, her face wreathed in smiles. She holds up a saucer full of shiny black shavings and glittering white crystals that she has found in the kitchen. The powerful potion has been sucking the moisture from me all day, until I feel as tough and salty as the strips of dried beef people chew on in Hong Kong.

'Black salt,' Reta says proudly, poking a finger in the speckled mess and stirring it about meditatively. 'Sea salt and black scratchings from my big soup pan, to keep us safe, darling.'

Subira smiles indulgently at her mother. 'If it makes you feel better.'

Reta glances at Alice, laying the table and sharing a joke with her son Kosey.

'It does,' she says, replacing the saucer on the kitchen windowsill and nodding to herself. From halfway up the stairs, gripping the banisters and peering out, as if from a prison cell, I grimace at the necromancer.

Reta, unlike me, is in her element. She cooks large meals, stirring her cauldron with glee, revelling in having so many to look after. She washes and irons and cleans, delighting in the fresh scents that are choking what little life there is out of me. She throws away the ingredients of old spells and speedily prepares new ones. And when I am not fighting for survival indoors, I am being dragged all over London by Subira and Kosey. Like their mother, they both seem fascinated by the similitude between Alice and their cousin Kesia.

'In this early evening light,' Subira says wonderingly, 'you could be her reflection.' We are sitting on a park bench—well Subira and Alice are. There is barely any room for me, so I am perching on one of the curved cold metal arms. Kosey is leaning his back against the trunk of a nearby oak tree, surveying us contentedly. Alice laughs doubtfully. 'No, really, you are so very like her. Even the way you talk—nothing for ages and then an excited rush,' Subira says, patting Alice's arm insistently. 'Kosey, doesn't that remind you of Kesia, the way Alice speaks?'

Kosey nods. He looks at Alice and I see a fond protective gleam in his eyes.

'You could be her twin,' he says. He covers the short distance between us, graceful as a cat, and gives a lock of Alice's hair a playful tug. 'If you weren't white that is.' They all laugh and the coldness inside me expands into ice.

Alice is not a reincarnation of their dead cousin, Kesia, someone for them to care for and pet as if she was their dog. They do not know Alice at all, the dark landscape that lies just beyond the horizon. They have excavated no more than a few inches of my host, whereas I have unearthed every cursed treasure. I am at home with Alice in a way they can never be. If they realised what demons lurk behind the innocent large eyes that look so very like their cousin's, they would run from my host. However tenuous my hold, I am still in possession of Alice. If they breach her walls they will find me waiting for them.

On one of these outings an idea surfaces. I am not sure whether it comes from Subira, or Kosey, or even, disappointingly, from Alice. It hangs over us this idea, like an indistinct whirling mass of grey cloud, before suddenly it shapes itself. Alice is going to stay in Paris for a time with Kosey. Now the small house is full of plans. Kosey talks excitedly of France, of the flat he has in Paris, how vibrant the city is, how wonderful the art galleries, of how much my host will love it there. The bright curtains in Reta's small house are drawn tight against the advancing darkness. Alice sits in the middle of the settee, Kosey one side, Subira the other. They are leafing through a photograph album, pointing, giggling, telling family stories, talking of cousin Kesia, of how much they miss her. Reta is humming happily as she brings in a tray of coffee and cake. They draw closer in the circle of cosy light. Tomorrow I am going to Paris. Hunkered down beside the front door, a draught knifing through me, a gelid mantle settling over my ectoplasm, I feel a sharp stab of homesickness for the island, for the flat on The Peak, and for *my* Alice.

Myrtle 1980

'Mrs Safford, your letters,' Ah Dang says, holding out a small silver tray with the post piled neatly on it. Last week, she just bundled the letters on the breakfast table. I told her it wasn't good enough. She was to bring them to me on a tray as she had always done, and that was that. I am still at breakfast, taking my time enjoying my coffee. Ralph has dashed off to work. The flat, apart from the amahs of course, is gloriously empty.

'Hmm . . . thank you, Ah Dang,' I say, scooping up the wad of letters. Ah Dang nods and shuffles off. She has slowed down considerably recently and, though always given to plumpness, has put on even more weight. Her hair is streaked with white too and some days she doesn't even bother to plait it. If it wasn't so hard to find staff at the moment, I would probably dismiss her. I flick through the letters, a bill from my tailor it looks like, an invitation to a reception at Government House, a postcard from Beth and Nigel holidaying with the family in the Caribbean. I sigh longingly and glance at the last letter, airmail, postmarked France. And now I look more closely at our address, hand-written. I freeze. I recognise the style, the tilt, the looping letters, the distinctive swollen 'a'. It is from Alice. I cup my mouth and smother a cry. I rise too quickly from my chair and it rocks on its back legs, then comes down with a thud.

In an instant I slough off the five years since Alice went missing. Revisiting my daughter's life and its effect on all of us is like diving from a safe rock into boiling seas. It is the spring 1975 and we are sitting in the front room of the red brick house in Ealing. Three of us are present, Ralph, myself and a young policewoman, WPC Atherton. Mother is not with us. In the short time it took for Ralph and I to arrange our trip to England, my mother had a tragic accident. She fell down the stairs and hit her head. She died. Indirectly I hold Alice responsible. I know my mother was very worried about her, that she was preoccupied and no doubt consequently careless.

As I sit in the drab little room and listen to the

constable talk, my mind keeps drifting off. There is so much to do, so much to arrange—the funeral, the guests, the flowers, the food, the drink. Whether to bury her or have her cremated? When I finally succeeded in getting Albert's attention, he seemed to favour burial. I am thinking about headstones, marble or granite, and what might be a fitting epitaph for my mother, when I notice that Ralph is close to tears.

I make an effort to concentrate on what the constable is saying, but as far as I can tell it is good news. She has visited Alice's bedsit in Ealing and met with another lodger, a Miss Roper, who saw our daughter only yesterday. She says that it looks as though Alice has been keeping a dog and flouting the landlord's rule forbidding pets. I raise an eyebrow. What a surprise, I think, as Ralph makes a curious little bleating sound. The policewoman looks up at him sharply. Then she goes to great pains to explain that in all probability this is why Alice has quit her lodgings. And no, she says, her voice steady and reassuring, she does not know where Alice is currently staying. Apparently she did not pass on that information to Miss Roper, only gave her a letter of notice and the rent she owed. When Ralph keeps demanding what the police are doing to find his daughter, WPC Atherton gently informs him that Alice is nineteen and, in the eyes of the law, an adult. She has committed no offence, and hard as it may be for us to accept, she is free to go where she pleases. Seeing Ralph's face crumple and his eyes brim over, she adds hastily that she is sure we will hear from our daughter very soon. I concur, unfortunately. As soon as Alice needs something

345

she is bound to be in touch. But I am wrong. Ralph hires a private detective at great expense and I hold my breath, fully expecting him to arrive on our doorstep any day with Alice in tow. But the Alice-free months keep sliding by and the detective explains ruefully that the trail has gone cold. Then Alice-free months turn into blissful Alice-free years. Until now that is.

I summon Ah Dang from the kitchen and tell her I am not feeling well, that I am going to lie down for a bit, that I am not to be disturbed. She nods and her eyes slide down to the letter grasped in my hand, then, seeing the warning on my face, she quickly averts them. Once inside the bedroom, I fetch the key from my dressing table drawer and lock the door. Then I sit at my desk by the window, pick up the horn paperknife we bought in Aden, slide it under the letter flap, slit it and draw out Alice's letter. It is May, a fine day with sunlight slanting through the bars. I can see knots of cloud, the edges teased into gold by the rising sun, bowling along in the arc of blue. A shadow flickers over my face as a bird skims past. A swarm of flies hover in the air a few feet from the window. They do this, gather high in the air in the cool of early morning, before setting off to feast on whatever putrefaction they can find. Their faint buzz is audible through the open window. I drop my gaze and read.

> 'Dear Father and Mother,
>   I wanted to write just to let you know I am
> fine and living in Paris. I am very sorry if I
> have caused you pain and worry. It was never
> my intention to do so. The way I disappeared

without letting anyone know where I went, I know it was wrong. Unforgiveable maybe, but I hope not. All I can say is that it felt as if everything was crashing down on me, that if I didn't hide I would be crushed. I think of you both most every day, and of the flat on The Peak, and Hong Kong. Sometimes it feels so hollow this separation.

I have some exciting news that I just have to tell you. I am getting married. I expect you won't be able to believe it any more than I can. His name is Carl, Carl Napier. I am going to be Mrs Napier. Isn't it wonderful? So many exciting things have happened to me. I made friends with a wonderful family in London, the Okellos, and their son Kosey asked me if I would like to return with him to Paris where he lived. He said it was a beautiful city and that I would love it there. And I did. I do. We weren't romantically involved, if that's what you're thinking. He was just like . . . well, a big brother. But it was through him that I met Carl. They are in business together exporting luxury foods. It's only a small company but Carl says it's growing fast. Anyway Kosey introduced me to Carl and we began seeing each other. It wasn't serious at first. For a long time we were just good friends. But over the last year all of that changed. Still, when he asked me to marry him I couldn't believe it. I think you'd approve. He is very handsome, with green eyes and sandy gold hair. He's old fashioned really, likes to look after me.

I have a job now too. I work in a

restaurant. It's called Ramirez, after the owner, Pierre Ramirez. He seems very pleased with me. I started in the kitchen doing anything that was needed really, endlessly peeling and chopping vegetables, and washing up so much that I had dishpan hands for a while. But now I am serving tables. I speak French too. I took lessons at a college. I felt like I was back at the Island School again. It was hard work, but because I was having to speak it every day I soon picked it up. Carl and I live in a lovely airy third floor flat on the Boulevard de Ménilmontant. It reminds me sometimes of the flat on The Peak. Of course it's nowhere near as special, but it's home for me now. We are nearby the fascinating Père Lachaise Cemetery, named after a Jesuit priest. It's simply vast and hundreds of famous people are buried there, painters and writers and politicians. I know it sounds a bit macabre but I love it, walking along the many paths, looking at the graves and the tombs. Some of them are like miniature houses, only without windows and some them are so grand, mansions, carved out of swirling marble and speckled granite with gold lettering. It's like a really peaceful park, with beautiful trees and benches to sit on in the shade, and birds and flowers. I have to admit Carl doesn't like me going. He thinks it's very strange that I should enjoy the company of the dead so much.

We are getting married next month. Of course I know how busy you are and that you won't be able to make it. And besides, I realise I have no right to expect it after everything that's happened. But I just thought you'd like know. I hope you are both well. I picture you at home on The Peak. You're wearing a beautiful dress, Mother, that whispers as you glide down the corridor, and lots of jewellery and that perfume you love, Je Reviens. I close my eyes and I can smell it, heavy and spicy. And Father has just got home from work and slipped off his jacket. He's in the lounge staring at his cabinet of snuff bottles and ivory figurines. Oh, and night is falling with the sky a great mess of colour.

I've put my address at the bottom of the letter. I would love it if you wrote back. But if I don't hear I'll understand why.

I miss you both and love you very much, Alice.'

I reread the letter carefully and then I go to the kitchen where Ah Dang is already preparing lunch, beating batter for the fish to be dipped in. I ask for a saucepan and matches.

'You want to do some cooking, Mrs Safford?' Ah Dang asks, surprised, rinsing her hands under the tap.

'No.' Ah Dang stands poised, waiting for me to explain. I say nothing, just cross to the unit of open shelves where the pots and pans are kept. I select one, snatch up the matches from the lacquer box they are kept in and return to my bedroom. A few minutes later and I have quite a nice blaze going. If it was a cold day just think what a comfort it would be.

Bear—1986

I am floating in liquid blackness. It is very peaceful. The blackness purls about me. It is like the sigh before sleep. I hang on the ebb and flow of that sigh. I am inanimate. Here is where I stop, like falling in a well but knowing you will never reach the bottom. I am dormant, my being in a state of stagnancy. And a voice, a small voice, a voice that I thrill to, a voice that once when I had a heart made it dance, comes to me. It is Alice's voice. It says:

'Don't go, Bear. Stay with me a while longer.'

And so I wait. I do not go forwards. I do not go backwards. I wait for the voice to summon me.

What I notice first is that the black is not so black any more. It is while I am thinking about this that the black becomes the dark brown of rich earth. And before I have time to consider the significance of this it has transmuted to drab grainy greyness, like a faulty television screen. At first the grey appears even, an unending uniform fuzziness. Then the lines form, some vertical, some horizontal. They fill with light, dove-grey light. Two become more pronounced than the rest, stretching before me. The space between them glows like the mother-of-pearl I saw inside shells on the beaches of my island home. It glints invitingly. It is a path and I am moving stealthily down it. To either side of me are blocks, some tall and upright, some long and narrow, and some with triangular roofs. These last are like little houses. They have doors but no windows, and must be black as a starless night inside. Scattered among the houses are stone people, a few with wings, their hands folded as if in prayer. I feel the wind scourging me. I hear the fiery whoosh and crackle of leaves. My path is bordered with tree trunks, straight and forbidding as iron bars. My eyes slide upwards, see them flow into fluid manes, undulating and tossing in the breeze. I move on. Above me the sky is like a length of silk, the colour of it shifting from deep navy to the metallic blues of slate and steel. I feel the drag of an ivory moon bowling through the night.

I do not know where I am, only that something is propelling me forwards. On and on I go, one track leading to another like the tree branches that surround me. It has been raining and sweet wet smells rise up from the damp earth, the mizzle still falling, glistening in the moonshine. Now I break into a trot, a growing sense of urgency quickening my pace. I round a bend and stop abruptly. Another scent permeates the air, a familiar scent, the scent of sadness. My head rotates slowly seeking the source. Beside me is a large rectangular marble box nestling in grass, and huddled on the top of it hugging her knees is the Chinese girl. She nods in greeting. I leave the path, pick my way carefully around it and come upon Alice. She is curled up in the shadow of the structure cast by the moon, though her long hair spills out into the gilded light. She is asleep, but it is a poor kind of rest. Her breath misting the air comes erratically. She whimpers and moans, and gulps now and again as if out of breath. She wears no more than a skirt and cotton blouse, and her pale skin is pricked with the cold. I lie by her side and nudge her. Automatically her arm encircles me, though still she sleeps. I have no breath so we cannot find a shared rhythm. But she must find some comfort in my presence for very soon her respiration deepens and she quietens.

'Bear. Bear.' Alice speaks my name from deep in her dreams.

'Welcome back,' says a voice from above. I swivel my head and roll my eyes upwards to see the Chinese girl peeping over the edge of the marble block. 'I wondered when you'd show up. I expect the others will be along sooner or later.'

'It's nice and peaceful here,' I comment sleepily.

Again she nods. 'Cemeteries usually are.' Then she settles down on her back, one arm draping down over us. 'I far prefer it here with the moon and the stars and the dead of course, than back in the flat with Carl. He's a brute, but you know that already don't you, Bear? That's why you're here.'

In this way I pass the night with Alice and the Chinese girl. Once a cat, white and black, hunting through the night, happens upon us. I bare my teeth and snarl. It freezes, its hair standing on end, and emits a low growl in response before scampering off. And once a tiny shrew pauses to nudge my spectral muzzle with its long dark snout. Its spray of silver whiskers twitch, then, like the cat, it too is paralysed for a second, before it scurries away into a forest of grass. As the moon fades and sinks and the sky shakes off the night, I slip out from under Alice's arm to stand watch over her still sleeping body. The Chinese girl rouses herself and stretches. She peers down at me.

'You going now?' she says.

Far off I can hear a city waking up, the birds, the traffic, the aeroplanes, all growing braver, challenging the silence.

'I think so. I'm tingling a bit. That's a sure sign.'

But only when the dew starts to sparkle and a faint ribbon of primrose yellow hugs the horizon do I feel myself start to fade properly. Again, though I will myself to stay with Alice, the absolute blackness engulfs me. It seeps into me and I am unable to resist its sweetness. This time the limbo seems short-lived. The blindness melts away and I find myself materialising on a busy street corner with people rushing past. I stare about me in confusion and then down the road I see Alice. She has fallen and is being helped up by a large man with a bushy brown moustache. She looks stricken, face streaked with tears, her cheeks blotched red, her lips chewed raw.

The Chinese girl stands close by her, while overhead the monkey swings on a telegraph wire. I sidle up to Alice and nod at the Chinese girl.

'I can't have children. I'm spoiled inside,' Alice mutters over and over under her breath when the man has gone.

I track them home, but before I can make myself comfortable indoors I am smothered by the raven-black ocean. But there is no peace in it, only a whine to its voice that has me thrashing about, desperate to find my way back to Alice.

'You filthy whore . . . I had a right to know . . . I'm your husband . . . You should have told me the truth . . . How can I believe anything you say now? . . . I don't want you working in that place any more . . . How can you call it rape, you were drunk . . . What other lies have you told me? . . . You're my wife, you do as you're told ... Where have you been? ... It's not right wandering around graves day after day ... This place is a tip ... For Christ's sake, what's the matter with you? ... I don't want you going to that awful cemetery any more. Do you hear me, Alice?'

The snatches of speech jump out at me, pouncing on me in the swirl of thick sooty dye. They jar on my sensitive ears. And with them come terrible visions. Once a hand splits the ocean, flying through space and striking pale flesh with a crack. Once the blackness fractures into a mass of fine hair. I feel the grip tightening on it, yanking it back, the jab of pain in her neck that makes her wince and cry out, the stinging sensation in her scalp as strands are torn out. Once the murk roils about me, sloshing forward and back, again and again. As he shakes her, vicariously I feel the confusion and growing disbelief, along with the swimming sensation of light-headedness, the black roses blossoming before the eyes. And once the blanket grows threadbare, and I become sodden with light, I am crouching at Alice's feet ready to spring. There is a man with light-coloured hair grasping her shoulder. His fingers dig into her flesh until she begs him to let go. He is shouting at her.

'Whore! Liar! You fucking liar!' Cloudy flecks of his spittle land on her face, on her bruised upper lip, on her hair, in her eyes. She flinches, tries to wrench free, to pull her body away from his. But he is too strong for her. I smell his rage. It is of the killing kind, a bitter rancorous stench that will not abate until her blood stains his hands. He clenches his fist and draws back his free arm. The impulse that sends it flying towards Alice's soft womb is murderous. Hackles up, muscles bunched, muzzle drawn back into a savage grin, auroral razor sharp teeth bared, I spring. I bring him down as a lion would his prey, nail him to the floor. My claws rake his flesh. My jaws are clashing scissors ripping into his mouth, peeling back his upper lip until the bloody laceration vanishes into a nasal cavity already blocked with clots of thick blood and dark mucus. Then I am upon his arm, my gnashing teeth tearing through the fabric of his shirt. I am shredding the softness to a pulp, feeling his blood pumping out warm and wet, seeing the shaking limb bloom in glistening reds and purples.

He is limp as a rag, eyes closed against me, when finally I back off to skulk in the shadows. Alice is standing by the window. I think she is motionless, but when I study her more carefully I see that her head is moving. She is shaking it fractionally. Now, as well as the smell of sadness, her face is wreathed in sorrow. The man on the floor stirs. He is lying in his own sticky blood and seems unable to believe it. One hand moves to the red mash of his mouth. He gurgles in a shocked breath. He scrabbles to a sitting position and groans. Again with tentative fingers he explores the tattered bloody shirtsleeve, the bite wounds on his arm. His cold green eyes grow round and wide with terror. Alice's head is to one side as she surveys him.

'I'm sorry,' she says quietly, almost to herself.

He staggers to his feet. His blood splashes on the wooden floor as he moves away from Alice, out of the room, out of the flat. The door slams and the stillness laps back in. Alice opens the French

355

doors and steps out onto the tiny balcony. She rests her hands on the metal railing. Beside her stands the Chinese girl, barefoot, in her army jacket. Out of the corner of my eye I see something wiggling on the floor where the drawn curtains fall in soft folds. A moment later, and a tiny shape the colour of autumn leaves dashes over to join Alice outside, shimmying up the balcony railing. I steal out of the gloom and shuffle over to them scenting the crisp night air. There is a brilliant flash of green and yellow and the budgie swoops out of the darkness and alights on Alice shoulder, clawing at a strand of her hair. Alice glances down at me and I feel the leash tighten between us. I do not think I will be returning to oblivion for some time. I pad over to the Chinese girl.

'I'm back,' I say, nosing a ghostly bare calf.

She turns to me. 'Mmm, so you are,' she smiles. She looks sidelong at Alice, busy plucking a loose thread from her lavender cardigan. Now she pulls and it starts to unravel from the bottom of the sleeve.

'It may be a long night,' the Chinese girl says.

Pierre—1986

'Forget her,' advised my restaurant manager, Eugéne, snapping a finger at the new waiter, Bernard. His thin lips twitched into a smile when the nervous lad dropped the handful of forks he was carrying and they clattered on the floor. 'I always told you the English girl would be trouble.

356

And I was proved right, non? You can't rely on her anymore. Most of the time she's drunk and what a sight! She's putting the customers off their food. Her hair all messy, her clothes dirty. She's bad for business.'

I sighed regretfully. We had all guessed that bully, Carl, was at the root of her problems. Hadn't we seen the bruises? But after all, he was her husband. If she wouldn't leave him there was nothing anyone could do. Eugene read my thoughts.

'She made a bad marriage. She was young, naïve. It happens,' he said with a shrug. 'But she is not your responsibility,' he added, his tone now grave. 'However sorry you feel for her, she is not worth the ruin of your restaurant.'

I knew he was right, that I must dismiss Alice and forget her. Still, I was delighted to learn from one of the waitresses some months later that she was going to divorce Carl.

Secretly, I harboured the hope that once it was all settled, Alice would return to work. Until the trouble with her husband she had been doing so well. I had really begun to believe she had a future at Ramirez. She seemed such a lonely young woman, with no family here to support her. Sometimes, when service was over, I would sit at my usual table in the window, hoping to see her. But the only thing looking back at me day after day was my own reflection, a short plump man overly fond of his food, his eyes set too close together, a prominent nose and a little twist of a moustache.

Myrtle—1986

Ralph grips the wire fencing that cages in the veranda, just as Alice did all those years ago. Back then, our daughter told me she was pregnant, putting all our lives in jeopardy. Now, my husband says, 'Alice. I wonder where she is?' And I wonder, will I never be rid of her? 'I think of her, that this very second she is somewhere eating or sleeping or maybe—' He breaks off and laughs softly. 'Maybe even holding a child. You know it is possible that Alice has a family of her own by now.'

I pat him on the back. Oh yes, yes it is, Ralph. Only the letter I received last week told me that her marriage hadn't worked out. Such a pity, but hardly a surprise. Still, apparently this Carl fellow held out for a good five years. In, my view, he deserves a medal.

'I should have tried harder,' Ralph sighs, pressing the side of one cheek into the fencing.

'Tried harder?' I query. It is a summer's evening and the ice is melting in my whisky. But if I go inside and sit down now, it might appear . . . well . . . heartless.

Ralph fixes me with those lucid blue eyes of his. 'Tried harder to find her.'

'You did your best,' I console him, giving his arm a squeeze. 'You couldn't have done more. The police. A private detective. All that money you—'

'Money!' Ralph pushes away from the veranda railing and starts to pace the length of it. 'I'd have spent ten times that much, a hundred times, whatever it took, if it brought her back.'

'Of course, of course,' I say soothingly 'That's not what I meant. Just that you did all you could. You know Alice and I had our differences. There's often a bit of friction between mothers and daughters, isn't there? But I miss her as much as you do.'

'I know I'm not the only one suffering,' Ralph concedes with a backwards flap of his hand. 'I'm being so selfish. She's your daughter too.'

'Mm . . . so she is.' I glance at my whisky through the lounge doors. Would Ralph notice if I slipped in and fetched it? Ralph, who has his back to me, wheels round.

'Sometimes I just can't bear it, the God-awful pain of missing her, as if a limb had been severed. And, just like they say, feeling it there some days but having to accept it's only an illusion.'

'Oh . . . I know. It's dreadful, darling.' Ralph moves away from me again and slumps against a corner post of the veranda. He has sweat patches all over his shirt. He should shower and change. He'd feel so much more comfortable. 'Do you think she's altered very much?' he asks the night.

Not at all, I muse dryly. The letter, Alice's second letter, was a chaotic outpouring, full of errors and smudges and inkblots. No doubt she had been crying. Her marriage hadn't worked out. According to her, Carl had become possessive, jealous, unreasonable, didn't want her to have any life of her own. Apparently she had pushed him over the edge and the poor man had become violent. *"I am so unhappy. I rang Uncle Albert. I didn't tell him where I was or worry him with this. I just needed to hear his voice. I wish I could come home but I expect that's not possible any more."*

359

That's what she wrote. How very familiar it all sounded. Horribly so, actually. Then there were some confused ramblings about spending the night in a cemetery, how she felt safe there, and about a dog attacking Carl and him having to go to hospital for stitches. God, the sordid images it conjured up.

'She'd be ten years older now,' Ralph says wretchedly, rubbing the dome of his head on the metal post. '1986. It's ten years almost to the day that she went missing.'

'Oh darling, must you torture yourself like this?' I say. But I am slightly off key, sounding more baffled than solicitous. Thankfully awash with emotion, Ralph does not seem to notice.

'Is her hair the same colour, the same length? Has she put on weight? She could have done with that. Far too thin. What about her clothes? Do you think she has a job?'

Not for much longer, if that letter is anything to go by, I muse darkly. Missing shifts and turning up drunk at that restaurant she was working at? Wasn't that what Mother said had happened at that supermarket in Ealing? Some people never change, do they? Ralph breaks down, sobbing. I cross to him and stroke his back. He swings about and collapses onto me, tears flowing freely now, his chest heaving.

'There, there, Ralph.' I feel the wetness inching onto my hand-embroidered silk collar but resist the urge to disentangle myself. 'You must try to be brave,' I urge. Ralph nods his head against me, pathetically.

The last thing my daughter wrote was that she thought they would divorce, that like everything else in her life her marriage had failed. What a surprise! It reeked of self-pity. Always the victim, that's Alice. Well, she isn't finding her way back here, not if I can help it. Life on the island these days is hard enough without coping with all her traumas again. Hong Kong is not the same any more. The children have married and gone, Nicola and Harry settling in England and Jillian going to America, of all places. I thought I'd enjoy the peace but in fact I miss them. The way things are, well, it's unsettling.

Anyone would think the Chinese were already in charge. You just don't get the respect any more. And would you believe it, Ah Dang told me last month she had decided to retire, said she was getting too old to work. I was aghast, after everything we've done for her, she deserts us when we need her most. I told her I couldn't find anyone to replace her at such short notice, if at all. No one wants to be an amah now. They all think they can do so much better. I explained with admirable patience that it is not as easy as she might think finding good amahs. She nodded at that, with a funny glint in her eye I didn't like at all. And then she had the cheek to say couldn't Mrs Safford manage with just one servant, Ah Wei? No, Mrs Safford could not, I told her. So grudgingly she agreed to hang on till the end of the year, or until I found someone, whichever came sooner. And do you know, I think she expected me to be grateful. Whatever happened to loyalty?

Once Ralph retires, I have no idea where we'll be living. The last thing I need in my life right now is Alice. Ralph's sobbing has subsided. I lead him into the lounge, sit him down and place the

361

tumbler of whisky in his hand.

'Have a drink, Ralph, it'll make you feel better,' I direct him. While he sits nursing his whisky, I toss back mine, proving my theory. Immediately I feel more in control. My eyes flick over to Ralph, his body crumpled in the chair. Well, one us has to be. Alice's second letter went the way of the first. I glance through the open glass doors at a sky sequinned with stars. There's a new moon. It glows a purifying snow-white. On such a night as this, optimism is called for. I take a deep breath and make my wish.

'Do you think . . . do you think, Myrtle, that she'll ever come back to us?' Ralph says lifting his wet blue eyes to mine.

I hold his gaze and sigh plaintively. 'I want to say yes, darling, you know I do. But perhaps it's time to accept Alice has gone for good,' I whisper resignedly. As I turn away to freshen up my drink, I cannot resist a brief smile.

Pierre—1996

We are in a small fishing village in Brittany. We stroll along the harbour front, the wind whipping Alice's hair about, and flattening what little I have left. We find a small restaurant on the seafront. From our table we look out on the colourful fishing boats bobbing about on their moorings, their lacy brown and green nets piled on the decks. Beyond them, luring them on, sprawls their tempestuous mistress, the vast blue body of Atlantic Ocean. We order a seafood platter and, for me, a bottle of Chablis, chilled to perfection, for Alice mineral water. We gorge ourselves on the flaky white flesh of crab and lobster, on plump pink prawns, on slithers of grilled squid, on tangy golden-brown mussels, on round fat milk-white scallops with their half-moon orange corals, and on semi-pellucid oysters with the palest sensual hint of olive-gold in their wet gleam. I am drunk, not on wine, but on the sting of the salt breeze still lingering on my skin, on the colours, bold and primary, that rush at us through the little window, the blue and red hulls of the boats, the jagged spill of topaz yellow from the sinking sun, the sea banquet enchanting my palette.

I look across at Alice, the manager of my restaurant and my companion. She is laughing, her face intent on extracting the delicate meat from a lobster's claw, and I remember. I remember a bitterly cold January morning, the start of 1987, my breath misting the air as I hurried to my restaurant. I halted mid-stride at the sight of the restaurant sign, Ramirez, gold on black, and under it, hunched on the doorstep, a small woman shivering in a navy blue duffel coat. Alice. She scrambled to her feet at the sight of me. 'Hello Pierre. I'd like my job back,' she said without preamble, through chattering teeth, direct as ever: 'I can start straight away.'

She looked terrible. Her skin grey, dark sickles under bloodshot eyes, hair dull and tangled. I nodded and tried not to look too pleased. 'I see. Well . . . I don't know Alice. I have to—'

'I know I let you down before and I'm sorry,' she hurried on. 'But that's all sorted. I'm . . . I'm divorced now, living . . . living by myself. I thought

363

I was doing quite well before . . . before the break up.' She paused and bit her lip pensively. 'I'd really like another chance, Pierre.' I shrugged, then folded my arms. 'You don't want me back, do you?' said Alice, her face blenched and her shoulders caved in.

'What I want, Alice, is for you to step out of the way so that I can open the door to my restaurant. Then we can get inside in the warm and you can make us both a cup of coffee, hmm?' Alice met my eyes and grinned.

I am not going to pretend the early weeks were easy. Alice turning up to work in ill-fitting garments, the colours at war with each other. Alice struggling to chop vegetables without taking a finger off, her brow a tight 'v' of concentration. Alice trying to check off deliveries, the words and figures before her clearly a jumbled blur. Alice struggling with her now rusty French, so frustrated I thought she would dissolve into tears. But gradually she came back to me. Her pride in her work returned, and along with it her reliability, her confidence and her sense of fun. And when Eugéne left to run a restaurant in the South France where his family lived, Alice got the job. She soon exceeded my highest expectations, rewarding my faith in her.

I am no longer a young man and my health is not good. I smoke too much and I eat too much. Alice scolds me continuously about these vices. But these days it is the simple pleasures I enjoy. Sitting at a street café in the sunshine, sipping an espresso and relaxing with a cigarette, strolling around the Louvre with Alice at my side, staring in wonder at the paintings, attending a concert together, savouring an excellent meal, drinking a fine wine. Pierre Ramirez, a man who lived too well. It is a good epitaph, non?

Ghost—1997

I slip into each corner of the room in turn to see if the view is at all improved from another angle. Then I hover just above the bed in which Mr Ramirez is dying. But it makes no difference. Of course his death is not nearly as dramatic as mine, though with all Alice's weeping and the wailing, you would think it was. I tell her, he is an old man, and that anyway he brought this on himself. I draw her attention to the countless times she warned him to give up smoking those cigarettes. But Alice disregards my logic and remains distraught.

The budgie is absent from this death scene, as is the monkey. But I have spotted the dog's glittering feathery tail poking out from under the sick bed. If the officious nurse, her huge breasts rising with every indignant breath she takes as she bustles about, could see him, he'd be ousted. She's fretting about germs though it hardly seems worth it. Put plainly, Mr Ramirez is going where germs are of absolutely no concern at all.

He is sucking greedily on his oxygen now, fed from a tank through a tube, then a mask, into his suffocating body. In and out it goes, in and out, with an ominous rattle. That is the death rattle. We all recognise it. The grumpy nurse, head to one side, checking the pressure dial listens attentively, then sighs her acceptance. I shall miss the pernickety old boy. After all he did take Alice back to work at his restaurant when we fell on hard times. What's more he had an inhibiting effect on our ghostly menagerie, and that is quite an accomplishment. They didn't quite vanish but they kept a much lower profile, like naughty children when a parent arrives.

Alice is clasping his fingers now, and if I slip into her I can feel they are quite cold, and as stiff as if rigor mortis had begun to set in already. She is muttering her thanks, and tears keep squeezing out of her ducts and trailing down her pale cheeks. Such a show of anguish—what a pity he can't hear a thing. It is June, and a summer shower is drumming softly on the windowpane. But, peering out at the gleaming Paris pavements I judge it will soon pass.

Mr Ramirez has left my host his restaurant, so he must have thought very highly of her. But even this when I remind her of it, does not comfort Alice. The dying man gives a gravelly sigh that seems to fill the room. Then I observe his locked fingers unfurling ominously, as if giving a last stretch. Something in the room stops beeping. Alice bursts into tears proper, and the nurse seizes her by the scruff of her neck and hoists her out of the way. She is busy with a stethoscope prodding and pushing and listening for some time, before finally she stands back and shakes her head, her long face lugubrious. At the very moment that Alice collapses, I am distracted by Pierre Ramirez's spirit rising up in creased white pyjamas, and starting to float gently out of the room. The dog peeps out from under the bed, flattens his ears and gives a low throaty moan.

'Oh for goodness sake,' I mutter. 'By now you really should have got used to the company of ghosts. In reply, Bear-as-Was bares his teeth half-heartedly and slinks back under the bed.

As for me, I waylay Mr Ramirez as he glides through the closed window.

'Aren't you going to put up a fight?' I demand scornfully. 'Some little show of outrage.'

He shakes his ghostly slicked-down locks with such force that they fly up in wispy curls.

'You do fully comprehend what this means, Sir?' I ask, clasping my ethereal hands before me.

Again he nods his head and turns his face away. The nurse clatters about like some old cleaning woman. You'd think out of common decency she could give us a moment's peace. Alice sobs and the dog snarls. It is pandemonium. The solution, I decide, is to ask Mr Ramirez to delay his departure and join our number.

'As you can see Alice is inconsolable,' I persuade with my chipped smile, arms stretched wide in a gesture of welcome. 'Perhaps if you joined us, the "undead", for a short while, it might soften the blow.'

Mr Ramirez turns back to me and I am struck immediately by his incandescent face, now a beacon of unearthly light. 'Won't you join us?' I wheedle. But yet again Mr Ramirez shakes his head and I see he is leaving! He casts one backward look over his opalescent shoulder. The expression I glimpse makes me feel that it is me and not him missing out on something. For the first time, I find myself wondering if perhaps remaining here, fastened to my host, clinging onto life with every fibre of my being, is not as clever as

I first thought. Is it possible that far from cheating death, the only spirit I have cheated of that otherworldly uplifting light is me?

And this is not all that disturbs my emanations. Only a matter of days after Mr Ramirez's exit, my host and I are sitting together on the small settee in our Paris flat. She is sniffing and periodically dabbing her nose and eyes with a hanky. The dog is slouched on the floor snoring noisily. One flame-red leg rotates against the floorboards, the scrabbling silver claws clicking like a typewriter. I suspect he is chasing ghostly rabbits in that great field in the sky. The monkey is skating on the coffee table, executing little pirouettes and every so often smacking its fish lips together in satisfaction. Aware it has an audience, it gives an improvised pyrotechnic display, a shower of tangerine spangles shooting out of its dented head. Meanwhile the decapitated budgie makes jerky progress along the top of the settee back, like the mindless cack-winged bird it is. You would think, without its beak it could not do much damage. But its destructive powers, now employed shredding cushions with its talons, are awesome. But I am distracted now by the images on the screen: before us is home, our home, the island of Hong Kong. In that instant I realise how much I've missed it.

'It's finally come,' Alice mutters under her own real breath. 'The hand back of Hong Kong to China.' I turn to my host. Her face is pensive, her mouth drawn, her eyes clouded. She looks all of her forty-one years. 'June the 30th 1997. The British are leaving and the Chinese are arriving.' Her lips barely move. I slide into Alice and feel the goose bumps all over her flesh, and the hairs standing up on the back of her neck. Her throat is constricted, as if someone has her in a stranglehold. And there is a wound inside so raw I can hardly bear to share it with her.

We listen to Prince Charles, in his admiral's white uniform, make a speech, while the skies spill fat drops all over him. Solemnly we follow the descent of the Union Jack, as it is lowered from its flagpole for the last time. We see the black arch of heaven blaze with a lavish display of fireworks.

'They're making sure we have a good send off,' Alice says, in a reverent tone. 'There are lots of important people there. Look, Chris Patten. He is the last governor of Hong Kong, the 28th. Was the last governor of Hong Kong,' she corrects herself.

Then Alice scans the rows of dignitaries at the ceremony. I know she is looking for just one man. It is not the last governor of Hong Kong. It is not even the future King of England. It is her father, with those piercing blue eyes that used to light up every time he saw her. Her eyes are trained with fierce concentration on the changing televised picture, hands pressed together in front of her, little fingers crooked. We see footage of the People's Liberation Army crossing the border from China, in their buses and open trucks, rolling into the New Territories, Kowloon, and Hong Kong island

'It is the end of empire,' says Alice quietly. That night, we are both dreadfully homesick. The dark is pierced by the dog's plaintive howls, and the monkey's falsetto bawling, and the sound of ripping, as the budgie rends apart what remains of the curtains. At least the restaurant provides some diversion for my host. While Alice works, the dog, the monkey and the budgie stand sentry the door.

But the seed planted that day takes root. Time and again we catch ourselves daydreaming, my host and I, visualising our island basking in the South China Sea. We stare out of windows, blind to the busy Paris streets and the River Seine sliding inexorably towards the ocean. Instead, we conjure up a mountain range of skyscrapers clinging to the waterfront, their dizzying peaks nearly lost in the pipe-clay clouds. We see the thousands of windows throwing back the dazzling glare of the summer sun. Then, after sunset, we envision their long bellies glittering in electric shades of orange and red, purple and blue, pink and yellow and green, sending arrows of light quivering and zig-zagging across the stippled black waters of Victoria Harbour.

Our ears are full of the never-ending cacophony of traffic, slithering through clouds of exhaust fumes, and the ding of tram bells, packed carriages rolling noisily up and down the length of the island. Alice breathes in air thick with remembered smells, fair and foul: the crisp scent of dawn, refuse and spices, the heady fragrance of orchids, all mingled with the aromas of food sizzling and popping in woks. But most of all, we recall The Peak, and the two of us standing as one on top of the world, gazing down the dusty green slopes into the jewelled depths of the sea.

Ralph—1999

My mind has become a sponge. Most of the time I fall through the holes. The onset of this porous condition was gradual. It started after my retirement, when I had already begun to feel that it was no longer my island, but nevertheless could not bear to leave it. The embryonic signs were present when we said our goodbyes to the flat on The Peak and moved into the Girl Guides' Headquarters, my last British bolthole. It seemed safe, to retreat to rented rooms in this remaining outpost of Her Majesty the Queen. The date of the handover was fast approaching. The mood on the island was changing. I felt like a guest who has overstayed his welcome. And yet I could not bring myself to go home. Home! Is it my home? England? Arguable. So the Girl Guide Headquarters seemed the obvious choice. An English oasis surrounded by increasingly foreign territory.

In the large meeting hall there was a portrait of Her Royal Highness Queen Elizabeth the Second on the wall. It was placed in such a way—centrally and high up—that it dominated the room. She struck a regal pose, Her Majesty, standing in an imposing dress with a full skirt, a royal-blue sash over the glittering bodice, a splendid crown sitting atop her brunette curls. Alongside her, placed respectfully lower down, were portraits of Sir Robert Baden-Powell and his wife Olave, founders of the scouting and guiding organisations.

Here I was able to recapture, for a short while,

security and a sense of the familiar. But despite this, I knew that beyond these walls all was crumbling, all was changed, all was depolarising. I, who was awarded the OBE for services rendered to Her Majesty the Queen, had become obsolete. Dressed in dazzling white, gold buttons shining in a neat row on my jacket front, I knelt before the then governor of Hong Kong, Sir David Trench, and became an Officer of the British Empire. He had been wearing full regalia too and looked even grander than I. He had smiled warmly, his eyes full of pride. His pewter hair, burnished in shafts of citrus light, was made steel. It had been a job well done and I knew it. I had steered a course through typhoons and landslides, through riots and 'flu epidemics, through influxes of refugees, through the trickle of swimmers prepared to pit their lives against the rigours of the sea for their freedom, and through periods of unimaginable transition.

When Mao Tse-Tung spearheaded his Cultural Revolution, and incited the Red Guards to embark on their trail of destruction and terror, I had been staunch. I had kept a clear head, standing erect in China's long shadow, and waving the union flag on Her Majesty's island enclave, never balking. I had claimed this small territory for Queen Elizabeth the Second of Britain, let those who challenged her authority do so at their peril. However foolhardy, this was what I did. And for these deeds and more I was given an illusory post—I was made an officer of her vanishing empire.

It was the spring of 1970, an unseasonably hot day, I recall. The interior of Government House felt pleasantly cool. My shoes tapped on the tiled floor of the ceremonies' room. Alice had been there, and Harry, and Myrtle, of course. My wife wore a white hat, with white feathers that curled around her face. She wore a dress with a pleated skirt, the fabric patterned with small white and pale yellow checks, white lace gloves and white shoes, while Harry wore a short-sleeved white shirt and white shorts. Alice was wearing a pink cotton dress sprigged with white flowers. She was wearing ankle socks and they were white too. Surely our audience was snow-blinded by the profusion of whiteness. Alice's long, brown hair was drawn back in a ponytail, making her eyes look even larger than usual. I opened the dark leather box afterwards and showed her my medal.

'See, Alice,' I said, 'your father is an Officer of the British Empire.' She stared at me with those big eyes of hers, slipped her hand into mine and held it tightly.

Eventually, after my retirement, we bought a flat in Quarry Bay and moved out of the Girl Guide Headquarters. We ignored entreaties from Nicola that it was time to return to Britain, staving off the inevitable I suppose. The British flag, my flag, was lowered on the colony of Hong Kong for the last time on the night June 30th 1997 amid torrential rain. I followed it as it slid down the high flagpole where it had fluttered for one and a half centuries. British rule had come to an end, and so I felt had I. Already the advance guard of the People's Liberation Army were triumphantly crossing the border from China into Hong Kong. Now the Union Jack was being superseded by another flag, five yellow stars spiked against a red background, the Flag of the People's Republic of China, while the Chinese national anthem, March of the Volunteers, swelled in the gleaming wet of the night. And with it, I knew, would fly the new Regional Flag of Hong Kong, the delicate white petals of the Bauhinia blakeana flower, standing out against its familiar crimson background. The island that marked the boundaries of my life was to be reabsorbed into its mother country, and all that I had known was evanescing. I had already lost Alice, and now I was to lose my island home.

'Alice,' I said, the voice in my head heavy with despair, 'they have come for Hong Kong. What shall I do?'

'You knew that sooner or later we would have to give it back,' Alice replied solemnly. 'It was never *ours*.'

Later that night, we visited friends who lived on Mount Austin on The Peak. Standing on their balcony, and staring out across the blurred mountain slopes, while above my head the sky shuddered and blossomed with fireworks, a thought struck me. In some place, in some pleat of time, there would be Alice and there would be Hong Kong, always. Alice roaming The Peak with Bear, while the sun shone, and the rain fell, and the mist swirled about. For a long time I stood on the balcony and stared out to sea.

The island was undergoing a process of vicissitude. Daily, it mutated into an increasingly alien organism. I disliked going about now. I, who had once been the honoured guest at the feast, found myself queuing for a table. Some friends left, relocating to Britain, to America, to Australia, to Canada, scattering to the far ends of the earth, and with them went my prestige. Once I was worth everything, now I needed to be worth *something*.

Myrtle had her whisky. I think, more than anything, that blunted the transmogrification for her. Her greatest trial, as she often told me, was the nigh on impossible task of finding staff to cook and clean for us.

'What has happened to all the amahs?' Myrtle would complain frequently. 'How am I expected to cope without help? It really is *too* bad. Nobody wants a job in service now. I shall never manage, Ralph.'

But we did limp on with a series of unsuitable Filipino maids, who I suppose did their best. But they were no longer content and that was apparent. The compensation for us was a kind of camaraderie among the old retainers who remained behind, those of us who had served our Queen in this little outcrop of the British Empire and, now it was gone, would go down with comportment and the appropriate gravitas, waving our outdated flags. The young—oh they would weather the changes as the young always do, but we were dinosaurs and we knew it, all of us putting off the moment when we would lumber back to Britain, as out of place there as we now were here.

And as I said, it was around this time that I began to forget. It started with the odd word. You know what you want to say, the blasted thing is on the tip of your tongue, but it just won't come. Never mind, you tell yourself, later it will surface from the deep recesses of my mind. Only it didn't. I grew adept at substituting other words, at changing a sentence once begun, so I did not have to embarrass myself, floundering on the rock of some fugitive word. Finally we succumbed to Nicola's entreaties that we return to England.

375

'It's high time you came home. I'd love you to buy a place near us in Sussex. I'm on the lookout for something special. Besides, you can't stay over there forever. I imagine the island is quite altered now with the Chinese in charge. After all, Father, you *are* British,' she reminded me, 'so isn't it time you lived in Britain?'

Myrtle was reconciled. The novelty of a Hong Kong where she was no longer queen bee, had worn off long ago. 'It will be lovely to spend some time with the children,' she coaxed me.

I made no response to this. I felt that in leaving Hong Kong I would be deserting Alice. I knew this was a nonsensical argument, entirely without foundation. Alice had vanished in England, and the chance of her having returned to Hong Kong in the intervening years was negligible. In the early days I had done everything I could to find her. The police had not been interested at the time. They had said she was an adult, that it was up to her if she wanted to keep in touch. In the end I had hired a private detective, a Mr Morris Cowie, a short, rotund, pedantic man, with a pointed nose and disconcerting weasel eyes. He maintained that, despite considerable efforts on his part, the trail had gone cold. You have to understand that this was not the age of computers and databases. The world seemed an altogether vaster place than it does today. Some years after she disappeared, Albert insisted he had had a call from her. But I wasn't so sure. After his mother's death Albert absented himself entirely in his plays and musicals, no longer, it seemed, able to distinguish between acting and reality. Nevertheless, I like to think it was true about the 'phone call.

I let things slide. That's what I must live with. I tell myself that there was little I could have done. I try to believe it. But the truth is it was just easier that way, to let her go. Age is a great leveller. It reduces everything to the mundane. It dulls the pain. But despite this, I believe I failed my youngest daughter. The burden weighs heavily on me now.

Nicola took us to view Orchard House outside Uckfield during our annual leave in Britain in 1998. It seemed overly large the house, Edwardian, stylish, full of period features, but the garden was rather too sprawling. We'd never had a garden, well . . . not one of our own. The gardens belonging to the flat on The Peak were communal, and all taken care of, except Peter Everard's treasured patch of course. Why should we want the millstone of a garden dragging us down, and one of such massive proportions as well, at our time of life? There seemed no logic to it. But as Myrtle appeared smitten with it, I went ahead with the purchase.

It was during that trip to England that Albert died. He fell in front of a tube train during the rush hour. One onlooker said it was a deliberate act, that he threw himself onto the line just as the train hurtled into the station. He told the police he was convinced it was suicide, said Albert was humming at the time. A song from *South Pacific*, he said. 'I'm Gonna Wash That Man Right Outa My Hair.'

The following year we packed up our lives in wooden tea crates. Chris Patten had sailed out of Victoria Harbour for the last time on the royal yacht *Britannia*. We followed in his wake on a

Chinese cargo vessel, the *Jade Empress*. I thought a cargo ship might be a more genteel way of travelling than one of those awful ocean liners. This seemed entirely fitting to me. Manufactured in Hong Kong. Now we were being exported abroad.

Myrtle—1999

I am sitting on a tea chest in the tiny flat in Quarry Bay. Our lives have been crated up. In a matter of weeks we will be back in England and living in Orchard House. The island was once such a gracious place to be. The old values stood for something. There was a sense of purpose, of direction. And now, as far as I can see, the Chinese are going to do their damnedest to wreck all that we have achieved for them. Oh, they'll skim off the cream, naturally, and take all the credit, while we are made to scurry back to England like whipped dogs. It makes my blood boil just thinking of it.

Is it really nearly two years since the handover ceremony? I suppose so. I recall it was a washout and the Chinese officials revelled in it, as if the gods themselves refused to mark our going with the panache we deserved. Speaking for myself, I can't quit the place soon enough. The humiliation of it and the smug delight of the locals that you meet at every turn. We couldn't get a table the other night at the Sea Palace. I told them who I was.

I said, 'This is Myrtle Safford, wife of Ralph Safford OBE. We have been coming to your restaurant for years.'

'Very good. I know who you are, Mrs Safford. But I'm afraid we have no tables for Saturday.'

'I don't think you understand—' I began. And he interrupted me. He *interrupted* me!

'I'm sorry, we are fully booked on Saturday, Mrs Safford. Perhaps some other night would suit?'

'No, it wouldn't. I'll go elsewhere. And you can be sure we won't be dining at your establishment in the future,' I said and slammed down the phone. Well, of course we wouldn't. Like so many others, we were joining the exodus abroad.

And it wasn't an isolated incident either. My tailor, the man to whom I had taken my business for years, told me he was too busy to run up a few winter dresses for me to take back to England. In Cloth Alley last week, when I tried to bargain, the stallholder laughed in my face.

'I offer you a fair price,' he said. 'Take it or leave it.' And he shrugged. So what choice did I have but to buy the silk from him? Even if it was overpriced. Glancing back I swear I saw him smirking at me. And yesterday a Chinese man pushed past me and took my taxicab. Well, I expect the place will fall apart after a few years without the British organising things. Then they'll be sorry.

Ralph is out buying luggage for the journey. The few pieces we have were in a sorry condition. He set off early. Just as well or he might have intercepted the mail. Since his retirement, I've had to be eagle-eyed about getting to the post before he sees it. I look down at the letter one last time.

'*Dear Father and Mother,*

I don't know if this will be forwarded on to you. Father will have retired by now. You might not even be in Hong Kong anymore. You certainly won't be living in the flat on The Peak. Perhaps you've moved back to England already. It was selfish of me to pour out all my troubles to you when I wrote last, and I'm sorry for it. I just had no one to turn to. I was so unhappy and I missed you so much. But I'm divorced now and I put all that heartache behind me long ago.

I watched the hand back of Hong Kong on the television in '97 and ever since it has preoccupied me. It broke my heart. Not Hong Kong being given back to the Chinese, that was as it should be. But seeing the island again. As the camera scanned the crowds, I kept thinking you might be there. I looked and looked but I didn't see you.

My friend Pierre died that same year. If you received my last letter you'll remember he owned the restaurant where I work. It was very sad. He had been ill for a little while. I don't know how to fill the void left by him. He willed me his business. At first I thought I couldn't manage it alone, but I'm coping quite well.

I expect you're both feeling empty too, seeing the island go. It's strange isn't it? I think about it all the time now. It comes to me in great waves and then I recall the big things: the shape of the mountains on The Peak silhouetted against the night sky, the crescent curve of a beach, the endless moods of the sea. And sometimes it's the tiniest details that prick at me when I least suspect it, being woken by the heat of the sun, the feeling of ice cold water sluicing down your throat on a burning hot day, rose velvet light lancing through a veined scarlet petal.

I would like so much to see you both. I really believe things might be different now between us. Please can we try? If you don't want that, maybe we could just talk. A few words, that's all, I promise. I've noted down my telephone number next to my address at the bottom of the letter. Sometimes I think I have forgotten the sound of your voices, the music of them, and that frightens me. Then, they come unbidden into the silences inside me. You, Mother, chattering on the telephone, sounding so wonderfully regal and authoritative. And Father, the way you'd insist with a groan to the pedlars that came to the door that you had enough rugs, or fabric, or china, or whatever else they were selling. And then, minutes later, be gleefully showing us your purchases.

So many years have passed. I expect an awful lot has changed. I'm a middle-aged woman now, not the girl who ran away. Perhaps I am only considering myself. Perhaps this is too distressing for you now. Perhaps you don't want to be bothered by it. And of course that's your choice. If I don't hear, I'll understand. In any case, I needed to tell you that I love you, Alice.

The letter was forwarded first to the Girl Guide

Headquarters and then to the flat in Quarry Bay. It seems wherever we go, Alice will find us. I treat it with the contempt it deserves. Mutia, our Filipino maid, is puzzled when I bring the pan of ashes into the kitchen for her to wash up. But she says nothing.

When Ralph comes home at lunchtime with a new set of suitcases, he sniffs the air and frowns. 'Do I smell burning, Myrtle?' he says.

'It's the toaster. Faulty wiring. I think we should sling it out,' I reply easily, opening a window and letting the draft clear the air. 'I've told Mutia to unplug it.'

'Best not to use it again,' Ralph advises. 'Far too dangerous.'

'Exactly what I thought,' I agree.

Ingrid—1999

'Zandra, that's your third glass of wine.'

'Oh so what! Christ, do you *have* to be so anal, Mum?'

We were at a party to welcome home Ralph Safford, Lucy's brother. He had lived in Hong Kong most of his life I was given to understand by the elderly lady I cared for, Lucy Holiday. Now he had returned to England to settle down in Orchard House with his wife, Myrtle. I was in the kitchen, fetching Aunt Lucy a tumbler of water. I guessed the raised voices were coming from the next room.

'You're getting drunk. Making a spectacle of yourself. You don't want to go the way of your—'

'Oh Jesus, not that again. The way you keep

dredging her up. It's like a monster in a fairytale. I'm not a kid any more, Mum, so you're wasting your time.'

'I'm being serious, Zandra. These things can be carried in the genes. You want to be careful.'

Curious, I thought. Perhaps the Saffords have a dipsomaniac relative? 'Look, all I'm doing is having a bit of fun. For fuck's sake, leave me alone.' I heard a door slam, turned, and came face to face with Nicola Salway. She was Ralph's second daughter, I recalled, and Salway was her married name.

'Oh, it's you, Ingrid,' she said, somewhat ungallantly. 'I suppose you heard all that.'

I shrugged, hands spread, as if to say I couldn't really help it. 'I was just fetching Aunt Lucy some water. I think she's had a little wine and it's made her dizzy,' I explained raising the glass in my hand.

'Ah, I see,' said Nicola, her voice decidedly lacklustre. 'Zandra's such a handful. It wouldn't be so bad if her father shouldered half the burden but, oh no, he's far too busy for that.' She sighed in annoyance. She was wearing a dusty mauve pantsuit with a pleated flower-print scarf pinned at her shoulder with a large gold brooch. The sunlight, shafting through the kitchen window, picked out the amber shades in her bangs. 'Why don't people warn you what it's like bringing up teenagers?'

She sighed and I smiled understandingly. 'It's a lovely party,' I mollified. 'And what a splendid house too.'

'Do you think so?' She sounded mildly pleased.

'Yes, quite splendid.' I tucked a loose strand of hair behind my ears and glanced out at the sunlit garden—the walkway shadowed by the pergola with its tumble of blush-pink roses, the buzz of lazy bees, the wavering butterflies, the buffet table weighed down with food and drink, the clusters of people all laughing and talking, and Lucy, red-cheeked and tipsy, propped up in her chair by a large bush of sage-green hebe. 'Quite a challenge for your parents to look after though,' I observed idly. I was surprised by Nicola's defensive reaction.

'They needed a big place. My parents are accustomed to lots of entertaining.'

'I see. Lucy did say something about your sister staying with them for a bit.'

'That's right,' Nicola said cagily. 'At least in a place this size they won't get on top of each other.'

'True,' I agreed. But in reality I was thinking about upkeep, heating and cleaning, and how Orchard House, however grand, was the last place an elderly couple would want to be ensconced.

'Anyway, if you'll excuse me, I must see to our guests.'

'Of course,' I said. 'And I must take Lucy her glass of water.'

I waited a moment, then followed Nicola through the door that gave from the kitchen onto the garden. In my absence, someone had given Lucy another large glass of wine, and she had nearly polished it off by the time I arrived.

'Lucy, ought you really to have had that?' I admonished with mock gravity, lifting it out of her hands.

'I feel . . . I feel . . . I feel—' Lucy waved her fragile hands about expansively, as if searching for the word.

'Drunk?' I supplied disapprovingly, realising I

384

was beginning to sound much as Nicola Salway had with her daughter minutes earlier.

'Not at all,' Lucy said hoarsely. 'Actually I feel rather . . . rather . . . ' She tailed off, burped softly, then took a deep breath, and resumed. 'Rather wonderful.' I gave a little shake of my head, looking down at my rebellious charge. Lucy leaned heavily on one arm of her chair, raised up her vivid blue eyes to meet mine and flirtatiously fluttered her sparse lashes.

'Can I have another wine, Ingrid? Try the red this time?'

'I really don't think it's a good idea,' I advised. 'What about a nice drink of water?' I held the glass before her nose to which her face-powder had adhered in patches. The tip wrinkled in disappointment, but she let me bring the cup to her lips. Ten minutes later she announced she was feeling sick and thought perhaps we should go home. She did look very flushed, her eyes over-bright and her forehead when I felt it rather hot.

'Oh Lucy, I did tell you not to have any wine. You know it doesn't agree with you,' I reprimanded her, wheeling her towards our host to make her apologies.

Although Lucy, unlike Zandra, did not tell me to stop being so anal, I caught the flash of defiance and repressed a giggle at her septuagenarian schoolgirl spirit. Ralph Safford seemed a little confused as we said our goodbyes, as if he was having a hard time placing his sister. I had heard so much about this man, now with his hunched shoulders and his potbelly and straggly whiskers. The striking blue eyes were clearly a family trait.

'Come and see me again soon . . . ah—' He

385

seemed about to go on but his brow suddenly furrowed as if he was trying hard to remember his sister's name. There was something almost desperate about the request, a sense that he was trying hard to find some familiar anchorage in this foreign harbour he had unwittingly sailed into.

For most of the journey to Lucy's Hailham home she slept, though for the last ten minutes she was suddenly wide-eyed and preternaturally alert.

'My brother Ralph is very forgetful these days. He used to have such a sharp mind,' Lucy declared portentously. 'It's very tragic.' Glancing across at her my lips twitched. Lucy's own memory seemed haphazard at best. 'You know, I don't think he ever got over it,' she added.

'Got over what?' I asked, my mind elsewhere. I had just come to a crossroads and was concentrating on pulling out safely.

'What happened . . . well over the years it ate away at him,' Lucy added fingering her belt.

'Oh Lucy, don't undo the strap,' I pleaded, knowing this habit of hers only too well by now.

'I don't like it. I feel trapped,' Lucy maintained pugnaciously, slipping the catch. 'That's better. Now I can breathe. He worshipped her, you see,' Lucy volunteered, her mind leapfrogging again.

'Who?' I was feeling a little tired myself. 'Ralph worshipped who?' We had just turned into the High Street.

'Al-ah!' I braked suddenly as a child dashed out in front of the car. Lucy, unbelted was shunted forwards in her seat.

'Lucy, are you all right?' I asked, looking aslant. Mercifully, there was no one behind us and we had been doing less than 30mph.

'No broken bones I don't think,' Lucy piped up but I could see she was shaken.

'Now perhaps you realise how important it is you keep your safty belt fastened, Lucy,' I said. I leant over to double check she was unhurt and refasten it, simultaneously scowling at the child now safely across the road and pulling faces at us. We had stalled. There was a lengthy pause as I fired the engine and accelerated away once more. 'Who did Ralph worship?' I prompted again. But Lucy seemed not to hear me.

'Shall we have fish fingers for tea,' she suggested brightly. 'All that wine has given me a fearsome appetite.'

Ralph—2003

A sense of transience persisted long after our arrival in Britain. I found myself eagerly anticipating my return home to the sunshine, where once I had lived in a flat on The Peak and been King of the Castle. Here, on this cold, desolate isle, it seemed I was no better than the dirty rascal. On the heels of this came the unpleasant thought that home, my home, had gone, that here I was to stay, here to die and, no doubt, here to be buried. The holes in my sponge brain were widening all the time, and the world about me was becoming a bewildering conundrum. Shortly after we moved into Orchard House, Jillian and her husband arrived, along with their son, Amos. The trouble was that they simply did not go. Then one day, don't ask me how, they were a permanent fixture, along with the furniture and the curtains.

But by then my thoughts had solidified into ingots of dull metal. They were exhausting to heave about. It seemed so much easier to simply set them down. Nicola suggested that she and Jillian might take care of our bills to lighten the load.

'You don't want to be worrying about paying bills at your age, Father. We can take care of it,' she reassured. And then I think she took me to a doctor. In any case she made me sign something she insisted would make life a good deal less complicated.

But it didn't, because one day a man came with boxes that he dumped in the hall, and he wanted me to sign something too. Then I was filled with terror, because I suspected he might want money as well my signature. You see I wasn't sure . . . sure of the value of the coins and notes I had, for the numbers on them were all tangled up and illegible.

'That is the Queen,' I remember telling the man. I jabbed a finger at the picture of Her Majesty on the note in my hand. There was no mistaking the value of her. 'She is the Queen of Hong Kong. Her name is Edwina, and I am an officer in her empire. What do you think of that, eh?' I barked.

But he just looked at me as if I was insane, and thrust a clipboard at me. 'Just sign 'ere mate,' he told me. But what was my name? I couldn't remember my name. Perhaps, I thought desperately, if I scribbled something on his form, he would think that it was my signature. But then he was pushing a pen towards me, and I wasn't sure how I should hold it, in the middle or at both ends. 'All I need is a signature mate.'

He was impatient, and he smelt of sweat and orange peel.

Suddenly I felt bellicose. How dare this man invade my house with his boxes, and try to make me do things against my will. 'Why don't you smile?' I berated him. 'You can smile can't you?' He didn't know what to say to that. Sure enough I had him there. 'What's the matter, you miserable little worm? I am Queen Edith's officer. Perhaps I should fetch my sword? I expect you'd grin soon enough with that pointing at you. Get out of my house!' That's when Myrtle and Jillian appeared, with Amos in tow, and everyone began shouting. The man with the boxes told Jillian that she should lock me up.

'What have you done now?' demanded Jillian, when the man had gone. 'What did you say to him? He probably won't make any more deliveries here.'

'Good!' I told her. Then I shoved the note with the portrait of the Queen at her. 'He didn't know his own Queen, Queen Eleanor the Second. I told him that I was her officer. Once I had a sword. Did you know that? I should have cut off his head. That would have served him right.' Myrtle started crying, so I patted her on the back. Everyone was so tense these days. Sometimes I thought it would be better if I left them to it.

I know a secret. I have told no one my secret, but I will tell you. Orchard House is shrinking. It is reducing. I explain this carefully to Larry one morning. I am sitting in an armchair, and I lean in towards him. He is lounging on the settee.

'When I arrived here it was a large house,' I

389

confide in an undertone to my son-in-law. I make an effort to keep my voice steady. I do not want to alarm him unnecessarily. 'Now there is no space anywhere. I am being hemmed in, besieged. There are piles of papers all over the floor and,' here I beckon him closer with a curling finger, 'they are spreading. Soon they will infiltrate the entire house. We need to call someone, to alert the authorities.'

But Larry remains infuriatingly calm. He shakes his head slowly, and greasy strands of yellow hair fall over his eyes. When he pushes them back I see he is grinning. It is an unattractive, mirthless grin.

'Oh, they're just a few of my papers, old boy,' he tells me airily. 'I'll see to them when I can.'

I am about to tell him to pick up his fucking papers and get out, when I stop. I bite my fist. I am not sure anymore whose house it is. Maybe it is I who should get out? But then where would I go? A staccato series of explosions brings my head up fast.

'The soldiers are on parade. I should be there,' I tell Larry. He rises languidly, and stretches.

'No, Ralph, old boy, it's just Amos jumping up and down the stairs. It's a new game he's got.' As he speaks, he sets down another pile of papers near the chair where I sit.

'How would you like some fish and chips for lunch, Ralphy boy?' he offers, tucking a straggle of hair behind a large ear.

'I don't like fish and chips.' I am firm.

'Oh yes you do,' he overrides me.

'No I fucking don't!' I thunder back.

'I'll get you a nice bit of cod,' he tells me, turning for the door.

'I've wet myself,' I bellow after him, vindictively.

I would like to bend down, take up the pile of papers, and fling them in the air. But it hurts too much to stoop these days. I cast a malevolent eye over them. I can feel my heart leaping in my chest. Once my heart pounded. It was a mighty organ, and the boom of it was invincible. I think of the steady, heavy clunk of a grandfather clock, and the light runaway tick of an alarm clock. The latter best describes my heart now. What's more, I feel the alarm might go off at any moment. I allow myself a few minutes' reminiscence. You are entitled to one or two lapses when you are old. I bring to mind my last boat, *Ruby Red*. I am sitting at her helm, gripping the rudder in my hand, while the sail fills out and billows in the wind. My nostrils flare with the salty spume. I am scudding over the waves and steering my own path.

Myrtle comes into the room. She is wearing an orange and pink kaftan and some beads. She looks as if she is dressed for a party. Perhaps we are going out.

'Did I hear Larry say that he was getting fish and chips?' she asks, settling herself down on the settee with a newspaper.

'I hate fish and chips,' I tell her, my tone defeated.

'I know you do. We both do,' she empathises, knotting her beads around her fingers.

Then, 'Is Alice buried in the garden?' I say. 'Is she buried in the apple orchard?'

Myrtle closes her eyes. I guess that she must be feeling as tired as I am.

'You see the apples . . . the apples have gone rotten, Myrtle. They should have been picked but they have been left, and now they are riddled with wasps and worms. They are putrid with decay.' Again I pause. I concentrate very hard, tracing a swirling pattern on the upholstered arm of my chair. I refuse to let this thought elude me. 'Alice will . . . not . . . like that, you see,' I say measuredly. 'Being buried under all that . . . rotten fruit.' The smell of apples, sweet and buttery, permeates my nostrils, and I feel a strand of golden hair brush my face. 'Amanda?' I say, my voice thick with wonder and the joy of recognition. 'Oh . . . Amanda!'

I am jolted out of my reverie then by Myrtle. She expels the air from her lungs with a harsh grating noise. Looking up, I see her shudder involuntarily. In the silence that follows I swear I hear the buzz of angry wasps.

Nicola—2003

I finally managed to lure Father and Mother back to Britain, persuading them to buy Orchard House, just far enough away from my rural idyll for me not to be bothered on a daily basis, but within easy reach if there was an emergency. I solved Jillian's financial problems, all down to that deviant gambler she married, in the same stroke. How? By relocating them of course, all three. Jillian, Larry, and costly test-tube baby Amos. Goodbye America, hello Blighty. And not just Blighty, but Orchard House, big enough for all of them. They have free board and lodging, and I have live-in carers for the parents and a lot less to worry about.

Of course I'd like to help more, but what with a husband, a daughter, a home to run, I have very little free time. True, Desmond spends the week in London, but nevertheless I have to keep things spic and span for the weekends. Actually I'm not terribly sure what my husband does. I think he sells computers or something like that. I've never taken much interest in his employment. So long as the money keeps rolling in, it really doesn't bother me what he gets up to.

Brother Harry has plumped for Kent, and easy access to the Channel Tunnel, so he's no use at all when it comes to shouldering his share. He's living on one of those estates where all the houses are identical, not to my taste at all, along with his wife, Carmen, a nondescript little thing, and their two children Edgar and Tiffany. As for Alice, nothing has been heard or seen of her for well over two decades. She might as well be dead. Oh, there was that couple of call Uncle Albert claimed to have had several years ago. Poor Uncle Albert, falling under a tube train. What a way to go. Still, I wouldn't be surprised if he made it all up. About the phone call I mean. Honestly, he was raving mad, a performer living in his own production. The preposterous thing is, that Alice 'dead' seems to make her presence more felt than Alice alive, what with father constantly drivelling on about her.

It may sound heartless, but Father losing his grasp of reality has been an unexpected bonus. When, his tone irascible, he demands why Jillian, Larry and young Amos are still houseguests, we simply tell him it is by his express invitation. His

393

brow knits and he ponders this for while, before accepting it without demurral. Even more fortuitous, we managed to persuade him to give me and Jilly joint Power of Attorney. Harry was happy to leave us to it, though I have to admit we cut it very fine. He was just barely compos mentis when he signed on the dotted line.

'Success,' I recall telling Desmond later that evening over the phone. 'We now have joint Power of Attorney. Isn't that marvellous?'

'Mm . . . yes,' Desmond replied distractedly.

'Desmond, do you fully understand what this means for us?' I tried again.

'I think so. I suppose it—'

'You think so!' I interrupted crossly. 'It means that we now have complete control over father's estate . . . over his capital, Desmond.'

'I see. That's . . . good. Look, Nicola, I'm afraid I can't make it home this weekend. I'm snowed under. We have that new contract to work on and—'

'That's fine,' I told my husband sweetly. We said our goodbyes, that we would see each other the following weekend, and hung up.

I knew that Desmond intended to spend the weekend fucking prostitutes in London, that work didn't come into it. I knew too that he did this on a fairly regular basis. I had no problem with it. Why should I? Frankly, those whores saved me considerable effort, for, it has to be said, very little reward. It seems odd to me now, sitting in my immaculate home, surrounded by valuable antiques, creations that are vastly superior to the creatures who fashioned them, that sex once played a major part in my life. And, I suppose, looking back, I wasn't so different from a working girl myself then. It was part of the deal and I seem to recall I fucked with gusto. It empowered me. It brought me what I craved—mastery. Though it used to infuriate me when Desmond and I first met that he visited trollops in Wanchai.

'Don't come near me, you stink of sex. If you think you're screwing me after you've fucked your prostitutes, forget it,' I would rage at him as he crept guiltily into our flat.

He would grin then, as if he had been no more than a naughty schoolboy, and try to nuzzle closer. Truthfully, I did find something stimulating about him when he came in reeking of 'eau de slut'. I would wonder what she had done, what she had sucked, what she had used, what acrobatics she had performed? Though of the two of them, the whore was always infinitely more tantalizing. All the same, the prospect of what the seductive Suzie Wong might pass on to me via my husband was sufficient deterrent to curb my appetite for voyeurism.

These days, however, sex is no longer part of the deal. There is still a deal of course. There is always a deal. I keep the house impeccably clean and stylish, and bring up our daughter, an accomplishment in itself, and Desmond gives me lots of money. I have not aged too badly, a tendency to plumpness being my biggest downfall as the years slip by. However, the thought of sex with Desmond, flabby and pale as a raw chicken, with all the tugging, pulling and rubbing that it entails, quite simply revolts me now. Sometimes when I recline in the hall on my newly upholstered, wine-red velvet chaise longue, I fancy myself as a madam at the helm of a glamorous brothel. I sip a glass of chilled white wine and nibble on a chocolate, enjoying the fruits of Desmond's labours, while I visualise some other woman opening her legs for him, and putting up with all that panting and moaning and mess.

Lately the cottage is very silent. I am becoming increasingly aware of this stillness. I live in fear of shattering it. Our daughter Zandra was home briefly last night. She's not frightened of shattering anything. I think she may have inherited sister Alice's neurotic gene. She was drunk too. She broke an antique vase. She was trying to reach a book and she bumped it. She laughed when it rocked and I dashed forwards and tried to save it. It was one of a pair of Japanese Imari vases. They were very valuable. This morning when I came down, I found a small piece of the golden dog that sat atop the lid of one of the vases, lying under the corner of an armchair. I leant down to pick it up. I was feeling the sharp edge with the pad of an index finger when the phone rang.

'Father is playing up,' Jillian informed me peremptorily. 'You have to come. I can't cope.' I told her that as soon as I had finished cleaning the house I'd swing by.

The sun is shining today. It's already quite warm, although it's still early. The sunshine shows up the dust. That is the down side to it. There is such a lot of work to be done. I thought the house was spotless but the sun has put me right. Desmond is away again so that makes things a little easier. Still, the dirt behind the kitchen appliances kept me awake last night. You can't see it but you know it's there, nestling in crevices, coating surfaces, furring up walls. Bacteria. Germ transference. Cross-contamination. Multiplying all the while.

When I arrive at Orchard House later in the morning I step into an uproar. The place is a tip. There are bundles of dirty washing lying around, piles of books and papers, shoes and coats and towels strewn about the floor, and used crockery scattered throughout. All this fighting for space among an assortment of Chinese antiques of considerable worth. We must think about putting them in storage or, better still, selling them off. The smell of cigarettes hangs on the air too, one of Larry's vices. As does the smell of urine: Father's.

Father, who is standing at the dining-room table, propping himself up on a chair, looks decidedly damp about the crutch. Mother is sitting at the table, staring disconsolately at a plate of congealed fried fish and chips. She is wearing an orange and pink kaftan and a rope of amber beads. There is a tiny fly trapped in one of the beads. I know it is there. I've seen it. Mother told me it was very lucky. I'm not sure the fly would agree with her. Dotted around father's feet are several soggy chips. There is a lump of battered fish in the middle of the table. It has left a smeary trail on the polished wood surface.

The trail leads to father's plate. There is another lump of battered fish grasped in the hand father is not using for balance. The hand is raised as if holding a weapon seconds before an assault. Father is squeezing the fish so tightly that drops of oil are trickling down his wrist. As I near him, added to the smell of smoke and urine is that of fat and fish. Amos is lying on the settee, shoes muddy

397

and still on, playing some sort of handheld electronic game. The game emits a high-pitched beep from time to time, a hit, along with a deflated whine, which I presume signifies a miss. Larry is nowhere to be seen. What a surprise! Jillian is standing in the dining room doorway snivelling, and brandishing a tea-towel in her hand.

'Look what he's done to his dinner. Just look. He's thrown it on the floor,' bawls Jillian. 'I lovingly prepare dinner for him and see how he repays me.'

She has dyed her hair an alarming shade of mahogany red and, from the look of things, it is a recent job. There is a slight discolouration on the skin that borders her hairline.

'I hate fish and chips,' shouts father, letting fly his handful of squashed fish and batter. It sails through the air and strikes the wall above the dresser, sticking fast to the red and white flowered wallpaper.

'What do you mean, Father? You've always loved fish and chips,' I say, trying to keep my tone calm and pleasant. 'Now apologise to Jillian, and let's get this mess cleared up.'

Amos sighs rudely, as if we are disturbing his concentration.

'I will not,' bellows Father, eyes popping.

'He really doesn't like fish and chips,' Mother adds unhelpfully, pushing her own food round and round on the plate. 'Jillian knows he doesn't like it. We don't like going to bed at seven o'clock either,' she adds daringly.

'That's not true. You take yourselves to bed early because you say you're exhausted,' shrieks Jillian, so impassioned one would think she had been accused of murder, and perhaps such a scenario is not as far-fetched as it might first appear. 'I slave day and night to cook your meals and—'

'But Larry fetched this from the chip shop, and your father told him twice he didn't fancy fish and chips,' Mother carps, her face flushing.

'Well, then, I'm sure Larry didn't hear him,' retorts Jillian acidly, bunching up the tea-towel as if readying herself to enter the fray. 'Larry tries his best and all you do is pick on him.'

Now I sigh, for it is perfectly obvious to anyone who knows Larry that never once has he tried his best.

'I hate fish and chips,' yells Dad. Then, just for good measure, 'Larry is a dickhead!'

'See! See!' Jillian is beside herself now. 'He delights in abusing my husband. Don't think I'm going to make you scrambled egg. If you don't eat your fish and chips, you can starve for all I care. I have better things to do than run around clearing up after you.' Amos rises, kicks the settee in temper, and storms out of the room, pushing his way past his mother, who barely seems to notice him. 'I don't know how much more I can stand. You're driving me crazy. I shall have a breakdown!'

'Why don't you do as you're told the first time then,' hollers Father, now turning a deep shade of mulberry. 'You never fucking do as you're told!'

'If you're going to swear at me I'm leaving,' Jillian shoots back, tossing her head of startling red hair.

'Why don't we all calm down,' I suggest with valiant optimism.

Jillian moves to stand menacingly behind mother, looking as if she might like to smother her with the tea-towel. 'I'm tired. I am *so* tired,' she warbles.

I scratch my head. 'How about a sandwich, Dad?' He shakes his drooping head. His expression is woebegone, his complexion paling a chalky white, his sparse hair awry. He is unshaven, and his sideburns have almost met under his chin and formed a beard. There is a blot of ketchup on his cream shirt, over his heart. It looks like a bullet wound.

But there is life in him yet. Up comes his chin for a second skirmish. 'Where's Alice?' he fires pugnaciously, lifting his chair a few inches and slamming it back down. 'What have you done with her?'

'Christ! Not that again,' Jillian shrills, leaning over mother and whacking the table with the flat of her hand. A nervous tic jumps in Mother's cheek. 'Can't you shut up about Alice! Just fucking shut up!'

'Let's all be one big happy family again?' Mother offers pathetically. She mashes her fish meticulously with her fork, then with her knife spreads it thinly around her plate. We all look on with macabre fascination.

Jillian takes a deep breath, holds it for a second and then lets rip. 'We were never a happy family!' Then she turns smartly on her heels and flees the room.

'Where's the whisky? I want a whisky. Where has bloody Jillian hidden the whisky?' mother wails, rising and moving heavily to the dresser, starting to open drawers and cupboards and rifle through them.

So preoccupied am I in the hunt for the golden cure-all, and in assuaging mother's maternal anguish, that I do not notice Death sidle into the room. When I turn back, a bottle of whisky held victoriously aloft, Father is slumped in his chair, his eyes half-closed, his lips blue and trembling, beads of sweat breaking out on his cadaverous skin, one hand clawing his arresting heart.

Nicola—2005

I was right about the dirt. When the removal men came and started shifting the furniture I saw it. And not just behind the furniture, underneath it as well. To think I had sat in the lounge and watched television, with all that filth only feet away. I am moving to a new build in East Grinstead. I would have preferred a place in Eastbourne, but it was just too expensive. And Jillian and Larry are moving to Hastings, a small two up, two down. Of course I've had to downsize a bit myself, though I have no complaints about the divorce settlement. Desmond was very generous when it came to it. He didn't seem interested in any of the antiques either. I wonder if he realizes how much money they're worth. Still, he said he didn't want them. He said I could keep them. He said Selena didn't like old things. Oh, that's her name, Selena, Se . . . le . . . na. Much as I would have expected. Pretentious and unlikely to be her real name. I don't bear her any grudge now. Not really. In a way, I sort of admire her. She saw what she wanted and she took it. It's a laudable ethos in my opinion.

Don't misunderstand me. I did fight for my marriage. In the final months we spoke more than we had done for ages. I even tried to seduce him. Can you believe it? Not that it made any difference. Actually, I think he was shocked, couldn't scuttle away fast enough. Still, I'm a pragmatist. If our marriage was dead I wouldn't waste any more time trying to revive it. Every so often these rain clouds come along in life and threaten to bowl you over, don't they? I expect it happens to everyone. You can stand there and get wet, or go somewhere it's dry and sunny.

Having to sell Orchard House was another surprise. Of course I knew that eventually we would have to dispose of it, though I hadn't been anticipating the need for such an early sale. But I might have known that Larry, with his weakness for gambling, would be our downfall. I rushed over to Orchard House when I got Jillian's urgent summons. Larry was out and Amos was at school. Before we'd even sat down it all came out.

'We're in a dreadful mess,' Jillian sobbed, swaying on the soles of her slippered feet in the hall. 'Larry's been gambling. He's gambled away thousands, Nicola, on line. All our credit cards maxed up to the hilt. The final tally is over £100,000. The money from Dad went long ago. The debt collectors have been round. I don't know what to do!'

When she finished speaking, her mouth carried on working. I took her by the elbow and guided her into that dismal back room. God, it was in a state, and it stank too. I tried not to think about the germs flying about spreading disease. As I pressed Jilly down into a seat, having moved the clutter off it first, I noticed that several of the buckets used to catch the drips from the leaking roof were spilling over on to the carpet. She's a slob, I thought, remembering how lovely I had made it before Father and Mother moved in— pretty soft furnishings, everything gleaming, fresh, clean. Still, we all have different standards I suppose. And some of us, I reflected, reluctantly turning my focus back to my elder sister, now weeping uncontrollably, have none.

I've got to admit that when she first told me, I could cheerfully have wrung Larry's neck. Of all the irresponsible stupid things to do. But after I'd composed myself, and Jillian and I had shared a drink, I began to see that this situation might be salvaged.

'You despise me, I know,' Jillian said, staring glumly into her empty glass, having downed her drink in one.

Inwardly I sighed. What could I say? Why did you marry that useless pillock? Why did you blow a small fortune on trying to have a baby, when you could have picked up one at some adoption agency for free? Why didn't you keep a closer eye on your worthless husband, and put a stop to his nasty little gambling habit before it got out of hand? Oh,why didn't you just pull yourself together and make something of your life, instead of sitting back, like a useless victim, and letting everyone else do the work. Well, me in fact. Sometimes I wanted to shake Jilly till her teeth rattled. Nevertheless she was my sister, and even now, after all these years, hearing the desperation sound in her voice, I wanted nothing more than to find a solution to her

403

woes. Gradually, as I stared at the bowls and buckets full of rainwater, a plan formulated in my head.

'We'll sell the house,' I announced to Jillian, crouching in front of her and meeting her tearful eyes. 'After clearing your debt, we'll split the proceeds three ways. Luckily we put the house in your name, so it should be straightforward enough. Besides, I could do with a bit of extra cash at present, what with moving myself. And Harry will be glad of the additional funds too, with his youngsters growing up fast.'

'But where will I live?' Jillian wailed pathetically, her hands towards me, palms outwards, in a gesture redolent of the statues of the Virgin Mary we had met at every turn in the convent.

At that, I told her to snap out of it, that she must buy a new home in a less expensive location. 'If you have any sense you'll lose Larry, but if you choose to hang onto him, you had better take away his credit cards, because if he does this again Jilly, I'm telling you, you're on your own,' I advised her, my tone sonorous, in an effort to impress the gravity of her situation upon her. My sister produced a soiled tissue from an equally grubby sleeve and blew her nose noisily. Hunkered down on my heels, my hands resting on her knees, I rose rapidly and retreated a short distance, remembering that the common cold is an airborne virus. 'And Jilly, this will be the very last time I'll bail you out. It will have to be,' I added as an afterthought, wagging an admonishing finger at her. 'Once we've sold the house there will be no money left, and nothing I can do for you.'

Having heard my plan she revived. The two of us were just talking about opening a bottle of some sickly liqueur Jilly had hanging about from last Christmas, when my sister suddenly rocketed out of her seat. 'What about Mother,' she shrieked, gesturing towards the ceiling, where Mother mostly stayed these days in her upstairs bedroom. 'What are we going to do with Mother?'

On the instant, I decided that it would be impossible for me to take her. I was moving to a new build where everything was immaculate. I cannot tell you how much I was looking forward to a salubrious, uncontaminated home, where at last I could sleep at nights without worrying about bacteria. Mother and that sleek, minimalist look were incompatible. I understood from Jillian's endless whining that Mother was fast becoming unpredictable, and most recently obdurate.

'You know, I wouldn't be surprised if she's gone the same way as her brother. Uncle Albert was barmy, don't you remember? Always mumbling lines from some old play or musical, or singing,' Jillian suggested. I nodded, recalling mad Uncle Albert, and his endless repertoire. 'Even if this hadn't happened Nicola, I've been meaning to tell you that I didn't feel I could carry on for much longer. She's constantly wandering off. And half the time she just doesn't make any sense, going on about Hong Kong and Daddy and parties and people. And they're all dead. They've all gone.'

It was then, anticipating the care of Mother falling to me, Harry with his busy household not even being an option, that I began to ponder whether we could find a local carehome for her.

405

After all, she would be able to contribute her generous overseas pension towards the cost. Besides, with her deteriorating mental state, the council, I felt sure, had an obligation to look after her. The moment this idea struck me, I knew we had found the way forwards. Luckily, Mrs Diane Malloy from social services was sympathetic, having had personal experience in caring for an ageing relative. Doctor Hillman was also extremely helpful in confirming Mother's deteriorating mental condition. With their assistance I was able to secure her a place at Greenwood Lodge, a carehome for the elderly outside Brighton.

We also found a buyer for Orchard House fairly rapidly. The chap from Golders and Packman Estate Agency, Ray Clegg, a stocky man with stringy grey hair, rabbit's teeth, and no scruples at all, was confident that a period property like ours, in need of a bit of work, would be a buyer's dream. And he was right. Within the month we were under offer, having achieved an excellent price for the ramshackle old house too. Time has simply flown by since then. I had the best of intentions, but sadly I haven't managed to get over to Greenwood Lodge very much. I have rung regularly though, and the manager there, a Mrs Bowker, has been most understanding. Besides, I see little point in feeling guilty when she tells me Mother is doing just fine. In any case, I know Ingrid, Aunt Lucy's carer, has promised to visit, so there's no need to panic. After the removal men have come and gone I might try to call in.

It is a lovely spring day. The sky is deep rich blue ribbed with filmy white clouds, like a ladder arcing overhead. The wisteria is just out. The cottage thatched in pale green and tasselled with lavender-blue looks like something off the lid of a biscuit tin. I am standing in the kitchen. My hands are rubbed raw. There is the lingering smell of disinfectant in the air. I drink it in. I'd have hated the newcomers to think I was dirty. I am staring out into the back garden and there is a thrush, a mistle thrush, hopping on the clipped, green grass, looking for worms. Every so often it stops and swivels its small, grey-brown head, as if peering behind to see if anyone is following. It knows the worms are down there, burrowing through the crumbling earth, turning things over, mixing things up. It's biding its time.

I think suddenly of Zandra. Of course I love her very much but . . . well . . . she is so destructive. She's better off staying with her father. He's more patient with her than I am. Walter Scott should have written, oh, what a tangled web we weave when first we practise to conceive. Desmond says she's been nurturing a secret love of art all these years, that she wants to be an artist. He said something or other about her going to art college. Well, if he's prepared to fund it why not? Personally I've never rated all those arty-farty careers.

And now, as so often, inexplicably I think of Alice. She is in the gardens of the flat on The Peak. I see her flying through the air on the swing. She is soaring upwards, her long, brown hair trailing behind like the tail of a comet. In the rush of it she holds the mauve hills, and the shimmering sea, and the limitless expanse of blue sky. I want her to come back down, to stay with the rest of us earthbound mortals. I call to her but she can't hear me.

'One day,' she shouts from above, and her voice is seized by the streaming air, so that I have to strain to catch her words as they dash by, 'one day . . . I am going to go so high . . . so high . . . that I shall swing right over.'

Ghost—2006

He comes in when there are just a few stragglers finishing off their meals. Alice, sitting in the same corner that Pierre Ramirez occupied when he was alive, glances up. Their eyes meet. I know she is going to say that service has ended, that she is sorry, that she hopes very much the gentleman will return another day. Then she is rising, gasping softly, fingers splayed across her mouth. She is not certain yet, but I am. He moves towards her. He is older of course, his tight black curls threaded with grey. The shadows have deepened beneath his eyes, below his cheekbones. His brow is lined. There are crow's feet at the outer corners of his eyes. Deep furrows run from the base of his nose to either side of his mouth. But he is still a tall imposing figure. He wears a grey winter suit, a beige shirt, a red and silver striped tie. He moves gracefully for such a tall man. He reaches the table and speaks quietly.

'Hello Alice.'

Alice's fingers slip from her mouth, drop to her neck. She is wearing a heavy silver chain and rolls it back and forth between thumb and middle finger.

'Hello Kosey,' she says.

She offers him a coffee. When he declines she leads Kosey Okello to her office in the rear of the restaurant, says they can talk undisturbed there. Once inside she closes the door, gestures Kosey to take a seat across the desk from her, and sits herself. There is one large window giving onto the courtyard through which a weak trickle of grey light filters. It is January and already it is growing dark.

'It's good to see you after so long,' Alice tells him. She leans forward and presses a switch and the desk lamp blinks on. A pool of yellow light, reflected in the highly polished surface of the desk, lights up Kosey's features. 'You look well.'

'So do you, Alice,' Kosey says, returning her gaze. 'I asked around.' His eyes rove about the office. 'They say this place is yours now, has been for some time, that Pierre left it to you in his will.' He fidgets with a gold and blue enamel cufflink, adjusts the pin nervously.

'That's right, he did,' says Alice simply. Then in a lower voice, 'He was like a father to me in many ways.' I lean back against the wall, arms by my sides. I am suspicious, doubting already that this is merely a social call after so many years.

'Carl would have been livid. He hated you working here.' He gives a dry cough and smiles awkwardly. 'Have you heard from him, Alice?'

Alice shakes her head. She glances away, out of the window and remembers the cold green eyes, the furious face, the slaps, the kicks, the shoves, the dread. But now she does not feel afraid, she feels angry. Her back straightens. She holds her head up with dignity. 'What about you, Kosey?

409

Has Carl been in touch with you?'

'Not since he left the company, and that was over a decade now.' He lowers his gaze to the desktop, taking in a neat stack of bills, a pot of pens, a large leather diary, a circular glass paperweight with a swirling orange and red flower encased in it. 'I was very sorry it didn't work out for the two of you.'

Alice shrugs. She asks Kosey if he is married and if he has a family. Now Kosey smiles in earnest as he describes his French wife Lorraine, and his twin daughters Sophia and Zoe, who will be sixteen in May. He talks a little of his new business venture as well, exporting select French wines, how well it is going.

'And what about you,' he says at last. 'Are you married, Alice? Do you have a family?' Resting on her elbows, my host plaits her fingers together. She takes a moment before explaining that she never remarried and that she has no children. Then Alice and Kosey tumble into an uncomfortable silence. Distant sounds from the kitchens reach their ears, pots clanging, muffled voices, the clatter of a something falling to the floor.

'How is your sister and your mother?'

As Alice speaks, Kosey's hand slips into a jacket pocket. There is the faint crackle of paper.

'That's really why I'm here, Alice.' His head sinks and he draws his free hand across his brow. When he looks up there is the unmistakable dullness of grief in his brooding eyes. 'My mother is dead. Reta is dead, Alice.'

For the second time that afternoon Alice's hand cups her mouth. There is a box of tissues on the desk and she reaches for it now, although she is

410

dry-eyed. 'What happened, Kosey?' she whispers, drawing one tissue from the box.

Kosey Okello sighs sadly. His fingers stroke the desktop. 'Oh Alice, she was ill for some time, kept it to herself, you know. It was cancer. She was a nurse. She knew what to expect. She only told us towards the very end. I think Subira and me, we knew by then anyway. My mother said she didn't want any kind of fuss.'

'I'm so sorry. I will never forget how kind she was to me, Kosey, all those years ago, how kind you all were.' Alice's hands are busy shredding the tissue as she talks. Kosey nods.

'She wasn't very kind to me,' I remark, still leaning back against the wall. Alice responds by diving into the box and plucking out another tissue.

'My mother didn't forget you either, Alice. We found this while we were going through her things.' Kosey pulls a sealed envelope from his pocket and lays it in the centre of the table. The name 'ALICE' is written in capitals in black ink on the front of it. My host stares down, her eyes tracing the lettering, an expression very like wonder etched on her face. Long after Kosey has left she is still looking at it. But she doesn't open it until she is back in her flat, business over for the night. She is in bed. I am sitting cross-legged in one corner. Bear-as-Was is stretched out on the drawn coverlet at the bed end. The headless budgie has made a nest for itself in the overhead lampshade. And the monkey has finally settled under the duvet, leaving a few hairs, like shiny snippets of copper wire on the white pillow. Alice's side-light is on, the open letter in her trembling

411

hands, a gleaming metal paperknife in the other. We are all waiting. The monkey's head peeps out from under the duvet. The dog rolls into a sitting position. The budgie cranes its neck-stump over the edge of the frosted glass shade. And I lean forwards. We all want to know what Reta has to say for herself. Perhaps it is an apology for how she treated us.

'Dear Alice,
I am writing this at the same table where we sat and had tea together all those years ago. You have been with me so much recently. I sit in the spare room and remember the first night you slept there, how scared you were. I stand in the kitchen and I hear you laughing with Kosey. I look at the portrait of Kesia and it is your eyes I see. You are haunting me, Alice. I am sorry your marriage with Carl was not a happy one. Kosey is sure you are still living in Paris, that you run a restaurant there. I expect your father would be very proud of you if he knew. Does he know, Alice? Does he know where you are? Have you been to see him?
What bothers me, Alice, as I near the end of my life, is not the words I have spoken, but the words I have not spoken. When I lost my husband, when I lost Kesia, I felt so angry with myself. I left so many things unsaid and then it was too late. It is not too late for you, Alice. Go home and see your father.
With love always,
Reta.

Alice sleeps clutching the letter tightly in her hands. We ghosts nod at one another. Already I can feel growing in my host, the determination to return to England and visit her father. It seems that, despite being dead, Reta Okello still has the power to turn our existence upside down. Seven months later we leave Paris, arriving by train at London's Waterloo Station, on the first leg of our journey to see Ralph Safford. The others are overcome with excitement. They tumble pell mell down the escalator in a rush of yellow and green feathers, rust and ruby fur, and into the muggy tunnels of the London Underground. I slink behind, filled with the most terrible sense of foreboding. Not that I expected an intelligent considered response to our changing circumstances from a motley crew of fairground apparitions. But such an undignified arrival, with the monkey 'halloo-ing' hysterically, the dog dashing about barking and snorting, and the budgie pin-balling off the tiled ceiling and walls, well . . . it shows such a lack of breeding. I have nagged Alice incessantly about this insane plot of hers.

'Was it wise to dispose of the restaurant?' I asked.'Especially when it was doing so well.' And, 'Are you quite certain we will be welcomed back into the Safford family, after an absence that seems, even to me, a trifle prolonged?'

But, after receiving Reta's letter, Alice was intractable.

It doesn't take her very long to track down Harry. We go to an internet café in London. My host sits down before a screen, starts busily tapping on a keyboard, and before the dog has time to

413

pace the length of the room, finds what she is looking for. Then she speaks to someone on the shiny silver phone she keeps in her bag, and jots down a number in her diary. Finally she calls Harry and after a stilted conversation a meeting is arranged for Saturday at 3pm at his home in Kent.

'He wasn't pleased to hear from me,' mutters Alice.

We are making our way back to the hotel, our motley retinue barrelling alongside. 'Ghosts from the past, Alice, do not always have the warmest of receptions when they show up,' I explain tactfully. My host shoots me a sideways glance. I beam back angelically.

Harry—2006

It is the weekend. Carmen is dressmaking in the dining room. The fabric she has chosen, a slippery azure-blue silk, is draped over the dining-room table, as if the sky has collapsed on it. I glimpsed it through the open door half an hour earlier, making my way, coffee in hand, into my study. I am online reading *Which* reports on washing-machines, listening to the comforting 'grit-grit' of her sewing scissors as they slice around a pattern. It is mid-afternoon, and a feeling of euphoria is radiating outwards from the pit of my satisfied stomach. The lunch, traditional roast beef, puffs of crisp golden Yorkshire puddings, a selection of perfectly cooked vegetables, followed by apple pie, thick clotted cream and cinnamon custard, was excellent. Fifteen-year-old Edgar woofed it down, and sped off to the rec with friends to play footy. Tiffany, thirteen and going on twenty, stayed over at a friend's last night and has not yet returned home.

Dimly I am aware first of a drowsy warmth enfolding me, then a thin ringing noise piercing the silence. This gathers in volume until the blare of it is deafening, needles of pain stabbing my eardrum, making me dizzy. The screen before me blurs and I close my eyes, grateful that I am sitting down. I know something is about to occur. I am not a fanciful man, and yet I know this with absolute surety. The jangle of the ring tone jars on me like an electric shock. My eyes spring open, my hand shoots out automatically towards the ivory telephone, and then halts mid-air.

I think it is on the fifth ring that Carmen calls to me, but it may be the sixth.

'Are you going to get that, Harry, or shall I?' Her voice is slightly muffled, and I imagine her speaking through a mouthful of pins.

Almost simultaneously I reply. 'I've got it.' And I have. I am clasping the receiver and holding it to my tingling ear. The thrumming stills to a sweet silence. I do not break this with my usual cheery, 'Harry Safford here'. Whoever is at the other end is reluctant to speak too. For a moment, perhaps no more than a few seconds, we are both speechless. Then, there is the lisp of a gulped breath.

'Hello, Harry?' That's all she says. 'Hello, Harry?' That's all it takes. My heart pounds, the tang of coffee in my mouth sucks all the moisture from it. The blood pummels my ears, makes them burn.

415

'Hello Alice,' comes my reply. I picture her voice bouncing like a ball along shady time tunnels. I reach her, at the very end of the last tunnel, standing in a blast of brilliant sunshine. She is in the flat on The Peak of course. Where else? Her body rigid, her eyes trained on the barred windows, stripes of light and shadow falling across her face. From the other end of the line there comes a trembling exhalation, a cross between a sigh and a few beats of laughter loosely strung together. But if she is surprised that I know instantly who it is at the other end of the line, she never says so.

'I'm in London, Harry. I want to see you.' Another shuddering intake of breath. 'I want to see all of you.'

Staring down at the keyboard I spot a miniscule insect cresting the summit of the Home key. I wince, stroke the key with a fingertip, and crush it. It is so tiny that it barely leaves a smear. We falter on, Alice and I, slowly approaching that inescapable point where our two lifelines will converge. I am ashamed to say that if I could plot an abrupt change of direction, I would, in a heartbeat. I do not want to see Alice. I do not want this ghost from the past stalking me in the present, dragging unwelcome baggage from the island behind her. Neither, I feel positive, will Nicola, or for that matter Jillian. I skip around my missing sister's increasingly direct questions about our father. How do I tell this Rip Van Winkle that her adored father is dead, that whatever plans she has entertained of an emotional reunion this side of the grave are impossible.

Neatly, and, as our conversation tumbles on,

416

not so neatly, I sidestep my role of messenger. We siblings will tell her together, I decide grimly. The meeting is arranged for the following Saturday. I ring off.

'Everything alright?' sings out Carmen.

'Oh yes, absolutely fine,' I return brightly. What is the point in breaking with the Safford family's lifetime tradition now?

The subsequent calls, first to Nicola, and lastly, because I cannot face it, much, much later on to Jillian, have echoes of that earlier, discarnate communication with my long lost sister. We progress haltingly. Alice is back. Not for prodigal Alice do we wait with open arms, ready to kill the fatted calf, to celebrate her return with joy unbounded. Not for her will we cry "our sister was dead, but now she is alive! Alice was lost, but now she is found. Hallelujah!" At first, the news renders both Nicola and then Jillian incapable of speech. Gradually, suspicions, dark and a long while brooding, help them regain their composure. Soon they are able to form coherent sentences. What on earth does Alice want after all these years? There's no money left, if that's what she's after. And if it's not the money, it must be something else, that none of us have thought of. Besides, what good can possibly come of this repatriation? Finally, grudgingly, both Nicola and Jillian come to the same conclusion I have, we are *destined* to see Alice. We might as well get the pantomime over with.

The allotted day, that might have been set for world destruction, considering the growing dismay I experience as it approaches, dawns fair. The time scheduled for Alice's advent is 3pm. Both Nicola and Jillian arrive shortly after half past two. We three take up poses in the sitting room, like actors positioning themselves on stage just before curtain up. It is my guess too that each of us is suffering the equivalent of first night nerves. Nicola and Jillian each occupy one of the two armchairs. I sit uneasily between them, in a dining chair that I carried in earlier for the purpose. The sofa we leave conspicuously empty. If any of us sits there, we might rub shoulders with our revenant sister. We might even have to concede that she is real, flesh and blood, merely human.

The clock on the mantelpiece ticks loudly, as clocks will when you give them your undivided attention. Upstairs, Edgar's football thumps periodically on his bedroom floor and, in consequence, on the sitting room ceiling. Grey leaf -shadows thrown by a young golden ash rooted in our front lawn, flutter on the cream walls. Striations of moss green grass, gritty grey tarmac, rosy brickwork, tiled roofs, and bluebell skies, ribbon the windowpanes.

'What time did you say she'd be here?' asks Nicola, her tone deliberately careless. As ever, her clothes, a full midi skirt in oyster-grey, French navy blouse, brown leather ankle boots, finished off with floral silk scarf, look impeccable.

'3pm. She said she'd be here at 3pm,' I reply, a finger easing my shirt collar. It feels uncomfortably tight, pinching my neck. I would like to take off my tie, polyester, a harlequin design that I'm rather fond of. But somehow it seems essential that I be properly dressed for Alice's manifestation. This thought arrives with an astute partner. There is no prescribed style, formal or otherwise, for a tryst with a sister who has been missing for thirty years.

At the sound of a car Nicola turns expectantly to the window. I notice, not for the first time, that her hands look very red and sore. Eczema? Hadn't Mother said that Father had terrible eczema once? Yes, that's right, when we were young, that it ended his career in photography prematurely. I ponder on whether perhaps it is a hereditary condition. She sees me scrutinising her hands, and slips them self-consciously into her bell sleeves. Jillian gives an enormous sigh and makes much of looking at her watch, an unnecessary gesture with the clock directly in front of her.

It's . . . it's a quarter to three,' she says. She has a frog in her throat. She clears it and tries again. 'It's a quarter to three,' she repeats too loudly.

'Mm,' I affirm, with an upward lift of my chin.

Jillian plucks at her neck absently. It looks slack, not quite a turkey's but on its way. We are all getting older I'm afraid. And yet, the Alice I envision leaping out at us from the past is a teenager, hooking her dark hair behind her ears, her voice high, her eyes clear and large. Above us the football thumps. I gaze up and shake my head, grinning indulgently.

'Boys eh?' I comment with a breathy laugh.

'Hmm . . . not having a son I wouldn't know,' manages Nicola with a brief smile.

'Actually Amos is very good,' Jillian says sanctimoniously.

'Lucky you,' I rejoin with a disbelieving grin, thinking that young Amos is anything but. I am sweating under my suit jacket and would dearly like to strip it off. Jillian, I observe, is underdressed for the occasion, slouching in some

419

sort of sloppy, cotton-jersey affair, yellow and blue dots, a bit like pyjamas. Really, she might have made a small effort. I feel irritated as my eyes run over my eldest sister with distaste. Her hair looks greasy and untidy. In yet another reincarnation it is bluish black. Far from making her look younger, the stark funereal shade against her putty complexion puts years on. No make-up. Trainers. It is as if she intends our mythical sibling to see how unimportant this meeting is to her.

We all jump when Carmen pops her head round the door. She has changed into her best silk dress reserved for special occasions. The fitted bodice and full skirt in a small blue and green check pattern looks well on her slender frame. Her nut-brown, frizzy hair is caught up in a yellow velvet bow, and she has applied lipstick. I detect a waft of her subtle perfume too, and think ruefully that she has gone to more trouble for Alice, her sister-in-law, than her real sister has.

'No signs of Alice, the guest of honour, yet?' she inquires. Our heads all rise in unison at that, hearing the name spoken out loud.

'Not yet,' I say jovially. Jillian scowls thunderously. Nicola gives a pained sigh.

Carmen hovers for a moment clutching the side of the sitting-room door. 'Right-oh. I'll get on with preparing tea, then,' she announces gaily. She disappears and is back an instant later. 'You know, I've never met Alice. She was long gone by the time we got together, isn't that right, Harry?' My wife's voice climbs to a high-pitched trill when she is excited, as she is now. I give a fleeting smile and nod. Carmen's hazel eyes sparkle in anticipation. She searches our expressionless faces for an answering effervescence. Finding none she gives a small shrug. 'I expect you'll have lots to talk about,' she declares, her head nodding as if persuading us.

I am not so sure. My stomach rumbles noisily. I smile apologetically at my wife and at my sisters. Carmen takes this as her cue to hurry off to the kitchen. Once she has gone Jillian volunteers the time again, and again, some five minutes later. Talk is desultory. Schools. Holidays. Mother. Of Alice, the reason for this gathering, nothing is said. At quarter past three the front doorbell rings. We all leap up like jack-in-the-boxes, as if someone has simultaneously jabbed pins in our posteriors. We pile out of the sitting room and into the hall. It turns out to be one of Tiffany's friends from the Close, Sonia, a skeletal girl with delicate features, a nose-stud and a white streak in her shoulder-length dark hair.

'Is Tiffany in?' she demands in a bored monotone, as she casts mint-green eyes over us in mild surprise, Nicola to my right, Jillian to my left. Behind us, Carmen cranes forward interestedly. Even Edgar, clutching his football, stoops and peers down from the top of the stairs, his eyes concealed in a mop of tousled brown hair.

'Tiffany's gone swimming,' I furnish absently, stepping forwards and dodging Sonia, determined to discover where Alice is hiding.

'Oh okay,' mutters Sonia, viewing us all with puzzlement, as if doubting she has called at the correct address.

A young girl pedals past on a pink bike ringing her bicycle bell enthusiastically. Across the road Nancy Harben gives a neighbourly wave as she wrestles her green recycling bin back up her drive. A Siamese cat eyes us lethargically from her warm roost on a sunbathed doorstep. But of Alice there is neither sight nor sound. I am about to scuttle back inside and close the door on Sonia, when I hear the hum of an approaching car. We all do. We strain our ears to pick up every nuance of this vehicle's engine, as impressed as if it is a Tardis transporting Alice into the present.

'This is her now,' I tell my sisters on an amazed rising inflexion. Our eyes root on the entrance road to the cul-de-sac. Sonia, made curious by my heraldic announcement, pirouettes in her marmalade mini-skirt. She executes the move with praiseworthy alacrity considering her clumpy black boots, and follows our gaze. As the Tesco's delivery van rounds the bend, our shared sigh ascends and swells like a dense cumulus. Once again we take up our opening positions in the sitting room, still awaiting curtain-up. By half past three however the cracks are definitely beginning to appear.

'Where *is* she?' snaps Nicola, fiddling irritably with the fringe of her scarf. She throws herself about in her chair as if she is on a rollercoaster ride at the fair.

'I'm sure she'll be along shortly,' I soothe. I am on my feet and standing at one of the windows, spider's-leg fingers lacing and unlacing busily. Uncomfortably, I survey the short stretch of road, visible from my sitting room.

'For Christ's sake, this is typical of her!' cries Jillian, out of her chair and pacing before the mantelpiece.

Considering we have not seen Alice for thirty

years, my feeling is that none of us can say with any real confidence what our sister's typical modus operandi is.

'Are you sure she said three o'clock?' checks Nicola, hair mussed after her ride, feet tapping a military tattoo on the carpet.

'Yes,' I say uncertainly. In fact, suddenly I am not sure of anything. I rub the ball of my palms over my temples. A wave of tiredness sluices over me. I did not sleep well the previous night, and made several forays into the kitchen to sustain me. The result, acid indigestion, only served to prolong my wakefulness.

'Perhaps you should have put her off, Harry,' Jillian ventures critically.

Suddenly I feel ridiculous, sitting starch-stiff in a work suit on a warm Saturday afternoon in September, waiting for my vaporous sister.

'Good Lord, Jillian, what do you expect?' I fire, rounding on her. The grey shadow leaves quiver on the wall in a sudden breath of wind. Jillian raises her eyes to heaven, a gesture that further inflames my temper and sends it crackling into life. 'What would you have done then, eh? Told her to piss off for another thirty years?' I growl.

Jillian folds her arms, hands tucked protectively into her armpits. 'That might not have been a bad idea,' she admonishes quietly, her head wagging.

I march over to my chair and throw myself into it. It is reproduction Regency, and it creaks in protest. I remind myself that I am large and it is small, and must be treated more respectfully if I don't want it to buckle under me at a climactic moment. I determine to corral my emotion into speech alone, and sit forward charily. 'Brilliant, just brilliant, Jillian!' I hiss. 'Banish Alice. Tell her never to contact us again. That would solve everything, wouldn't it?'

'You never know till you try,' counters Jillian, with a stubborn thrust of her bottom lip. Somewhere far off an ice-cream van jingles irreverently.

'This isn't getting us anywhere,' Nicola breaks in. 'Harry's right. If he tried to put Alice off, she'd only have come back again at a later date. We need to deal with this now.'

The football thumps several times above us, followed by Carmen's voice distantly berating our son. His truculent reply is just discernible too.

'Well, maybe I don't want to see her. Isn't that my right?' Jillian is shouting. Her cheeks glow red, and her slate-blue eyes contract into pinpricks behind their lenses. 'She walked out on us without a moment's thought, didn't she?' She flounces towards the door blinking back tears. 'Haven't I got the right to walk out on Alice?' she yells flinging the door wide. And there, with the comic timing of a slick farce, is Alice!

'Look who I found wandering around the Close, all lost and forlorn,' Carmen twitters in a motherly tone. She beams like a shepherdess who has found her missing lamb and ushers Alice forwards. Our sometime sister steps timidly into the room. She is nearly invisible, camouflaged by the enormous bouquet of flowers she carries. The arrangement of tropical orange, red and sulphur-yellow flowers is so unnecessarily extravagant that it adds to the growing atmosphere of burlesque. And there is wine as well, and chocolates. Alice has all eventualities covered. Nicola and I are upstanding for our sister. Jillian, a few feet from the door, is riveted to the spot as if carved from stone.

'Alice. How . . . nice. How . . . nice to . . . to see you,' I stutter, crossing to where the bouquet sways. She pushes the gifts towards me, Alice, trying to purchase approval. Taking them, I feel a stab of remorse, remorse for the lost years that will never be recovered. 'For us? . . . how . . . nice, Alice. Wine and chocolates too. Aren't we spoilt?' A truism if ever I uttered one. Carmen dashes forwards and takes the presents from me.

'She was wandering about the Close looking abandoned. So fortunate I spied her from the hall window. I said to myself, I'll bet that's sister Alice, looking for us. Anyway, I'll go and put these in water and get the tea.'

In the moments that follow, while we surreptitiously study Alice, I speedily amend the mental picture I have formed of her over the years. Alice had taken on in my mind the proportions of some vengeful virago, malice bristling in every fibre of her being, bent on destruction. But the middle-aged woman who stands before us is petite, unexceptional, ordinary even. Her hair, though still tucked behind her ears, is cut into a bob, faded to a mousy brown. Her clothes are classic cuts in neutral shades. Her features are small and neat, the lines that have formed around her eyes, her mouth, that crease her brow, are not the grooves of a tempestuous nature, but the tracery of stoicism and quiet fortitude. I gesture Alice to the settee. Nicola and I retake our chairs. Briefly I lock eyes with Jillian, while she battles with the urge to flee this confrontation. At length, defeated, she too sits. And the clock ticks on.

425

'I'm . . . sorry . . . sorry I'm late,' opens Alice breathlessly, perched on the edge of the settee, as if frightened she might sully the covers. 'I got . . . lost.'

This last has me wrestling down the urge to guffaw with helpless laughter. Just a bit, comes my unspoken slightly hysterical rejoinder. I ponder the probability of double meanings presenting themselves for every sentence spoken on this momentous afternoon, and hope I can keep a straight face.

'Well . . . never mind. You're . . . you're here now,' I console out loud.

What follows is like wading through wallpaper paste. Just what do you say to a sister you haven't seen for thirty years, a sister who you thought might very well be dead, buried, a sister whose grave you have imagined on some lonely windswept cliff top more than once? What do you say to a sister who has come back to life, and not just any life but yours? So, how have you been keeping, Alice? It's incredible, thirty years and you haven't aged a bit. Tell us Alice, we'd love to know, your vanishing trick, how exactly does it work?

'So . . . where . . . have you been living, Alice?' Nicola voices courageously. However, her eyes are averted, fixed on the outspread fingers of her hands laid on the armrests of her chair. She looks fascinated, as if seeing them for the first time. Jillian is sitting very still, containing herself. Probably for the best, I muse wryly.

'I've been living in France. Paris actually.' Alice says.

'Oh really?' responds Nicola as if she doesn't

426

quite believe her.

'Yes. It's a beautiful city. The Eiffel Tower lit at night. The Seine. Wonderful art galleries too.' For a few minutes she describes Paris as if she is a travel agent selling a holiday.

As I listen, I imagine Alice buying her bread at a patisserie, Alice at the Louvre drinking in the enigmatic beauty of the Mona Lisa, Alice at the Moulin Rouge, staring wide-eyed at a froth of colourful petticoats, listening to the yips of the dancers with unconcealed delight. Alice looking up at a silvery moon, wondering . . . wondering if her father, across the English Channel, is stargazing too. I have visualised hundreds of Alices over the years. Alice on a sheep farm in Wales, her adoring sheepdog, a Bear double, prancing by her side. Alice in the North, pinched with cold, trudging down a snowy pavement leaving a trail of drab-grey footprints in her wake. Alice in Ireland, perched on a slab of rock on the Giant's Causeway, waiting for her fisherman husband to chug home. In my mind I have journeyed to locations the world over, and seen Alice in every imaginable setting and costume. And yet, the expression in her limpid eyes as she looks back at me is unchanged, one of all-pervading sadness.

'What did you do there . . . in France . . . in Paris?' Jillian asks as Alice's tour of the city comes to an end.

'I worked . . . um . . . in a restaurant.' Alice circles her shoulders waiting for our reaction.

'Sounds excellent,' I say, genuinely impressed.

'You were cooking?' asks Nicola in surprise, probably recalling Alice's poor appetite.

'Waiting tables?' Jillian speaks over her sister.

427

Alice, one hand on her knee, starts pleating the hem of her midnight-blue skirt.

'Well, both really. Cooking and waiting tables. Actually more chopping vegetables than cooking. I sort of worked my way up.'

'Ah?' Nicola sits forward interestedly.

'Up where?' Jillian says deadpan.

Alice talks of her mentor, Pierre Ramirez, the restaurant owner, how he trained her on the job and promoted her when he felt she was ready. I look into her anxious face and remember. Alice, I remember when I was sick, had a fever. I must have been very young, five, or perhaps six. Not much dialogue to the footage, just you dressed in a white apron. You wore a matching white scarf with a red cross painted on it, knotted at the back of your neck, under your hair. I lay in a rattan cot, far too small for me, limbs sticking out rebelliously, you tidying them back in, undeterred in your ministering.

'I am Nurse Alice,' you piped up authoritatively. 'I am going to make you better, Harry.' And you smoothed my hot forehead with a tiny cool hand, your dreamy brown eyes fixing mine. You mixed medicine on a trolley. You were a stork, one bare foot stroking the calf of the leg you stood on, concentrating on your apothecary's duties. In a small yellow bowl you mixed orange juice and sugar and jam painstakingly with a metal spoon. I heard it scrape and chink against the china. Then you held it to my lips while I sipped it. It was sticky and sweet and I can still taste it on my tongue now.

'So in the end you were the manager?' rejoins Jillian incredulously, as Alice finishes explaining how she worked her way up in the restaurant.

'Well done,' Nicola comments, her eyebrows raised, her hands miming applause.

'It wasn't quick. It took ages, years. I left for a bit and went back again.' Alice's tone is one of apology. 'There was so much to learn. I made so many mistakes.'

'Mm.' Jillian shoots me a meaningful look.

'Still, not bad going,' Nicola remarks with a trace of envy.

Alice has stopped pleating her skirt, and now fiddles with the hair behind her ears. 'I became close friends with the owner.' She coughs and clears her throat. 'When he died he left it to me.'

'What?' Nicola's ears prick up. 'The restaurant? The entire restaurant?'

'Mm, yes.' Alice nibbles on a nail.

'What about his own family?' I ask, picturing a tribe of irate Parisians shaking their fists at Alice.

'He didn't have any. Over the years we became close friends,' Alice tells us defensively, as if responding in court to prosecuting counsel.

'What kind of close friends?' Jillian says and there is a slanderous undercurrent in her voice.

'Oh nothing like that. He was like . . . like . . . well a bit like a father to me,' Alice falters. 'Losing him was awful,' she adds tremulously under her breath. None of us is inclined to break the silence that follows this statement. It is Nicola who finally tackles it.

'Well, well, he must have thought a great deal of you, Alice.' Her tone implies that this is nothing short of miraculous. Alice hangs her head. Another long hiatus follows. Then Alice questions each of us in turn about how we have filled in the missing years, leaving Jillian to last. I outline my job selling life-insurance, talk about Carmen, the children. Nicola mentions she is divorced, has moved fairly recently to East Grinstead, and that her daughter Zandra is hoping to attend art college. We sound a bit like one of those trailers for American TV programmes. Previously on the Saffords . . . Only our previously does not flow in quite the same way. We jounce and bump along like an old cart on a rutted track.

Alice turns to Jillian.

'What about you, Jillian?' she inquires diffidently.

Jillian shrugs. 'I'm married. Happily,' she adds emphatically. 'We're living in Hastings. We have a son, Amos, and he's—' She breaks off to say what is really on her mind. 'You could at least have rung to let our parents know you were safe. All you would have had to do was pick up the phone.'

Alice's head swings up and she flinches, as if someone has spooked her.

'I did write. I sent the letters to the flat on The Peak. Three of them.' We all exchange looks of disbelief at this. 'Well, perhaps they never arrived. I rang Uncle Albert as well,' she offers lamely. She takes in our accusatory stares. 'I did,' she adds softly. She rubs the side of her forehead, her fingertip massaging it with a circular motion, and wets her lips. 'I . . . I . . . it never seemed . . . it was just the wrong—' She limps to a painful stop. A television can be heard upstairs, excited dialogue followed by canned laughter.

'So . . . are you married?' asks Nicola.

And while Alice talks of a man called Carl and a marriage that I know will have been doomed, I am back on the first boat we owned, *White Jade*. We are anchored in a peaceful bay. Mother is reading the paper in the stern, sipping a glass of wine. Father is fishing close by. And we, Alice, sister and brother, are splashing in the cold, clear sea. We are watching the honeycomb light waver and fracture over our pale white bodies, making them elastic and fluid. Our vision is hazy with salt smart, the edges of our island life sanded smooth. We are owls blinking slowly at each other in tacit understanding. This idle space should be filled with our game, we agree. As the boat lifts and strains at its anchor mooring, we slide in turn behind the wooden stepladder. We grasp the sides of a framed square, our makeshift television screen. The sea slaps against the curved hull, and sloshes back into us. But we refuse to be thwarted.

We parrot advertising jingles, act out adverts, snatches of our favourite programmes. You giggle, sea spray dribbling from the corners of your mouth and I desperately try to keep a straight face, choking on a mouthful of salty water as I deliver a sloppy line.

'It didn't work out, the marriage,' Alice finishes wanly in the 'now', where there is no room for game-playing.

'Do you have any children?' Jillian asks.

And when Alice says no, inexplicably Jillian erupts in staccato questions. 'Why not? Didn't you want any? Too much responsibility? Too expensive?' Alice fidgets, coils a strand of hair tightly around a finger, uncoils it, starts again with the next finger. She mumbles about the time not being right, her career in the restaurant, other pressing commitments.

Do you recall how we played 'Kick the Can' on

the long, hot summer evenings, Alice? How the can would be placed with precision between the two rows of garages, over the rusty manhole-cover, the golden evening rays bouncing off it in jags of champagne light. I would squeeze behind the hedge and garage walls, my heart thudding madly, my face crimson and slick with sweat, gagging back hiccups of laughter. Brushstrokes of filigree cloud would tarnish as they slipped away into the night. The wind would sigh with contentment. Taking a deep breath, charged with adrenalin, at last I would dare to peep round the edge of the wall. For a second our eyes would meet, then I would break cover. We two would streak towards the can as if our lives depended on reaching it first, me to kick it, you to keep it upright at all costs. You nearly always outpaced me, with my big belly hampering me. Then your foot would slam down on the tin lid.

'One, two, three, Harry,' you would yell in exultation, 'you're out!' I would grind to a stop, my shoulders slumped in defeat. Then seconds later I would recover, and hands in pockets, swagger off, your victory cry echoing in my ears. 'One, two, three, Harry, you're out!'

And it was okay because it was my sister who'd beaten me, it was Alice. No shame in that. Pride, that's what I felt as I joined the others, swinging my legs on the low wall of defeat, under the rippling green fingers that fringed the palms.

'How is Father?' Alice breaks into my reminiscing.

Eyes slide guiltily away from her. The stillness expands. There is no means of softening this news. You cannot say, well, Alice, you must be brave,

Father is a little dead right now. Alice traces our conspiratorial exchanges, one to another. She ages in a second, her expression settling into stark lines of terror. Nicola coughs and fingers the pendant at her neck. It is a Chinese character fashioned in gold, Fu, symbolising good luck. It has an ironic glint to it. I close and reopen my eyes. I will tell her I decide, but Jillian is already talking.

'I'm sorry Alice, but he's dead,' she tells her baldly. Alice's head is on one side, her brow scrunched, as if she is trying to decipher the meaning of Jillian's words. Her hands saw at the air, seeking something tangible in it. 'Actually, Alice, now I come—'

'Jillian!' Nicola interrupts on a warning note.

'What?' Jillian speaks so sharply that her teeth clash. 'I'm just telling her the truth. Father's dead. It's a shame that Alice is too late. I'm sorry for it.' But you can tell she is not. Her voice has just the hint of jubilation in it. 'Surely she must have considered the possibility this might happen?' she continues. 'You've been out of our lives for thirty years, Alice, not a long weekend,' she debates reasonably. Alice nods dumbly and with a great effort draws herself up. Then I am up too, explaining that it was a heart-attack, quick, painless. Nicola interjects that she was there, with him, that he didn't suffer. I feel I should hold this chimerical Alice, wrap my arms around her trembling shoulders. I take a step closer but I am embarrassed. She feels like a stranger, not my sister. She is whey-faced and for a moment I think she might faint. An old-fashioned word that conjures up ladies in Empire dresses, backs of hands touching their flushed brows, comes to mind. Swoon. Alice swoons.

'Nooo!' It is like a sigh, like air leaking out of a slow puncture in a lilo. I hurry to prop her up, Nicola rushing to assist me. Awkwardly, one side apiece, we hold up this sibling wraith.

'Honestly, what did she expect!' mutters Jillian, contemptuous of the attention Alice is garnering. Nicola casts her a withering look.

Jillian shrugs, wearing her lack of repentance ostentatiously. 'It's not my fault, the way this has worked out,' she offers in her defence.

'When?' Alice asks, her lips barely moving, her voice no more than a thread.

'He died about three years ago, Alice,' fills in Nicola. We lower Alice back into her seat and retake our own.

'I'm too late,' she says, but not to us, to herself.

'Well, you could go and see his grave instead,' Jillian says trenchantly. I shall be generous, and say that Jillian did not deliver this with cruel intent. But all the same Alice shrinks back on the settee. Where, I think, is Carmen with the tea and that fruitcake I saw her baking yesterday?

'I looked after him. So you needn't worry. I didn't desert him. I looked after them both,' Jillian bugles into the sudden quiet.

'But Mother's alive?' Alice says, only just managing to keep despair at bay.

'Oh yes,' I rejoin, 'She's still alive and kicking.' The chord of jollity I strike is inappropriately redolent of Santa Claus, after he's washed down his mince pies with one too many sherries. Rapidly, I adjust my pitch to one of sympathy, explaining about the care home we found, how pleasant it is, how well Mother has settled in.

'I'd like to visit,' says Alice, the way in a fairy story you might say, I wish it with all my heart. 'If it's alright with you,' she adds as an apprehensive afterthought.

Jillian pouts, but, before she can offer up her views on the request, Nicola is speaking.

'I don't see why not. I'm sure she'd love to see you and—' She breaks off, nettled to see the start of a ladder on her stockings. She picks at it and frowns, then begins afresh. 'Mother comes and goes, Alice. You mustn't be surprised. Let's just hope it's one of her lucid moments, eh?'

'It must have been nice to devote all your time to your career,' is Jillian's next barbed observation. 'I'd like to have had a career, Alice. But circumstances prevented it.'

Before Alice has time to respond, Nicola jumps in to say how felicitous our discovery of Greenwood Lodge was. She describes the attractive country setting and how well Mother has settled into the routine. But Alice's blank eyes show that she is not listening. While she is talking Carmen brings in the tea, together with her magnificent cake. After depositing the tray she scampers away, leaving us to catch up she says. For the next quarter of an hour, thankfully, we are all diverted, pouring, sipping and eating, especially me. And there are paste sandwiches too, with lashings of butter, just the way I like them, piled up on a plate, a sprig of parsley on the top. Carmen has made plenty for everyone so I quell my rising panic, though oddly my siblings seem reluctant to tuck in.

As we sit, the Safford children at their tea, I feel the hand of time whisking us back through the years, until we are there, ranged about the dining-room table in the flat on The Peak. Father is carving, and bloody juices coat the gleaming silver knife and dribble down the sharp blade. Mother is clasping her wine glass. The sunlight catching on the crystal planes creates a jewelled tessellation bewitching us all. Alice is chirpy, eager to please. Nicola's calculating eyes flit about, as she adds, divides, multiplies and subtracts the sum of all our misery, turning it to her advantage. Jillian sees her father's striking blue eyes soften as they sweep over her little sister. She glares at Alice. Her own eyes, flint-cold, narrow in hatred. And I concentrate every molecule I have on the food in front of me, on shovelling forkful after forkful into my mouth. Chew, chew and swallow, chew and swallow, barely time to breathe. But back then I had faith, unshakeable faith, that there would come a day eventually when the hole would be plugged.

The fuzzy television voice filtering down from upstairs is suddenly choked. An eerie hush descends. I feel a cold draught from somewhere slither under my collar. My mouth stops working on my bolus of cake crumbs. We all stare aghast as the teapot, the milk jug, the sugar bowl, the cake-stand, and the plate of sandwiches, Royal Albert China all, a gift from Carmen's parents, start to vibrate. What I notice first are the ripples on the lily-white milk pond. This is followed by the rapid tinkle of the lid quaking in the teapot's grip. The sugar bowl adjacent to it, repeatedly nudges its hot belly. The cake stand judders. The plate starts to slide on the glass-topped coffee table, just millimetres, but its laboured progress, nevertheless, can be clearly tracked. The empty plastic tray with its design of orange and yellow marigolds, leaning against the side of the coffee table where I set it, topples over onto the carpet.

I am on my feet, wheeling round, my eyes raking the room. 'Stay calm everyone, I'm sure it's nothing.'

'God Almighty, what's happening?' Nicola exclaims, rising from her chair.

'Harry, do you think it's an earthquake?' This last is Jillian, also standing now, clutching her cup of tea in one hand, head raised, scanning the ceiling worriedly. Only Alice does not move, I notice. Her expression is one of tragic resignation.

'No, no, surely not an earthquake. Not here,' I mumble.

If we were sitting on the runway at Heathrow airport as a jumbo jet roared past, its wingtip only feet away, the phenomenon would have had a simple scientific explanation. But we are not at Heathrow airport, we are at tea in the sitting room of No. 14 Victoria Close.

The large flat-screen television mounted on the wall to one side of the fireplace suddenly swings out on its supporting arms and bursts into life. A whirlpool of coloured pixels drains into a central black unblinking eye, accompanied by a painfully discordant din. Scraps of words, cries, exclamations, moans, a burst of Chinese opera, growls, wailing, chattering, announcements, the British National Anthem, the chirruping of a bird, a terrified scream, the clatter of Cantonese, gunshots, an explosion, a whimper, all slur into each other. The overhead Savoy pendant lamp starts swinging gently, then blinks on. Light glows through the misted glass shade, and almost immediately starts to flicker and crackle. As if in answer, the CD player's two speakers boom into life, thundering out music.

Nicola's hands are clasped, resting protectively over her hunched head. Jillian is pointing at Alice. 'She's doing this. Can't you see, Alice is doing this.'

Alice holds her arms out and shakes her head as if to prove she has nothing hidden up her sleeves. 'No. No. It's not me.'

'*I Am The Walrus*,' I mouth, 'The Beatles.' I recall, amid the furore, that I had listened to the album the previous night. 'I must have left it switched on.' Then all our heads snap up. The ceiling appears to be trembling. A small cloud of plaster dust puffs out from the light fitting.

'Christ!' gasps Nicola just as the curtains, sprays of lilac on a magnolia background, free somehow of their tiebacks, draw together. Then as we watch, grotesquely mesmerised, they swish open, and yet again they close, an encore in a puppet theatre.

Slowly Alice draws herself up, her eyes darting about the room. 'Stop it! Stop it now!' She twists her body and wriggles her shoulders as if wrenching herself out of someone's grip. We all duck as the overhead lightbulb explodes, the blackened splinters of glass pinging against the interior of its shade. In reply, the television gives a blinding flash, then dies. With a final agonised groan, The Walrus sinks in an ocean of white noise, before being swallowed completely. A whine from somewhere rapidly descends several scales to a deep guttural roar, as the curtains inch back letting in blocks of afternoon sunlight.

'Oh my God!' exclaims Jillian in a hushed tone. Glancing around I see the armchair she was sitting in leaning over tipsily, beyond the point of return, then thwacking heavily on its side. Jillian jumps, letting go the teacup she is holding. Warm liquid cascades all down the front of the strange blue and yellow sweatshirt she is wearing. The cup and saucer smash into pieces on the glass top of the coffee table. Jillian screams. She fixes Alice one last time, before she flees, sobbing. We hear her trainers squeaking as she runs across the hallway's wooden floor. The front door slams.

'I didn't do it,' mumbles Alice, first to Nicola and then to me. A car engine is gunned, fires, and tyres squeal in the drive as it speeds off.

Carmen appears looking stunned, the jaunty yellow ribbon trailing across her face, hair awry. Eyes bulging, she surveys the devastation in our lounge. 'What's . . . what's happened?' she stammers, eyes lifted to the brown wisp of smoke snaking out from the exploded ceiling light.

'It was an accident. We'll soon put it to rights,' I assure her, trying to arrange my face into a relaxed smile and failing miserably. My brow has been pinched into a deep frown for so long now that it aches.

'Don't worry, Carmen. It's only one cup and you can always get replacements,' Nicola consoles her sister-in-law, dropping to her knees. She starts to scoop up fragments of Royal Albert china from the table and the carpet. In the background, Alice is still protesting her innocence. Carmen takes in the spilt tea soaking into the rug and without a word dashes off. I am tracing with a forefinger the hairline crack I have spotted on the coffee table, when she reappears with a basin of soapy water and a sponge. She kneels and scrubs frantically at the honey tea-puddle on the cream Axminster. Alice leans over Carmen stammering how sorry she is, that she will pay for any damage.

'Do let me help you clear up?' she begs my wife's bobbing head.

'Good heavens no, you're a guest!' Carmen tells her, rocking back on her heels, closing with finality on an unmistakably manic note. She waves her away with a flapping hand. I am using a napkin to mop up the splashes of tea on the tabletop. Nicola rises and places the broken china carefully on the mantelpiece. Then she turns to examine a trail of drops that have plopped like fat pebbles between coffee table and the overturned armchair. She swivels and stares at Alice. Our sister has drifted apart from us, her skin leached to a whitewash. A sense of purpose settles on Nicola's face as she looks at Alice hovering by the open door.

'I'll give you the address and number of Mother's care home,' she says, finding her bag by her armchair. She fumbles in it and produces pen and paper. She scribbles something down. 'And the church, I've written down the address of the church where Father . . . where you can visit Father.' She hesitates for a moment. 'I'll give you my mobile too. And I'll speak to Mrs Bowker, the manager at Greenwood Lodge, tell her you're coming.' She scrawls her mobile number down too. I peer over her shoulder as she does this. She looks up and locks eyes with Alice. 'Alright Alice?'

'Yes, that's fine, Nicola,' Alice mumbles awkwardly. There is a pause of a few seconds.

'Anything else, Alice?' My voice is more abrupt

than I intend it to be.

'No, no . . . no nothing else,' Alice falters, one hand circling the wrist of the other, rubbing it as if to ease a pain. Another pause. Carmen looks up. Her cheeks are very pink, and there is a blot of tea together with a dusting of cream carpet fibres on the silk skirt of her dress.

'Then perhaps you should—' I begin but Alice interrupts.

'I'd better get going, Harry. Thank you so much for the lovely tea, Carmen.'

Carmen leaps up, sponge in hand. 'Do come and visit us again,' she says, but she makes no move towards her guest.

'Mm . . . that would be lovely,' says Alice quietly, then sighs desolately.

In tandem, rather I think in the style of a Laurel and Hardy silent movie, Nicola and I cross to Alice. Inexplicably, the clock on the mantelpiece begins to chime. It is 5:15pm. We march Alice to the front door. Nicola hands over the slip of paper. Alice nods. She looks like a famous actress who has just inadvertently revealed a shameful and unforgivable secret about herself on national television.

'Goodbye Alice,' we mutter, speaking in unison. We do not make another date. For the last time I stare into Alice's melancholic eyes. She gives a slight lift of her head, turns and walks sedately to her car. She reaches it just as the thirteenth chime rings out. As the reverberations fade, I see Alice as before, the termagant whose powers of destruction are apocalyptic. I close my front door on her before the engine even starts up.

'Harry, what happened in there? You saw it.

Heard it. So did Jillian. We all did.' She stands in the hallway, eyes wide with fear, her dry red hands fluttering about her, sketching abstract shapes in the air. Now she lowers her voice to a fierce whisper. 'There is something . . . something about Alice. It's Alice. Harry there . . . is something . . . something . . . ' she winds down like a clockwork toy and grinds to a halt with a gasp.

'I know, Nicola, I know,' is my rejoinder. Then I shake my head and put a finger to my lips, and Nicola nods in tacit understanding.

Now they're all gone, I'm feeling a wee bit peckish, hazarding a guess at the exact amount of paste sandwiches left over, and whether I'll be able to cram them all in. I expect I'll find an empty corner.

Ghost—2006

We hare down country lanes in the hire car, the dog complaining that he feels sick, the monkey sticking its deflated head out of the window and squealing dementedly as the wind rushes at its puckered, effulgent features. The budgie, a scintillating flash of butter yellow and bright green over our heads, supplies us with an air escort. Craning my ghostly neck around the raving monkey, I glance up, wince at the brilliant sun, then gaze into the blue mantle of sky that encompasses it. It is marbled with shifting translucent pearly wisps as transient as sea foam.

We park by a sheltered wooden gate and bundle out before a church built of mottled stones, in browns and greys and beiges, with a slate roof. It has high, arched, stained-glass windows, and a steeple that sits like a witch's hat over a bell-tower, a metal cross perched right at its pinnacle. And there is a clock on the side of the tower, with golden hands that glide slowly round its blue face. When we arrive people are filtering into the church. We steal past the great wooden doors, and down a verdant slope to a graveyard. Behind us we hear muttered prayers and muffled singing. We pass a huge tree, a wooden seat encircling its trunk. We walk through a sea of gravestones daubed in milky-green, mustard-yellow, rust-brown and ivory-white lichens. Some stand sentry, dominoes, bolt upright, marking the life-spans of unflagging spirits, others lean wearily towards the earth, worn down by wind and weather, and still more are cracked and crumbling, the names inscribed on them long since rubbed away.

But we pass on, to a distant stretch of paler green, set aside for those still smarting from the wound of death, their names scalded into marble and stone with fresh tears. We walk slowly down one row and up another. Right at the end of this we find a blackmarble tombstone with gold lettering upon it. There is an urn squatting on it, with large red and white plastic roses poked into its metal grid.

Alice reads:

443

In Memory
of
RALPH SAFFORD
1927 to 2003
Loving husband to Myrtle
Devoted father of Jillian, Nicola and Harry

Alice stands back and rereads the epitaph. For once, the dog, the monkey and budgie seem subdued. A blackbird, alighting on a tree close by, bursts into song. As the last notes melt away, it cocks its gleaming head, its yellow eyes swivelling curiously at us. Leaves rustle in the breeze. Beyond the boundary of the churchyard, I follow a mass of a dark cloud slipping silently over a field of waving golden grasses.

'My name is not there,' says Alice, her voice small and flat.

She is holding a dainty spray of daisies tied with white ribbon. She loosens the ribbon, picks the plastic roses from the urn one by one, casts them aside, and replaces them with the fragile flowers. I linger respectfully a few yards down the path, to give my host some privacy.

Alice hunches down by the side of the grave, her fingers raking the clipped turf. I am not sure how long she sits there, perfectly still, her face a blank page. But when at last she stands, her cottonwool legs very nearly crumbling under her, the service in the Church is over and the people have gone to their homes.

Greenwood Lodge, when we find it some time later, is an ugly Victorian villa set back from the road, with bits added onto it, like the Wendy houses children play in. The main building has a gabled roof and bow windows, and is painted a pale green. We are greeted by Mrs Bowker, a big, dark-skinned woman, who reminds me of Reta Okello. She has a mass of black, springy hair, anchored down with several shiny steel grips, and a way of laughing through her speech.

'Welcome, welcome. You must be Alice,' says Mrs Bowker, shaking Alice's hand vigorously. 'Your sister Nicola rang me and said you were coming.' She draws us into a rabbits' warren of corridors and shady rooms.

'It is so lovely for Myrtle to have a visitor,' she says, leading us through to the rear of the building, then into the 'dayroom', where she explains the home's residents are resting after lunch.

Alice is having a hard time taking anything in— not the shabby wallpaper, or the drab furniture, or the rumpled old faces that line the walls, faces from which confused eyes are horribly magnified behind spectacles thick as the bottoms of glass bottles. Nor is she really aware of the faint odour of urine, mingled with stewed vegetables, and stale bodies. The drone of the vast television does not register either. Alice starts to search the faces for her mother's, until Mrs Bowker, who has stopped to speak to a few residents, glances back and sees what she is doing.

'Oh no, dear, Myrtle is in the garden, sitting on the bench by the monkey-puzzle tree. She likes her own space I think, dear. Doesn't want to mix too much with the rabble.'

Mrs Bowker pushes open some French windows, and we are soon all tearing down the garden path, the headless budgie bringing up the rear with a flourish of its bright plumage. Then we

445

stride over a bumpy lawn of velvet moss, dandelions and molehills. Finally we thread our way through a few shrubs, and there, in a small clearing overlooked by a towering monkey-puzzle tree, is Myrtle Safford. Our first sight of her seems to wind Alice entirely. The dog too halts in his tracks, his planar head turning this way and that, as if he cannot believe the evidence of his own spectral eyes. Much as I might expect, the gremlin starts pointing rudely, shaking with laughter. And the budgie crashes into the monkey-puzzle tree, pricks itself on the spiky foliage, slumps to the ground, and immediately starts to thrash about as if in its death throes, hardly likely considering.

I am more composed, though believe me it is easy to see why Alice is so shocked. Gone is the fine lady we use to see sweeping down the corridors of the flat on The Peak. She is slumped on a wooden bench as if she had no spine to prop her up. Her face is bloated and her eyes puffy. She has not just double chins but treble ones. And the mane of rich dark hair has moulted, so that now her scalp is patterned with bubblegum-pink diamonds and crescents. The thick snake of a plait, that once upon a time she wound round and round her head and pinned into place, has shrivelled to a worm. Her slack skin is creased. She has dark red shadows in the hollows of her face. Now she wears glasses, the large rectangular lenses set in thick dark frames. And her eyes, which once flashed with pride, contempt and haughtiness, have grown small and dingy as the British pennies Alice has in her purse. Her hands, anchoring a brown and blue wool rug over her lap, are freckled with age-spots. She is still wearing a fine dress though, a black and white kaftan. But the hem looks scuffed with dirt, and sequins are trailing from a loose thread at the collar. A single diamante earring droops disconsolately from one of her earlobes. Strangest of all, squashy, fat, luminous-orange trainers hug her feet, together with thick aquamarine-coloured socks, printed with small red strawberries.

'How are you, Mrs Safford?' Mrs Bowker greets her. For the present Alice is struck dumb. 'I've brought a visitor. I understand you haven't seen her for a bit so this will be a real treat. See. It's Alice!' she says. She stands back to reveal my host, as if unveiling a long-anticipated work of art.

Slowly Myrtle looks up, eyelids contracting in the sunshine. Her movements are jerky, her head teetering so much on her neck that she looks the way she did sometimes in the evenings in the flat on The Peak. The sunlight, falling through the spiky branches of the monkey-puzzle tree, makes serrated patterns of light and shadow on the grass. Mrs Bowker waits a few seconds, while Mrs Safford's dull eyes flick over her daughter, taking her in.

Now she looks past Alice at Mrs Bowker. 'I want you to bring the tray out here, Ah Lee, with the bottle of whisky, the tub of ice, and tumblers. Do you understand?' she slurs grandly.

'Oh yes, Mrs Safford, right away,' Mrs Bowker tells Myrtle Safford brightly, winking at Alice. Then to us she says, lowering her voice to a whisper, 'I'll leave the two of you to get acquainted again. If you need anything, just shout,' she calls back over her shoulder.

Alice sits down on the empty wooden bench opposite her mother. I shoo the beasties away, determined that here my host will have the privacy denied her in the churchyard. They cooperate, albeit reluctantly, vanishing into a coppery-leafed bush. Alice clears her throat. She combs back her hair with her quivering fingers. She inches forwards on her seat, and tilts her head this way and that, in a vain attempt to get her mother's attention.

'Mother, it's me. Alice,' she says at last. Unconsciously, one of her hands finds the wooden arm of the bench, and runs forwards and back along it, as if she is stroking it. 'I've been away, Mother, remember. For a long time. For a very long time. Well . . . thirty years, Mother. I . . . I've come home now. I can come and see you, if . . . if you like? Would you like that?' She is hesitant at first. 'I've been living in France. I sent you letters, three of them. But perhaps you didn't receive them. Anyway that's where I was, in Paris. I was married for a time. I wrote and told you. Did you get my letters? Oh, it doesn't matter. I would have loved you to have come to my wedding. I thought of you, pictured you there. We . . . we lived in a big airy flat with views over the city. I think you would have liked him, Carl. I did. Well, I loved him of course . . . at first. It didn't . . . didn't work out though. But I was happy for while. For a while I was . . . I was happy.' She speaks as if she is trying to convince herself. There is a burst of birdsong, but I cannot see the bird anywhere. Beyond the monkey-puzzle tree is a tall fence. Not much can be seen over it,—a line of treetops, the roof of a building that may well be a barn, and still further away, on the rise of the next field, a handful of cows ambling about. Distantly I hear them lowing.

'My guests will be here soon,' Myrtle says, the light bouncing off her lenses as she glances about her. 'I must get ready. Where's Ah Lee? I think I'll wear the purple dress tonight. Do run along now, I'm far too busy to chat.' Her tone is dismissive. She closes her eyes.

Alice hesitates, fighting the impulse to obey and leave. Then she stops the stroking motion of her hand, balls her fist and raps the armrest firmly. She takes a huge breath as if she is about to dive into a deep pool. 'I've been to see Harry and Nicola, and even Jillian. You know, Mother, given time, I think we just might patch things up.' Alice's voice is brittle. 'They're doing very well, aren't they? They have families of their own now. Just think. Husbands and wives . . . and . . . and children. They have children. Funny isn't it? I . . . oh, I haven't got any children myself. Carl and I, well . . . we didn't have any in the end.' There is a catch in her voice. She lays the flat of her hand at the base of her throat and presses.

'Beth dear, I think I'm going to have to let that amah go. She hasn't brought the whisky yet. Whatever will my guests think.' Mrs Safford's eyes are still closed. She flaps a hand at a drowsy bee bumbling past. Alice stares down at the grass, and watches the progress of a trail of ants bent on shouldering a biscuit crumb.

Keeping her hand in place as if the gesture will steady her voice, she speaks. 'You'll never guess what, Mother. I can talk French.' She looks up into her mother's face, still searching for a sign of recognition. 'I wasn't very good at it when I was at the Island School. I only got a B pass in my O level. Do you remember? But now I can talk

449

French. Isn't that strange?' Alice waits a beat. Myrtle opens her eyes, and licks her lips with a lazy swipe of her tongue, in a way that reminds Alice of a lizard catching flies. Alice gives a soft whinny of laughter. 'I expect you'd like to know what I've been doing all these years. I put it in my letters. I so hoped you'd reply. But most likely they got lost in the post. It happens all the time. I ran a restaurant. Well, not at first. To begin with I just helped out in the kitchens. But in time Pierre promoted me. Oh, that's Pierre Ramirez. He owned the restaurant. He was my boss. He was very kind to me. You know he reminded me a bit of . . . of . . . well, anyway he was good to me. I watched the handover of Hong Kong on the television. I thought of you both there while the rain came down and everyone got soaked.'

The bird delivers another explosion of song, even more frenzied this time, as if its life depended on being noticed. 'He willed the restaurant to me, Mother. I put it all in a letter. But it must never have arrived. You'd have got in touch if it had, sent me a reply. Of course you would.' Her voice drops until it is barely audible.' It was so sad when . . . when . . . Pierre died. I was with him. I held his hand. I thought if I held his hand he wouldn't go, but he slipped away just the same.' Now her tone lifts perceptibly. 'I was the owner, Mother, can you imagine? Your daughter running a restaurant? I had staff, paid their wages.' Alice nods emphatically, like a child who knows they won't be believed. 'Mm . . . really, I was. If you'd seen me at work you would have been so surprised.'

Then suddenly she shakes her head as if trying

to wake herself. 'Imagine me being good at languages, and running a restaurant. Can you believe it, Mother?' Her delivery is speeding up, getting faster and faster as if she hasn't time to stop and breathe. 'I went to see a play in London. I did, Mother. I had some free time and I thought that I'd like to see a play. It was called *Moon for the Misbegotten*. It's a wonderful title for a play, isn't it, Mother? 'M' is such a generous consonant, don't you think? So warm and round. Like marshmallows, and mattresses. Murderers too, I suppose. I hadn't thought of that. And well, 'Misbegotten', that word, starting as it does with 'mis', that's significant I think. Because life is about missing all sort of things, isn't it? Then the 'begotten' part, to me that sounds like the words are tripping and falling down a flight of stairs, that they just can't stop themselves.'

Myrtle looks over Alice's shoulder. 'Ralph could never deal with the staff. Too kind by half. You have to be firm with these people. He should have got rid of Amanda too and he knew it. She became a liability, a threat to all of us. In the end I had to do it for him. I had to rescue him. The little bitch would have been our ruin if I hadn't stepped in. So I sorted it out once and for all. Would you like to know what I did? Is that why you're here, Beth?' The spread fingers of each hand rest on the arms of her glasses, adjusting their position.

'What . . . what did . . . you do, Mother?' Alice asks. There is a quaver in her voice, as though she is frightened to hear the answer. 'What did you do . . . do to Amanda?'

She lowers her hands into her lap. Her eyes glint behind their lenses and her mouth breaks into a secretive smile. 'I took care of it. I told her at the Boxing Day party. Outside the amahs' quarters. I said, "Would you like me to tell Phillip that you're screwing my husband? Or perhaps I should go and tell your children, tell young Oliver and pretty little Jemima that their mummy's opening her legs, not for their daddy but for Uncle Ralph." Oh that made her angry, spitting like the common alley cat she was. "I expect you'd like me to say making love. Is that what you think you're doing, Amanda? Oh no, darling, love's got nothing to do with it. Don't fool yourself. You're Ralph's whore, no more than that. I'm Myrtle Safford. I'm his wife. He knows his duty. He won't leave me. You are never to go near him again, Amanda. Do you hear me?"' Now her hands clench tightly in her lap as her voice rasps out. ' "If you do, I'll find out, and I'll destroy your family. I'll smash it apart, until your children can't look you in the face." ' She gives a rough, mirthless snort. 'She knew she couldn't stay away from my Ralph, knew she couldn't help herself.' Again she laughs, her flaccid mouth closing on the soft snigger. 'She knew what she had to do. She didn't waste any time. She got on with it. Poor Amanda, flying through the air like a trapeze artist, only no one caught her. She was no match for me and she knew it.'

No sound comes from Alice, but the tears brimming in her eyes spill over and slide down her pale cheeks.

'So you see, I kept the family safe. And Amanda wasn't the only one who tried to take my husband away.' Alice looks confused, scared. 'My own daughter. My own flesh. I took care of that too. Burnt those letters she sent. One, two, three . . .

whoosh. So pretty. I dealt with her.' Alice's hands move to cover her ears, then change course and, almost violently, wipe away her tears. 'Of course Ralph's dead now, so I don't have to worry about her any more.'

Alice shakes her head slowly from side to side. Then she is still, speaking quietly. 'I . . . I was . . . so sad to hear about Daddy, about him—I'm sorry he didn't get my letters. But he knew,' she says with dignity, 'he knew how much I loved him. Even if he didn't see the letters. I went to his grave, this morning. My name isn't there, Mother. My name, it isn't with the others. There's Jillian and Nicola and Harry . . . but not me. Alice isn't there. I'm not there, Mother. As if . . . as if I never was.' She stops and sucks in her mouth. There is a moth in her stomach. I sense it, a giant moth. Its wings are coated with sticky, black gum. It twists and buckles inside her. Its head is not furry and soft. It is as rough as the texture of shark's skin. She feels it nosing about, grating at her, feels the juices it writhes in turning to a burning acid. 'I was . . . was—' With the flat of one hand she strikes her mouth, as if trying to clear it of an obstruction. She sucks in a breath and her small chest rises with the effort of it. 'I tried, Reta, but . . . but I was just . . . just—' This time the air is sobbed in. 'I'm . . . sorry, that's all!' she finishes, sinks back on her bench, and folds. A long moment passes.

The bird is silent now. On an impulse, Alice drops to her knees before her mother.

'Look at me!' Her hands reach out and lightly touch the folds of Myrtle Safford's dress. Her mother's response is almost leisurely. She inclines her head, the gesture imperious, and gazes down

453

at her daughter. Just for a second the lenses of her glasses flash, blinding Alice, then their eyes meet. 'It's me, Mother. It's Alice!' Alice does not speak, she beseeches.

Mrs Safford leans forward in her seat. The movement sends her earring swinging. The sun catches on it, and light splinters and springs off it. She puts her head to one side and frowns, as if she is trying hard to remember something, someone. For a few seconds she studies Alice's features, like someone searching a map for a familiar landmark. Then she edges even closer. Her eyelids relax. Her face is empty. Alice can feel her mother's breath against her skin, can detect a trace of sourness in it.

'Who . . . who are you?' Myrtle Safford asks her daughter. 'I don't know who you are.'

Alice lifts herself up then, hypnotically climbing to her feet, her look glazed, seeing nothing at all. And that's when I catch it. It is just a flicker, deep down in Myrtle Safford's eyes, but it is unmistakable, the cold glimmer of recognition. Almost imperceptibly, the corners of her mouth twitch upwards, as if . . . as if she is acting, the way she did sometimes in the flat on The Peak, as if she knows the audience has been entirely taken in, as if she is enjoying her very own private joke.

Minutes later we leave, our entourage creeping out of the bushes and racing after us. But to my consternation Alice follows signs not to London but to Brighton and the coast. There is a harrowing stiffness in her posture. And I have sinister misgivings when she parks her car close to the seafront and climbs out. The day shrugs off its warmth as the five of us head down to the beach.

454

Alice crunches over the pebbles, looking neither to right nor left. The dog trots behind, nose to the ground in a heaven of sea scents. The monkey bounces off the pebbles like a ginger beachball, gurgling joyously on each bumpy impact. The headless budgie soars alongside the gulls, causing quite a stir. And I skitter after Alice, trying hard not to lose my airy footing on the uneven surface. At last we stand before a monstrous thing, like the skeleton of some great sea serpent that has washed up on the shore, and perished there.

'The old West Pier,' Alice mutters. 'There was a fire. It's all burnt out.'

Day-trippers still freckle the beaches—strolling adults, children at play, paddling and shouting, young lovers sharing a last kiss. The merry-go-round is winding down, the music fading away. The buzz of traffic is diminishing. A couple of dogs bark and rush into the breaking waves. They lollop out, spinning their coats, showers of droplets catching the light. A kite, a dash of red and yellow, tail dipping, sails high above us. A man bends to retrieve bats and a ball. A solitary voice cries out excitedly. Boats bob and dip in the blue arms of a capricious sea. Gulls loop and dive and screech, owning each kingdom in turn—the mounds of pebbles, the reaches of the wooden windbreaks, viridescent with lanky tresses of seaweed, the wide scope of changeable sky, the rough blanket of the sea. Sometimes they swoop, puncturing the blue-green drum with their hooked yellow beaks, emerging with some wriggling silver titbit, and streaking away to gobble it down in solitude, unhampered. But Alice is oblivious to all this, choosing rather to stand before the bones of the beast.

Suddenly I sense the sun has withdrawn its beneficence, and the sky has transformed itself into a scumble of mutinous grey. The pebbles that looked so bright in the golden sunlight, varnished with the surf, are all over salt dust, drab and monotonous. The sea breath grows frosty and murky. Seaweed ribbons sprawl like beached, lifeless snakes. The people have gone. The merry-go-round is still, its jaunty tune suffocated. The seagulls huddle together on the bones of the beast. The cold curls about me, reclaiming its own. I seek comfort in the solid beat of Alice's heart, slinking down into the elastic passages that wind through her body. I feel the beat of that munificent organ reverberating through her. I am held in thrall by the swell of her life-giving lungs. On I journey, pumped through oak-solid arteries that thin presently to a web of veins, and still further, coursing through her tiny capillaries, slim as hair gossamer thread, delicate as coral tips. Alice sits, hugging her knees. Bear-as-Was is by her side, smouldering eyes trained on her face, while the monkey whirs about my host's head, humming tunelessly.

I know there is ice settling in the marrow of my host's bones, that her skin is stamped with cold, that her red cotton dress is no protection against the fast approaching night. I stand guard, ghostly arms akimbo, while that doltish bird, deserting its new-found feathered friends, circles over us. Its puny body seems to have bloated suddenly, like a waterlogged corpse. It has swapped its bright plumage for a leathery bilious-yellow skin, encrusted with scurf. Suddenly it lumbers down, and while it hovers before Alice's milk-white face, the mess of clotted blood at its neck oozing like a sluggish stream, I detect the unmistakable stench of death hanging on the air. The monkey's droning builds and builds until Alice's head throbs with it. Her hands reach up to cup her ears, desperately trying to block out the dissonant whining.

Now the winged creature crashes to the pebbles, and with a sequence of clumsy belly-flops makes its way down to the sea's edge. The dog, coat ablaze, the monkey riding him like an impish jockey, races to the shoreline. They dart into the creaming waves, then rush back to us, barking and chattering invitingly. I scowl at all three in turn, saving my grimmest face for the dog.

'In life you hated the sea,' I spit at him. But the dog only nips at Alice's dress, tugging at it, while the monkey on his back performs some hideous parody of a belly-dance, rippling its glittering body and reeling Alice in.

Alice stands. No matter how hard I try to push her up the beach towards safety, she eludes me. She walks as if in a trance, over the pebbles to meet the furling tide. She bends, the sea catching at the heels of her sandals, lapping greedily at the soft, brown suede. She stares enraptured at the mashing foam and at the rolling crystal gyres of the incoming waves. I try to pull us back from the deep, try to skim over the smooth flat stones, drawing Alice with me. But I seem to have no stability, no point of gravity. I skid about as if I am a novice on a skating rink. The wind, now picking up, pierces us with sharp needles of rain. Alice wants to sink into the pebbles, huddle under their mass, have the weight of all those stones quilt her in, like clods of earth. Blackness descends, unstoppable, cloying. Alice slips off her sandals and steals towards the bones of the beast. I have no choice but to follow. Then I hear them, my ancestors, and know they are coming for me.

'Lin Shui! Lin Shui!' they implore, 'let us lead you to the other side of night.'

When I glance back at the deserted beach, I think I see a child, a golden-haired child clad in black rags, crouching behind a windbreak. Then I turn and Alice is wading into the icy water. The dog paddles at her side. The turgid bird, a few yards ahead, arrows down into the now cinereous depths. The monkey floats on its back, blowing black bubbles and winking roguishly. Alice's red dress spreads out and flowers about her. My host is a red hibiscus blossom and the sea lusts after her. She barely feels the gelid sludge pushing into the soles of her feet, the pressure of it sucking us down. Deeper and deeper she goes. Trails of icy brine net her numb limbs, dragging her down. Over us climbs the oppressive bars of the beast. It blocks out the moon. We slip silently between its slippery, charred beams.

The sea drinks Alice down into a tenebrous vortex. I wind myself around the slimy bones of the relic, catching at Alice as she falls. I burrow into the fray of seaweed and barnacle, into the spirals of lucid shells, and snag on the spiky black pins of sea urchins. In an instant the water is veined with moonlight. The tiny fish come then and nibble on us, their silvery mass moving like one organism. They are curious of me. They are curious of the others, the dark entities weaving through them, the shadows that are neither fish, flesh nor fowl.

458

They are curious of Alice dying among them.

Further and further we descend, until silt fingers rear up from the seabed to take her. I know, as I huddle down in the cavernous, cold depths, that this is the puissance of death, its touch sweetly savage. Alice's heart grows sluggish and prepares to beat its last. But I am not ready yet, not yet. Nor is my host. I seize hold of Alice by the jellyfish trails of her hair. I fill my spectral hands with it, and grip hard. I fix on the sea's skin stirring above us, and I heave, with all the living energy I can summon. Alice's body shifts. Again I heave. And again. The fingers disintegrate into muddy clouds, grudgingly relinquishing their mermaid prize. We rise, my host and I, through the icy currents, up and up, until in a splash of rage I wrench Alice from the fist of the sea, and cast her back on the pebble-strewn shore. She chokes and splutters. Her body spasms. The sodden sea breath pours out of her, and the element of air, of life, gushes in.

As our bedraggled little band makes its shivering way back up the beach, I meld with Alice.

'*Bù dào huáng hé xïn bù sǐ*, We have not come to the Yellow River yet, to the place of despair,' I tell her gravely.

And Alice must have been listening to me, because the following day she books us on a flight back to Hong Kong. We are going home.

Ghost—2006

The flight is unremarkable. The arrival . . . anything but! We do not touch down on the tongue of Kai Tak airport that used to lick out into the sea, but at Chep Lap Kok Airport on Lantau island. The Fasten Seatbelt sign snaps off. As Alice gathers together her hand luggage, there is a frisson of excitement pulsing between us. We are on the move, and much, much more important, we are home. We elbow into the throng making its way towards the open cabin door. Alice pauses at the top of the portable steps, and takes a deep breath of sweltering mid-afternoon air. I feel it instantly, a geyser of life force jetting up from the tips of her toes, energising every cell. For me, arriving on the island has the opposite effect. It is as if Alice's oxygen, that vital gas that once buoyed me up, has metamorphosed into a deadly, boiling lava. I feel it dousing my spirit, petrifying me until . . . until what? Until I am no more than a stony imprint in time! From this moment on, however gradual, I know I am wilting, and Alice is growing steadily stronger.

But this is only the first sign that Hong Kong may not be the oasis I was expecting. My negative reflections end abruptly when something catches my eye. It is the maniacal monkey, scrunched up tightly, twinkling in the unforgiving sun like a globe of rusty metal-filings. Then, startling us all, it launches itself, in the fashion of a kamikaze pilot, down the steps.

The *bump, bump, bump* of its staccato progress is accompanied by an exhilarated *Yaaaah*! This explosive tremolo turns out to be its final aria. As it bounces off the last step and onto the asphalt, there is a sudden Boom!, accompanied by a shower of auburn sparks. We rush down to investigate but incredibly all that remains of the demented anthropoid is a tiny pile of dirt. Closer inspection reveals this to be nothing more than soot, soon dispersed by a gust of fuel-tainted air. It seems the monkey has detonated like a simian grenade. A quick look back confirms that the dog at least appears unscathed. Although, having witnessed the alarming spectacle, I note he is picking his ghostly canine way down the steps with the utmost care. And that is when another coruscation draws my attention. Flattened against each of the aircraft cabin windows in turn are an iridescent green torso and two variegated grey wings. Clearly the budgie cannot find its way out of the aircraft cabin. But Alice is hurrying on, and I do not intend to be left behind.

'Sorry, but it's every ghost for itself from here on,' I call up from the dusty asphalt to the headless budgie. 'Besides, this island never was your home. If you stay put I'm sure they'll fly you back to Britain.' I shrug my regret to show I am not completely lacking in emotion. The dog snatches one cringing glance at a 'plane window curtained with a spray of budgie feathers. Then, with a yelp, he races after us, in his panic very nearly knocking Alice over. As we go through Immigration, a Chinese officer glances at the stamp in Alice's passport that reads 'Hong Kong Citizen'. On the strength of that he waves through the three of us.

461

From here we take an express train to the Hong Kong Island terminus. And all the while our eyes grow wide as dollar coins, for the country we remember has become a mighty dragon whose life-blood never stops flowing.

As far back as I can remember it was busy, but now it is frenetic, the pace of life at a sprint. We have never seen so many people, all rushing somewhere, glancing down at their watches, clasping mobile phones to their ears, grasping suitcases and briefcases and bags fit to burst with bright things from markets—vegetables, fruits and flowers, bottles, parcels and packages. Truly, I had forgotten how noisy the sound of Cantonese and Mandarin can be, as people shout and gossip, and negotiate and bargain, and give directions, and argue, and make up.

There are trains and trams and buses and cars and lorries and motorbikes and bicycles, all jostling one another, winding along roads, through the tunnels and over the bridges. Victoria Harbour has become a vast moving collage of cargo ships, junks, ferries, sampans, pleasure-cruisers and police patrol boats. Girdled about us is the sea, the jade-green bangle of the sea, offering up the three of us to cerulean skies and a fiery sun. It is hard to believe the sleepy little island of Hong Kong I first came to with father all those years ago ever occupied this same spot. We are carried along like a cork bobbing on water until we find ourselves walking, as if in a dream, by the waterfront. We stare up open-mouthed at the crowd of spangled giants, skyscrapers, sleek and silver, defying gravity with nonchalant ease.

We find a hotel that looks out over the harbour,

across to the Ocean Terminal and Kowloon. And the very next day we start to search for somewhere to live. I imagine us finding a fine house on The Peak, but what we finally end up with is a Pokfulam flat no bigger than a broom cupboard. Alice is philosophical.

'It has a view and we can watch the sun set. That's what counts,' she insists.

But another shock lies in store. Alice decorates, she furnishes the flat, and we settle in. She starts to have Mandarin lessons and, as the year turns the corner, to think about finding employment, for the money from the restaurant, she says, will not last indefinitely. Day by day her vitality grows, as mine wanes. Spring arrives and the temperatures start to soar. Since our arrival the dog has whined incessantly about the heat, until I am quite out of patience with him. So it comes as no surprise when he takes up his familiar refrain on a fine day at the start of June.

'I am *soooo* hot!' he grumbles, standing in the minuscule sitting room, inches from the whirring fan. 'I can't stand it. It's simply diabolical. I'm being cooked alive.'

I am lolling on the settee, my now customary exhaustion leaving me a semi-invalid. Alice is in the kitchen, washing up and whistling cheerily.

'Oh do give it a rest,' I drawl fractiously at the dog. 'Why must you always complain? You seemed to have no problem with the hot climate when you were alive.' In a weak gesture of protest I waft the air with a pearly hand .

'But you don't understand,' grizzles the dog through his now somewhat dull, dish-brown muzzle, 'I am *soooo* hot I think I may be melting.'

463

'Don't be such a hypochondriac,' I mutter contemptuously, shifting my phantom limbs into a more comfortable position. Experience has taught me that these lesser apparitions are prone to exaggeration. I try to grab a moment's respite to reinvigorate myself, but when I look up the dog is nowhere to be seen. With a supreme effort I levitate off the settee and seek out poor roasting Bear-as-Was. There is no sign of him. On the floor however, below the fan, is a sticky brown mess and, from it, a trail of acrid smoke spiralling towards the ceiling. Acrid smoke tainted with a distinct whiff of old dog!

'Bear! Bear-as-Was, is this some kind of practical joke?' I demand, poking a cloudy finger cautiously in the burnt-almond gunge. There is no reply. All is quiet. Seconds later, Alice bustles in, tweeting like a spring bird, cloth in hand. She pauses over the glistening puddle on the wooden floor. Two lines pinch together above the bridge of her nose, as if she has a vague recollection of something. Then she gives a dismissive shrug and without a moment's hesitation she wipes up Bear-as-Was, trots back into the kitchen, and washes him away down the plughole.

Ghost—2007

I am struggling to keep pace with Alice now and she knows it. I hobble after her like an elderly relative, longing for nothing so much as peace. Together we watch the sun set from the small veranda of the Pokfulam flat. It is like standing beneath a waterfall of mutating lights—gold and red and copper, tumbling into purple and blue and green, only to drown minutes later in cauldron-black. Alice, I know, is thinking about tomorrow. I am thinking too. I am thinking that I no longer want to say, 'Not yet. I am not ready yet.'

One sultry night I hunch at the end of Alice's bed, studying my host as she sleeps. The cicadas chirrup, as they did through the long nights we spent together in the flat on The Peak. Alice's breathing is easy, effortless. There is a bloom upon her cheeks. Her eyes flicker under their closed lids, and I wonder if she is dreaming of the future, a future she must face alone? Sensing me watching her, tuning in to my monologue of thoughts, as I have to hers for a lifetime now, she stirs and sits up. As she does so, she is made silver-white in a spill of moonlight, like . . . like a ghost. Her hair is mussed up. She yawns widely, pushes back her sheet and hugs her knees. She is wearing a baggy, cotton pyjama top that swamps her. For a long moment we face each other. Unconsciously I realise I am mirroring her, lost in my army jacket, clutching my own misty knees. From far off comes the sound of a motorbike buzzing like a wasp, approaching then receding. A car engine turns over, the coughing slurring until it finally grinds to a stop. A door slams.

'Alice,' I start, 'Alice it's—'

'Don't,' Alice ambushes me. 'Don't say it.' Her voice is hushed but pertinacious.

Another long moment drags by. It is strange, I muse, looking at my host, how well I have learnt her—the changing light in her eyes, the line of her nose, the curve of her mouth, the lift of her brow, the way her little finger crooks when she is uneasy, as it does now. I follow the rise and fall of her chest, and I can feel it too, the rushing in of the air, the release of it.

'Alice,' I try again, 'it's time.'

'No!' says Alice. 'No! You're wrong. It's not, not yet. Stay with me a while longer?' she implores. Her eyes are liquid. Her hands tremble slightly, only very slightly, and her heart beats wildly. 'How will I manage without you?' she mumbles, as if to herself. 'I can't manage without you. I just can't. If you leave, I'll be adrift. I'll be alone.'

'Alice, I am so very tired,' I tell her. 'So weary of this world. Let me go Alice, please.'

Alice nibbles a fingernail, then rakes back her hair and forces out a smile.

'It'll change. You see if it doesn't.' She reaches her hands entreatingly towards me. In return, all I can offer is a barely visible ripple of my gossamer fingers. Slowly, Alice's hands drop. She looks away to the window, to the first pale tendrils of the approaching dawn. 'How will I cope . . . how, without you by my side?' she murmurs to herself.

I manage just the trace of my broken-toothed smile. 'Oh Alice, you will do very well. It wasn't me, you know, dragged along by the rushing river.' The curtain blows in a breath of wind, and the moonlight shivers like a little sea stirred. 'I was always on the bank, out of the current, running to keep up. You're the one who endured, not me.' Alice's fingers interlace, and there is challenge in her unblinking eyes. 'I fished you out a couple of times when it looked as if you might go under,' I allow in a ghostly undertone, wearing this new-found modesty like an ill-fitting garment. 'That's all.'

Now Alice fixes on an expanse of white wall. When she turns back to me her face is resolved. 'I want to come with you,' she says. But her eyes are hooded, hiding the truth.

I shake my head. I do not speak, I simply share the weight of ploughing on, here, in this element of air, how painful it is for me now. By the second I become more drenched in the desire to eschew this half-life.

'Ah Alice, let me go?' My susurration falls away, a silken sigh.

Alice presses her lips tightly together for answer, and her face seems to close down. I feel the way I imagine an old dog feels, kept hanging on, not for its delight but for the comfort of its owner. I never considered when I latched on to Alice that I would need her blessing to sever the tie. I was so busy hanging onto life, not for one moment did I entertain the possibility that I might have a surfeit of it. It is as if I am fastened to her by a thread. Only a thread, but it serves as well as an unbreakable chain. Only Alice can release me, set me free and let me rise up to where the clouds are hemmed with gold, where the ink-black sea is infinite, spinning with chatoyant, timeless stars. Life has become a drudge, not a joy, and all the while I am kept under close surveillance by my hawk-host.

On 1st of July we watch the ceremony marking the tenth anniversary of the historic handover of Hong Kong to the Chinese at the Convention and Exhibition Centre. Throughout the weekend there are colourful parades and swirling dragon dances. The sky cascades with fireworks. We note the

467

conspicuous absence of the bad British fairy from the feast, excluded from the proceedings by Beijing. We see also the pro-democracy protests that follow, where tens of thousands march in Causeway Bay and Wanchai. The people are demanding better pay and more justice. They explain they want the right to vote in their own chosen leaders, a promise not yet delivered. And they describe the new flag of Hong Kong, the representation of the white Bauhinia blakeana flower, standing out against a red background.

'This is *our* flag,' they say, and their eyes shine with patriotism.

The images crowd in upon me now, a cluster of smoky islands, scattered like amethysts in a spinach-green sea. Boat people, clambering with the agility of spiders over the rigging of giant junks as they nose out of Aberdeen harbour, brown-patched sails, plumped-up pillows in the wind. Stooks of rickety shacks thatching the hillsides. The pomp and ceremony of the British—crisp, snowy linen, white helmets, gold tassels, gleaming swords, and men keeling over backwards under a scorching noon-day sun.

A kaleidoscope of exotic produce—golden mangoes, bunches of prickly russet lychees, the mottled sage-green skin of pomelos, the Lincoln green frills of bok choi restrained by their elegant, veined, white stalks, clusters of tiny buttercup-yellow blossoms frothing among the Chartreuse fingers of choi sum. Warrens of cloth alleys, packed tight with bolts of every imaginable fabric, mesmerising the eye with whorls of colour, seducing the eye with their seductive voile kisses. Bench stalls buffeted by wind and weather,

468

through to emporia several stories high, crowded with painted porcelain, and carvings, from musk-scented cedars to the dark glossy limbs of blackest ebony, cool jade in frosty white, through celadon, and darkening to that most highly prized emerald green.

Birds clucking and cooing, pecking frantically at the wicker mesh of their basket-cages. The sweet, pervasive taint of garnet-red raw meat, banded with thick yellow fat, emanating from carcasses dangling from huge blue-grey hooks; stone floors blotched liver-brown, drains running red with blood. Steam, rising like genies from bowls of tangled noodles, at makeshift restaurants on street corners. A swaying, apricot-coloured paper lantern suspended from a bamboo cane, its leaping flame casting mysterious shadows, as you seek for the pearl of the moon among a fold of crushed velvet night. Young Chinese men, muscles taut, clambering up towers of glazed buns. Tiny girls dressed in shimmering silks and satins, their faces works of art, their hair braided and looped, adorned with shiny diadems, perched up high like miniature goddesses on festival floats. Ears blasted with the cacophany of lighted firecrackers. Lacy pink blossoms of peach trees, standing quivering in bud, rows of shy princesses ready for the Chinese New Year.

Walls of fire, leaping and licking down the blackened flanks of charred hillsides. Typhoons pounding the island to its very foundations, their screams reverberating at its core. Shoulders of mud sliding down precipitous slopes, loosened by torrential rains, gobbling up whole buildings. Opalescent, milky bodies, stealthily wrapping

469

themselves about the island's high peaks. Wizened brown faces split in wide, gold-toothed grins. New-minted babies' faces, topped with sheaves of crisp black hair, breaking into gummy toothless chuckles. I swell with love for my dramatic, invincible, resilient home. It has been tossed and turned by history, shaken by the rigours of nature, and has emerged thriving, vibrant, and ever more magical. All this I turn over, knowing that soon I must leave.

One evening bonfires are lit all over the island. It is the fifteenth day of the seventh moon, the lunar month in the Chinese calendar; the ghost month. Red, yellow and blue flames flay the encroaching gloom, appeasing the restless spirits of the dead. It is the festival of Yue Lan when Hungry Ghosts roam the island. Death—sudden, violent, premature—has cheated them of life's bounty, and of the funeral rites that would have secured their peace. And so, once a year, when the gates of the dark kingdom are flung wide, the restless spirits surge back, bent on filling their bottomless bellies with all life dared to withhold. Paper offerings—model homes, cars and money—blaze. Plates are piled high with food for the dead. The air is laced with the heavy scent of incense, and prayers are muttered fearfully by old and young alike.

How can I tell Alice, as she watches the celebrations enraptured, that the air is thick with ghosts, with snatching shadow hands, and greedy, covetous eyes? How can I explain the drag of them, the craving I have to slough off my host, and dance my fury with demons on the world's edge? How can I make her understand I want to stalk the

470

island's shores, where the sea's husky chords lure men to watery graves? Silently I watch my ancestors weave wildly among the living, brushing warm flesh with their last glacial, stagnant breaths.

While Alice sleeps, her head pillowed on her hands, I stand on the small veranda. The hot night air throbs with phantoms, swooping and diving, twirling, scuffling and thrusting, brawling, grabbing, clawing and wailing at the living. They reach towards me with their scrolling glassy fingers.

'Come. Join us Lin Shui. Slip away and leave the living to their clumsy workings,' they murmur, their siren song dipped in honeydew.

Again and again they call, catching at my army jacket, tempting my febrile spirit until it jerks and tugs to be away. All that binds me is a thread; no more than that, a single thread fastening me to Alice. But it is enough. Soon they are gone, leaving me behind.

The Ghost—2007

'Let's walk today,' persuades Alice. 'The weather is splendid. It will rejuvenate us.' She dismisses my empty laugh, and strides off, pulling at my leash, so that I have no choice but to follow. For once she does not choose to stroll about The Peak. Instead we take a taxi to Aberdeen harbour, also known as Heung Gong Tsai or Little Hong Kong.

These days the waterfront is crowded out by towering apartment blocks. And yet the land almost seems to extend gawky limbs into the sea, so chequered is it with houseboats and sampans, a floating village. There are banks of Chinese junks, their hulls protected with black tyre circlets. Makeshift tarpaulins in glaring greens and blues, draped over wooden frames, provide relief from the growing heat of the rising sun. The air is pungent with the scent of salt and refuse and fuel, alive with the shouts and cries of the boat people, with the noise of chugging engines, and slapping, splashing water, and the ceaseless murmur of traffic.

Where once there had only been the Sea Palace and the Tai Pak, gently swaying on their moorings, now they compete for custom with the mighty Jumbo restaurant, and many other smaller businesses. Against a background sponged with the shifting hues of the sea comes the panorama of browns, the gradient of charred crusts to mellow biscuits, claimed by the fleets of wooden vessels. Day and night, boat-dogs, yellow, cream, brown and black, dash up and down patrolling these floating homes, or lie semi-comatose panting in a patch of shade, lulled by their rolling waterbeds.

Everywhere foaming sprites burst from the ruche of sea, sluicing the sides of the boats as they snake through the busy channels. They are shaped from nothing more solid than salt water and air, rise up and are dashed to bits, only to be instantly reborn in dazzling white froth. And overlaying this are the slashes of red signs, from where Chinese characters stand out in gleaming gold relief, drawing in customers. Washing flaps from poles and rigging. The smells of cooking and washing rise as one on the warm air currents. This Little Hong Kong was my home, where I lived and worked and slept and dreamed. 'Was', not 'is'. It is Alice's home now, not mine.

For a while longer we wander about drinking in all manner of sights and sounds, a glut for the senses. Alice is about to hail a taxi when we glimpse the child, an urchin, dressed in skimpy black rags, skin shining like varnished cedar, wispy hair a shade of the purest gold, on fire with the sun's touch. A distant memory lifts and stretches, before clouding over. Then he is streaking past us, his bare feet slapping on the paving stones, glancing back over his shoulder. Dark eyes flash arrestingly, his thin mouth splits in a wide, mischievous grin, white teeth aglitter.

'Follow me if you dare,' he seems to say.

And we find ourselves shouldering our way through the crowded streets, hungry for another glimpse of the entrancing child. We turn a corner, and there he is again, just yards ahead of us, small, brown hands beckoning us on, a stream of laughter bubbling from his lips, setting the tiny Adam's apple, no bigger than a cherry stone, bobbing up and down. The silvery sound seems to transcend all others. He does not speak and yet we both hear it.

'Catch me if you can! Catch me if you can! Catch me if you can!' The chant fills the air. Then off, off he races, and we speed after him. Even now I feel it, every brief sight of him infusing me with a sparkling zest. There he is across the street, his head wagging cheekily, his hair tinsel-gold, the lustre of those magnetic eyes urging us forward. There he is, peeping out from behind a market stall. Follow him as he dodges a chain of nursery children trustingly reaching up to grip the giant

473

hands of their carers. He's turning into a deserted alley, puffs of dust rising in his wake. And now he's darting up the path that skirts the necropolis, the city of the dead, the Chinese Permanent Cemetery. He's winking at us, an elfin creature, speeding round the solemn, ashen monuments in giggling, giddy hoops, arms outspread. We stumble after him, echoing his laughter, my face bleached lace, Alice's, rosy-cheeked with her exertions.

Some of the graves have mounted upon them touched-up photographs of their dead occupants. Dabs of florescent pink daub the gaunt cheeks; clothes, so drab in life, grown toxically brilliant in death. And I see, as we rush past, desperately seeking our elusive pixie, that their tallow faces are ridged with broad smiles, that their glossy eyes are full of promise. Into the sudden stillness comes a soughing threnody, as their stiff lips shape my name.

'Lin Shui! Lin Shui! Lin Shui!'

The susurrus murmurs, like thousands of grass snakes, slithering at our heels. As we track our fairy child, Alice is panting, fighting for breath. Her chest hurts as if it would burst. Her heart batters at her ribcage A wave of nausea starts to engulf her. But I—oh, I am new made, moving with the ease of the sunlight playing over us. Then the grass becomes scrub, and the scrub a rutted path, climbing steeply, and I know where it leads. It leads up the mountain, up to The Peak. It is Alice who drags her feet now, head circling to gaze back the way we came, and it is my spirit that forges ahead, carried like goosedown on the hazy air. The ragged child is always just beyond us, as the sun throbs down, leaching the blue in its kiln to

474

a blazing albescence.

Then we are upon it, and it is as ordinary as meeting with an old friend, clasping them to you and feeling the years peel away. It is, of course, the place where I died—almost died—where a shred of me clung tenaciously to life, worrying at it ever since. Alice, coming up behind me, gulping frantically for breath, suddenly senses it. She jars to a stop and recoils.

'So far and no more,' the child flutes into the torrent of light. I spin and so does Alice, and he is there; not on the path, but hunched in the branches of a tall tree, that reaches up to us from the olive tangle below. And I know him now. It is the child who crouched with me beneath the mantle of the morgue, the child I glimpsed on Brighton beach. It is the angel of death. Not a bleach-boned skeleton in a hooded cape, grimacing and clutching a glinting scythe, but a small boy with hair of spun gold, glazed cedar skin and eyes as deep as infinity. But to Alice he is an alien. She bristles at the sight of him, knowing he has come to claim his own.

'That's where my body snagged; there, below the child. It's only an ancient wound in the bark now, but then there was a sturdy branch. For a time I sat beside my corpse, watching my blood spill into the wide greenness far below. Then I broke it, the branch, so she fell and was hidden, burying my shame from . . . from . . . from them.'

I glance up and see the air is teeming with the wavering wings of myriad gilded butterflies, where once there were only swarms of bloated carrion-flies. All this I communicate to Alice in the excited tones of a child showing a parent the very spot

475

where they enacted a scene to make all proud. The urchin chuckles. He seems to rise until the tips of his bare feet balance on his branch. His crown of gold hair is brushed from above by a bracelet of green leaves. Then he is circling his arms outwards, opening them to me in invitation.

And I want so much to go that the pang of longing seems all there is of me. But still I am shackled to Alice, standing desolate at my side. I guide her tenderly to an overhang of rock a few feet above the path. And there we sit, my host and I, above us the branches of a small fir tree affording some shade. The soft breeze ruffles the fists of dark green pine needles above our heads. Alice sighs, and such a sigh that had I a heart I know it would have broken in two. I merge with Alice, and the voice, clear and calm in her head, is mine.

'My father was a teller of stories, Alice. When we returned from a night's fishing, the sun rising, and me squinting at it with tired eyes, the salt drying on my skin, I would draw my quilt onto the deck of *Heavenly Sea*. I would let my body sink into it, the sun a balm to my exhausted muscles. Then Father would produce his small clay pipe and pack it with strands of tobacco. And when it was lit and drawing well, he would sit cross-legged at my side, and in his deep, melodious voice he would tell his tales.

'My favourite was of the Chinese daughter of a rich warlord. Her father bought her a small white bird in a beautiful gilded cage. She watched the bird flit about all day and it enchanted her. In the evenings she would knot a tiny silk thread about the little bird's stalk leg. Then she would walk in her cool green garden, captivated to see it hop and flutter before she jerked it back to her.

'As the days passed the bird fell into an impenetrable despondency. It hunched into itself on its golden perch, it black-bead eyes jaded as they raked its prison. And the girl knew that if she did not set it free, one day it would pass away, and she would find it stiff and cold lying at the bottom of its cage. So one evening, when she went for her walk, she paused on a wooden bridge that arced over a narrow babbling silver stream. She bent to the bird, hopping miserably at her feet, and with the tiny silver scissors she kept tied at her waist, she snipped the thread. For a moment the bird hesitated, its head cocked, eyes held by the severed cord. Then suddenly it stretched its wings, lifted into the air and vanished into the dark canopy of trees. Although the girl pined for a time, that time passed. And eventually, despite thinking fondly of the little bird, she missed it hardly at all.'

I slide out of Alice and am there by her side. Her expression is bleak. She interlocks her crooked little fingers in her lap, then tries in vain to pull them apart.

'It was the story I loved best. What I imagined as I drifted off to sleep, with the deck of *Heavenly Sea* rocking very gently under me, and Little Hong Kong stirring and wakening around me, was how it felt, that first moment, as the bird rose up, flying free.'

I can hear, as well as feel, Alice's painful breaths shuddering in and out. The child crouched in the tree is quiet now, as if he too is waiting for the moment of release. The cicadas trill. In the undergrowth below us, insects burrow. The fallen leaves rustle. The grasses swish. An Asian Koel takes flight, the light possessing its jewel-red eye, the stroke of its blue-black wings finding their rhythm. A few more long beats. Alice inhales the fragrant pine-sap. Shadows dance on the pale canvas of her skin. I sense her little fingers growing fluid, see them fork apart. Alice turns to me. In our locked eyes two spheres meet.

I slip into her, feeling the heat of her one last time. She hugs herself, though she knows you cannot hold onto something as insubstantial as air.

Her breathing grows shallow. The beat we have shared quickens as if readying itself for separation. I draw myself from Alice and her arms slacken.

'Who will catch me now when . . . when I fall?' she mumbles brokenly.

She does not blink. She makes no sound. Her eyes fill. They are rimmed with mercurial light. They brighten and rupture, and the silver tears course down her cheeks. She buckles, bringing up her knees, trying to find purchase for her feet on the craggy rock face. Then, with the slowness of a flower opening, her face lifts to me. She sniffs. The collar of her dress is sodden with spent tears. But now her eyes blaze with something else.

'It has been extraordinary sharing my life with you!' The smile begins in Alice and ends in me, as everything always has.

Keeping her eyes fixed on mine, she nods her assent. The thread snaps and I hesitate. But the butterflies are closing in and the boy has become a golden eagle, outstretched wings seared with fire. I have been a long time 'undead'. Gripping onto water, that's what it is like, holding on to life when its substance has fled. It is hard work and I want so much to play, to let it all go. Then I am riding the eagle of death. I am there, clasping onto him as he ascends, higher and higher, out of time, my ghost liberated, sailing into the setting sun. I have one last fleeting impression of Alice. See, she is there on the path far below, the splash of her red dress moving upwards towards The Peak. The last thing I notice is a detail, nothing more, but I mark it. It is the carriage of her shoulders. Surely they are straighter, more open. If I didn't know better, I would say that a weight has been lifted from Alice.

EPILOGUE
Ghost

I am dead, fully dead. Resting in peace. No half-life now, no turning back. What's done is done. For surely you understand the dead, the 'fully dead', cannot return to life. I expect, being alive, you would like me to tell you what it's like to be without a fleshy husk, to know the vessel that contained you has long since been eaten away by worms and returned to the primordial dust from whence it came. I should imagine you want to know where your spirit is when it no longer roams the earth. How, you ask, does it go with the dead? We have our tomorrows, you say, but what do they have to compensate?

Where I am, the most I can do is assure you that there is no hunger or thirst, no pain or sorrow, no disease or injustice, and no yearning. But what of pleasure, you want to know? Is this death of yours an endless round of pleasure? My answer to that is human pleasure, much like pain, has a shelf-life. Oh, I am above such temporal treats now. My sybaritic death style must sustain me for . . . well . . . for an eternity. Whereas you poor mortals know nothing you have will last. You scurry about endlessly trying to satisfy your desires, ironically counting yourselves lucky to be alive. It is not my intention to make you jealous, but the truth is that I am basking in empyreal radiance.

Naturally you would like to know how Alice has got on without me. I do visit from time to time. Oh

480

yes, of course I do. We all do. Even the dead can be curious occasionally, although I must explain that when I drop in, it is not the way it used to be. Ellipses between our worlds occur every once in a while, and when they do I drift by and there is Alice. But, as I say, it has all changed. She is no longer conscious of me. Even if I had a voice she would be deaf to it.

But I have encountered her several times—in a market filling her basket with Chinese pears, buying a spangled Garoupa fish, choosing a bunch of yellow chrysanthemums, chattering in Mandarin to the stallholders. Oh yes, Alice seems to have mastered the language. Her pronunciation is a little idiosyncratic but on she goes, blissfully unaware of her solecisms. So sweet! She works part-time in a Sichuan restaurant, gives lessons in French conversation, and is taking classes in Chinese painting. She writes to Nicola at least once a month and every now and then she'll telephone her for a chat. I eavesdropped on the last call. It seems Alice's siblings are surprised that she's made her home in the new Hong Kong. Oh yes, Alice is very industrious these days. Once, roaming about the island, I found her sitting on the prow of a small boat, kicking at the sea spray with her bare feet and scattering salty diamonds over the swell. One might almost have said she looked happy, if that isn't too strong a word.

The last time I saw her was in her flat. It was late in the evening, and she was curled up on the plump cushions of her rattan settee reading a book. Suddenly the ceiling light started to flicker. Alice's head snapped up, and when the light snuffed out completely she got herself in the most dreadful panic. It wasn't me though. Poor Alice was quite overcome with emotion as she hunted in a kitchen drawer for a new bulb. I wanted to tell her that long gone are the days when I am the cause and I have an effect. But of course my lips are sealed now. Overall, Alice seems surprisingly contented, and I am genuinely pleased about that. She deserves to come at last to a peaceful plateau, after what has been, for the most part, a fairly treacherous climb. Besides, didn't I say I am at rest, so why would I begrudge my one-time host the same calm shallows?

I am not being mendacious when I say this. It is perfectly true: almost all of the year I am as tranquil as a slumbering infant, halcyon, serene . . . that is until the seventh month in the lunar calendar, the ghost month, the festival of Yue Lan. I'm not greedy. I don't hog the entire month the way some of my ghostly colleagues do. Three days is quite sufficient for my needs, the three days that precede the fifteenth, the feast of Yue Lan. At that appointed time I leave Yinjian, the world of darkness. I burst out of its gates, and inside me— oh there is such a hunger, such an emptiness eating away at me, that I will do anything to fill it.

As I roar to the earth, skim over the South China Sea, corkscrew in tight hoops above the island, I see that I have company to share the sport: three Hungry Ghosts also bent on filling the chasm hewn out of them by death. There is a galloping mastiff, a massive beast, his eyes, scorching grape coals, his rat-tailed fur red as Mars, snapping voracious jaws at the clouds, his blood-stained muzzle flecked with acid-yellow foam. There is a monkey with a mighty pendulum-like gait, skin withered as a dried sour plum, but agile as a cobra when it's time to strike. It has grown, this monkey, to the proportions of a great ape. Its pleated flesh is bald and scabby, but for a few stray patches of fur, oxblood, tipped with bronze. Its rotten, yellow teeth are bared, while its sticky fingers, finished with razor-sharp claws, excoriate the skies. And there is a bird too, huge as a vulture, but headless, gore dripping from its ragged neck. Sparse, bilious-green feathers spike its torso, huge glaucous wings lash into a cyclone the air it tears through. And all the while, its fish-hook claws seek for fleshy purchase.

We hell-raisers rampage about the island, consuming everything in our paths. So light your bonfires, let your infernos compete with the stars. Hurry to put upon the crackling pyres your offerings—your model houses and cars and boats, your furniture, your clothes, your televisions and radios, your computers and your mobile 'phones—all fashioned out of crisp paper, stiff card and matchstick wood. Gold and geranium-red, silver and leaf-green, kingfisher-blue with copper trim, a shower of living colours to feed our flames. Throw on your wads of money, packs of 'hell notes', and see us guzzle them up with our fiery, blistering tongues. Burn your incense and your joss sticks. Do not stint. Take handfuls of them, and shake them at the heavens till the trails of smoke grow thick as fog, blinding our smarting, rapacious eyes. Shut up your doors, close your windows tight, hold close and closer still your babies, with their juicy papaya plumpness, soft and yielding to our primed fangs. Keep your children safe indoors, under your watchful eyes.

And whatever you do, stay away from the sea and its restless, pounding, bloodthirsty surf. Or, believe me, we will have you. Never doubt it! We will gorge ourselves on the foolish ones, the ones who scoff, the ones who swim out of their depth, who wander the beaches at night, who brave their rickety, fragile boats. We will drag them down to the sludgy tar on the ocean bed, feast on their distended meat, devour their waterlogged hearts and season their marrow with sea salt before sucking them dry.

Oh, I almost forgot. On the last night of Yue Lan make sure you lay a place at the table for the absent ones. Starve yourself and pile *our* plates high. Serve us tender slices of chicken, chunks of spicy pork, slithers of succulent beef, shreds of crispy duck, bowls of fluffy white rice and glistening noodles. Heap cakes and sweetmeats upon the altar, build towers of luscious fruits, labour without rest to slake our epicurean appetites. Hope upon hope that you manage to reform us this time. That, cleansed, our spirits will be released to the pure lands. That we will not come back in a twelve month to gorge ourselves on your riches, to feed on your families, to pick you to the bone. Pray that we will not curse you, and bring the fury of the damned down upon your brittle human heads.

No one takes the festival of Yue Lan more seriously than Alice, when the Hungry Ghosts roam the earth. She takes armloads of paper offerings to her Chinese friends, and feeds them to the starving fires. For three full days she shuts herself up in her Pokfulam flat, closes the windows and locks the doors, refusing to answer the ring of the doorbell or the hammer of a closed fist, no matter whom the caller claims to be. Meticulously she lays four places at her table and, while she fasts, in each sets down plates filled with tempting delicacies. She burns incense and chants prayers to appease the restless spirits. She takes immense care. It is almost as if someone or something has warned her of the dangers.

All children have nightmares. The fisherman's daughter I used to be was no exception. There were times when she would waken with a cry and sit up gasping for air. Her almond eyes would be round with terror, her brow dewed with sweat, her lips trembling. When her father came to her and asked her what was wrong, her reply was always the same. 'The ghosts, the Hungry Ghosts had come for me, Father. The sky had grown dark with them. They blotted out my sun. They tried to take my breath from me, to thrust their icy fingers into my body and draw it out. I was so afraid.'

'Was your mother among them?' her father would ask his daughter with a gentle smile, smoothing back the hair from her dampened forehead.

'I don't know. I think so, Father,' she would answer, trying hard to remember.

'Then you have nothing to fear.' When Lin looked searchingly into her father's dark eyes he would nod reassuringly and add, 'Some Hungry Ghosts can be guardian angels, my daughter. They will hold hell at bay for all eternity to keep you safe.'